Natural Eye Care, Inc.

3 Paradies Lane, New Paltz, New York 12561

Tele: (845) 255-8222

Website: www.naturaleyecare.com

E-mail: info@naturaleyecare.com

W0008349

Our Mission

Our mission is to help support healthy vision by providing guidance along the holistic nutritional, dietary and lifestyle path. Our strategies and recommendations are based on peer review studies and optometrist Marc Grossman's 38+ years of patient experiences. Our website www.naturaleyecare.com offers information for helping educate yourself in over 40 eye conditions including macular degeneration, glaucoma, cataracts, dry eyes, blepharitis, etc. We consider supporting healthy vision in relation to the health of the whole body.

Ask about Dr. Grossman's new whole food, organic, GMO-free eye formula, **Advanced Eye and Vision Support formula** now available online or by telephone (845-255-8222).

We provide the following services:

- Free phone and e-mail nutritional and lifestyle consultations
- Free monthly newsletter by email
- Specific nutritional and lifestyle recommendations by eye condition
- Website that keeps abreast of the latest developments in holistic approaches to supporting healthy vision.
- For Pets - holistic eyecare and general care

The Authors

Dr. Marc Grossman is a leading holistic optometrist, and has been in practice since 1980. He is the author of *Magic Eye Beyond 3D* (with Magic Eye Inc., 1996), *Greater Vision* (2001), *Natural Eye Care: A Comprehensive Manual for Practitioners of Oriental Medicine* (2002), *Natural Eye Care: Your Guide to Healthy Vision* (2007), and now, an updated, revised, and greatly expanded second edition of *Natural Eye Care: Your Guide to Healthy Vision and Healing*. He founded the Rye Learning Center in 1980, a multidisciplinary center for learning problems, in 1996 co-founded Integral Health Associates in New Paltz, New York, and in 1999 co-founded Natural Eye Care, Inc.

Dr. Grossman lectures nationally on topics such as Natural Vision Improvement, Vision and Nutrition and Chinese Medicine and Vision Care. He also teaches workshops nationally for a variety of different health care professionals.

Michael Edson is the co-founder and president of NaturalEyeCare.™ Michael is a New York State Licensed acupuncturist and co-author of *Natural Eye Care: A Comprehensive Manual for Practitioners of Oriental Medicine* (2002) and *Natural Eye Care: Your Guide to Healthy Vision* (2007, 2nd Ed: 2018). He is currently working on a new book, *The Memory Book: Self Help and Caregivers Guide to Brain Health.* His hobbies include the practice of Qi Gong, traveling, hiking, tennis, golf, movies, reading and chess.

For more information, you can visit their website at www.naturaleyecare.com or call 845-255-8222.

Disclaimer

The information contained in this book is intended to be educational, and is not for diagnosis, prescription, or treatment of any eye conditions or disease, or any health disorder whatsoever. This information should not replace competent optometric, opthalmologic, or medical care. The authors are not liable for any use or misuse of the materials or products contained within this guide.

The products recommended in this book are based on the opinion of Dr. Grossman and his years of experience as an optometrist. Many of the products mentioned in the Appendix can be purchased on naturaleyecare.com, or may be available at your local health food store. Individual results will vary when targeted supplements are taken.

The statements contained in the guide and on the website have not been evaluated by the Food and Drug Administration. The material and products presented are not intended to diagnose, treat, cure or prevent any disease.

NATURAL EYE CARE

Your Guide to Healthy Vision and Healing

Second Edition

Marc Grossman, O.D., L.Ac. and Michael Edson, M.S., L.Ac.

Natural Eye Care, Inc., New Paltz, New York

Important Information

This book is for anyone interested in wholistic and proven approaches for strengthening eyes and vision. It is not intended as medical advice. Its intent is solely informational and educational. Please consult an eye doctor should the need for one be indicated.

LIBRARY OF CONGRESS CATALOGING IN PUBLICATION DATA

Natural Eye Care: Your Guide to Healthy Vision and Healing, 2nd Ed.

By Marc Grossman, O.D. L.Ac. and Michael Edson, L.Ac.

Edited by Jennifer W. Miller

P. 799 Cm. 8.5" x 11"

Includes appendix and index

ISBN: 978-0-692-07431-2

1. Eye—Diseases—Alternative treament—Encyclopedias. 2. Eye—Care and hygeine—Encyclopedias.

I. Title

RE21.G76 2018

617.7-dc21   cip

Contributors: Andy Rosenfarb, N.D., L.Ac., Jody Toyonaga, O.D., C.N.P., Sam Berne, O.D., Daniel Orlansky, Mark Fillipi, D.C., Ami Ranani, O.D., Damon Miller, M.D., Scott Forman, M.D., Ron Wish, M.D., David Nidorf, M.D., Brett Bevell, Jason Elias, M.A, L.Ac., Dipl. O.M., Phyllis R. Freeman, Ph.D.

Jody Toyonaga, O.D., C.N.P., Contributing Editor

Copyeditor & Indexer: Kathaleen Kelly

Design & Illustrations: PrairieComm.net

Cover, Yoga Illustrations: TheTurningMill.com

Printed in the United States.

CONTENTS

FOREWARD

The world is changing. Our concepts of Western medicine have shifted over the past 10–20 years with a vast amount of new research coming out regularly that supports the benefit of lifestyle, diet, and targeted supplementation. The reductionist mentality of referring only to each symptom often isolates the person from the health condition, defining them in terms of diagnosis and specific medications for that diagnosis.

The wholistic and Eastern medicine approach seeks to look at each person as a unique individual where treatment strategies can often vary from person to person, even with the same diagnosis.

It has been my privilege and pleasure to work with Dr. Grossman the last couple of decades, and he has opened my eyes to perceiving vision problems in a new light. Dr. Grossman believes that changes in our eyesight do not happen in a vacuum, rather they have roots in our total being, including our genetic makeup, the food we eat, our exercise routine, management of stress levels and emotions, exposure to airborne toxins, as well as general belief systems about ourselves and the world around us. Each of us is unique, and we literally take in the world around us through our senses, primarily our vision. How we take in the world is often a reflection of who we are and which symptoms and health conditions we experience.

Using their combined background in optometry, nutrition, Traditional Chinese Medicine, herbal medicine, and Qigong, Marc Grossman, OD, L.Ac. and Michael Edson, MS, L.Ac., along with contributing doctors and health care practitioners, offer readers specific natural strategies for supporting and protecting healthy vision. This includes those genetically at risk for certain eye diseases, as well as patients working with their eye doctor to manage eye conditions, which include macular degeneration, glaucoma, retinitis pigmentosa, Stargardt disease, rod-cone dystrophy, cataracts, eye floaters, computer eyestrain, and dry eyes. This exceptional book will open our eyes to the power that lies within us to help take control of our vision and overall health. It will reconnect us to the basic truth that the body's own natural wisdom and ability to heal can be supported through the right nourishment, through our belief system, diet, exercise, and targeted herbs and supplements.

Natural Eye Care: Your Guide to Healthy Vision and Healing offers a bridge where Western medicine, Western nutrients, and Eastern healing wisdom come together to help the whole person heal and, just as importantly, stay healthy.

Jason Elias, M.A., L.Ac., Dip. O.M., co-author of:
The Five Elements of Self-Healing, Feminine Healing
The A-Z Guide to Healing Herbal Remedies
The Memoir: Kissing Joy as it Flies: A Journey in Search of Healing and Wholeness

PREFACE

Natural Eye Care: Your Guide to Healthy Vision and Healing offers a unique approach to supporting healthy vision from early childhood to mature age, with the understanding that healthy vision relies on overall health and emotional health. Filled with wisdom and insight of both ancient and modern-day healing methods, this book integrates the full range of alternative therapies as they apply to vision and vision disorders.

This book will help you make sensible, researched, and clinically based decisions to support vision. Chapters are devoted to a wide range of eye conditions and issues that include macular degeneration, glaucoma, cataracts, dry eyes, eye floaters, computer eyestrain, and much more, with recommendations that include Western herbs, nutritional supplements, Chinese medicine, and additional therapies. You will learn about the underlying causes of common visual problems and be given tools and techniques to develop your own eye health strategies. If a particular problem, cluster of symptoms, or changes in vision occur, please consult your eye doctor.

Natural Eye Care: Your Guide to Healthy Vision and Healing shows people how to become active participants in their own vision care, giving back the power and responsibility they have so trustingly handed over to their eye doctors. The primary goal of this book is to offer a practical approach to vision care, based on the underlying philosophy that emphasizes prevention and support. In doing so, we celebrate the healing power within all of us and the mind/body's inherent potential for self-healing.

Patients come in, year after year, with their eyesight worsening. For example, many eye care professionals just give stronger and stronger prescriptions that help weaken the eyes instead of eye exercises and lifestyle recommendations to help strengthen vision. Something is wrong with this picture. Diet, exercise, lifestyle, and targeted supplements should be a critical part of the discussion of how to maintain healthy vision, even with such eye conditions as macular degeneration, glaucoma, and retinitis pigmentosa. The peer-reviewed research is abundant in demonstrating these alternatives. They are listed in this book by eye condition.

This guide will educate readers about their vision difficulties, explain how to prevent vision disorders, and explore ways to help preserve vision for those with vision disorders. It will enable the individual to be a more informed consumer when it comes to vision care. Medication and surgery may sometimes be necessary or even appropriate treatment strategy, but nutrition and lifestyle choices always play an essential role in helping support healthy vision.

Doctors in China have reached out to the West to borrow the modern medicine we can offer. We in the West can, in turn, benefit from the ancient wisdom of the East. By combining the medical approaches of the East and West, along with other alternative health modalities, we may be able to achieve better health with less cost and greater success in helping patients preserve vision.

Natural Eye Care: Your Guide to Healthy Vision and Healing is dedicated to the belief that a common ground can be created in which the strengths of modern-day Western medicine are united with the preventive approach of other healing modalities.

PART ONE

UNDERSTANDING THE EYE

1. BASIC ANATOMY AND PHYSIOLOGY

Parts of the Eye

The Eyeball

Within the skull, the space in which the eye is located are bones collectively called the **orbit.** The eyeball, the optic nerve, the eye muscles, and the nerves of the eye are all found within the orbit. The floor and inside walls of the orbit are very thin and can be fractured easily by trauma.

The **eyelids** are located on the outside of the eye, on top of and below the orbit. They protect the eye from injury and excessive light. The eyelids also help keep the cornea moist.

The **eyeball** is contained within the center of the orbit. It is only 2.5 cm in length and is attached to a series of six muscles, which move the eyeball in all directions. These are called the **extraocular muscles.** Eyeball movements help focus light on the fovea (where 20/20 sight is possible).

The **conjunctiva** of the eye is a thin clear membrane that covers the **sclera** (the white of the eye).

The white tissue of the **sclera** is an external coat over five-sixths of the eye. Eye muscles are connected to the sclera. The transparent structure called the **cornea** covers one-sixth of the eye.

The Front of the Eye

The **cornea** is the key optical component responsible for refraction of approximately 80% of light that enters the eye. It is an unusual tissue in the human body, both because it is clear and because it has no blood vessels. The cornea is the clear window through which we actually see. The cornea also has many pain fibers; therefore, the primary symptoms of any corneal problem are pain, light sensitivity, as well as under- or over-production of tears. The **lens** lies protected, behind the cornea.

Directly behind the cornea is a clear, watery-like fluid called the **aqueous humor.** This fills the front part of the eye between the lens and the cornea. The aqueous humor fluid is produced by the **ciliary body** that contains the ciliary muscle.

Behind the aqueous humor is the **lens** of the eye. This is a flexible structure that, like the cornea, is transparent and has no blood vessels. It is another key part of the refractive system of the eye.

The lens fine-tunes focus through the process of accommodation. This is done, not by changing the position of the lens in the eye, but by changing its shape. The lens is not completely solid but is built up of thin layers, like an onion. It is suspended and held by a membrane called the **zonule.** When the lens is called upon to see objects that are near, tension is placed upon it, and the radius of its curvature is reduced. When the lens sees objects that are more distant, the tension is relaxed, and the radius of its curvature increases.

The **ciliary muscles** control the shape of the lens. When the ciliary muscle contracts, the lens thickens, which allows the individual to focus the image of an object onto the retina. As that object moves away from the eye, the ciliary muscle relaxes, the lens becomes thinner, and the focusing system relaxes, allowing the individual to be able to see the image clearly at a greater distance.

The **vitreous humor** is found behind the lens. It is a jelly-like, colorless, transparent gel that contains a meshwork of collagen fibers. It consists of 99% water and forms four-fifths of the eyeball. In addition to transmitting light, the vitreous humor holds the retina in place and provides support for the lens. It tends to liquefy with age, and its separation from the retina can lead to retinal tears and vitreous detachments.

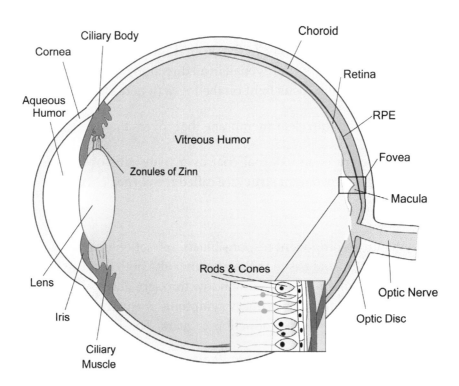

Three Concentric Layers

Let's return to the front of the eyeball to learn about the final structure contained in the eye. The eyeball has three concentric coats: the **iris**, the **choroid,** and the **retina.**

The **iris** is the colored part of the eye and is located between the cornea and the lens. An individual's eye color depends on the amount and distribution of pigment within the iris. The pupil is located in the middle of the iris and is a circular hole that changes in size as the iris's muscles expand and contract in response to light. The pupil acts like an aperture on a camera. The size of the iris changes to regulate the amount of light entering the eye through the pupil.

The **ciliary body** lies between the iris and the choroid. Its role is to secrete aqueous humor. It also contains the ciliary muscle that controls the focusing of the lens of the eye.

The **choroid** is a dark brown membrane that extends from the ciliary body to cover the entire back of the eye. The choroid contains the blood vessels needed to deliver nutrients to the retina.

The **retina** is the most internal layer of the eye. This layer is a very thin, delicate membrane. The term "retina" means "net" or "cobweb" and relates to the appearance of blood vessels within the retina. The retina consists of an outer pigment cell layer and an internal neural layer. In the back of the retina there is a circular depressed area called the **optic disc**; this is where the optic nerve enters the eye and where its fibers spread out in the neuronal layer of the eye. Because the optic disc contains only nerve fibers and no photoreceptor cells (rods or cones), it is insensitive to light. This is the part of the eye responsible for creating the blind spot that we all notice, most often when we drive.

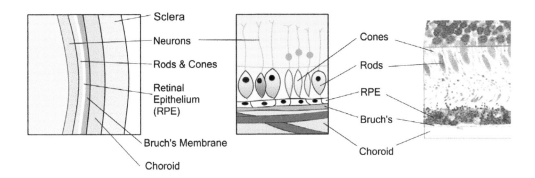

Photoreceptors

Both the **rods** and the **cones** are light receptors. Each is named for the simple geometric shape it resembles when seen under a microscope. Cones are found in the central part of the retina, the area that receives the brightest light. This is important because cones can function only in fully lighted conditions. When functioning properly, they give us the ability to see details and most important, perhaps, the ability to see colors. There are about 7 million cones in the human eye.

The rods are located in the periphery of the retina. Here they receive less direct light, which is important to their function, as they discern no specific colors, only shades of gray. They also discern the image far less clearly than do the cones. Rods cannot see objects better than 20/400—the size of the largest "E" on the eye chart. Rods supply peripheral vision and our ability to detect motion. There are about 120–130 million rods in the human eye.

The Macula

Central vision is controlled by the **macula**, which is located just beside the optic disc. Its center contains the **fovea**. Because the fovea is tightly packed with cone receptors, it is the section of the eye with the most precise detailed vision, allowing us to see most clearly and with greatest detail.

2. HOW THE EYE WORKS

The Path of Light

Through the Front of the Eye

Vision begins with light arriving at the eye and entering through the cornea, the eye's clear transparent "window." The cornea is actually the first layer where light starts to become focused. Here light is bent toward the center of the eye, on its way to the retina.

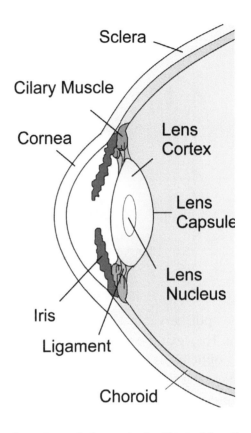

Light continues to the iris (the colored part of the eye), which contains muscles that dilate and constrict the pupil (the black hole). The pupil gets smaller in bright light and larger in low light, and thus regulates the amount of light entering the eye.

Light instantly passes onward to the lens. Similar in function to the cornea, the lens furthers the process of focusing light onto the retina at the back of the eye.

The lens is made up of transparent cells and changes its shape, depending on the distance on which it is focused. When we look at something far, the lens flattens, reducing the amount of focusing needed to place the light rays onto the retina. When we look at something close, the lens shortens and widens in order to bend the light so that it focuses onto the retina. This changing of shape is facilitated by the action of the **ciliary muscles**. As we get older, the lens of the eye loses its flexibility to focus (causing presbyopia). The lens is where cataracts (a loss of transparency of the lens) are found.

To the Retina

After passing through the lens, the path of light continues through the vitreous humor before finally reaching the retina, which is the nerve cell layer of the eye. The retina works like film in an older model camera. Photochemical reactions take place, which involve rod cells (approximately 120–130 million of them) used for night and peripheral vision, and cone cells (approximately 7 million) used for day vision, color vision, and detailed sight.

Through this multiple-step process, sight is instantly focused on the macula, near the center of the retina. The macula is the source of your most detailed vision. In the center of the macula is the fovea where the most precise sight occurs. When we look at something, we unconsciously turn our eyes so that the light falls on the fovea of each eye.

To the Brain

Like an old-fashioned camera, the image received by the retina is upside down and reversed, and the brain must make sense of it. Electrical impulses created by light energy in the retina are conducted to the brain as nerve impulses via the optic nerve.

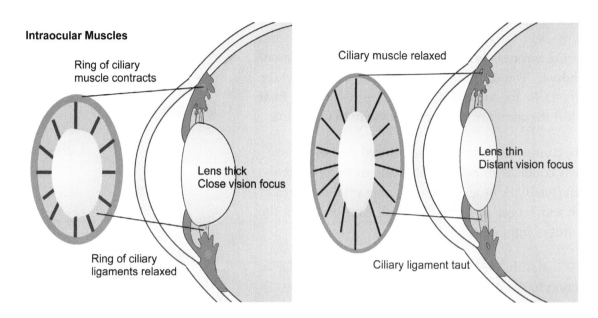

The optic nerves, each consisting of over a million nerve fibers, are the main "trunk lines" of the eye. They exit the eyeballs from the back of each eye and join together at the base of the brain at the optic chiasm. Here, the nerve fibers cross, and the visual impulses go to the optic tracts (channels) that end in the lateral geniculate bodies in the mid-brain. From there, the visual impulses pass along optic radiations, which end in the occipital cortex at the back of the brain. Here, as far as we know, the impulses connect with other areas of the brain, and we can then begin to interpret the meaning of the light energy that we receive through our eyes. Thus, we are given vision.

The Eye in Action

How the Intraocular Muscles Work

When the eyes look at a distant object, the ciliary muscle relaxes. The resulting pull on the suspensory ligaments (zonule fibers) causes the entire lens to flatten, enabling it to focus light from distant objects onto the retina.

When we look at objects near by, the ciliary muscle contracts, and tension is released on the zonules. The two surfaces of the lens capsule again become fatter, more convex, allowing the light from near objects to focus on the retina.

The ability of the eyes to focus at different distances by changing the shape of the lens is called "accommodation" or the "accommodative process." In summary, the flatter the lens, the better you see at a distance, and the fatter the lens, the easier to see up close.

How the Extraocular Muscles Work

Through a dual link-up, when you relax the extraocular muscles, you are also indirectly relaxing the ciliary muscles of your eyes, and vice versa. You relax the extraocular muscles when you gaze into the distance. When you put tension on these muscles, such as when you look at a book close-up, you are contracting the ciliary muscles of the eyes.

There are also muscles around the sides of the eyeball: above, below, to the side, pulling straight back, or pulling at oblique angles. These muscle movements change the shape of the entire eye. The eye is like a balloon, constantly being "pushed," "squished," "stretched," and shaped ever so slightly to allow the eye to focus light on the proper point of your retina. Excess tension on the extraocular muscles may cause a distortion in the shape of your eye.

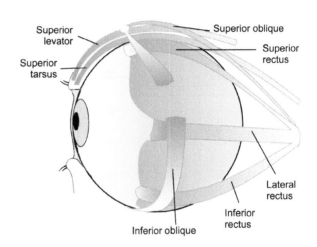

When the eyeball is shaped normally, the light that enters will focus on the retina. When the eyeball too long, then the light will focus in front of the retina, causing myopia (nearsightedness) and making distant objects blurry. When the eye is too short, the light will focus behind the retina, causing hyperopia (farsightedness), which makes it harder to see near objects.

The eye reshapes itself through the contraction and relaxation of rectus extraocular muscles. If the oblique muscles contract, the eye is squeezed at the equator, which makes it longer and causes temporary nearsightedness. If the two pairs of rectus muscles contract (for example, the medial, lateral, superior, and inferior rectus muscles), the eye is squished back into the eye socket, possibly causing temporary farsightedness. Remember, a nearsighted or farsighted eye only shifts a fraction of a millimeter to bring objects into focus.

Why Eye Exercises?

Through a combination of exercising and relaxing the extraocular and ciliary muscles, you can empower the eyes to improve. Like other muscles in your body, these muscles learn to become more and more flexible. When we wear our eyeglasses constantly, our eye muscles tend to lose their flexibility; *thus, it is often true that you need to return to the eye doctor one to two years later after getting new eye glasses for a stronger prescription.*

3. CONVENTIONAL APPROACH TO VISION

Patients go to their eye doctors year after year with worsening eyesight. They are typically told that this is a normal part of the aging process and that nothing can be done to prevent visual decline. Those diagnosed with diseases such as glaucoma may be put on a lifetime of medications. The following are common examples of conventional treatment or advice.

- Eye care professionals increase their patients' prescriptions year after year as needed, and they explain that weakening vision is just part of aging, even in children.
- People with cataracts, which include nearly all adults over the age of 65, are told there is nothing to prevent the growth of cataracts, and therefore they must wait until the cataract "ripens" (gets more opaque), and then have it surgically removed.
- In the past, most patients with macular degeneration were told there was nothing that could be done, that they would most likely lose vision, and in some cases, go blind. Since publication of the AREDS studies (2001, 2003, and 2013), an increasing number of eye doctors are recognizing the value of nutritional supplementation.
- Patients with early stages of glaucoma are either immediately placed on medication for a lifetime, or told to wait and see if the condition worsens. In the meantime, the patients are not given any of the preventative measures that could be taken.

Something is Missing

Where is public awareness of much needed prevention, education, and rehabilitation? There are many peer-reviewed studies that clearly show that many eye conditions can respond to proper diet, lifestyle adaptations, and nutritional supplementation, and that people can preserve their vision. Leaders in the complementary health care professions can readily expand their role into one of helping people maintain their invaluable gift of sight.

Medication and surgery are sometimes necessary, and in acute cases, they can preserve vision. The role of modern Western medicine in saving lives and vision is remarkable. But medicine as practiced today lacks the wholistic and preventive emphasis that may obviate the need for surgery and medication.

A Common Ground

Natural vision care is not intended to replace conventional treatments, but to serve as valuable adjuncts to standard care and as needed. We don't need to choose between the benefits of Western medicine or complementary medicine. The breakdown or malfunction of the body machine arises from the condition of the whole body.

Complementary medicine supplements Western medicine. There is a common ground that unites the strengths of modern day Western medicine with the advantages and strengths of other healing methods.

4. A COMPLEMENTARY APPROACH

Complementary medicine, or wholistic medicine, recognizes the body as a single, whole, complex, and organic unit. It recognizes the body's tissues and organs as interrelated and mutually dependent. Through a variety of health modalities and through use of the body's natural healing processes, it is possible to support the overall balance of the physiology and provide therapy and nutrition that brings support to vision and illness.

Our approach to vision care considers a wide variety of influences on vision health. Nutrition, lifestyle and habits, diet, and alternative therapies may be combined to address health concerns in a wholistic manner and support healthy vision in a natural way.

Nutrition

Because many vision conditions are caused by, or aggravated by, nutrient deficiencies, nutrition plays an essential role in protecting our vision. Some conditions, caught early, such as macular degeneration, are manageable or even preventable by attending closely to nutrient needs. Other problems are not resolved by nutrients alone, but they can act in a strong complementary role to support and often improve vision. In other cases, even if there is not a lot of research on the subject, it is possible that certain nutrients may be helpful because they are known to address an underlying issue. Inflammation and poor circulation are major factors in many vision conditions.

The Nutrition chapter of this book discusses different nutrients, their applications to eye conditions, and research that support their use.

Diet

The standard Western diet tends to lack essential phytonutrients that support the health of the retina, as well as other nutrients such as adequate amounts of omega-3 fatty acids and a wide range of amino acids, minerals, vitamins, and vitamin-like nutrients. The standard diet features processed foods, non-whole grains, fats, sugars, and some types of meat that may aggravate inflammation in the body. Inflammation is an underlying, or sometimes a direct cause of many health issues, such as arthritis, in addition to having a negative impact on vision health. We recommend an anti-inflammation diet, based on a combination of the Mediterranean and alkalizing diet. These diets and information about other popular diets are included in Chapter 7.

Lifestyle

Bringing our attention and helpful changes to our habits can make a great difference in our vision health. Very simple things like wearing UV-blocking sunglasses, getting sufficient exercise, eating a healthy diet, and stopping smoking are fundamental essential must-dos. In each chapter about different vision conditions, we discuss important lifestyle points and tips.

Genetics

Although we can't change the genetics we were born with, nutrients, diet, and lifestyle can help. The study of epigenetics shows that environmental factors cause changes in gene activity, which may lead to a healthy life or may cause disease. Advances in stem cell technology and various implantable devices are beginning to increase the quality of life, even for people with genetically based vision conditions.

Additional Therapies

One effective approach toward improving vision is through acupuncture, which has been found to succeed in treating a wide range of visual conditions, including glaucoma, cataracts, macular degeneration, optic neuritis, and optic atrophy.

Traditional Chinese Medicine views each individual as unique; for example, cataracts may arise due to different imbalances for different individuals. Consequently, the treatment approach may be different for each patient for the same diagnosis.

In the Appendix, and where relevant in the eye conditions chapters, we discuss additional therapies that may be useful.

PART TWO

THE FUNDAMENTALS OF HEALTHY VISION

5. THE ROLE OF ANTIOXIDANTS

Our body is under constant stress due to the creation of free radicals. Oxidative stress, resulting from the presence of free radicals, is implicated directly or indirectly in many vision and health conditions. Some researchers consider oxidative stress to be the root of all (non-genetic driven) health conditions. With respect to vision, it is a factor in deterioration of the macula,[1] the cornea,[2] the photoreceptors,[3] retinal microcapillaries,[4] and the optic nerve.[5] Even for those prone to genetic diseases, free radicals can significantly worsen health conditions.

What are Free Radicals?

Free radicals (prooxidants) are atoms that lack a particle called an electron, and as a result, they are very unstable. In the atom, electrons exist in pairs; it is the unpaired electron that creates instability in an atom, turning it into a free radical. In the free radicals' attempt to become stable, they attack other cells as they try to "steal" an electron. This attack harms the cells' delicate membranes and DNA structure and makes them a target for disease.

There are two types of free radicals (prooxidants): **reactive oxygen species** (ROS) and **reactive nitrogen species** (RNS); they play both toxic and beneficial roles. Low or moderate levels of free radicals support cellular messaging and the immune system,[6] as when they are purposefully created to neutralize viruses and bacteria.

Free radicals are created when a chemical bond is broken. This occurs naturally in normal metabolism, but the over-generation of free radicals can result from excess sugar intake, processed foods, fried foods, trans-fatty acids, charred food, cooked and processed meats, or excess alcohol. Environmental factors such as cigarette smoke, radiation, pollution, and herbicides can also create free radicals, as can chronic stress.

When prooxidants steal electrons from healthy cells (oxidation), the health of cells is impacted. The common visible signs of oxidative damage can be seen in aging skin changes and ocular changes such as the development of cataracts. Of course, oxidation is just one cause of these eye conditions. Poor circulation and lack of essential nutrients getting to the eyes are examples of other causes.

Causes of Free-Radical Generation

Endogenous. Free radicals are created from within the body due to inflammation, aging, immune cell activity, mental stress, excessive exercise, inadequate blood supply, infection, or cancer.[7]

Exogenous. Free radicals are generated by outside factors such as environmental pollution, smoking, alcohol, heavy metals, some prescription drugs, solvents, and foods (such as sugars, smoked meats, and trans fats). Ultraviolet sunrays promote oxidation. If you stare at the sun (do not do this), the UV rays "oxidize" retinal cells at the back of the eyes, resulting in a loss of central vision.

Benefits of Free Radicals

Low to moderate levels of free radicals have a place in a healthy body and visual system. They are essential to the immune system; they are involved in the activation of several cell-signaling pathways that govern cellular activity and coordinate the pathways' activities. They are essential for symbiotic behavior among all cells to support health.[8] Errors in signaling result in conditions like autoimmune diseases when the immune system attacks the body.[9]

What is Oxidative Stress?

Oxidative stress develops when production of free radicals in cells exceeds the ability of antioxidants to stabilize them.[10] Oxidative stress is probably at the root of most health conditions, because it has the capacity to damage all cell structures. It is implicated in a wide range of chronic and degenerative diseases.[11]

Effects of Oxidative Stress

- **Inflammation**. Inflammation is both a cause and result of oxidative stress. Oxidative stress and inflammation easily induce each other.[12]
- **Impair nutrient function**. Too many free radicals react with fatty acids and proteins within cells and impair their function.[13]
- **Cell membrane damage**. Membranes of lipids are highly vulnerable to oxidative stress, and damage to them in the brain may be important in understanding Alzheimer's disease where accumulation of beta amyloid may be a protective response to oxidative stress.[14]
- **Mitochondrial damage**. Much of the free radical damage is done to the energy producing mitochondria in cells, which causes mutations or premature cell death.[15]
- **DNA damage**. Within cell mitochondria, damage due to oxidative stress results in DNA-strand breaks and lowered ability of DNA to replicate. Some forms of cancer are traced to this malfunction.[16]

How do Antioxidants Help?

Antioxidants neutralize free radicals by donating an electron to unstable atoms. In that way, they inhibit oxidation of molecules. After being neutralized, the free radicals will no longer attempt to damage cells, and therefore they become less harmful to the body.

- The body makes some of its own antioxidants, including glutathione, superoxide dismutase, and coenzyme Q10. Glutathione and superoxide dismutase are known to neutralize the full spectrum of free radicals.
- Selenium, riboflavin, vitamin C, cysteine, glycine, and glutamine are needed to produce glutathione.
- Nutrients such as vitamins C and E and beta-carotene are also antioxidants.
- Fruits, vegetables, some herbs and spices, and mushrooms provide a wide range of antioxidants.

As we age, decreases in antioxidant levels in the eyes is believed to be a major factor in the decline of vision. For example, the destruction of retinal cells can occur slowly over many years, due to exposure to UV sunlight or from a gradual degradation of the antioxidant defense system.

Antioxidant Classification

Antioxidants may be divided into three groups:

- Enzymes: (glutathione, superoxide dismutase)
- Phytonutrients: (bioflavonoids, carotenoids, polyphenols, indoles)
- Vitamins/Vitamin-like: (vitamins A, C, E, CoQ10, alpha-lipoic acid, for example)

Evaluating Antioxidants' Effectiveness

One problem for researchers is that sometimes certain antioxidants reduce oxidative stress, and sometimes they don't. The explanation appears to be that for effective "anti-oxidation" the nutrient needs to address **both oxidative stress and inflammation at the same time.**[17]

When cells experience oxidative stress, biomarkers are produced; increased levels warn of a problem. Biomarkers are biochemicals that increase when stressed conditions prevail. Their levels can be measured by scientists as they evaluate ways to combat oxidative stress.

Bilberry is an example of a nutrient that reduces oxidative stress[18] and also reduces inflammation.[19] In one study, researchers wanted to find out whether bilberry extracts could help reduce levels of a biochemical marker for oxidative stress. In this case, the researchers were looking at enzyme levels that increase as a defense of oxidative stress. The enzymes are called heme-oxygenase (HO)-1 and glutathione S-transferase-pi (GST-pi). They were measured in human retinal-pigment cells that had been grown in the lab.

Before exposure to chemicals that would increase oxidative stress, the cells were exposed to 25% enriched bilberry extractions. They were then exposed to H2O2 (hydrogen peroxide). Under a stressed situation like H2O2 exposure, the normal concentrations of glutathione are reduced and free radicals increase. The scientists found that early exposure to the bilberry extract reduced the development of free radicals in the cell tissue, even though the toxicity of H2O2 was not affected. After 4 hours of exposure to H2O2, the defense enzyme levels increased, suggesting that such exposure to the extract had stimulated defense mechanisms against free radicals.[20]

Antioxidants and Vision Disorders

Oxidative stress and inflammation play critical roles in the start and progression of many eye diseases, including macular degeneration, glaucoma, cataract, macular edema, and diabetic retinopathy that, if untreated, lead to progressive loss of vision and blindness.[21] [22] [23] Growing evidence indicates that supplementing with targeted antioxidant and anti-inflammatory nutrients may have a role in the prevention and treatment of these age-related eye disorders.[24]

Doctors and eye care professionals often overlook the power of antioxidants, despite the many peer-reviewed research studies confirming the essential need for such nutrients for eye and overall health. However, you can take steps to increase antioxidants available in your system.

Antioxidant Building Blocks

If given the right building blocks, your body can manufacture certain antioxidants. Glutathione, superoxide dismutase, alpha-lipoic acid, CoQ10, and vitamin D can be made in the body. Other antioxidants must be ingested, including resveratrol, carotenoids, astaxanthin, lutein, zeaxanthin, mesozeaxanthin, vitamin C, bilberry, and vitamin E.

Your Body Manufactures These

Glutathione and superoxide dismutase. Why are glutathione and superoxide dismutase called super antioxidants? These substances can neutralize the full range of free radicals. Other antioxidants neutralize specific types of prooxidants. Low levels of glutathione are linked to cataracts, macular degeneration, and other age-related diseases. Our body manufactures glutathione, but it is limited by the rarity of cysteine in our diets. Cysteine is an example of a co-factor, a substance that is needed to complete a biochemical transformation.

Glutathione Cofactors

- **Cysteine** is a required amino acid in glutathione production. The best dietary sources of cysteine are from cruciferous vegetables such as broccoli, Brussels sprouts, cabbage, kale, and bok choy. Supplements may be needed. Glutathione pills and capsules are poorly absorbed. Intra-oral and sublingual forms are much better absorbed.
- **Other cofactors** that help the liver produce more glutathione include the amino acids cysteine, glycine, glutamine, alpha-lipoic acid, selenium, and vitamin C.

Alpha-lipoic acid (ALA) is not considered an essential nutrient, but it is a powerful antioxidant. It also converts glucose into energy and helps "recycle" glutathione. ALA appears to have a direct effect on ocular tissue metabolism.[25]

Coenzyme Q10 (CoQ10) supports all cellular activity, muscle health, and heart health. Healthy individuals naturally produce sufficient CoQ10. However, a genetic flaw, advanced age, low fat intake, side effects from statin drugs, and other reasons can cause a deficiency. Some doctors routinely prescribe CoQ10 for statin drug users. If tests reveal a deficiency, supplementation is needed.

Vitamin D is a membrane antioxidant; it protects membranes against oxidative damage. Your body can create vitamin D from enough sun exposure. However, people in northern climates or those who do not spend enough time outdoors, may have a deficiency. Milk is vitamin D-fortified to help calcium absorption, but this may not be enough. Make sure your milk is fortified with vitamin D3, not D2 (which is not as beneficial and can be toxic in large doses). Seniors require four times the amount of sunshine to get the same amount of vitamin D as a 20-year-old.[26] The accepted normal range for vitamin D levels runs from 20 to 50 nanograms per milliliter.

Carotenoids are a class of antioxidants, critical to eye health, that include beta-carotene, astaxanthin, mesozeaxanthin, zeaxanthin, lycopene, and lutein; they are found in brightly colored fruits and vegetables. The eyes require relatively large amounts of carotenoids for healthy vision maintenance. The macula (part of the retina where we get our most detailed vision) gets its yellow color from zeaxanthin and lutein, which protect it from damage from UV and blue light exposure.

Vitamin C is highly concentrated in the eye. It, along with beta-carotene and zinc, enhances lutein absorption, which is important for preventing macular degeneration. It reduces inflammation and swelling that are prevalent in uveitis patients. Vitamin C somewhat lowers intraocular pressure (glaucoma) and supports connective tissue health (vitreous floaters and detachment). While most other mammals can manufacture this nutrient, humans cannot. A diet rich in various fruits and vegetables will provide plenty of vitamin C.

Vitamin E is a major fat-soluble antioxidant. It also helps eliminate toxins, treats hardening of the arteries, helps to recycle glutathione, and enhances brain functioning.

Resveratrol is a delicious antioxidant. This nutrient is found in blueberries, raspberries, mulberries, lingonberries, senna, and the skin of grapes. Think red wine, dark grape juice, and bowls of berries. Resveratrol has neuroprotective properties, supports the immune system, reduces inflammation, supports heart health, encourages a healthy insulin balance, and supports mitochondria function.

Wholistic Approach for Good Health

By themselves, antioxidants are not sufficient for good health. You can't ingest a lot of supplements to bring the body into balance. Other lifestyle factors are essential: getting regular exercise, managing stress, not smoking, not excessive use of alcohol or drugs, meditation, and having a balanced diet.

Also See

Chapter 6, Inflammation and Oxidative Stress

Chapter 7, Vision Diet

Chapter 8, Nutrients

Chapter 10, Self Help and More

---

[1]Blasiak, J., Petrovski, G., Vereb, Z., Facsko, A., Kaamiranta, K. (2014). Oxidative stress, hypoxia, and autophagy in the neovascular processes of age-related macular degeneration. *Biomed Res Int,* 2014:768026.

2Cejka, C., Cejkova, J. (2015). Oxidative stress to the cornea, changes in corneal optical properties, and advances in treatment of corneal oxidative injuries. *Oxid Med Cell Longev,* 2015:591530.

3 Tsuruma, K., Yamauchi, M., Inokuchi, Y., Sugitani, S., Shimazawa, M., et al. (2012). Role of oxidative stress in retinal photoreceptor cell death in N-methyl-N-nitrosourea-treated mice. *J Phrarmacol Sci,* 118(3):351-62.

4 Kowluru, R.A., Kowluru, A., Mishra, M., Kumar, B. (2015). Oxidative stress and epigenetic modifications in the pathogenesis of diabetic retinopathy. *Prog Retin Eye Res,* Sep;48:40-61.

5 O'Hare, D.R.L., Barlett, C.A., Maghzal, G.J., Lam, M., Archer, M., et al. (2014). Reactive species and oxidative stress in optic nerve vulnerable to secondary degeneration. *Exp Neurol*, Nov;261:136-46.

[6] Pham-Huy, L.A., He, H., Pham-Huy, C. (2008). Free Radicals, Antioxidants in Disease and Health. *Int J Biomed*, Jun;4(2):89-96.

[7] Ibid. Pham-Huy. (2008).

[8] Wikipedia. Biochemical Cascade. Retrieved May 17 2018 from https://en.wikipedia.org/wiki/Biochemical_cascade.

[9] Ibid. Pham-Huy. (2008).

[10] Yokota, T., Kamimura, N., Igarashi, T., Takahasi, H., Ohta, S., et al. (2015). Protective effect of molecular hydrogen against oxidative stress caused by peroxynitrite derived from nitric oxide in rat retina. *Clin Exp Ophthalmol*, Aug;43(6):568-77.

[11] Ibid. Pham-Huy. (2008).

[12] Biswas, S.K. (2015). Does the Interdependence between Oxidative Stress and Inflammation Explain the Antioxidant Paradox? *Oxid Med Cell Longev*, 2016:5698931.

[13] Khasari, N., Shakiba, Y., Mahmoudi, M. (2009). Chronic inflammation and oxidative stress as a major cause of age-related diseases and cancer. *Recent Pat Inflamm Allergy Drug Discov*, Jan;3(1):73-80.

[14] Axelsen, P.H., Komatsu, H., Murray, I.V.J. (2011). Oxidative Stress and Cell Membranes in the Pathogenesis of Alzheimer's Disease. *Physiology (Bethesda)*, Feb;26(1):54-69.

[15] Biswal, M.R., Ahmed, C.M., Ildefonso, C.J., Han, P., Li, H., et al. (2015). Systemic treatment with a 5HT1a agonist induces anti-oxidant protection and preserves the retina from mitochondrial oxidative stress. *Exp Eye Res*, Nov;140:94-105.

[16] Han, Y., Chen, J.Z. (2013). Oxidative stress induces mitochondrial DNA damage and cytotoxicity through independent mechanisms in human cancer cells. *Biomed Res Int*, 2013:825065.

[17] Ibid. Biswas. (2015).

[18] Milbury, P.E., Graf, B., Curran-Celentano, J.M., Blumberg, J.B. (2007). Bilberry (Vaccinium myrtillus) anthocyanins modulate heme oxygenase-1 and glutathione S-transferase-pi expression in ARPE-19 cells. *Invest Ophthalmol Vis Sci*, May;48(5):2343-9.

[19] Miyake, S., Takahashi, N., Sasaki, M., Kobayashi, S., Tsubota, K., et al. (2012). Vision preservation during retinal inflammation by anthocyanin-rich bilberry extract: cellular and molecular mechanism. *Lab Invest*, Jan;92(1):102-9.

[20] Ibid. Milbury. (2007).

21 Levkovitch-Verbin, H. (2015). Retinal ganglion cell apoptotic pathway in glaucoma: Initiating and downstream mechanisms. *Prog. Brain Res*, 220:37–57.

22 Kowluru, R.A., Mishra, M. (2015). Oxidative stress, mitochondrial damage and diabetic retinopathy. *Biochem. Biophys. Acta*. 1852:2474–2483.

23 Dib, B., Lin, H., Maidana, D.E., Tian, B., Miller, J.B., et al. (2015). Mitochondrial DNA has a pro-inflammatory role in AMD. *Biochem Biophys Acta*, 1853:2897–2906.

24 Rhone, M., Basu, A. (2008). Phytochemicals and age-related eye diseases. *Nutr Rev*, 66:465–472.

[25]Filina, A.A., Davydova, N.G., Endrikhovskiĭ, S.N., Shamshinova, A.M. (1995). Lipoic acid as a means of metabolic therapy of open-angle glaucoma. *Vestn Oftalmol*, Oct-Dec;111(4):6-8.]

[26] Kruse, J. (2013). Epi-paleo Rx: The prescription for disease reversal and optimal health. New Orleans, LA: Optimized Life, PLC.

6. INFLAMMATION AND OXIDATIVE STRESS

Inflammation is the means by which the body's immune system responds to injury. It does so in order to maintain stability and heal damaged tissue. When the body is exposed to intrusion of toxins, foreign materials, pollutants, UV radiation, or a host of other infiltrators, various components of the cell oxidize. Oxidation causes stress and this phenomenon is called oxidative stress. The body's natural response to this imbalance is to activate the immune system, which results in inflammation. The role of inflammation and oxidative stress are intertwined and are causes of eye conditions and other diseases, ranging from dry eye syndrome to cancer. Oxidative stress and inflammation can induce each other; sometimes oxidative stress causes inflammation; sometimes inflammation causes oxidative stress.[1]

The body protects against excessive oxidative stress caused by free radicals (prooxidants), by means of antioxidants. Free radicals are atoms that are missing an electron, and consequently, are unstable. Antioxidants supply the missing electron and restore stability.

Over the last 30 years, research has established why and how imbalances in the relative levels of prooxidants and antioxidants result in oxidative stress. High levels of free radicals cause damage to DNA, lipids, and proteins. These three are the fundamental building blocks of cells with a wide variety of tasks.[2] They are the building blocks of carbohydrates (e.g. simple sugars like glucose that supply energy, transport proteins, and permit cellular recognition).[3] Oxidative damage stimulates an immune response that, in turn, causes inflammation.[4] If the levels of oxidative stress are chronic, then inflammation is also chronic and health issues and vision disorders develop.

Measuring Inflammation

Scientists are able to identify the presence of inflammation hidden within the body by measuring biomarkers. Biomarkers are indicators of a problem; they can be biochemicals or changes in structure that are seen via imaging techniques. Biomarkers are proof that inflammation is present, and to some extent, what vulnerabilities are present.

Imaging biomarkers. Doctors can look at physical changes or abnormalities as evidence of dysfunction. Some abnormalities can be seen in an eye exam, others require special equipment. For example, to assess the degree of inflammation in the retina that is due to diabetes, doctors look at intra-retinal reflective retinal spots (a fancy term for pockets of fluid under the retina), subfoveal neuroretinal detachment (retinal detachment at the focus point of the retina), and increased foveal autofluorescence (the natural release of light by cell tissue).[5]

Biochemical biomarkers. Biomarkers can also be chemical. Elevated levels of biochemical biomarkers are linked to inflammation. For example, in conditions involving the surface of the eye, such as blepharitis, dry eye syndrome, conjunctivitis, and allergic reactions, interleukins (IL-1beta and -6) and matrix matalloproteinase (pro-MMP-9) are measured.[6] Interleukins and another biomarker, interferon-y (IFN-y), are used to distinguish between inflammatory and age-related cataracts.[7] Blood work can identify systemic inflammation through markers, including erythrocyte sedimentation rate (ESR), C-reactive protein (CRP), and plasma viscosity (PV).

Biochemical biomarkers also indicate oxidative stress. Examples include serum total oxidant status (TOS), the level of free radicals in the blood, and total antioxidant status (TAS). When oxidative stress is present, the level of TOS increases, but TAS does not. In other words, oxidation increases, but the remedy, antioxidants, does not.[8]

Biomarkers of exposure. Toxins present in the body are also considered to be biomarkers. High levels of lead in the body are a good example.

Inflammation's Role in Vision Disorders

Inflammation over time can affect the health of the body and eyes in many ways, including negatively affecting circulation, digestion (poorer absorption of nutrients), joint damage, and increased free-radical activity. Common eye problems that directly result from chronic inflammation include uveitis, scleritis, iritis, macula edema, Sjogren's syndrome, central retinal vein occlusion, diabetic retinopathy, macular edema, retinopathy, and macular degeneration.

Take dry eye as an example. A review of more than 450 studies, 200 of which look at dry eye syndrome in humans, reports that inflammation has a central place in the development of dry eye. The authors conclude that chronic immune-system dysfunction leads to a cycle of chronic inflammation, along with natural and adaptive immune responses, and that anti-inflammatory treatments can be beneficial.[9]

Cycle of Inflammation

Dry eye syndrome is a good example of how inflammation manifests in vision conditions. If we look at the cycle of irritation and inflammation in dry eye syndrome, the most common complaint brought to eye doctors, we see that the problem is a repeating cycle.

Uveitis describes several different conditions involving inflammation of the uvea of the eye. It may arise from problems in the eye itself or as a symptom of diseases of other parts of the body. It can be short in duration (acute), or continue for a long time (chronic). It may develop as a result of an autoimmune condition, trauma, bruise, infection, tumor, or due to environmental or other toxins.[10] The resulting inflammation, if untreated, can destroy tissue, leave scars, lead to eye conditions such as glaucoma, cataracts, optic nerve, and retinal damage, and even result in blindness if left untreated.

Macular degeneration. The retina features unique structural and functional properties and is therefore able to tolerate antigens (a toxin or other foreign substance that induces an immune response, such as an increase in the production of antibodies) without causing an immune system response. However, over the years, the retina is exposed to low levels of ongoing oxidative stress. This stress continues and increases as we age, resulting in a state of chronic low-level immune-system activity called parainflammation. If the eye remains healthy, this response is able to maintain stability and healthy functioning. But in patients with macular degeneration, this response is not regulated and contributes to damage to the macula.[11]

Diabetic retinopathy. Having both diabetes and high blood pressure creates the risk of development and advancement of diabetic retinopathy. It is becoming increasingly evident that chronic inflammation and oxidative stress are major factors.[12]

Myopia. Nearsighted people are at higher risk for many vision disorders, including retinal detachment, glaucoma, and cataracts. Oxidative stress may help explain changes in the eye that create the increased risk. Oxidative stress, linked to damage associated with insufficient oxygen, changes the regulation of neural messaging. Free radicals damage the retina, vitreous, and lens, and they contribute an increase to the risk of retinal, vitreous, and lens problems.[13]

Reducing Inflammation and Oxidative Stress

We can reduce inflammation and oxidative stress to protect our vision.

Antioxidants in our diet and supplemental nutritional support provide ingredients for fighting excess inflammation and oxidative stress. These include enzymes, phytonutrients (lycopene,[14] lutein,[15] and astaxanthin,[16]), and vitamin and vitamin-like compounds.

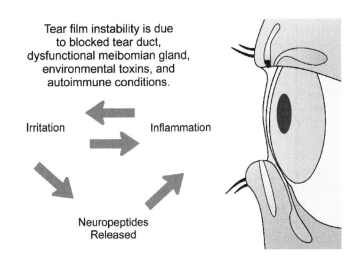

Tear film instability is due to blocked tear duct, dysfunctional meibomian gland, environmental toxins, and autoimmune conditions.

Irritation

Inflammation

Neuropeptides Released

Other nutrients and spices that help reduce inflammation include omega-3 fatty acids[17] (such as fish oil), holy basil, turmeric (curcumin), ginger, MSM, CBD oil, cayenne pepper, cloves, rosemary, sage, black pepper, green tea, and spirulina.

A well-balanced diet, combined with good eating habits, promotes the best possible absorption of nutrients. The Vision diet (see Chapter 7) is an anti-inflammatory diet. It is based upon the Mediterranean diet and is an alkalizing diet.

Moderate daily exercise not only supports our muscular system and physical strength, but it supports every system of the body, including the visual system, circulation, respiration, digestion, the immune system, brain functioning, and hormonal balance.

Managing stress and anxiety are also important, as these have been found to contribute to chronic inflammation.

Lifestyle habits are important; for example, it can make a significant difference if you stop smoking and wear ultraviolet-blocking sunglasses.

Also See

Chapter 5, Antioxidants

Chapter 7, Vision Diet

Chapter 8, Nutrients

Chapter 10-4, Eye Exercises

Chapter 12, Drugs

[1]Biswas, S.K. (2015). Does the Interdependence between Oxidative Stress and Inflammation Explain the Antioxidant Paradox? Oxid Med Cell Longev, 2016:5698931.

[2]Muro, E., Atilla-Gokcumen, G.E., Eggert, U.S. (2014). Lipids in cell biology: how can we understand them better? *Mol Biol Cell,* Jun 15;25(12):1819-23.

[3] Cooper, G.M. (2000). The Molecular Composition of Cells. *The Cell: A Molecular Approach, 2nd ed.* Sunderland (MA): Sinauer Associates.

[4] Kruk, J., Kubasik-Kladna, K., Aboul-Enein, H.Y. (2015). The Role Oxidative Stress in the Pathogenesis of Eye Diseases: Current Status and a Dual Role of Physical Activity. *Mini Rev Med Chem,* 16(3):241-57.

[5]Vujosevic, S., Torresin, T., Bini, S., Convento, E., Pilotto, E., et al. (2017). Imaging retinal inflammatory biomarkers after intravitreal steroid and anti-VEGF treatment in diabetic macular oedema. *Act Ophthalmol,* Aug;95(5):464-471.

[6]Acera, A., Rocha, G., Vecino, E., Lema, I., Duran, J.A. (2008). Inflammatory markers in the tears of patients with ocular surface disease. *Ophthalmic Res,* Oct; 40(6):315-21.

[7]Chen, W., Lin, H., Zhong, X., Liu, Z., Geng, Y., et al. (2014). Discrepant expression of cytokines in inflammation- and age-related cataract patients. *PLOS One,* Oct 10;9(10):e109647.

[8]Toprak, I., Kucukatay, V., Yildirim, C., Kilic-Toprak, E., Kilic-Erkek, O. (2014). Increased systemic oxidative stress in patients with keratoconus. *Eye (Lond).* Mar;28(3):285-9.

[9] Wei, Y., Asbell, P.A. (2014). The core mechanism of dry eye disease is inflammation. *Eye Contact Lens,* Jul;40(4):246-56.

[10] Facts About Uveitis. Retrieved Jul 31 2018 from https://nei.nih.gov/health/uveitis/uveitis.

[11]Chen, M., Xu, H. (2015). Parainflammation, chronic inflammation, and age-related macular degeneration. *J Leukoc Biol,* Nov;98(5):713-25.

[12]Duarte, D.A., Silva, K.C., Rosales, M.A., Lopes de Faria, J.B., Lopes de Faria, J.M. (2013). The concomitance of hypertension and diabetes exacerbating retinopathy: the role of inflammation and oxidative stress. *Curr Clin Pharmacol,* Nov;8(4):266-77.

[13]Francisco, B.M., Salvador, M., Amparo, N. (2015). Oxidative stress in myopia. *Oxid Med Cell Longev,* 2015:750637.

[14]Giovannucci, E., Ascherio, A., Rimm, E.B., Stampfer, M.J., Golditz, G.A., et al, (1995). Intake of carotenoids and retinol in relation to risk of prostate cancer. *J Natl Cancer Inst,* Dec 6;87(23):1767-76.

[15] Kijlstra, A., Tian, Y., Kelly, E.R., Berendschot, T.T. (2012). Lutein: more than just a filter for blue light. *Prog Ret Eye Res,* Jul;31(4):303-15.

[16]Lee, S.J., Bai, S.K., et al, (2003). Astaxanthin inhibits nitric oxide production and inflammatory gene expression by suppressing I(kappa)B kinase-dependent NF-kappaB activation. *Mol Cells,* Aug 31;16(1):97-105,

[17] Calder, P.C., (2015). Marine omega-3 fatty acids and inflammatory processes: Effects, mechanisms and clinical relevance. *Biochem Biophys Acta,* Apr;1851(4):469-84.

7-1. DIET AND VISION: HEALTHY EATING

Second only to the brain, the eyes are the most physiologically active organ in the human body. They require a great deal of ongoing, high-quality nutrition to keep them functioning well. The body naturally generates some important eye nutrients, but most are attained through the foods we eat.

This chapter includes the following:

- Healthy Eating
- General Dietary Recommendations
- The Alkalizing Diet
- The Mediterranean Diet
- The Vision Diet (including phytate reduction, soaking, and sprouting)
- Other Diets

Let's address the overall importance of what we put in our bodies. A human being has trillions of living cells in his/her body, each with a specific function. Each cell needs on-going nourishment to function at peak performance. An enormous amount of peer review research supports healthy eating as a way to significantly reduce the risk of many health problems, including heart disease, eye disease, and even dementia.

The preservation of the "essence" of healthy food also needs to be considered with respect to how we prepare food. Many vegetables, for example, may be eaten raw (if digestion is strong); others can be lightly steamed. Over-cooking or over-processing food destroys many of its nutrients, and according to some, destroys its "living" energy that replenishes our own energy. We turn food into energy to exist, to absorb nutrients, to neutralize free radicals, and to eliminate toxins.

Reaping the Benefits of What You Eat

Additionally, there is one crucial concept that is important to understand about good nutrition: health is determined not only by **what you eat** but **by what you absorb.** So, paying attention to how you feel after you eat, to the quality of your digestion, and to your elimination will give you clues as to how well you are assimilating your food and its nutrients.

First, we'll summarize some general dietary recommendations. Then we'll discuss two fundamental diets that are the basis of the Vision diet: the Mediterranean diet and the Alkaline diet. We'll discuss the Vision diet in detail. We will provide overviews of other popular diets.

General Dietary Recommendations

Key Components of the Vision Diet

The Vision diet is a healthy diet for both eyes and body consisting mainly of plant-based foods, along with small portions of preferably organic, animal products, such as free-range, grass-fed meats (for non-vegetarians). A plant-based diet, along with exercise, and maintenance of proper weight reduces the incidence of a range of health conditions, including chronic diseases, heart disease, type II diabetes,[1] and the incidence of cancer by 30–40%.[2][3]

Vegetables and Fruits

The largest percentage of the diet, in terms of quantity, should be vegetables and fruits, preferably lots of dark leafy-green vegetables and other colorful vegetables and fruits. These are rich in antioxidants, especially lutein and zeaxanthin, which are the colored pigments that your eye needs to function well. **These nutrients protect plants that contain them from sun damage and impart the same protection to our eyes, functioning as internal sun filters**. Even if you don't like vegetables such as collard greens, kale, and spinach, you can add them to soups, puree them in green drinks, juice them with other fruits and vegetables, or add them to other greens in salads. Many studies report, for example, that the nutrients found in these healthy vegetables lower the risk of developing macular degeneration, as well as other eye conditions, heart disease, and brain diseases.

In Quest of a Vision Diet

The Vision diet is based on an alkalizing diet and the Mediterranean diet. It is an anti-inflammatory diet that includes a lot of fresh vegetables and fruits, whole grains, olive oil, nuts, and seeds; it limits red meats, fried foods, and sweets. It focuses on the nutrients that support vision health, primarily carotenoids, essential fatty acids, vitamins, and enzymes.

---

[1] World Cancer Research Fund. (2007). Food, Nutrition, Physical Activity and the Prevention of Cancer: A Global Perspective. Washington, D.C. American Institute for Cancer Research.

[2] Glade, M.J. (1999). Food, nutrition, and the prevention of cancer: a global perspective. *Nutrition*, Jun; 15(6):523-6.

[3] Ibid. World Cancer Research Fund. (2007).

7-2. ALKALIZING DIET

The Vision Diet is an alkalizing and anti-inflammatory diet high in essential nutrients. We recommend favoring alkaline foods for everyone with an inflammatory condition (including heart conditions, arthritis, multiple sclerosis, lupus, diabetes, and digestive disorders of any kind), but even more so for anyone with chronic eye problems (even if not inflammatory), such as glaucoma, macula edema, uveitis, macular degeneration, retinitis pigmentosa, and Sjogren's syndrome.

Acidic diets, like the standard American diet, include high amounts of processed food, refined carbohydrates, poor-quality oils, and high levels of salt, which promote inflammation.

The pH scale ranges from 0 (acid) to 14 (alkaline), and a pH of 7 is considered neutral. The alkalizing diet is based on the understanding that a healthy body is slightly alkaline, somewhere around 7.365 pH. In the body, the pH can usually be measured by saliva pH and urine pH.

The issue in considering whether a food is acidic or alkaline is not the pH of the food itself, but the manner in which the body metabolizes the food. Foods that tend to cause inflammation in the body are acidic; foods that reduce inflammation are alkaline. Your body's digestive system's short-term goal is to maintain that 7.365 pH, regardless of the potential long-term result.

When there is excess acidity in the body, a condition results known as "long-term, diet-induced acidosis." It has a "significant, clinical, long-term pathophysiological effect."[1] Acidosis triggers overstimulation of cortisol production. The adrenals and other glands are stressed with continued high levels of cortisol, and chronically high levels of cortisol in the body are linked to autoimmune conditions,[2] heart disease,[3] digestive problems,[4] and some cancers.[5] Acidosis is also implicated in kidney problems.[6]

How Food pH is Determined

When we look at charts for alkaline/acidic foods, the results vary, sometimes greatly. One reason for this variation is the way most food pH analyses is done. PRAL (potential renal acid load) consists of taking a food, heating it until it is reduced to ash, and then measuring the pH of the remaining ash. This method may not be accurate because many sugars and yeasts quickly burn off before the entire sample is reduced to ash. The resulting analysis misclassifies many foods, such as sweet fruits like bananas, as alkaline.[7]

Because most sweeteners tend to increase inflammation, we favor a non-PRAL method of evaluating food pH. This approach was developed by researcher Robert Young who assessed foods as acid forming or alkaline forming, based on exhaustive blood testing. For example, this approach categorizes foods like many dried fruits (concentrated sugars) and sweet fruits as more acidic. In our juicing recipes, you will see that we recommend a higher proportion of vegetables and a smaller proportion of sweet fruit.

Alkaline / Acid Food Charts

Alkaline foods should be 80% of your diet and acidic foods the remaining 20% of your diet. The goal here is not to completely avoid acidic foods, but to limit them. You'll notice that most of the alkaline foods are plant based, e.g. vegetables and fruits.

The alkaline foods (80% of your diet) include:

- Vegetables and salads
- Citrus and less sweet fruits
- Some grains, legumes and seeds
- A few oils, especially olive oil
- Fresh herbs and spices

The acid foods (20% of your diet) include:

- Meat and seafood
- Dairy
- Sweet fruit
- Non-fresh vegetables
- Some flavorings
- Common cooking oils (limit these) and margarine (should be completed avoided).
- Sweeteners
- Alcohol, caffeinated drinks, and soft drinks
- Candy and snack foods

Resource. See the alkaline and acid food charts in Appendix 11.

---

[1] Pizzorno, J., Frassetto, L.A., Katzinger, J. (2010). Diet-induced acidosis: is it real and clinically relevant? *Br J Nutr,* Apr;103(8):1185-94.

[2] Montero-Lopez, E., Santos-Ruiz, A, Gonzalez, R., Navarrete-Navarrets, N., Ortego-Centeno, N., et al. (2017). Analyses of hair and salivary cortisol for evaluating hypothalamic-pituitary-adrenal axis activation in patients with autoimmune disease. *Stress,* Aug 30:1-8.

[3] University of Rochester Medical Center. Stress Can Increase Your Risk for Heart Disease. *Health Encyclopedia.* Retrieved from https://www.urmc.rochester.edu/encyclopedia/ content.aspx.

[4] Body Ecology. Fighting Adrenal Fatigue and High Cortisol Levels? How to Improve Your Energy. Retrieved from https://bodyecology.com/articles/fighting-adrenal-fatigue-and-high-cortisol-levels-how-to-improve-your-energy.

[5] Moreno-Smith, M., Lutgendorf, S.K., Sood, A.K. (2010). Impact of stress on cancer metastasis. *Future Oncol,* Dec: 6(12): 1863-1881.

[6] Adeva, M.M., Souto, G. (2011). Diet-induced metabolic acidosis. *Clin Nutr,* Aug;30(4):416-21.

[7] Bridgeford, R. (2017). The Definitive Acid & Alkaline Food Chart. Retrieved Nov 18 2017 from http://www.liveenergized.com.

7-3. MEDITERRANEAN DIET

The Vision diet also stands on the Mediterranean diet, an alkaline diet. We recommend this diet for most people. It has been well researched with fairly consistent results with respect to, not only vision, but to other health conditions. The Mediterranean diet may be summarized this way.

- High in vegetables and some fruit (particularly those low in sugar).
- Emphasizes whole grains, legumes, and nuts.
- Uses herbs and spices, instead of salt, to flavor foods.
- Replaces butter with high quality, first-cold-pressed extra virgin olive oil.
- Fish and poultry are recommended not more than twice a week, and red meat twice per month.
- A glass of red wine (preferably organic) with dinner is even permitted.

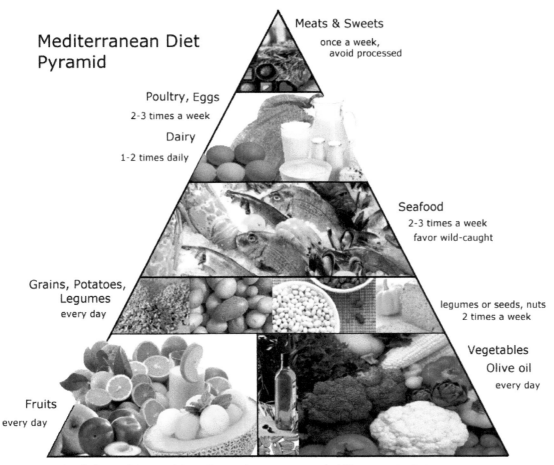

Mediterranean Diet Pyramid

Meats & Sweets once a week, avoid processed

Poultry, Eggs 2-3 times a week

Dairy 1-2 times daily

Seafood 2-3 times a week favor wild-caught

Grains, Potatoes, Legumes every day

legumes or seeds, nuts 2 times a week

Vegetables Olive oil every day

Fruits every day

Fresh Fruits & Vegetables: Every day, every meal, 1/2 cup cooked, 1 cup raw

These foods are high in antioxidants and nutrients that help fight against the risk of eye disease and support healthy vision. They also reduce heart disease, certain cancers, diabetes, and cognitive decline. Heart disease and diabetes are two major contributing causes of eye disease.

Mediterranean Meal Plan

- **Primary foods.** The Mediterranean diet is based on vegetables, fruits, nuts, seeds, seafood and olive oil. It includes whole grains, legumes, vegetables with herbs and spices for flavorings.
- **Secondary foods**. Poultry, eggs, cheese, and yogurt are taken in moderation.
- **Rare foods**. Rarely, eat red meat.
- **Avoid.** Don't eat sugars, processed food, refined (white) grains and breads, refined oils as well as anything labeled "low fat," or drinks that are labeled "diet."

Research

Studies have shown that the Mediterranean diet significantly reduces the risk of heart disease, cancer, and the incidence of Parkinson's and Alzheimer's disease.[1] One study shows that adherence to a Mediterranean diet is associated with reduced risk of progression toward advanced macular degeneration (AMD).[2] In a study across Europe, researchers examined 5,060 people over age 65. Throughout the previous twelve months, their diets were evaluated, as well as the incidence of AMD (both wet and dry forms) and a related condition, geographic atrophy. They found that those people most closely following a Mediterranean diet had the lowest rates of both forms of AMD, especially the lowest rates of the advanced wet form of AMD.[3]

---

[1] Mayo Clinic. Mediterranean diet: A heart-healthy eating plan. Retrieved from http://www.mayoclinic.org/ healthy-lifestyle/nutrition-and-healthy-eating/in-depth/mediterranean-diet/art-20047801.

[2] Merle, B.M., Silver, R.E., Rosner, B., Seddon, J.M. (2015). Adherence to a Mediterranean diet, genetic susceptibility, and progression to advanced macular degeneration: a prospective cohort study. *Am J Clin Nutr*, Nov;102(5):1196-206.

[3] Hogg, R.E., Woodside, J.V., McGrath, A., Young, I.S., Vioque, J.L. (2017). Mediterranean Diet Score and Its Association with Age-Related Macular Degeneration: The European Eye Study. *Ophthalmology*, Jan;124(1):82-89.

7-4. OMEGA-3 AND OMEGA-6 BALANCE

Essential fatty acids play an important role in vision health. We'll talk about omega-3 and omega-6 fatty acids in detail in the nutrients section later in this book.

The ratio of omega-3 and omega-6 fatty acids in our diet is important. Ideal dietary levels of omega-6 to omega-3 fatty acids are believed to be 1:1 to 4:1; however, the typical American diet now provides a ratio of about 10:1 to 20:1. To achieve a better fatty acid balance we need to favor omega-3s (from fatty fish, grass-fed eggs, and grass-fed dairy. Flaxseed also is a great source.

It is believed by scientists that the genetic patterns of evolving human beings developed when they had a diet with a ratio omega-3 to omega-6 of about 1:1.[1] The onset of modern agriculture over the last few decades and the increase of packaged and processed nutrient-deficient foods, toxic chemicals, antibiotic use, and stressful lifestyles has resulted in a dramatic increase in autoimmune diseases and chronic inflammatory conditions. The consumption of oils rich in the omega-6 linoleic acid (soybean, corn, safflower, and sunflower) has steadily risen in the United States, resulting in an increased ratio of omega-6 to omega-3 fatty acids in the American diet.

This change has been associated with an increased risk of such chronic inflammatory diseases as atherosclerosis, cardiovascular disease, rheumatoid arthritis, irritable bowel syndrome, diabetes,[2] [3] as well as obesity and waist circumference.[4] These systemic inflammatory conditions often result in chronic eye inflammation, such as uveitis, macular edema, diabetic retinopathy, macular degeneration, glaucoma, and even cataracts. Systemic inflammation contributes to poor circulation, which is implicated in compromised delivery of essential nutrients to the eyes.

Note. Certain omega-6 fatty acids such as those found in black currant seed oil, evening primrose oil, or borage oil do have natural anti-inflammatory properties and are therefore recommended.

---

[1] Simopoulos, A.P. (2002). The importance of the ratio of omega-6/omega-3 essential fatty acids. *Biomed Pharmacother,* Oct;56(8):365-79.

[2] Patterson, E., Wall, R., Fitzgerald, G.F., Ross, R.P., Stanton, C. (2012). Health implications of high dietary omega-6 polyunsaturated fatty acids. *J Nutr Metab,* 2012:539426.

[3] Ibid. Simopoulos. (2002).

[4] Torres-Castillo, N., Silva-Gomez, J.A., Campos-Perez, W., Barron-Cabrera, E., Hernandez-Canaveral, I., et al. (2018). High Dietary Omega-6:Omega-3 PUFA Ratio is Positively Associated with Excessive Adiposity and Waist Circumference. *Obes Facts,* Aug 10;11(4):344-353.

7-5. PHYTATE REDUCTION

Phytic acid is known to dietary experts as an "anti-nutrient." Phosphorus is stored in seeds and grains in the form of phytic acid. In the body, phytic acid binds minerals in the digestive tract, making them less bio-available. It is found mostly in whole grains and beans.[1]

Phytic acid slows absorption of iron, zinc, and less so of calcium. In addition, phytic acid also neutralizes some enzymes needed to properly digest these foods. This is true only within individual meals and not for overall digestion and absorption.[2] For those people with imbalanced gut bacteria or those with a nutrient deficient diet, especially vitamin A and D deficiencies, the phytic acid present in grains, legumes, nuts, and seeds can seriously deplete them of essential nutrients, such as calcium, zinc, magnesium, iron, and copper. Phytic acid also inhibits the thyroid (decreases TSH)[3] and induces metabolic and hormonal changes.[4]

Phytic acid content varies greatly, depending on the food and the conditions in which it is grown. Foods grown in high-phosphorous fertilized soil tend to have higher phytic acid concentrations than foods grown in naturally composted soil.[5]

Since everyone is affected by the effects of phytic acid, it is a reasonable idea to return to the food preparation traditions of soaking and sprouting foods, especially if digestion is an issue. Brazil nuts, brown rice, raw cacao, oats, and pumpkin seeds have some of the higher phytic acid levels, and they should be properly prepared before eating, or else kept to a minimum, especially if you are prone to tooth decay, bone density loss, mineral deficiencies, or are generally not well.

There are three methods of removing phytates from foods: soaking, sprouting, and fermentation.

Resource. For a more thorough description on how to neutralize phytate from foods, see the Weston A. Price website, "Living with Phytic Acid."

Soaking

For the average healthy person with a nutrient rich diet, here is a simple way to reduce phytates from your diet.

Soak all nuts, seeds, legumes, and grains in warm un-chlorinated water. You can add about a tablespoon of something acidic to each cup to be soaked.[6]

- For grains, soak 7–8 hours or overnight.
- Soft nuts, such as walnuts, pecans and cashews only need about four hours of soaking.
- Grains, such as oats and corn, require longer soaking. Adding freshly ground rye flour or sourdough rye culture and some lemon juice or yogurt can help; keep in a warm place overnight. For each cup of grain, add a tablespoon of something acid, such as yogurt, raw apple cider vinegar, lemon juice, whey, or kefir.
- Rinse in the morning before cooking.

- You can add unrefined salt into the water when you soak nuts to activate enzymes that neutralize enzyme inhibitors.
- Nuts that will be eaten later can be dehydrated on the lowest heat possible in the oven until completely dried. It is best to stir them occasionally and make sure they do not get burnt.

Resource. See the Soaking and Sprouting Guide in Appendix 12.

Sprouting

Sprouting takes health benefits to the next level. Some benefits include the production of vitamin C, an increase in B vitamins and carotene levels, further reduction of phytic acid, neutralization of enzyme inhibitors, and the production of many enzymes to aid in digestion.[7][8][9]

- You can sprout any grain, seed, or legume, and also raw almonds.
- Other nuts, as well as pumpkin, flax, chia, and hemp seeds cannot be sprouted.

Seeds, nuts, and grains need to be soaked before sprouting; but don't soak them too long. The amount of soaking depends on the hardness of the seed. Some take as little as 20 minutes while others take 8–12 hours.[10]

There are commercial sprouters available, or you can use the following procedure.

- Put the soaked grains, seeds, or legumes into a mason jar, cover with a cheese cloth, and tilt at a 45-degree angle to ensure all the water drains.
- Keep the jar somewhere where it will be exposed to air.
- Rinse the sprouts with fresh water, at least twice a day.
- After 1–4 days, you will see the start of the sprouts.
- Rinse with fresh water, drain very well, and store in the refrigerator.

You will want to use your sprouts within 2–3 days.

Resource: For more information on sprouting, refer to *Nourishing Traditions* by Sally Fallon.

Fermentation

There are many traditional ways to ferment food. You may already be familiar with some of them, such as tofu (fermented bean curd) or sourdough bread. Fermentation means converting some of the starches or sugars in a food to alcohol or organic acids without the presence of oxygen. The process not only preserves food, but in many cases, it makes it more digestible. Here are some examples:

- **Legumes and grains:** tofu, soy sauce, tempeh, bread, Rejuvelac (a traditional Eastern European fermented drink made from sprouted wheat berries)
- **Liquids:** beer, sake, wine, brandy, mead, kombucha, vinegar

- **Fruits and vegetables**: pickles, sauerkraut, kimchi, as well as chocolate[11]
- **Dairy**: cheese, creme fraiche, yogurt, kefir

[1] Andrews, R. Phytates and phytic acid. Retrieved Apr 18 2018 from https://www.precisionnutrition.com/all-about-phytates-phytic-acid.

[2] Arnarson, A. (2017). Phytic Acid 101: Everything You Need to Know. Retrieved Apr 18 2018 from https://www.healthline.com/nutrition/phytic-acid-101.

[3] Mohamed, T.M., Salama, A.F., El Nimr, T.M., El Gamal, D.M. (2015). Effects of phytate on thyroid gland of rats intoxicated with cadmium. *Toxicol Ind Health,* Dec;31(12):1258-68.

[4] Szkudeslski, T. (2005). Phytic acid-induced metabolic changes in the rat. *J Anim Physiol Anim Nutr (Berl),* Dec;89(11-12):397-402.

[5] Niknamian, S. (2016). High Untreated Phytic-Acid in the Diet, May Lead to Mineral Deficiencies, Specifically, During Pregnancy. *J Multi Eng Sci Tech,* Oct;3(10):5765-69.

[6] Chaudhary, N. Soak Your Nuts Grains & Legumes. Retrieved Apr 18 2018 from http://myindianroots.blogspot.com/2015/03/soak-your-nuts-seeds-grains-legumes.html.

[7] Chavan, J.K., Kadam, S.S. (1989). Nutritional improvement of cereals by sprouting. *Crit Rev Food Sci Nutr,* 28(5):401-37.

[8] Godman, H. (2017). Are sprouted grains more nutritious than regular whole grains? *Harvard Health Blog,* Nov 6.

[9] Devi, C.B., Kushwaha, A., Kumar, A. (2015). Sprouting characteristics and associated changes in nutritional composition of cowpea (Vigna unguiculata). *J Food Sci Technol,* Oct;52(10):6821-7.

[10] Sprout People. Soaking. Retrieved Apr 18 2018 from https://sproutpeople.org/growing-sprouts/sprouting-basics/soaking/

[11] Yes, chocolate is fermented. It must be fermented, dried, and roasted to produce the chocolate flavor.

7-6. THE VISION DIET

A Plant-Based Diet

We believe that this is a healthy diet for both eyes and body, because it consists mainly of plant-based foods, along with small portions of preferably organic, consciously produced animal products, such as free-range, grass-fed meats. Vegetarians on a strict plant-based diet need to routinely check their levels of certain nutrients that are difficult or not possible to obtain from plants and supplement where deficient. Be particularly careful of vitamin B12, zinc, and iron.

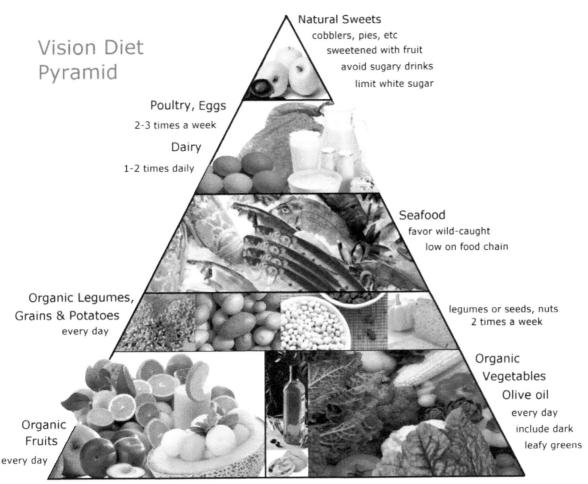

Vision Diet Pyramid

Natural Sweets
cobblers, pies, etc
sweetened with fruit
avoid sugary drinks
limit white sugar

Poultry, Eggs
2-3 times a week

Dairy
1-2 times daily

Seafood
favor wild-caught
low on food chain

Organic Legumes,
Grains & Potatoes
every day

legumes or seeds, nuts
2 times a week

Organic
Vegetables
Olive oil
every day
include dark
leafy greens

Organic
Fruits
every day

Fresh Fruits & Vegetables: Every day, every meal, 1/2 cup cooked, 1 cup raw

Putting It All Together

Vision diet incorporates the following principles:

- **The Alkalizing diet** avoids the foods that cause inflammation, including high amounts of processed food, refined carbohydrates, poor-quality oils, and high levels of salt.

- **The Mediterranean diet** is alkaline in nature and avoids processed and refined foods; it is rich in vegetables and fruit.
- **Balanced omega-3 and omega-6**.
- **Phytate reduction** to enhance better absorption of nutrients.

Go Organic

Evidence is increasing that the nutritional value of fruits and vegetables is closely linked to the quality of the soil they are grown in. Evidence is also increasing that non-organic foods are not the same as organically grown foods. Non-organically grown foods contain residues of herbicides and pesticides.[1] Organic food contains statistically higher levels of polyphenols that are important for health.[2] For example, organically grown tomatoes have 79% more quercetin,[3] organic tomato juice contains much more beta-carotene, rutin, flavonoids, and quercetin compared to non-organic. The differences in nutritional constituents of tomatoes may vary according to growing season; the organic crop of a different season may have higher levels of vitamin C and quercetin.[4]

A meta-analysis of research on organic compared to conventional dairy products found that the organic dairy products contained significantly higher amounts of protein, ALA, omega-3 and omega-6 oils, and other nutrients;[5] there was also a higher ratio of omega-3 to omega-6.[6] Other research suggests that organic foods may be higher in vitamin C, iron, phosphorus, and magnesium, and many organic foods may have higher levels of anthocyanins, flavonoids, and carotenoids.[7]

One more thing. Organic farming delivers greater ecosystem services and environmental benefits,[8] making it the most sustainable farming method,[9] critically important in this era.

Favor These Foods

Pure Water

Drink plenty of pure water every day, preferably spring water. Nutritionists recommend half an ounce to an ounce per pound of body weight. But you should drink what seems normal and natural. Water is essential for almost every cell activity. Being even slightly dehydrated reduces your metabolic efficiency. Chronic dehydration can lead to problems like kidney stones.[10] If you feel hungry much of the time, it might be that you are a little dehydrated. As a bonus, if you are trying to lose weight, drinking a glass of water before meals will help you feel more "full."

Drink 1/4 cup of water at a time (when not exercising). This is the amount of water the kidneys easily absorb and process at one time. Excess water intake will stress the kidneys.

Recommended. In general, try to keep water near you and sip it from time to time.

Caution. Tap water may include the following toxins: arsenic, aluminum, fluoride, pesticides, over-the-counter drugs, and/or disinfectant byproducts. Recommended home filters include reverse osmosis filters, ion exchange filters, or granular carbon and carbon block filters. If you use a filter that removes all minerals, such as for distilled water and RO (reverse osmosis), you should consider adding minerals. Only a few drops are needed per gallon of water.

Carotenoids from Vegetables and Fruits

The largest percentage of the diet in terms of quantity should be vegetables and then fruits. Focus on lots of dark leafy-green vegetables, other colorful vegetables, and a few fruits daily. These vegetables are rich in carotenoids, especially lutein and zeaxanthin, which are the colored pigments that your eyes need to function well.

Carotenoids are the pigments found in plants, where they function as internal sunscreens, protecting the plants from solar radiation. Carotenoids are antioxidants that help protect the body from oxidative damage. They are found throughout the body, but are highly concentrated in our eyes. When their level in eye tissue is low, then the risk of eye disease increases; for example, many studies report that these carotenoids found in vegetables significantly lower the risk of developing macular degeneration (as well as heart and brain disease).[11]

Even if you don't like vegetables such as collards, kale, and spinach, you can add them to soups, puree them in green drinks, juice them with other fruits and vegetables, or add them to salads.

Some people need to avoid nightshade-family vegetables and fruit that can cause inflammation; these include tomatoes, white potatoes, eggplant, okra, pepper, goji berries, tomatillos, and sorrel.

Recommended. Aim to have 1/2 cup cooked or one cup uncooked vegetables at almost every meal, every day. Be sure to include dark leafy-green vegetables.

Whole Grains for Protein, Fiber, and Minerals

Whole grains supply protein, fiber, minerals, and some B vitamins (not B12). No single grain is healthier than any other.[12] Each grain supplies a unique blend of nutrients; therefore, enjoy a wide variety of whole grains. There is a good deal of debate as to whether organic and non-organic grains are equivalent, but there has been evidence that the quality of the soil in which grains are grown makes a difference.

Whole grains are complex carbohydrates. They take a little longer to digest and help you maintain an even energy balance. They break down into glucose slowly. The slower the rate at which glucose is created, the more stable is your blood sugar. Food combining proponents recommend that grains be eaten with healthy fats and vegetables. Grains are best digested in an alkaline environment.[13]

Researchers report that whole grains, as opposed to processed (white or hulled) grains, help keep you healthy and able to ward off conditions such as high blood pressure and heart disease.[14]

Recommended. We recommend that you eat whole grains every day and vary your selection. Markets now offer a wide selection of different types of grains. Try them all.

Legumes

Legumes are a great source of protein, carbohydrates, fiber, minerals, and vitamins. They are higher in protein than other vegetables and generally low in fat. They're a good source of B-vitamins (but not B12) and contain antioxidant phytonutrients such as isoflavones and lignans. They partner well with whole grains because they are low in an essential amino acid, lysine.

Recommended. We recommend at least 1/2 cup of legumes, at least two times a week, preferably served in the same meal with whole grains. Soak them, if possible, to reduce phytates.

Herbs and Spices

Use herbs and spices to completely or partially substitute for salt or sugar. They contain many phytonutrients such as carotenoids and polyphenols.

Recommended. Use herbs and spices daily for all meals. If you can, grow them fresh.

Nuts and Seeds for Healthy Fats, Protein, Vitamins, Minerals

Nuts and seeds provide healthy fats, protein, vitamins, and minerals, including vitamin E, zinc, and essential fatty acids critical for retinal health; for example:

- Pecans contain more than 19 vitamins and minerals, and research has shown they may help lower LDL cholesterol and promote healthy arteries.[15]
- Walnuts provide high amounts of anti-inflammatory plant-based omega-3 fats, along with high amounts of copper, manganese, molybdenum, and biotin; they also contain powerful free-radical scavenging antioxidants.
- Pistachios are high in lutein, beta-carotene, and gamma-tocopherol (vitamin E) compared to other nuts (all excellent nutrients for eye health).
- Seeds such as sunflower seeds are rich in vitamins and minerals, including vitamin E, copper, B vitamins, manganese, selenium, phosphorus, and magnesium, which support heart health and the immune system.
- Pumpkin seeds offer a wide variety of nutrients, including zinc, magnesium, manganese, copper, and protein.
- Almonds contain plenty of vitamin E, magnesium, and protein, and help lower blood pressure and cholesterol levels while promoting weight loss and reducing hunger.

Recommended. We recommend a few nuts or seeds daily. Vary the kind of nut or seed for good balance.

Other Protein

For vegetarians, good protein sources include fermented soy products such as tempeh, which per ounce provides more protein than beef. For non-vegetarians, fatty fish like salmon (wild only) provide essential omega-3 fatty acids in addition to protein. Smaller fish like herring and sardines are lower on the food chain and tend to contain lower levels of heavy metals than the larger fish like tuna.

Reduce These Foods

A characteristic feature of most of the foods we suggest you limit or avoid is their ability to create inflammation in the body. As discussed earlier, scientists are coming to understand that systemic inflammation is a contributing cause to eye disease and to most chronic health conditions such as heart disease, diabetes, lung issues, bone health, depression, cancer, and emotional disorders.[16]

Similarly, these foods increase oxidative stress in the body. Overload of free radicals causes oxidative stress and plays a major role in the development of chronic and degenerative illness such as cancer, autoimmune disorders, aging, rheumatoid arthritis, cardiovascular and neurodegenerative diseases. Oxidative stress is implicated in age-related macular degeneration and cataracts.[17]

Refined Carbohydrates

Avoid or minimize refined carbohydrates such as the white versions of bread, pasta, rice, and sugar. Most of their food value is removed when the nutrient-rich outer husks are removed in processing. Furthermore, they deplete the body of essential enzymes and minerals needed to break down these foods. For those prone to chronic inflammatory conditions, these foods are quite acidic (as opposed to alkaline) and exacerbate body and eye inflammation.

In the past, carbohydrates were classified as either simple (such as sugar and fructose) or complex (such as those that contain fiber, vitamins, and minerals). More recently, the glycemic index has become more relevant because it rates foods by how quickly they break down into sugar in the body. It ranks carbohydrates on a scale from 0 to 100, based on how quickly and how much they raise blood sugar levels after eating.

Glycemic Index

A high glycemic index diet increases the risk of macular degeneration,[18] [19] [20] diabetes,[21] heart disease,[22] [23] and obesity.[24] [25] [26] A glycemic index of 70 or above is considered high.[27]

Another study suggests that a low glycemic index has anti-inflammatory benefits.[28]

Low glycemic index foods have an index of 55 or less. These foods include lentils, cashews, kidney beans, black beans, garbanzo beans (used to make hummus), oranges, apples, almonds, walnuts, peanuts (though these can be inflammatory and should be avoided for anyone with an inflammatory condition), carrots, bran cereals, all leafy-green vegetables, quinoa, millet, wild caught fish, free-range beef, and eggs.

Medium glycemic index foods have an index of 56–69 and include whole grain breads, rice cakes, oatmeal, brown rice, and whole grain pasta.

High glycemic index foods have an index of 70–100 and include all refined carbohydrates (white flour, rice, pasta), sugars, refined breakfast cereals, baked potato, pretzels, French fries, couscous, millet, muesli, sugar sweetened soft drinks, fruit juices, melons, pineapple, corn tortilla, sweet corn, rice, Udon noodles, and sugar added salad dressings.

Recommended. Favor whole grains over refined grains.

Note. The glycemic index of food on your plate depends on several factors. For example, you can decrease the glycemic level by adding lemon juice or by increasing the proportion of low glycemic food in a meal. The longer starches are cooked, or the riper the fruit, the higher their index.[29]

Sweeteners

With consumption of soft drinks and candy, Americans consume an enormous amount of sugar, the equivalent of more than seven tablespoons daily. This amount of sugar is about 355 calories. We are in the midst of a crisis of obesity in the U.S. and the consumption of sweet foods is part of the problem.

Furthermore, sweeteners **of all kinds** contribute to inflammation. Sugar is one of the most acidic foods, and excess sugar in one's diet is considered a leading contributor to disease, such as type 2 diabetes, cardiovascular disease, high blood pressure (hypertension), dementia, and cancer.[30] Numerous research studies have linked a number of these health conditions to eye diseases, such as cataracts, glaucoma, and diabetic retinopathy; studies have also linked diets high on the glycemic index with macular degeneration.[31] [32] [33]

Balancing blood sugar

When you eat or drink something sweet, it gives a quick surge of energy. However, the consequence of glucose entering the bloodstream so quickly is that the body's ability to maintain stability is compromised.

With some attention to our diet, we can help balance blood sugar. This is especially true in type 2 diabetes (adult onset), which sometimes can be managed by diet alone. It is rarely true of type 1 diabetes (juvenile onset).

Recommended. Limit your sweets and avoid sugary drinks and sodas. In general, an alkaline diet will be a low sugar diet and will be anti-inflammatory. Avoid aspartame and other chemical sweeteners (foods labeled "diet"). Avoid high glycemic index foods.

Fried Foods

Fried foods provide almost no nutritional value and present digestive challenges. This is especially true of foods containing trans-fatty acids, which can cause diarrhea. Fried foods and foods containing trans-fatty acids substantially increase free radicals in the body that cause the breakdown of healthy cells.

Excess intake of fried foods is tied to increased risk of diabetes and heart disease. One study found that people who ate fried food at least once per week had a greater risk of type 2 diabetes and heart disease, and the risk increased as the frequency of fried food consumption increased. On a per-calorie basis, trans fats appear to increase the risk of chronic heart disease more than any other micronutrient.[34] In one study, the participants who ate fried foods 4–6 times per week had a 39% increased risk of type 2 diabetes, and those who ate fried foods seven or more times per week had a 55% increased risk.[35]

Recommended. Limit fried foods, especially deep-fried foods.

- Avoid man-made fats (corn oil, safflower oil, trans fats, and hydrogenated vegetable oils, including canola oil).
- Avoid trans-fatty acids. These are oils that have added hydrogen incorporated to turn their liquid state into a solid, e.g. margarine. Avoid hydrogenated oils, trans-fatty acids, and saturated fats, which also disrupt the digestive process.

Processed Foods

Breads, frozen meals, canned foods, and other foods that have been created in "food factories" tend to be loaded with artificial sweeteners, flavor enhancers, and a host of preservatives.

Many such chemicals have been gradually phased out as the food industry yields to scientific research, proving their detrimental-to-health qualities. A good example is the use of many different chemicals used to color food.[36]

But there are a number of food additives that are banned in Europe that are still permitted in the U.S. These include, but are not limited to, Olestra, brominated vegetable oil, BHA/BHT, azodicarbonamide, rBGH or rBST hormones, and neonicotinoid pesticides.[37]

New chemicals are created frequently as substitutes for those that are no longer permitted. When you are in the grocery store about to buy pre-prepared foods, look at the label. If the food label includes any number of unidentifiable chemicals, you would be wise to avoid it or do some research. And if the first three ingredients are a refined grain, sweetener, or hydrogenated oil, it is best to pass it by.[38]

Recommended. Cook from scratch whenever possible. Many healthy meals take no longer to prepare than frozen meals and are considerably better for you.

Additives

Processed foods all contain additives. These are ingredients that are designed to keep food from spoiling, to supply an inexpensive source of flavor, or to provide texture. Some of these additives include the following:[39]

High fructose corn syrup. High fructose corn syrup is one of the worst culprits. This sweetener causes intracellular depletion of adenosine triphosphate (ATP). ATP is the primary biochemical that delivers energy throughout the body. When a cell needs energy, the process of breaking down ATP releases energy. High fructose corn syrup causes nucleotide turnover (these are the structural components of compounds such as DNA). It increases generation of uric acid that may have a critical role in causing diabetes and obesity.[40]

There are a number of sweeteners that are chemically similar to high fructose corn syrup that may be labeled as fructose, invert sugar, honey, evaporated cane juice, sugar, and sucrose.[41] Even when used in moderation, these are a primary or contributing cause of cardiovascular disease, cancer, liver failure, and tooth decay.[42] They are implicated in metabolic syndrome,[43] memory problems,[44] and much more.

Phosphates. Many food additives contain phosphates, which increase danger for those with kidney disease and may contribute to heart disease, bone loss, and other chronic conditions.[45] These are often added as flavor enhancers. Phosphates that occur naturally in food are fine; the body absorbs them incompletely. However, added inorganic phosphates can significantly increase the blood phosphate level. The main problem is damage to the blood system, causing malfunctioning of tissue that lines the blood vessels and the accumulation of plaque.[46]

Sulfites. When added as a preservative, sulfites attack B1, especially under acid conditions.[47]

Emulsifiers. These help oil and water-based liquids stay mixed together in foods. When you add a bit of mustard to your vinaigrette, you are adding an emulsifier. Early research reports that lab animals given chemical emulsifiers added weight, added fat, had poor blood sugar control, and had more severe elimination problems. These artificial emulsifiers include gums, polysorbates 60 and 80, lecithin, and carboxymethylcellulose.[48]

Hidden allergens. Potential allergens are hard to identify because they are undeclared, and they are the biggest cause of food recalls. Baked goods are the biggest source. The most common hidden allergens are milk, wheat, soy, and sometimes nuts.[49]

Recommended. If you buy pre-prepared foods, read the label carefully, and avoid those with a long list of additives, preservatives, artificial flavorings, and colorings.

Caffeine

Caffeine may present challenges to the eyes. Caffeine is a stimulant found in cocoa beans, coffee beans, black and green tea. Smaller amounts of caffeine intake have been found to have potential health benefits, e.g. coffee contains antioxidant phenols and reduces the risk of developing neurodegenerative disease and other health conditions, including type 2 diabetes mellitus and liver disease. Studies are mixed, but some show a small amount (organic) is healthy.

At the same time, on the negative side, coffee can increase serum homocysteine and cholesterol levels and therefore has adverse effects on the cardiovascular system.[50] One study showed that participants who reported drinking three cups or more of caffeinated coffee per day were at a higher risk of developing exfoliation glaucoma.[51] However, another review of people who drink 3–4 cups of coffee a day (300–400mg of caffeine) suggested that there is little evidence of health risk and some evidence of health benefit.[52] These benefits were associated with cardiovascular disease, coronary heart disease, and stroke, when compared with those not drinking coffee.[53]

Chinese medicine perspective on coffee

Coffee is yang in nature. It regulates Liver Qi (energy) and clears the Gallbladder, resulting in its ability to protect against formation of gallstones and alleviating constipation. Coffee moves Qi and Blood, invigorates, and disperses (meaning that it has a diuretic effect and helps move energy and fluids in the body).

The benefits and risks of drinking coffee for eye and general health can depend on each person's constitution and the environment they live in. For people living in a cold environment, coffee can be very warming. For those living in a hot environment, it may create too much heat. Excessive amounts of coffee will agitate the liver yang. Symptoms can include headaches (typically on one side of the head or in or above the eyes), breaking blood vessels on the outside of the eyes (sclera), elevated eye pressure (IOP), red eyes, visual disturbances, ocular migraines, possible changes in eyesight, ringing in the ears, dizziness, dry mouth, heavy feeling, insomnia, and increases in blood pressure. It can stimulate internal wind with symptoms that can include the following: pain that moves around, itchy skin conditions, dizziness/vertigo, tremor or spasms, sudden appearing rashes, sudden onset of headache or migraine with vertigo, or possibly sudden onset of disease.

For people that are yang deficient (low in energy and generally cold overall), moderate amounts of coffee can be therapeutic to warm the body and stimulate yang. Excessive amounts can eventually have the opposite effect by depleting the adrenals.

Coffee is warm, sweet, and bitter. The slight sweetness of coffee also makes it mildly tonifying and nourishing. The primary bitter taste has the action of drying and dispersing. It can also clear heat, which helps balance out the very warm nature of coffee. It reduces the risk of colon cancer as it moves Qi and Blood in the large intestine.

In traditional Chinese medicine, food is divided into five natures: cold, cool, neutral, warm, and hot. Coffee brings warmth and heat to the body. So, a person who tends to have too much heat should avoid coffee or keep it at a minimum. Common symptoms of chronic heat include feeling hot, sweating all the time, being grumpy, having a swollen tongue, and often being constipated.

Coffee can be helpful for those who tend to be cold and/or damp. Common symptoms of having a cold constitution include being pale, having cold hands and feet, sensitivity to cold temperatures, feeling weak, and having poor circulation. Dampness tendencies include being overweight, particularly around the stomach, distended stomach, sticky mouth, greasy tongue, swelling, water retention, loose stool, and/or nodule masses (lymph nodes).

Recommended. Limit yourself to one cup of coffee, tea, cocoa daily, and it is best unsweetened.

Alcohol

Alcohol reduces protective glutathione levels because it interferes with liver functioning. Although red wine has been touted for its antioxidant benefit and heart health, "moderate" consumption has been associated with an increased risk of breast cancer.[54] Heavy drinking increases the risk of many diseases, including heart disease, anemia, cirrhosis, depression, seizures, hypertension, immune system suppression, nerve damage, and pancreatic disease.[55]

Most alcoholics are malnourished; the metabolism of alcohol by the liver prevents the proper digestion of proteins, and vitamins. This is especially true of vitamin A,[56] which is essential for good vision. In addition, toxins and free radicals that interfere with fat digestion are created when alcohol is broken down in the liver.[57]

Recommended. Limit alcohol consumption to one glass of red wine daily.

In Summary, the Vision Diet Recommendations

We recommend the Mediterranean Diet and the Alkalizing Diet.

- **Pure water.** Sip throughout the day.
- **Fresh vegetables and fruits**. 1/2 cup cooked or 1 cup raw, every day, every meal, more vegetables than fruits, include dark leafy greens.
- **Olive oil.** Use first cold-pressed extra-virgin olive oil in a dark bottle.
- **Whole grains, legumes, starch**. Every day, potatoes only once or twice a week.
- **Nuts and seeds.** A few each day, if more than a few, then twice a week.
- **Seafood.** Not more than 2–3 times per week, favor wild-caught.
- **Dairy.** Not more than once a day.
- **Poultry, eggs.** Not more than 2–3 times per week.
- **Natural sweets**. Cobblers, pies sweetened with fruit.
- **Go organic.** Know what you are putting into your body.

Avoid Harmful Ingredients that impact your health negatively.

- **Limit sweets**, particularly white or refined sugar. Avoid artificial sweeteners such as aspartame.
- **Limit alcohol** to one glass of red wine daily; alcohol reduces the protective glutathione levels, because it interferes with liver functioning (the liver produces glutathione).
- **Cut down on caffeine** in coffee and tea to one cup a day, for most people.
- **Read the labels** when you buy processed foods. Avoid artificial sweeteners, flavorings, colorings, MSG, and fat blockers like Olestra.
- **Slow down on the fast foods** and reduce or eliminate deep-fried foods.

---

[1] Zalecka, A., Bugel, S., Paoletti, F., Kahl, J., Bonanno, A. (2014). The influence of organic production on food quality - research findings, gaps and future challenges. *J Sci Food Agric,* Oct;94;(13):2600-4.

[2] Ibid. Zalecka. (2014).

[3] Mitchell, A.E., Hong, Y.J., Barrett, D.M., Bryant, D.E., Denison, R.F., et al. (2007). Ten-Year Comparison of the Influence of Organic and Conventional Crop Management Practices on the Content of Flavonoids in Tomatoes. *J Agric Food Chem,* Jul 25;55(15):6154-9.

[4] Hallmann, E., Lipowski, J., Marszalek, K., Rembialkowska, E. (2013). The seasonal variation in bioactive compounds content in juice from organic and non-organic tomatoes. *Plant Foods Hum Nutr,* Jun;68(2):171-6.

[5] Palupi, E., Jayanegara, A., Ploeger, A., Kahl, J. (2012). Comparison of nutritional quality between conventional and organic dairy products: a meta-analysis. *J Sci Food Agric,* Nov;92(14):2774-81.

[6] Ibid. Palupi. (2012).

[7] Crinnon, W.J. (2010). Organic foods contain higher levels of certain nutrients, lower levels of pesticides, and may provide health benefits for the consumer. *Altern Med Rev,* Apr;15(1):4-12.

[8] Reganold, J.P., Wachter, J.M. (2016). Organic agriculture in the twenty-first century. *Nat Plants,* Feb 3;2:15221.

[9] Strasser, C., Cavoski, I., Di Cagno, R., Kahl, J., Kesse-Guyot, E., et al. (2015). How the Organic Food System Supports Sustainable Diets and Translates These into Practice. *Front Nutr,* Jun 29;2:19.

[10] Clark, W.F., Sontrop, J.M., Huang, S.H., Moist, L., Bouby, N. et al. (2016). Hydration and Chronic Kidney Disease Progression: A Critical Review of the Evidence. *Am J Nephrol,* 43(4):281-92.

[11] Guest, J., Grant, R. (2016). Carotenoids and Neurobiological Health. *Adv Neurobiol,* 12:199-228.

[12] Whole Grains Council. Grains Compared (chart), Retrieved from https://wholegrainscouncil.org/sites/default/files/thumbnails/image/GrainsComparedAll3.jpg

[13] Elkaim, Y. Food Combining Rules: The Complete Guide. Retrieved from https://yurielkaim.com/food-combining-rules/

[14] Bechthold, A., Boeing, H., Schwedhelm, C., Hoffmann, G., Knuppel, S. et al. (2017). Food groups and risk of coronary heart disease, stroke and heart failure: A systematic review and dose-response meta-analysis of prospective studies. *Crit Rev Food Sci Nutr,* Oct 17:0.

[15] Morgan, W.A., Clayshulte, B.J. (2000). Pecans lower low-density lipoprotein cholesterol in people with normal lipid levels. *J Am Diet Assoc,* Mar;100(3):312-8.

[16] Szalay, J. (2015). Inflammation: Causes, Symptoms & Anti-Inflammatory Diet. *LiveScience.* Retrieved from https://www.livescience.com/52344-inflammation.html.

[17] Pham-Huy, L.A., He, H., Pham-Huy, C. (2008). Free radicals, antioxidants in disease and health. *Int J Biomed Sci,* Jun; 4(2): 89–96.

[18] Chiu, C., Milton, R.C., Gensler, G., Taylor, A. (2007). Association between dietary glycemic index and age-related macular degeneration in nondiabetic participants in the Age-Related Eye Disease Study. *Am J Clin Nutr,* July; (86):180-188.

[19] Hitti, M. (2007). High-Sugar Foods May Affect Eyesight. WebMD. Retrieved Apr 18 2018 from https://www.webmd.com/eye-health/macular-degeneration/news/20070713/high-sugar-foods-may-affect-eyesight.

[20] Hitti, M. (2005). Healthy Diet May Help Seniors' Vision. WebMD. Retrieved Apr 18 2018 from https://www.webmd.com/eye-health/news/20051227/healthy-diet-may-help-seniors-vision#1

[21] de Munter, JS, Hu FB, Spiegelman D, Franz M, van Dam RM. (2007). Whole grain, bran, and germ intake and risk of type 2 diabetes: a prospective cohort study and systematic review. *PLoS Med,* 4:e261.

[22] Beulens, J.W., de Bruijne, L.M., Stolk, R.P, Peeters, P.H., Bots, M.L., et al. (2007). High dietary glycemic load and glycemic index increase risk of cardiovascular disease among middle-aged women: a population-based follow-up study. *J Am Coll Cardiol,* 50:14-21.

[23] Halton, T.L., Willett, W.C., Liu, S., Manson, J.E., Albert, C.M., et al. (2006). Low-carbohydrate-diet score and the risk of coronary heart disease in women. *N Engl J Med,* 355:1991-2002.

[24] Anderson, J.W., Randles, K.M., Kendall, C.W., Jenkins, D.J. (2004). Carbohydrate and fiber recommendations for individuals with diabetes: a quantitative assessment and meta-analysis of the evidence. *J Am Coll Nutr,* 23:5-17

[25] Ebbeling, C.B., Leidig, M.M., Feldman, H.A., Lovesky, M.M., Ludwig, D.S. (2007). Effects of a low-glycemic load vs low-fat diet in obese young adults: a randomized trial. *JAMA,* 297:2092-102.

[26] Maki, K.C., Rains, T.M., Kaden, V.N., Raneri, K.R., Davidson, M.H. (2007). Effects of a reduced-glycemic-load diet on body weight, body composition, and cardiovascular disease risk markers in overweight and obese adults. *Am J Clin Nutr,* 85:724-34.

[27] WebMD. How to Use the Glycemic Index. Retrieved May 30 2018 from https://www.webmd.com/diabetes/guide/glycemic-index-good-versus-bad-carbs#1

[28] Buyken, A.E., Goletzke, J., Joslowski, G., Felbick, A., Cheng, G., et al. (2014). Association between carbohydrate quality and inflammatory markers: systematic review of observational and interventional studies. *Am J Clin Nutr,* 99(4): 2014;813-33.

[29] Ibid. WebMD. How to Use the Glycemic Index.

[30] Doheny, K. (2012). Americans Sweet on Sugar: Time to Regulate? WebMD. Retrieved from https://www.webmd.com/diet/news/20120201/americans-sweet-on-sugar-time-to-regulate#1

[31] Chiu, C., Milton, R.C., Gensler, G., Taylor, A. (2007). Association between dietary glycemic index and age-related macular degeneration in nondiabetic participants in the Age-Related Eye Disease Study. *Am J Clin Nutr*, July; (86):180-188.

[32] Hitti, M. (2005). Healthy Diet May Help Senior's Vision. WebMD. Retrieved Apr 18 2018 from https://www.webmd.com/eye-health/news/20051227/healthy-diet-may-help-seniors-vision#1.

[33] Hitti, M. (2007). High-Sugar Foods May Affect Eyesight. WebMD. Retrieved Apr 18 2018 from https://www.webmd.com/eye-health/macular-degeneration/news/20070713/high-sugar-foods-may-affect-eyesight.

[34] Mozaffarian, D., Katan, M.B., Ascherio, A., Stampfer, M.J., Willett, W.C. (2006). Trans fatty acids and cardiovascular disease. *N Engl J Med*, Apr 13; 354(15):1601-13.

[35] Cahill, L.E., Pan, A., Chiuve, S.E., Sun, Q., Willett, W.C., et al. (2014). Fried-food consumption and risk of type 2 diabetes and coronary artery disease: a prospective study in 2 cohorts of US women and men. *Am J Clin Nutr*, Aug;100(2):667-675.

[36] Association of Food and Drug Officials. Food Color Additives Banned in the USA. Retrieved from http://importedfoods.afdo.org/food-color-additives-banned-in-the-usa.html.

[37] Seattle Organic Restaurants. Top 10 foods, additives and preservatives that are banned in many countries except US. Retrieved from http://www.seattleorganicrestaurants.com/vegan-whole-food/foods-banned-in-other-countries-but-we-eat-in-us.php.

[38] Bjarnadottir, A. (2015). How to Read Food Labels Without Being Tricked. Healthline Newsletter. Retrieved from https://www.healthline.com/nutrition/how-to-read-food-labels#section3.

[39] WebMD. Food Additives: What's Hiding in Your Food? (2017). Retrieved from https://www.webmd.com/news/breaking-news/food-additives/food-additives-infographic.

[40] Johnson, R.J., Nakagawa, T., Sanchez-Lozada, L.G., Shafiu, M., Sundaram, S., et al. (2013). Sugar, uric acid, and the etiology of diabetes and obesity. *Diabetes*, Oct;62(10):3307-15.

[41] Ibid. WebMD. Food Additives.

[42] Hyman, M. (2011). *5 Reasons High Fructose Corn Syrup Will Kill You*. Retrieved from http://drhyman.com/blog/2011/05/13/5-reasons-high-fructose-corn-syrup-will-kill-you/.

[43] Legeza, B., Marcolongo, P., Gamberucci, A., Varga, V., Banhegyi, G. (2017). Fructose, Glucocorticoids and Adipose Tissue: Implications for the Metabolic Syndrome. *Nutrients*, Apr. 26;9(5).

[44] Noble, E.E., Hsu, T.M., Liang, J., Kanoski, S.E. (2017). Early-life sugar consumption has long-term negative effects on memory function in male rats. *Nutr Neurosci*, Sept 25:1-11.

[45] Ibid. WebMD. Food Additives.

[46] Ritz, E., Hahn, K., Ketteler, M., Kuhlmann, M.K., Mann, J. (2012). Phosphate Additives in Food--A Health Risk. *Dtsch Arztebl Int*, Jan;109(4):49–55.

[47] Thiamine. Wikipedia. Retrieved from https://en.wikipedia.org/wiki/Thiamine.

[48] Ibid. WebMD. Food Additives

[49] Ibid. WebMD. Food Additives

[50] Gokcen, B.B., Sanlier, N. (2017). Coffee Consumption and Disease Correlations. *Crit Rev Food Sci Nutr*, Aug 30:1-13.

[51] Pasquale, L.R., Wiggs, J.L., Willett, W.C., Kang, J.H. (2012). The Relationship between Caffeine and Coffee Consumption and Exfoliation Glaucoma or Glaucoma Suspect: A Prospective Study in Two Cohorts. *Invest Ophthalmol Vis Sci*, Sept. Vol.53, 6427-6433.

[52] Nieber, K. (2017). The Impact of Coffee on Health. *Planta Med*, Jul 4.

[53] Gulland, A. (2017). Scientists wake up to coffee's benefits. *BMJ*, Nov 22;359:j5381.

[54] Brooks, P.J., Zakhari, S. (2013). Moderate alcohol consumption and breast cancer in women: from epidemiology to mechanisms and interventions. *Alcohol Clin Exp Res,* Jan;37(1):23-30.

[55] Freeman, D. 12 Health Risks of Chronic Heavy Drinking. Retrieved April 18 2018 from https://www.webmd.com/mental-health/addiction/features/12-health-risks-of-chronic-heavy-drinking#1

[56] Lieber, C.S. (2003). Relationship between nutrition, alcohol use, and liver disease. *Alcohol Res Health,* 37(3):220-31.

[57] Ibid. Lieber. (2003).

7-7. OTHER DIETS

Other diets may be worth exploring. Every individual is different, and the dietary needs of one person can be vastly different from another. For ease, we have broken the diets into two primary categories: omnivorous and plant-based. Simply, the omnivorous diets include animal products while the plant-based diets include little.

Omnivorous Diets

The Atkins Diet

The Atkins diet is a popular low-carbohydrate, high-protein weight-loss diet created by the late cardiologist Robert Atkins, M.D. The diet, which advocates consuming only high amounts of proteins and fats, such as meat, poultry, seafood, eggs, butter, oils, and cheeses, along with high-fiber vegetables, at first promotes rapid weight-loss through the metabolic process called ketosis, which is the burning of fat, rather than carbohydrates for fuel. As the diet progresses, foods like beans/legumes, fruits, and whole grains can be added.

The diet is extremely strict in staying away from starchy and sugary carbs, including bread, pasta, chips, cookies, and candy. It recommends a wide range of vegetables. One advantage of the Atkins diet is that it prohibits most, if not all, foods with gluten, which tend to be high in carbs. People on Atkins, therefore, eat less gluten than people who eat the standard American diet.

Eye Health Risks/Rewards

The advantage of the Atkins diet is particularly good for people sensitive to gluten, helpful in controlling body weight, and possibly helpful in reducing acid reflux (GERD), acne, headaches, heart disease, cancer, diabetes/metabolic syndrome/insulin resistance, and dementia.

The disadvantage of this diet is that a high protein diet is not ideal for many people, and the diet does not focus enough on eating the right, healthy oils and staying away from those that should be avoided.

If the body is chronically depleted of carbohydrates, it exposes the liver to additional stress, as the liver produces glucose from fats and proteins instead of carbohydrates.[1] Toxic amounts of ammonia can be produced, and the immune system can become compromised. Proteins are said to not metabolize "cleanly." A byproduct of protein metabolism is ammonia, which is not thoroughly eliminated through urine. Adequate intake of water is also essential since protein metabolism requires water to break down amino acids and to process and eliminate nitrogen.

While the diet has proven effective for weight loss, opponents have gone as far as to condemn it as outright dangerous because of its high level of saturated fat intake, which has been linked to everything from high cholesterol and kidney problems to cancer.[2] In addition, a goal of rapid weight loss is neither safe nor sustainable.

Blood Type Diet

Designed by Dr. Peter J. D'Adamo, this diet is based on the theory that the foods we eat react chemically with our blood type, and therefore, can either improve health or make a person more susceptible to certain disease. He states that blood type is a key genetic factor, and as such, is a factor in both health and disease.

He notes, for example, that people with blood type O can efficiently digest protein and fat, but their metabolism of carbohydrates tends to produce fats and triglycerides. Consequently, they have a lower risk for heart disease but a higher risk for developing stomach ulcers and thyroid disorders. In addition, type O is prone to the "fight or flight" response, resulting in emotional imbalances, including bouts of excessive anger. Type O's benefit from regular brisk exercise as a tonic for the entire system.[3]

Eye Health Risks/Rewards

The Blood Type diet could be effective because the foods recommended attempt to address underlying issues by blood type, thereby supporting overall health in a more individualized way. This diet might result in, for example, reducing emotional stress for Type O people and improving digestion, which both support health vision by providing more essential nutrients available for eye health. It may be that eating incorrectly for one's blood type may increase inflammation, a key contributing cause of eye disease. One example is that type O people can safely eat chicken without increasing inflammation, but with type B and AB people, chicken increases inflammation.[4]

One risk is that strict adherence to the diet may ignore other factors that influence vision health, such as genetics, environmental concerns, and so forth. A comprehensive review of the literature found no evidence to support the validity of the blood type diet.[5]

This doesn't mean that the diet doesn't work, but it may not work for everyone. For example, another study found that adherence to the type A diet was associated with lowered BMI, blood pressure, cholesterol, triglycerides, insulin, and other biomarkers. It found similar improvements for diet AB (except BMI), and the type O diet was linked to lower triglycerides. These researchers, however, concluded that while the diets were favorable for some people, **those results were not associated with blood type.**[6]

Metabolic Typing Diet

Designed by William L. Wolcott, this diet addresses biochemical individuality. The same foods and their nutrients can have different effects in different bodies. Metabolic means the chemical processes that occur within a living organism in order to maintain life. Metabolic typing regards an individual's genetics as the key factor in the digestion and "processing" of foods and utilization of nutrients.[7]

The assumption is that one type of diet can help prevent disease in one person, while the same diet may promote disease in another. The Metabolic Typing diet analyzes many different aspects of a person's physiological makeup, including blood type, in order to specify a diet appropriate for that person's biochemical and metabolic tendencies. While there are three "basic" metabolic type categories: the protein type, the carbo type, or the mixed type, adjustments need to be made in coming up with the best diet.[8]

Eye Health Risks/Rewards

Similar to the blood type diet, the Metabolic Type diet can be effective because the diet is more individualized by body type, which maximizes the nutritional benefits of the foods recommended according to metabolic type, thereby supporting overall eye and body health.

One of the diets for the protein type is rich in organ meats and saturated fats and is thus more likely to increase the risk of heart disease and other conditions.[9] Although the diet can be helpful for weight loss, research is lacking as to the long-term effectiveness and safety.[10]

The Ornish Spectrum Program

More of a lifestyle program than a diet, this program emphasizes a low-fat, low-sugar, plant-based diet, along with regular exercise, stress reduction, and social support through relationship building. Although cardiologist Dean Ornish, designed the program specifically for heart health, he says the program works to improve health for anyone; and research has shown that it can reverse heart disease, type 2 diabetes, and even early-stage prostate cancer.[11]

The nutrition part of the diet consists of fruits, vegetables, whole grains, and legumes (organic soy in particular) with an emphasis on whole unprocessed foods. In its strictest form, animal protein is limited to egg whites and nonfat dairy foods, and there are no added oils. Less than 10% of calories come from fat. The diet starts with complex carbohydrates, fruits, and veggies. That makes it high in fiber and low in calories. Critics take issue with the low-fat component of the program and note that stages of the diet could be considered restrictive.

Eye Health Risks/Rewards

The beneficial dietary aspect of this program is that it is rich in vitamins, minerals, antioxidants, and fiber, and it is low in saturated fats and cholesterol, especially compared to high-protein/low-carb diets. Additionally, because the focus includes lifestyle actions toward improving heart health, the Ornish Spectrum program will not only boost circulation, which is crucial for eye health, but will also reduce stress, which is integral for resolving numerous eye disorders.

However, the diet tends to be lower in other nutrients that are predominantly found in animal foods, such as vitamin B12, iron, and zinc, as well as omega-3 fatty acids. For this reason, Dr. Ornish recommends supplementing with a multivitamin as well.[12]

Paleolithic Diet

This program is based on the hunter-gatherer diet of protein from lean meats, fruit (not too much and particularly those low in sugar, such as berries), and vegetables. There is essentially no dairy or grain in this diet. When you are following the Paleo diet, you eat foods that were hunted or gathered far in the past, such as meats, fish, nuts, leafy-green vegetables, regional vegetables, and seeds.[13] Here's the modern version of the diet

- Consume organic and range-fed meats and wild caught fish.
- To obtain minerals, eat the animal bone marrow, and consume the organs.
- If you consume grains, they should be minimal and unrefined, including cereals, breads, and pastas (preferably soaked and sprouted).
- Add abundant organic vegetables and moderate amounts of organic fruit.
- Add additional carbohydrates for those who need them (athletes, physical laborers, etc.). These include complex carbohydrate-containing vegetables such as winter squash, carrots, and potatoes.
- Certain nuts, seeds, and legumes are recommended (roasted pumpkin seeds, soaked flax meal, almonds, peas, dried lentils, green beans, and edamame). Additional protein can also be obtained from soy products such as organic tofu, natto, tempeh (higher in protein by weight than meat), and miso.
- Eat algae, sea vegetables, and spirulina—rich sources of minerals and antioxidants.

Eye Health Risks/Rewards

This diet has the potential to be very healthy. It can be high in antioxidants with a focus on fruits and vegetables, nuts and seeds, lean meats and fish, and oils from fruits and nuts, such as olive or walnut oil. It is important to understand that the Paleolithic diet contains approximately three times more plants than our typical Western diet today. It is also a good anti-inflammatory diet.

For vision, the primary risk of this diet is that it may not include enough vitamin D, calcium, and carotenoids like lutein and zeaxanthin. And the high levels of saturated fats increase the risk of heart disease.[14] Risks also come from wild game that may contain disease. For example, a Canadian study found that chronic wasting disease, a problem for deer herds, could be transmitted to primates.[15] A rare bacterial disease from eating rabbit meat is tularemia, rabbit fever.[16]

South Beach Diet

The South Beach diet was created by cardiologist, Dr. Arthur Agatston and dietician, Marie Almon. It focuses on the control of insulin levels and the benefits of consuming unrefined or complex carbohydrates versus simple carbohydrates, which can cause rapid spikes in blood sugar levels that result in cravings and other deleterious health effects.

Dr. Agatston believed that low-fat regimens were not effective over the long term for preventing heart disease. It was initially designed to help patients lower their risk of developing heart disease, but it rapidly became popular as a diet for losing weight. The South Beach diet focuses on selecting the "right" carbohydrates, including whole grains, specific fruits and vegetables, and fats such as canola oil.[17]

There are three phases in the diet with the goal of reaching one's ideal weight, and then keeping that ideal weight by maintaining healthy eating and lifestyle habits encouraged in the program.

The diet differs from the Mediterranean diet, most substantially in the first two phases where it emphasizes lean proteins and non-starch vegetables. This means no fruit or fruit juices, sugar, or alcohol, but also no "starches," such as bread, rice, potatoes, pasta, baked goods, etc. In the third, or maintenance phase of this diet, these types of foods can be added back in, so long as guidelines are met surrounding them, and the person continues to drop 1–2 pounds per week, until their ideal weight is achieved.[18]

Eye Health Risks/Rewards

The South Beach diet is high in antioxidants with the focus on intake of fruits and vegetables, lean meats, healthy oils, and whole grains. It focuses on the "right" carbohydrates, based on their glycemic index and on other foods that help fight against the risk of eye disease. Its potential to reduce weight, lower high blood pressure, and reduce blood fat and cholesterol levels also support healthier vision. Heart disease and diabetes (obesity is a risk factor) are two main contributors of eye disease and vision loss.

This diet, however, recommends canola oil as one of the good oils. Because canola oil can easily become rancid due to improper manufacturing, exposure to heat, and improper packaging, we do not recommend it or other vegetable oils except olive oil. Best oils are first, cold pressed, extra virgin olive oil, coconut oil, and organic, grass-fed butter or ghee (last two are best for cooking as they have a high temperature threshold).

Plant-Based Diets

Vegan and Vegetarianism

All vegetarian diets promote the value of consuming plant-based foods as one's primary source of nutrition. Technically, a vegan diet would not include animal foods or products containing animal sources. However, because of the rise in interest in health and plant-based diets in the U.S., and to reflect our nation's shift in consciousness away from consuming certain types of animal products, many variations of the plant-based diet have been named. Below is a list of "vegetarian" diets in order of least plant-based to the most.

Caution. It is important for those on a strict plant-based diet to routinely check their levels of nutrients that are difficult to obtain from plants and to supplement, if and when required. These nutrients include, but are not limited to, vitamin B12, zinc, and iron. Vegetarians also need to make sure they are getting enough protein.

- **Pollo-vegetarians** eat poultry but omit red meat.
- **Pesco-vegetarians** add fish to their diet, but do not typically consume other meats. This diet is common in Asia, where hundreds of millions live on rice, fish, and vegetables.
- **Lacto-vegetarians** eat dairy products (but not eggs) along with other plant-based foods.
- **Lacto-ovo vegetarians** consume eggs and dairy products with other plant-based foods.
- **Vegans** abstain from eating animal products, including honey: plant-based foods only.
- **Ethical vegans or total vegetarians** not only live solely on plant-based foods, but also abstain from using products derived from animals, such as silk, leather, and wool.

The Vegan Diet

Veganism is more than just a diet. People who adopt the lifestyle may not do it for health reasons only, but for social, environmental, and ethical reasons. As noted above, a vegan does not eat anything that is animal based, including eggs, dairy, and honey. It is also common for vegans to avoid using any animal products (or those products tested on animals), out of concern for the welfare of all living creatures; these people may describe themselves as ethical vegans.

Resources for vegans and vegetarians are abundant today. If interested in exploring this lifestyle, you might start by downloading the free *Vegetarian Starter Kit* at the Physician's Committee for Responsible Medicine (http://www.pcrm.org/ health/diets/vsk), or going to the Vegan Kit at www.vegankit.com, or visiting the Vegetarian Resource Group at www.vrg.org.

Eye Health Risks/Rewards

The advantage of the vegan (and vegetarian) diet is an overall lower risk of disease. Numerous studies show that eating animal fats and proteins raises a person's risk of developing lifestyle diseases, such as cancer, diabetes, arthritis, hypertension, heart disease, obesity, and a number of other conditions.[19] It is well documented that a whole-food, plant-based diet provides an abundance of nutrition and is crucial for reducing inflammation, a precursor to disease.

A vegan diet is rich in antioxidants, focusing on fruits and vegetables, seeds and grains, and soy products for protein (tempeh is one of the best sources). Avoiding animal products supports a healthier planet, since the raising of animal products involves much environmental pollution.

However, vegans must supplement with B12. Vitamin B12 is an essential vitamin for eye health. The body builds up large reserves of vitamin B12 over time, and people who lack it in their diets may not experience the serious symptoms of a B12 deficiency for many years. It is critical for proper brain and nerve cell functioning. Without B12 supplementation, vegans are at risk for deterioration of the fatty layer surrounding the nerve cells in the eye. In addition, vegans may be short on iron, calcium, vitamin D, zinc, and omega-3 fatty acids; they need to pay attention to these nutrients, along with getting adequate protein.

Raw Food Diet

The Raw Food Diet, or raw foodism, involves consuming foods and drinks that are not processed, are completely plant-based, and are ideally organic. At the foundation of the diet is the belief that organic raw foods, or nearly raw foods, provide the best and highest nutrition for the body. They accept as true that nature has given each food a perfect combination of nutrients that, in its whole and unadulterated state, provides the purest fuel for the body.

Proponents note that cooking alters or destroys vitamins, minerals, and enzymes, which are the essential life force of the food. Enzymes allow us to fully and easily digest and assimilate a food's nutrients without relying as much on our own digestive enzymes. For this reason, raw foods are also referred to as "living foods." The theoretical result is a well-running digestive system, which frees up energy for other activities, including fighting off illness and disease. Raw foodists generally say that at least 75% of their food intake consists of uncooked foods. A significant number of raw foodists are also vegans, which means they do not eat or drink animal-based products.

There are four broad branches of raw foodism:[20]

- **Raw vegetarians** eat mostly raw fruits, vegetables, nuts and seeds, grains (sprouted, some cooked), and the only animal products consumed are eggs and dairy.
- **Raw vegans** eat no animal products, and most foods are consumed raw.
- **Raw omnivores** eat both plant-based and animal-based foods, but most are consumed raw.
- **Raw carnivores** eat only raw meat products in combination with plant-based foods.

Foods in a raw diet include beans (typically soaked and sprouted), dried fruits, fresh fruits and vegetables, freshly made fruit and vegetable juices, grains (sprouted), legumes, nut milks, nuts and seeds, and other organic, or natural, foods which have not been processed, such as sea vegetables. Purified water is also a must, rather than tap water.

Health Risks/Rewards

This diet is rich in antioxidants, focusing on fruits, vegetables, nuts, seeds, grains, and nut milks. A disadvantage is that the diet is not good for everyone. This is particularly true from the metabolic type perspective if the body type fares better with animal products.

It is also true from the Chinese medical perspective if the body type tends to be damp and cold. For example, a raw diet would not be good for people who tend to be cold, have sluggish digestion, and are overall "damp" (often seen with a white, damp coating on the tongue). It would also not be good for people living in colder, damp climates. And for those with a lighter, airy body type (ayurvedic vata body type with cold and dry attributes), large amounts of raw food can cause digestive issues.

Some cooking helps to break cell walls making digestion easier for certain nutrients.

Caution. In addition, vegans need to pay careful attention to levels of B12, iron, and zinc since these are not easily obtained from raw foods.

Macrobiotic Diet

The Macrobiotic diet is both a food and lifestyle philosophy based on whole, pure, unprocessed foods following Taoist principles of yin and yang balance. The diet consists of whole cereals and grains supplemented with beans (such as lentils and peas) and vegetables (lightly steamed, boiled, or sautéed with a small amount of unrefined, cold pressed oil), with very little meat, though some fish may be included. Perhaps the most unique qualifier of the macrobiotic diet is its emphasis on the consumption of Asian vegetables such as daikon, sea vegetables such as seaweed, fermented foods such as Japanese miso and natto (fermented soybeans), pickles, and fermented sauerkraut.

Typically, animal products are eliminated from this diet, as well as coffee, alcohol, refined carbohydrates, fruit juices, tropical and semi-tropical fruits, food additives, spicy foods, and preservatives. Nightshades are also avoided, which include eggplant, white potatoes, tomato, okra, peppers, tomatillos, goji berries, and sorrel.

Eye Health Risks/Rewards

The advantage is that this diet keeps sugar to a minimum, eliminates refined carbohydrates, and follows mostly an organic vegetarian diet. Eating all produce fresh eliminates many of the dietary factors that contribute to heart and chronic disease, while maintaining a diet high in antioxidants.

But it may be too low in diet fat for some people. Furthermore, it is difficult to maintain enough levels of protein. It is low in calcium and dairy and too low in fat that is needed to absorb fat-soluble vitamins (vitamin A, vitamin D, vitamin E, vitamin K). The macrobiotic diet also requires a great deal of daily planning.

The McDougall Program

The McDougall Program is also more of a lifestyle plan than just a diet. Created by physician, and nutrition expert John A. McDougall, M.D., the program is a 100% plant-based (vegan) diet that includes whole grains and whole-grain products (such as pasta, tortillas, and whole-grain bread), a wide assortment of vegetables and fruit, plenty of spices, and usually only small amounts of sugar and salt to enhance the flavor; it also emphasizes regular exercise, as simple as a daily walk.

What sets this program apart from other plant-based programs is the exclusion of all oils, including olive oil, safflower oil, and corn oil. McDougall notes, "Oils are nothing more than liquid fats that increase obesity, which in turn, depress the immune function and contribute to the most common chronic diseases."

Eye Health Risks/Rewards

The dietary aspect of the program is rich in vitamins, minerals, antioxidants, and fiber, with similar benefits to the Dean Ornish diet.

The disadvantage for some is that this diet eliminates healthy oils, which have been shown in many research studies to help reduce heart disease, support brain and joint health, reduce inflammation, and support eye/retinal health. Furthermore, for some people, gluten is an inflammatory protein. Also, the protein contained in corn is a highly cross-reactive protein, which means that for some individuals, corn can be as proinflammatory as gluten. Very low consumption of beneficial omega-3 oils found in olive oil, fish, nuts, and seeds can contribute to health problems.

Also See

Chapter 8, Nutrients

[1] Greenfield, B. The Hidden Dangers of a Low Carbohydrate Diet. BenGreenfieldFitness. Retrieved from https://bengreenfieldfitness.com/article/low-carb-ketogenic-diet-articles/the-hidden-dangers-of-a-low-carbohydrate-diet/

[2] WebMD. High-Protein, Low-Carb Diets Explained. Retrieved from https://www.webmd.com/diet/guide/high-protein-low-carbohydrate-diets

[3] D'Adamo, P.J. Blood Type and Your Health. Retrieved from http://www.dadamo.com/txt/index.pl?1001.

[4] D'Adamo, P. (2015). Inflammation and the Blood Type Diet. Personalized Living. Retrieved from http://northamericanpharmacal.com/living/2015/08/inflammation-and-the-blood-type-diet.

[5] Cusack, L., De Buck, E., Compernolle, V., Vandekerckhove, P. (2013). Blood type diets lack supporting evidence: a systematic review. *Am J Clin Nutr*, Jul:98(1):99-104.

[6] Wang, J., Garcia-Bailo, B., Nielsen, D.E., El-Sohemy, A. (2014). ABO Genotype, 'Blood-Type' Diet and Cardiometabolic Risk Factors. *PLoS One*, 9(1): e84749.

[7] Jockers, D. What is Your Metabolic Type? Retrieved from http://drjockers.com/what-is-your-metabolic-type/.

[8] Ibid. Jockers.

[9] Wong, C. (2017). The Metabolic Typing Diet. Verywell. Retrieved from https://www.verywell.com/the-metabolic-typing-diet-89876.

[10] Healthline Newsletter. Metabolic Diet Review: Fact or Fiction? Retrieved from https://www.healthline.com/health/metabolic-diet-review-fact-or-fiction#changing-your-metabolism2.

[11] Redford, G.D. (2014). Ready to Ditch Your Low-Fat Diet? Not So Fast. AARP Newsletter. Retrieved from https://www.aarp.org/health/healthy-living/info-2014/dean-ornish-low-fat-diet.html.

[12] Berkeley Wellness. (2015). Ornish: Still Best for Heart Health? Retrieved from http://www.berkeleywellness.com/healthy-eating/diet-weight-loss/article/ornish-still-ultimate-diet.

[13] Mayo Clinic. Paleo diet: What is it and why is it so popular? Retrieved from https://www.mayoclinic.org/healthy-lifestyle/nutrition-and-healthy-eating/in-depth/paleo-diet/art-20111182.

[14] UC Davis Health. (2015). Is the paleo diet safe? Retrieved from http://www.ucdmc.ucdavis.edu/welcome/features/2014-2015/06/20150603_paleo-diet.html.

[15] Smith, P.A. (2017). Macaque study heightens concerns about human susceptibility to CWD. Retrieved from http://www.jsonline.com/story/sports/columnists/paul-smith/2017/06/28/macaque-study-heightens-concerns-human-susceptibility-cwd/430046001/.

[16] Illinois Department of Public Health. Tularemia. *HealthBeat*. Retrieved from http://www.idph.state.il.us/public/hb/hbtulare.htm

[17] Nordqvist, C. (2014). What is the South Beach diet? Medical News Today. Retrieved from https://www.medicalnewstoday.com/articles/7380.php.

[18] Ibid. Nordqvist.

[19] Nordqvist, C. (2017). Vegan diet: Health benefits, risks, and meals tips. MedicalNewsToday. Retrieved from https://www.medicalnewstoday.com/articles/149636.php

[20] Nordqvist, C. (2017). Nine most popular diets rated by experts 2017. Retrieved from http://www.medicalnewstoday.com/articles/5847.php#raw_food_diet.

8-1. NUTRIENT FAMILIES

Why are nutrients essential for vision health? These nutrient groups protect our eyes against UV radiation, blue light, and oxidative stress; they protect blood vessel and membrane integrity; they strengthen the immune system, remove waste products, enhance neuron pathway signaling, and protect the retina, lens, and optic nerve from damage.

Phytonutrients

Phytonutrients come from plant pigments and are divided into groups based on their chemical composition which is related to their color: yellow, red, orange, purple, or blue. As a group, the phytonutrients act as solar radiation filters to help protect plant cells. Plants also use phytonutrients to absorb light and convert that light to energy.

- **Carotenoids** are phytonutrients with special attention to the vision carotenoids: lutein, astaxanthin, zeaxanthin, mesozeaxanthin, and lycopene. Their function in the plant world includes coloring, fragrance to attract pollinators, and protection against oxidative stress.
- **Bioflavonoids'** functions include coloring to attract pollinators, symbiotic relationships with other plant forms, provide UV protection, and protect against disease. They include flavanols such as rutin, flavanones such as hesperidin, and anthocyanins such as bilberry.
- **Polyphenols** are complex plant chemicals with functions that include growth processes, hormonal adjustments, and protection, such as from UV light and microbes; curcumin, resveratrol and catechins are examples.

Vitamins and Vitamin-Like

Some vitamins and vitamin-like biochemicals also act as antioxidants. These include vitamins A, C, E, CoQ10, and alpha-lipoic acid. In addition to reducing oxidative stress, they have specific roles in protecting vision. For example, vitamin A helps to protect cornea transparency and is an essential component of rhodopsin, an eye protein needed for low-light vision. It helps to prevent night blindness and poor night vision and protects against a number of vision conditions.

Enzymes

Enzymes are a major class of antioxidants that act as catalysts to quickly stimulate essential body functions. They aid in metabolism, digestion, respiration, cardiovascular functioning, immune system functioning, and processes that make vision possible. Most enzymes are types of protein created naturally by our body from dietary protein. They interact with specific minerals, such as copper, zinc, iron or manganese to produce specific effects or to create essential biochemicals.

Enzymes that are valuable for vision health include superoxide dismutase (SOD), serrapeptase, and nattokinase, along with the following: amylase, which breaks apart complex sugars into smaller molecules like maltose; lipase, which breaks down complex fats into smaller fatty acids and glycerol; pepsin, which breaks down proteins in foods, into smaller peptides; lactase, which breaks down milk sugar called lactose; cholecystokinin, which causes the gallbladder to contract and release bile; and trypsin, which breaks down protein so it can be made into amino acids. The pancreas produces amylase that helps digest carbohydrates and lipase that helps digest fat.

Essential Fatty Acids

Essential fatty acids are as essential to good vision as vitamins, and minerals. They are an integral component of nerve cells, cell membranes, and hormone-like substances. They include omega-3 and omega-6 fatty acids. Omega-3 fatty acids are a specific type of essential fatty acid that reduces inflammation, is essential to retinal health, and lowers risk of chronic diseases, such as heart disease. Some omega-6 fatty acids are beneficial for vision health and reduce inflammation (borage and black currant seed oil); others increase inflammation (excess in processed grain products).

Amino Acids

Amino Acids are the building blocks of protein. Without complete proteins, some or much of the nutritive value of protein is lost. Therefore, it is important that your diet include complete protein, meaning all 20 amino acids are necessary. We produce some aminos naturally, we derive others from food sources. This is possible through food combinations. Classic combination examples are wheat and dairy, corn and beans, and rice and beans; one of each combined group possesses some of the amino acids that the other does not (or the other possesses in small quantities only). *Diet for a Small Planet* is the classic cookbook that discusses complete proteins.

Cysteine, glycine, and glutamine are especially important amino acids for healthy vision because they help build glutathione, which is essential for eye and overall health. The amino acid taurine is a potent antioxidant that helps remove waste from the retina (and supports cognitive function and neuron integrity). N-acetyl-carnosine, composed of several amino acids, is helpful for lens health and potentially prevents or improves cataracts.

Minerals

Our bodies need trace amounts of many minerals. They are essential nutrients that are critical for bone structure, energy production, nerve function, muscle function, retinal health, and the immune system. For example, zinc supports the immune system and is responsible for cell growth, wound healing, and digestion of carbohydrates.

Herbs

Herbs have been used traditionally for centuries, not only for common health conditions but also for vision disorders. They are effective as whole foods that bring the subtle balances and synergies of components into play through the knowledge acquired by herbalists over 100s of years. For example, cineraria maritima has long been used as an effective homeopathic remedy for early to moderate stages of cataract.

8-2. PHYTONUTRIENTS: CAROTENOIDS

Carotenoids are powerful plant-based antioxidants. They are fat-soluble pigments that give fruits and vegetables their color, mainly yellow, orange, or red. Animals and humans cannot create carotenoids directly; they need to get them through food. Carotenoids are best consumed with a fat in order for the body to absorb them better.

In humans, carotenoids maintain cell health throughout the body by neutralizing free radicals (single oxygen atoms that can damage cells by reacting with and destabilizing healthy cells). Carotenoids have strong cancer fighting properties, are anti-inflammatory, boost the immune system, and support healthy circulation. Some carotenoids are known as vitamin A precursors that can be converted to vitamin A.[1] There are more than 700 types of carotenoids, but we are most interested in alpha-carotene and beta-carotene, beta-cryptoxanthin, lutein, zeaxanthin, mesozeaxanthin, astaxanthin, bilberry, and lycopene, found in the Western diet.

Carotenoids fall into two groups: xanthophylls that contain oxygen in their chemical makeup and carotenes that do not contain oxygen. Photosynthesis is the process through which plants convert light to energy; the xanthophylls, which are yellow in color, absorb blue, violet, and ultraviolet light; the carotenes, which are orange, also absorb blue, violet, and ultraviolet light. The capacity of these carotenoids to absorb blue and violet light becomes an essential part of the defense mechanism of the eye. These two groups of carotenoids are found throughout the body, but are concentrated in the macula of the eye and to some extent in the eye lens and are essential for general growth and vision in dim light.

Some carotenoids called provitamins, in the liver turn into retinol, the most common form of vitamin A. These are alpha-carotene, beta-carotene, and the xanthophyll beta-cryptoxanthin.

Xanthophylls

The important role of xanthophylls is that they absorb blue, violet, and ultraviolet light. These wavelengths of light penetrate all the way to the back of the retina. They are short wavelengths. The shorter a wavelength, the greater the energy it possesses, and so these blue to ultraviolet wavelengths have the potential of damaging the retina, resulting in oxidative stress to the retina and its center, the macula. Only two xanthophylls, lutein and zeaxanthin, accumulate in the retina (though mesozeaxathin is found in the macula for supporting central, detailed vision).[2]

Lutein

Lutein accumulates in the retina, including the macula (mostly in the periphery of the retina), which is responsible for detailed vision. The macula is yellow because of the yellow color of lutein and zeaxanthin; it is able to absorb oxidizing blue, violet, and ultraviolet light.

Antioxidant. The retina is constantly exposed to oxygen and light, resulting in oxidative stress and phototoxic stress. Lutein[3] does not have a direct role in the process of sight. Rather, its powerful antioxidant ability protects the macula by absorbing damaging blue, violet, and ultraviolet light[4] that causes stress and free-radical activity. It further accomplishes this by supporting macular pigment thickness,[5] the eye's defense against damaging UV and blue light.

Biomarker role. In 2016, researchers identified lutein as one of the carotenoids that makes an excellent biomarker for observing women's dietary intake. In other words, the levels of lutein in the blood indicate the degree to which nutrients are actually absorbed by the body and used by cell tissue.[6]

Immune response. Lutein is more than merely a filter for the sun's UV radiation. A 2012 research study found that it modulates immune responses as well as inflammation, including inflammation in the eye, such as that manifested in uveitis, laser-induced choroidal neovascularization, retinal ischemia, and diabetic retinopathy.[7]

Cataract. Lutein helps protect against oxidative stress and inflammation that contribute to cataract development,[8] [9] especially when it is combined with omega-3 fatty acids.[10]

Diabetic retinopathy. Along with zeaxanthin and other important carotenoids, lutein plays a central role in protecting the retina against oxidative stress, inflammation, and neurodegenerative damage.[11]

> **Lutein, Zeaxanthin, Mesozeaxanthin Combination**
>
> Researchers found that a moderate dose of 13.3mg combined carotenoids, comprised of:
>
> - 83% lutein (11mg)
> - 10% zeaxanthin (1.33mg)
> - 7% mesozeaxanthin (.93mg)
>
> was more effective than higher doses in enhancing macular pigment, even though higher doses were reflected in serum blood levels.[1]

Macular degeneration. Abundant research has brought these phytonutrients into the mainstream of vision care.[12] [13] The landmark studies that came to the attention of many conventional eye doctors were the Age-Related Eye Disease Studies (AREDS).[14] There were two studies: AREDS (2001), AREDS2 (2006), and the AREDS update in 2013, which laid out protocols for macular degeneration treatment that include carotenoids, vitamins, and omega-3 fatty acids.[15]

Lutein lessens the risk of damage from age-related macular degeneration (AMD). Diets rich in lutein reduce AMD risk by 57%.[16] Treatment with lutein helps thicken the protective pigmented layer of the retina;[17] retinas with AMD have 30% less lutein than healthy retinas.[18]

Lutein is even more effective when coupled with the carotenoids, zeaxanthin and mesozeaxanthin. Lutein also reduces the risk of progression (by 25–30%) of the dry (early) form of macular degeneration into the more severe (wet) form, choroidal neovascularization.[19]

Other eye disorders. Lutein is somewhat helpful in preventing and managing central serous chorioretinopathy[20] and uveitis.[21] In retinitis pigmentosa research, lutein improves the visual field and may also improve visual acuity by improving macular pigment thickness.[22] [23] Combined with zeaxanthin and black currant extract, lutein protects against eye fatigue.[24]

Related disorders. Lutein may also be helpful in fighting atherosclerosis by improving circulation; lutein levels in the blood are tied to artery wall thickness,[25] [26] and may help to reduce accumulation of plaque by preventing oxidation of fats in the bloodstream.[27]

Source. The best source of lutein is kale and then spinach. Other good sources include turnip greens, summer squash, Brussels sprouts, orange foods (such as corn, pumpkin, paprika, yellow-fleshed fruits), pecans, and avocado.

Lutein is also available through enriched eggs. A small study found that lutein from enriched eggs was absorbed more easily than lutein from spinach or supplements.[28] In addition, the lutein that comes from red and orange foods supports macular pigment density more than that from spinach or supplements.[29]

Caution. People with cystic fibrosis may not very well absorb lutein from supplements.

Mesozeaxanthin

Mesozeaxanthin is a carotenoid in the lutein family and is found in the center of the macula where we get our most detailed vision. It is the most powerful of the three antioxidants in the macula, but is most effective in combination with the others, lutein and zeaxanthin.[30]

Vision health. A 2016 study showed supplementing daily with mesozeaxanthin, along with lutein and zeaxanthin, significantly increased macular pigment[31] (found to be compromised in those with macular degeneration). Another earlier study came to a similar conclusion.

Source. It is found in microalgae and sea creatures that consume the algae, such as trout, salmon, shellfish, and krill. It is found in the skin of trout, sardines, and salmon.

Zeaxanthin

Zeaxanthin is concentrated in the macula where it is fights oxidative stress. Like lutein, it is a yellow pigment that absorbs blue light. It improves central vision function in a number of ways.[32]

Antioxidant. It has similar properties to lutein; it is a retinal pigment and potent antioxidant.

Glare recovery. One of the diagnostic tests for macular problems (as distinct from optic nerve problems) is the glare recovery test in which the subject is exposed to bright light, such as the eye doctor's ophthalmoscope; the recovery time is measured according to how long it takes for visual acuity to return. Zeaxanthin, lutein, and mesozeaxanthin make up most of the macular pigment and are essential for good recovery from glare.[33]

Stem cell support. Researchers demonstrated that pretreatment with zeaxanthin was helpful in supporting transplanted stem cells.[34]

Macular degeneration. A number of studies found that a high intake of zeaxanthin lowers the risk of dry AMD advancing to the more serious form, wet AMD.[35] It does so by increasing the density of the macular pigment that protects the retina from damaging solar radiation.[36] One study focused on zeaxanthin alone, and found that zeaxanthin is more effective than lutein in protecting against oxidative stress from ultraviolet light exposure.[37] Another study found that zeaxanthin improves vision in elderly patients with early macular degeneration, according to both eye charts and reports of better night vision.[38]

Source. The best source of zeaxanthin is kale and then spinach. It is found in orange and red foods such as saffron, orange peppers, paprika and paprika peppers, goji berry, corn, oranges, and tangerines. Other vegetables such as collards, mustard greens, romaine lettuce, broccoli, kiwi fruit, peas, and chard contain a lot of zeaxanthin.

Astaxanthin

2011[39] and 2015[40] reviews of previous and ongoing research point to the wide range of benefits of this potent antioxidant, including excellent tolerability and safety factors. Astaxanthin lowers levels of free radicals in people who are smokers or overweight; it blocks oxidative damage to DNA, acts as an anti-inflammatory agent, supports tuberculin immunity, lowers triglycerides, increases blood flow and good HDL cholesterol, supports brain functioning with improved cognition and nerve stem cell growth, improves visual acuity,[41] reproductive health, and more.[42]

Astaxanthin is a fat-soluble carotenoid that is similar to beta-carotene, but a slight structural difference creates a radical biological difference. One unique quality is its ability to cross the blood/brain barrier,[43] which means that it has the capacity to deliver antioxidants directly to the brain, as well as to the eyes and nervous system. This explains its presence in the retina.

Antioxidant. Astaxanthin destroys the unstable reactive-oxygen species (ROS) molecules, commonly known as free radicals, and wards off their constant attack towards all parts of the body.[44] When tested against a wide variety of ROS and RNS (nitrogen-reactive species) molecules, astaxanthin was one of the most effective in free radical scavenging. Its antioxidant ability is ten times more powerful than beta-carotene,[45] lutein, or zeaxanthin, and from 60–500 times stronger than vitamin E.[46] [47] It must be taken through food or in supplement form since it is not made by the body.

Inflammation. Astaxanthin is also a powerful anti-inflammatory agent and pain reliever. Because inflammation is at the root of many eye conditions, this ability to reduce inflammation is extremely beneficial. It is able to block COX-2 enzymes, which cause the pain and inflammation behind various forms of arthritis.[48]

Mitochondria support. In the lab, astaxanthin was found to protect embryos against heat-stress, apparently by direct action supporting mitochondria, the energy-producers of the cell.[49] It also protected against the cell death of epithelial cells in vivo and in vitro, by supporting the mitochondrial signaling pathway.[50]

Cataract. Researchers found that astaxanthin reduced biomarkers that indicated oxidative stress and reduced cataract formation in diabetic animal models; the effect was greater when combined with pine bark extract (flavangenol).[51]

Eye fatigue. In a number of different studies, researchers found that astaxanthin was useful in reducing fatigue, sore dry eyes, blurry vision, and recovery from intense visual stimulation.[52] [53] In computer users, astaxanthin was found to significantly improve accommodation amplitude, which refers to the ability of the eye to change focus as distances change.[54] [55] [56] [57] [58]

Macular degeneration. Astaxanthin slows oxidative damage and protects the photoreceptors.[59]

Retinal injury. Investigations of the antioxidant effectiveness of astaxanthin in the eye are just beginning but are already very promising. Studies indicate that astaxanthin can be effective at ameliorating retinal injury[60] [61] and protecting photoreceptors from light-caused cell degeneration through its antioxidative capacity and through its activation of a by-product, Nrf2.[62]

Related disorders. Astaxanthin may offer support for the kidneys, protecting against renal tubular oxidative damage.[63] Additional research has pointed out that astaxanthin could be useful for prevention and treatment of neuronal damage, as in Alzheimer's disease,[64] Parkinson's disease, spinal cord injuries, and other types of central nervous system injuries.[65] It is able to cross the blood-brain barrier (unlike beta-carotene) and become available to the nervous system.[66]

Source. Sources include red yeast Phaffiarhodozyma (used in Asian cooking), salmon, shrimp, trout, and other pink seafood that eat the red algae Haematococcus.

Beta-cryptoxanthin

Beta-cryptoxanthin is another xanthophyll carotenoid that is a precursor to vitamin A.

Eye conditions. Unlike lutein and zeaxanthin, beta-cryptoxanthin is not concentrated in the retina or macula; it is found in blood plasma along with other carotenoids. It provides antioxidant support to cells and DNA.[67]

Related conditions. There has been a limited amount of research on this antioxidant. Patients who consume the most beta-cryptoxanthin are 24% less at risk for lung cancer.[68] Another study associates beta-cryptoxanthin as well as lutein and zeaxanthin with lower cancer risk.[69]

Beta-cryptoxanthin appears to help reduce conditions caused, or complicated, by inflammation, such as rheumatoid arthritis and polyarthritis (40% lower risk compared to controls).[70] As in the cancer studies, these researchers found that the greater the consumption of beta-cryptoxanthin, the lower the risk of inflammatory conditions. Researchers suggested that just a modest increase in beta-cryptoxanthin daily, such as in orange juice, could help limit arthritis incidence. Orange juice should be limited, however, due to its high level of sugar content.

High blood pressure, high blood sugar, and high cholesterol, as well as too much waist fat characterize metabolic syndrome. Consumption of carotenoids, including beta-cryptoxanthin, lowers the risk.[71]

Source. Beta-cryptoxanthin is found especially in red bell peppers and yellow squash, such as butternut. It is also found in fruits such as papaya, mango, oranges, and in yellow foods, such as corn, bell peppers, and yellow dairy (egg yolks and butter).

Carotenes

Beta-carotene

Beta-carotene is the carotene best able to convert into vitamin A (retinol) at twice the rate of alpha-carotene and beta-cryptoxanthin. Beta-carotene is the most abundant carotene found in plants; it gives orange foods their color; in fact, the word carotene comes from the Latin word for carrot.

Antioxidant. Of the carotenes, beta-carotene is second only to lycopene in its antioxidant capacity. It was one of the first antioxidants studied by scientists in order to develop an understanding of the mechanisms of free radical scavenging by carotenoids.[72]

Cataract. Early studies suggest that beta-carotene may provide protection against cataracts; some of these studies include multiple nutrients in addition to beta-carotene. Two studies in 2001 found that people with the highest blood concentrations of either beta- or alpha-carotene were 30–50% less likely to develop nuclear cataracts, which are those located in the central part of the lens.[73][74] But a 2013 meta-analysis (a review of a number of research studies) contradicts that. The reviews evaluated 13 studies involving nearly 19,000 patients. They reported that changes to lens opacity due to beta-carotene were not statistically significant; so, more research is needed here.

Night blindness. In pregnant and postpartum mothers, supplementing with either vitamin A or beta-carotene improved, but did not eliminate, night blindness.[75]

Other eye disorders. Researchers find that the carotenoids, including beta-carotene, generally support better vision. Higher intakes of beta-carotene from food, when coupled with reductions in cholesterol intake from food, appear to reduce damage from oxidative stress-related eye disease.[76] Teenagers with cystic fibrosis with low levels of alpha- and beta-carotene have poor night vision.[77]

Related disorders. High blood pressure, high blood sugar, and high cholesterol, as well as too much waist fat characterize metabolic syndrome. These imbalances are lowest in men who consume the greatest levels of beta-carotene.[78]

Source. The best sources for beta-carotene are red chili peppers, dark green lettuce, spinach, and kale. Good food sources include cantaloupe, mangoes, papaya, carrots, sweet potatoes, and pumpkin.

Note. Several flawed and debunked studies in the past, suggested that both former asbestos workers and people who smoked had a greater risk of lung cancer if they took beta-carotene as a supplement, rather than through food. Supplementing with beta-carotene is now known to reduce the risk of lung cancer for both smokers and ex-smokers.[79]

Caution. Beta-carotene is possibly unsafe if taken in large doses for a long time, although its vitamin A precursor status does not increase the risk of vitamin A toxicity. There is some concern that beta-carotene may interfere with healing after angioplasty.[80] Furthermore, beta-carotene can decrease effectiveness of some medications, such as those for lowering cholesterol.[81] Other medications and alcohol can decrease absorption of beta-carotene.

Alpha-carotene

Alpha-carotene is another precursor to vitamin A, though it creates only half as much vitamin A as beta-carotene.

Antioxidant. Alpha-carotene supports vision health by creating vitamin A, which is needed for low-light vision and cell health. Alpha-carotene's contribution to vision health is much the same as that of beta-carotene.

Diabetic retinopathy. Diabetics have a high risk of developing diabetic retinopathy. Patients with highest levels of alpha-carotene intake are less likely to develop type 2 diabetes. In one study men had a 48% reduced risk and women, 39%. However, intake of all antioxidants was not significant as a risk factor.[82]

Related disorders. Alpha-carotene has been associated with a lower risk of premature death. In a study of over 15,000 U.S. adults, those people with the highest levels of alpha-carotene in their blood have the lowest risk of death from all causes.[83] Researchers found similar lower risks for lung cancer[84] and cardiovascular disease.[85] The study concludes that fruit and vegetable consumption is directly linked with avoiding premature death.

Source. The highest levels of alpha-carotene are found in pumpkins and carrots. Yellow-orange winter squash varieties have high amounts, as do green vegetables, such as broccoli, green beans, peas, and spinach. Other vegetable sources include turnip and beet greens, collards, lettuce, avocado, and parsley.

Lycopene

Lycopene is bright red in color and found in red fruits and vegetables, but not all red foods contain lycopene. Although it is a carotene, it is not a vitamin A precursor, nor does it behave as vitamin A in the mechanics of vision. But it is a precursor to beta-carotene (goes through 2 cycles in the body to convert to beta-carotene). In order for it to be absorbed by the body, it has to combine with fats, and it is best utilized when cooked in the presence of fat.[86] It may be that supplements are more effectively absorbed than food, especially if the food source is raw.[87]

Antioxidant. Lycopene is the most powerful antioxidant in the carotene family. Researchers describe it as the "most efficient biological carotenoid singlet-oxygen quencher."[88] Some researchers feel that its benefit comes indirectly from the lycopenoids produced by lycopene, rather than its own antioxidant capacity.[89]

Inflammation. Lycopene is protective against nerve inflammation[90] caused by oxidative stress. Free radicals cause oxidative stress, which in turn damages and inflames healthy nerve cells. It is possible that this finding will point towards more effective therapies for optic neuritis and other eye conditions that involve inflammation of the optic nerve.

Diabetic retinopathy. Patients with diabetes have significantly lower levels of lycopene.[91] Diabetic retinopathy is a common complication of type 2 diabetes.

Macular degeneration. Researchers have reported that low levels of lycopene are associated with a higher risk of age-related macular degeneration.[92]

Related disorders. Lycopene appears to decrease side effects of cancer treatment drugs that damage the kidneys.[93] A study of nearly 50,000 men found a lowered risk of prostate cancer in men with high levels of lycopene in their diet (tomatoes). The greater the amount of lycopene in their diet, the greater the protection.[94]

Oxidation of low-density lipoprotein (LDL) is associated with increased risk of atherosclerosis and heart disease. Lycopene, found in high amounts in tomatoes, reduces LDL oxidation,[95] [96] though it does not reduce cholesterol levels. This benefit is amplified when lycopene is consumed through whole tomatoes or accompanied by alpha-tocopherol, a type of vitamin E.[97] Additionally, tomato extract reduces platelet clotting, reducing the risk of cardiovascular events[98] [99] and stroke (by 55–59%, compared to controls).[100] [101]

The diets of nearly a thousand patients were evaluated with respect to 13–16-year fracture records. Patients who had consumed the highest levels of carotenoids during that period had the lowest levels of fractures. Lycopene consumption was responsible for a slightly greater protection from hip fracture.[102] At issue in bone structure integrity is bone resorption. This means that bone deteriorates, and the composite minerals are released into the blood. A study in post-menopausal women found that lycopene supplementation helped reduce the biomarkers that indicate the presence of oxidative-stress and bone resorption.[103]

Source. Guavas have the most lycopene, followed by red watermelon and tomatoes, especially cooked or sun-dried. Other vegetables include sweet red peppers, asparagus, red cabbage, and carrots. Fruits include papaya, pink grapefruit, and mango.

Caution. If taken with anticoagulant drugs, lycopene can increase the risk of bleeding. It also interacts with blood pressure medications, the immune system, sunlight sensitivity, and some gastrointestinal drugs. Some people are allergic to lycopene.

---

[1]Szalay, J. What are carotenoids? Retrieved on Nov 2 2017 from http://www.livescience.com/52487-carotenoids.html.

[2]Widomska, J., Zareba, M., Subczynski, W.K. (2016). Can Xanthophyll-Membrane Interactions Explain Their Selective Presence in the Retina and Brain? *Foods*, Mar;5(1):7.

[3]Semba, R.D., Dagnelie, G. (2003). Are lutein and zeaxanthin conditionally essential nutrients for eye health? *Med Hypotheses*, Oct;61(4):465-72.

[4]Krinsky, N.I., Landrum, J.T., Bone, R.A. (2003). Biologic mechanisms of the protective role of lutein and zeaxanthin in the eye. *Annu Rev Nutr*, 23:171-201.

[5]Koushan, K., Rusovici, R., Li, W., Ferguson, L.R., Chalam, K.V. (2013). The Role of Lutein in Eye-Related Disease. *Nutrients*, May; 5(5): 1823–1839.

[6]Lampe, J.W., Huang, Y., Neuhouser, M.L., Tinker, L.F., Song, X. et al. (2017). Dietary biomarker evaluation in a controlled feeding study in women from the Women's Health Initiative cohort. *Am J Clin Nutri*, Feb;105(2):466-475.

[7] Kijlstra, A., Tian, Y., Kelly, E.R., Berendschot, T.T. (2012). Lutein: more than just a filter for blue light. *Prog Ret Eye Res*, Jul;31(4):303-15.

[8]Olmedill, B., Granado, F., Blanco, I., Vaquero, M. (2003). Lutein, but not alpha tocopherol, supplementation improves visual function in patients with age-related cataracts: A 2-year double-blind, placebo controlled study. *Nutrition,* Jan;19(1):21-4.

[9]Manayi. A., Abdollahi, M., Raman, T., Nabavi, S.F., Hablemariam, S., et al, (2015). Lutein and cataract: from bench to bedside. *Crit Rev Biotechnol*, Oct;36(5):829-39.

[10] Padmanabha, S., Vallikannan, B. (2018). Fatty acids modulate the efficacy of lutein in cataract prevention: Assessment of oxidative and inflammatory parameters in rats. *Biochem Biophys Res Commun,* Jun 2;500(2):435-442.

[11] Neelam, K., Goenadi, C.J., Lun, K., Yip, C.C., Au Eong, K.G. (2017). Putative protective role of lutein and zeaxanthin in diabetic retinopathy. *Br J Ophthalmol*, May;101(5):551-558.

[12] Parisi, V., Tedeschi, M., Gallianaro, G., Varano, M., Saviano, S., et al. (2008). Carotenoids and antioxidants in age-related maculopathy: multifocal electroretinogram modifications after 1 year. *Ophthalmology*, Feb;115(2):324-333.e2.

[13] Piermarocchi, S., Saviano, S., Parisi, V., Tedeschi, M., Panozzo, G., et al. (2012). Carotenoids in Age-related Maculopathy Italian Study (CARMIS): two-year results of a randomized study. *Eur J Ophthalmol,* Mar-Apr;22(2):216-25.

[14]National Eye Institute. (2013). NIH Study provides clarity on supplements for protection against blinding eye disease. Retrieved June 10 2017 from https://nei.nih.gov/news/pressreleases/050513.

[15] AREDS, AREDS2: (2001, 2006, 2013) Antioxidants & Macular Degeneration. Retrieved on Oct 15 2017 from http://www.naturaleyecare.com/study.asp?s_num=105.

[16] Seddon, J.M., Ajani, U.A., Sperduto, R.D., Hiller, R., Blair, N. et al, (1994). Dietary carotenoid, vitamins A, C, E, and advanced age-related macular degeneration. *JAMA*, Nov 9;272(18):1413-20.

[17] Landrum, J.T., Bone, R.A., Kilburn, M.D. (1997). The Macular Pigment: A Possible Role in Protection from Age-Related Macular Degeneration. *Adv Pharmacol*, 38:537-56.

[18] Ibid. Landrum. (1997).

[19] Ibid. Landrum. (1997).

[20]Sawa, M., Gomi, F., Hara, C., Nishida, K. (2014). Effects of a lutein supplement on the plasma lutein concentration and macular pigment in patients with central serous chorioretinopathy. *Invest Ophthal Vis Sci,* Jul 29;55(8):5238-44.

[21]He, R.R., Tsoi, B., Lan, F., Yao, N., Yao, X.S., et al. (2011). Antioxidant properties of lutein contribute to the protection against lipopolysaccharide-induced uveitis in mice. *Chin Med*, Oct 31;6(1):38.

[22]Bahrami, H., Melia, M., Dagnelie, G. (2006). Lutein supplementation in retinitis pigmentosa: PC-based vision assessment in a randomized double-masked placebo-controlled clinical trial]. *BMC Ophthalmol,* Jun 7;6:23.

[23]Sandberg, M.A., Johnson, E.J., Berson, E.L. (2010). The relationship of macular pigment optical density to serum lutein in retinitis pigmentosa. *Invest Ophthalmol Vis Sci*, Feb;51(2):1086-91.

[24]Yagi, A., Fujimoto, K., Michihiro, B., Goh, D., Tsi, H. (2009). Effect of lutein supplementation on visual fatigue: A psychophysiological analysis. *Appl Ergon*, Nov;40(6):1047-54.

[25]Dwyer, J.H., et al. (2001). Oxygenated Carotenoid Lutein and Progression of Early Atherosclerosis: The Los Angeles Atherosclerosis Study. *Circulation*, Jun 19;103(24):2922-7.

[26]Zou, Z., Hu, X., Huang, Y., Xiao, X., Ma, L., et al. (2011). High serum level of lutein may be protective against early atherosclerosis: the Beijing atherosclerosis study. *Atherosclerosis*, Dec;219(2):789-93.

[27]Howard, A.N., Thurnham, D.I. (2017). Lutein and atherosclerosis: Belfast versus Toulouse revisited. *Med Hypotheses,* Jan;98:63-68.

[28] Chung H.Y., Rasmussen H.M., Johnson E.J. (2004) Lutein bioavailability is higher from lutein-enriched eggs than from supplements and spinach in men. *J Nutr*, Aug;134(8):1887-93.

[29]Estevez-Santiago, R., Olmedilla-Alonso, B., Beltran-de-Miguel, B., Cuadrado-Vives, C. (2016). Lutein and zeaxanthin supplied by red/orange foods and fruits are more closely associated with macular pigment optical density than those from green vegetables in Spanish subjects. *Nutr Res,* Nov;36(11):1210-1221.

[30]Li, B; Ahmed, F; Bernstein, P.S. (2010). Studies on the singlet oxygen scavenging mechanism of human macular pigment. *Arch Biochem Biophys*, Dec 1;504 (1): 56–60.

[31] Ma, L., Liu, R., Du, J.H., Liu, T., Wu, S.S. (2016). Lutein, Zeaxanthin and Meso-zeaxanthin Supplementation Associated with Macular Pigment Optical Density. *Nutrients*, Jul 12;8(7):E426.

[32] Herman, J.P., Kleiner-Goudey, S.J., Davis, R.L. (2017). Dietary Supplements Improving Macular and Visual Function. *Adv Ophthal Vis Syst,* Dec;6(1):00166.

[33] Stringham, J.M., O'Brien, K.J., Stringham, N.T. (2016). Macular carotenoid supplementation improves disability glare performance and dynamics of photostress recovery. *Eye Vis (Lond),* Nov11;3:30.

[34] Liu, Y., Xiong, Y., Xing, F., Gao, H., Wang, X., et al. (2017). Precise Regulation of miR-210 is Critical for the Cellular Homeostasis Maintenance and Transplantation Efficacy Enhancement of Mesenchymal Stem Cell in Acute Liver Failure Therapy. *Cell Transplant,* May 9;26(5):805-820.

[35] Richer, S.P., Stiles, W., Graham-Hoffman, K., Levin, M., Ruskin, D., et al. (2011). Randomized, double-blind, placebo-controlled study of zeaxanthin and visual function in patients with atrophic age-related macular degeneration: the Zeaxanthin and Visual Function Study (ZVF) FDA IND #78, 973. *Optometry,* Nov;82(11):667-680.e6.

[36] Ibid. Richer. (2011).

[37] Delcourt, C., Carriere, I., Delage, M., Barberger-Gateau, P., Schalch, W., et al. (2006). Plasma Lutein and Zeaxanthin and Other Carotenoids as Modifiable Risk factors for Age Related Maculopathy and Cataract: the POLA study. *Invest Ophthalmol Vis Sci,* Jun;47(6):2329-35.

[38] Ibid. Richer. (2011).

[39] Kidd, P. (2011). Astaxanthin, cell membrane nutrient with diverse clinical benefits and anti-aging potential. *Alt Med Rev,* Dec;16(4):355-64).

[40] De Jesus Raposo, M.F., de Morais, A.M., de Morais, R.M. (2015). Carotenoids from Marine Microalgae: A Valuable Natural Source for the Prevention of Chronic Diseases. *Mar Drugs,* Aug;13(8):5128-5155.

[41] Sawaki, K., Yoshigi, H., Aoki, K., Koikawa, N., Zaumane, A., et al. (2002). Sports performance benefits from taking natural astaxanthin characterized by visual acuity and muscle fatigue improvement in humans. *J Clin Ther Med,* 18(9)1085-1100.

[42] Ibid. Kidd. (2011).

[43] Ibid. He. (2011).

[44] Maher, T.J. (2000). Astaxanthin, Continuing Ed Module., New Hope Institute of Healing.

[45] Goto, S., Kogure, K., Abe, K., Kimata, Y., Kitahama, K., et al. (2001). Efficient radical trapping at the surface and inside the phospholipid membrane is responsible for highly potent antiperoxidative activity of the carotenoid astaxanthin. *Biochimica Biophysica Acta,* 1512:251-8.

[46] BetaForce. Astaxanthin: The Most Powerful Natural Antioxidant Ever Discovered. Retrieved Apr 2 2018 from http://www.beta-glucan-info.com/astaxanthin.htm.

[47] Chiro.org. Antioxidants: Relative Singlet Oxygen Quenching Rates. Retrieved Apr 16 2018 from http://www.chiro.org/nutrition/FULL/ Antioxidants_Relative_Singlet_Oxygen_Quenching_Rates.html.

[48] Lee, S.J., Bai, S.K., et al, (2003), Astaxanthin inhibits nitric oxide production and inflammatory gene expression by suppressing I(kappa)B kinase-dependent NF-kappaB activation. *Mol Cells,* Aug 31;16(1):97-105,

[49] Kuroki, T., Ikeda, S., Okada, T., Maoka, T., Kitamura, A., et al. (2013). Astaxanthin ameliorates heat stress-induced impairment of blastocyst development in vitro: --astaxanthin colocalization with and action on mitochondria--. *J Assist Reprod Genet,* Jun;30(5):623-31.

[50] Song, X., Wang, B., Lin, S., Jing, L., Mao, C., et al. (2014). Astaxanthin inhibits apoptosis in alveolar epithelial cells type II in vivo and in vitro through the ROS-dependent mitochondrial signaling pathway. *J Cell Mol Med,* Nov;18(11):2198-212.

[51] Nakano, M., Orimo, N., Katagirim N., Tsubata, M., Takahashi, J., et al. (2008). Inhibitory effect of astaxanthin combined with Flavangenol on oxidative stress biomarkers in streptozotocin-induced diabetic rats. *Int J Vitam Nutr Res,* Jul-Sep;78(4-5):175-82.

[52] Astaxanthin (2002-2006) Reduces Eye Fatigue. Retrieved Nov 10 2017 from http://www.naturaleyecare.com/study.asp?s_num=272.

[53] Nagaki, Y, Hayasaka, S, Yamad, a T, Hayasaka, Y, Sanada, M, et al. (2002). Effects of astaxanthin on accommodation, critical flicker fusions, and pattern evoked potential in visual display terminal workers. *J Trad Med,* 19(5):170-173.

[54] Ibid. Nagaki. (2002).

[55] Nakamura, A., Isobe, R., Otaka, Y., Abematsu, Y., Nakata, D., et al. (2004). Changes in Visual Function Following Peroral Astaxanthin. *Japan J Cli. Opthal,* 58(6):1051-1054.

[56]Takahashi, N., Kajita, M. (2005). Effects of astaxanthin on accommodative recovery. *J Clin Therap Med*, 21(4):431-436.

[57] Ogami, S.K. (2010). Effect of astaxanthin on accommodation and asthenopia Efficacy identification study in healthy volunteers. *J Clin Ther Med*, 21(5):543-556.

[58]Iwasaki, T., Tawara, A. (2006). Effects of Astaxanthin on Eyestrain Induced by Accommodative Dysfunction. *J Eye (Atarashii Ganka)*, Jun;23(6):829-834.

[59] Otsuka, T., Shimazawa, M., Nakanishi, T., Ohno, Y., Inoue, Y., et al. (2013). Protective effects of a dietary carotenoid, astaxanthin, against light-induced retinal damage. *J Pharmacol Sci*, 123(3):209-18.

[60] Okazaki, Y., Okada, S., Toyokuni, S. (2017), Astaxanthin ameliorates ferric nitrilotriacetate-induced renal oxidative injury in rats. *J Clin Biochem Nutr*, Jul;61(1):18-24.

[61] Ibid. Otsuka, (2013).

[62] Inoue, Y., Shimazawa, M., Nagano, R., Kuse, Y., Takahashi, K. (2017), Astaxanthin analogs, adonixanthin and lycopene, activate Nrf2 to prevent light-induced photoreceptor degeneration. *J Pharmacol Sci*, Jul;134(3):147-157.

[63] Ibid. Okazaki. (2017).

[64] Chang, C.H., Chen, C.Y., Chious, J.Y., Peng, R.Y., Peng, C.H. (2010), Astaxanthin secured apoptotic death of PC12 cells induced by beta-amyloid peptide 25-35: its molecular action targets. *J Med Food*, Jun;13(3):548-56.

[65] Wu, H., Niu, H., Shao, A., Wu, C., Dixon, B.J. (2015). Astaxanthin as a Potential Neuroprotective Agent for Neurological Diseases. *Mar Drugs*, Sep;13(9):5750-5706.

[66] Zhang, X.S., Zhang, X., Zhou, M.L., Zhou, X.M., Li., N., et al. (2014). Amelioration of oxidative stress and protection against early brain injury by astaxanthin after experimental subarachnoid hemorrhage. *J Neurosurg*, Jul;121(1):42-54.

[67] Wikipedia. Beta-cryptoxanthin. Retrieved Sep 10 2017 from https://en.wikipedia.org/wiki/Cryptoxanthin.

[68]Männistö, S., Smith-Warner, S.A., Spiegelman, D., Albanes, D., Anderson, K., et al, (2004). Dietary carotenoids and risk of lung cancer in a pooled analysis of seven cohort studies. *Cancer Epidemiol Biomarkers Prev*, Jan;13(1):40-8.

[69]Voorrips, L.E., Goldbohm, R.A., Brants, H.A., et al, (2000). A prospective cohort study on antioxidant and folate intake and male lung cancer risk. *Cancer Epidemiol Biomarkers Prev*, Apr;9(4):357-65.

[70]Pattison, D.J., Symmons, D.P., Lunt, M., (2005). Dietary beta-cryptoxanthin and inflammatory polyarthritis: results from a population-based prospective study. *Am J Clin Nutr*, Aug;82(2):451-5.

[71]Sugiura, M., Nakamura, M., Ogawa, K., Ikoma, Y., Yano, M. (2015). High serum carotenoids associated with lower risk for the metabolic syndrome and its components among Japanese subjects: Mikkabi cohort study. *Br J Nutr*, Nov 28;114(10):1674–1682.

[72] Liebler, D.C., McClure, T.D. (1996). Antioxidant Reactions of β-Carotene: Identification of Carotenoid−Radical Adducts. *Chem Res Toxicol*, Jan;9(1):8-11.

[73]Gale, C.R., Hall, N.F., Phillips, D.I., Martyn, C.N. (2001). Plasma antioxidant vitamins and carotenoids and age-related cataract. *Ophthalmology*, Nov;108(11):1992-8.

[74]Jacques, P.F., Chylack Jr., L.T., Hankinson, S.E., Khu, P.R., Rogers, G., et al. (2001). Long-term nutrient intake and early age-related nuclear lens opacities. *Arch Ophthalmol*, Jul;119(7):1009-19.

[75] Christian, P., West, K.P., Khatry, S.K., LeClerq, S., Pradhan, E.K., et al (1998). Vitamin A or beta-Carotene Supplementation Reduces but Does Not Eliminate Maternal Night Blindness in Nepal. *J. Nutr*, Sep;128(9):1458-63.

[76] Braakhuis, A., Ramon, R., Yaghefi, E. (2017). The Association between Dietary Intake of Antioxidants and Ocular Disease. *Diseases*, Jan 30;5(1):E3

[77] Huet, F., Semama, D., et al, (1997). Vitamin A deficiency and nocturnal vision in teenagers with cystic fibrosis. *Eur J Pediatr*, Dec;156(12):949-51.

[78] Ibid. Sugiura. (2015).

[79]Shareck, M., Rousseau, M.C., Koushik, A., Siemiatycki, J., Parent, M.E. (2017). Inverse Association between Dietary Intake of Selected Carotenoids and Vitamin C and Risk of Lung Cancer. *Front Oncol*, Feb 28;7:23.

[80] WebMD. com, Beta-Carotene Side Effects & Safety. Retrieved Nov 18 2018 from https://www.webmd.com/vitamins-supplements/ingredientmono-999-beta-carotene.aspx

[81] Ibid. WebMD, Beta-Carotene Side Effects and Safety.

[82]Quansah, D.Y., Ha, K., Jun, S., Kim, S.A., Shin, S., et al. (2017). Associations of Dietary Antioxidants and Risk of Type 2 Diabetes: Data from the 2007-2012 Korea National Health and Nutrition Examination Survey. *Molecules*, Oct 5;22(10).

[83]Li, C., Ford, E.S., Zhao, G., Balluz, L.S., Giles, W.H., et al. (2011). Serum α-carotene concentrations and risk of death among US Adults: the Third National Health and Nutrition Examination Survey Follow-up Study. *Arch Intern Med*, Mar 28;171(6):507-15.

[84]Michaud, D.S., Feskanich, D., Rimm, E.B., Colditz, G.A., Speizer, F.E., et al, (2000). Intake of specific carotenoids and risk of lung cancer in 2 prospective US cohorts. *Am J Clin Nutr*, Oct;72(4):990-7.

[85] Ito, Y., Kurata, M., Suzuki, K., Hamajima, N., Hishida, H., et al. (2006). Cardiovascular disease mortality and serum carotenoid levels: a Japanese population-based follow-up study. *J Epidemiol*, Jul;16(4):154-60.

[86] Dhuique-Mayer, C., Servent, A., Descalzo, A., Mouquet-Rivier, C., Amiot, M.J., et al. (2016). Culinary practices mimicking a polysaccharide-rich recipe enhance the bioaccessibility of fat-soluble micronutrients. *Food Chem*, Nov 1;210:182-8.

[87] Linus Pauling Institute. (2016). Carotenoids: α-Carotene, β-Carotene, β-Cryptoxanthin, Lycopene, Lutein, and Zeaxanthin. Retrieved Jul 18 2017 from http://lpi.oregonstate.edu/mic/dietary-factors/phytochemicals/carotenoids.

[88] Di Mascio, P., Kaiser, S., Sies, H. (1989). Lycopene as the most efficient biological carotenoid singlet oxygen quencher. *Arch Biochem Biophys*, Nov 1;274(2):532-8.

[89] Erdman, J.W., Ford, N.A., Lindshield, B.L. (2009). Are the health attributes of lycopene related to its antioxidant function? *Arch Biochem Biophys*, Mar 15;483(2):229-35.

[90]Zhao, B., Ren, B., Guo, R., Zhang, W., Ma, S., et al, (2017). Supplementation of lycopene attenuates oxidative stress induced neuroinflammation and cognitive impairment via Nrf2/NF-κB transcriptional pathway. *Food Chem Toxicol*, Nov;109(Pt 1):505-516.

[91]Li, Z.Z., Lu, X.Z., Ma, C.C., Chen, L. (2010). Serum lycopene levels in patients with diabetic retinopathy. *Eur J Ophthalmol*, Jul-Aug;20(4):719-23.

[92] Mares-Perlman, J.A., Brady, W.E., Klein, R., Klein, B.E., Bowen, P., et al. (1995). Serum antioxidants and age-related macular degeneration in a population-based case-control study. *Arch Opthalmol*, Dec;113(12):1518-23.

[93]Mahmoodnia, L., Mohammadi, K., Masumi, R. (2017). Ameliorative effect of lycopene effect on cisplatin-induced nephropathy in patient. *J Nephropathol*, Jul;6(3):144-149,

[94]Giovannucci, E., Ascherio, A., Rimm, E.B., Stampfer, M.J., Golditz, G.A., et al, (1995). Intake of carotenoids and retinol in relation to risk of prostate cancer. *J Natl Cancer Inst*, Dec 6;87(23):1767-76.

[95]Agarwal, S., Rao, A.V. (1998). Tomato lycopene and low density lipoprotein oxidation: a human dietary intervention study. *Lipids*, Oct;33(10):981-4.

[96]Hadley, C.W., Clinton, S.K., Schwartz, S.J. (2003). The consumption of processed tomato products enhances plasma lycopene concentrations in association with a reduced lipoprotein sensitivity to oxidative damage. *J Nutr*, Mar;133(3):727-32.

[97]Balestrieri, M.L., De Prisco, R., Nicolaus, B., Pari, P., Moriello, V.S., et al. (2004). Lycopene in association with alpha-tocopherol or tomato lipophilic extracts enhances acyl-platelet-activating factor biosynthesis in endothelial cells during oxidative stress. *Free Radic Biol Med*, Apr 15;36(8):1058-67.

[98]Dutta-Roy, A.K., Crosbie, L., Gordon, M.J. (2001). Effects of tomato extract on human platelet aggregation in vitro. *Platelets*, Jun;12(4):218-27.

[99]Xu, X., Zhu, M., Hu, M. (2011). Effects of lycopene on blood cells and fibrinolytic activity in hyperlipidemic rats. *Wei Sheng Yan Jiu*, Sep;40(5):620-3.

[100]Hsiao, G., Wang, Y., Tzu, N.H., Fong, T.H., Shen, M.Y., et al. (2005). Inhibitory effects of lycopene on in vitro platelet activation and in vivo prevention of thrombus formation. *J Lab Clin Med*, Oct;146(4):216-26.

[101] Karppi, J., Laukkanen, J.A., Sivenius, J., Ronkainen, K., Kurl, S. (2012). Serum lycopene decreases the risk of stroke in men: a population-based follow-up study. *Neurology*, Oct 9:79(15):1540-1547.

[102]Sahni, S., Hannan, M.T., Blumberg, J., Cupples, L.A., Kiel, D.P., et al, (2009). Protective effect of total carotenoid and lycopene intake on the risk of hip fracture: a 17-year follow-up from the Framingham Osteoporosis Study. *J Bone Miner Res*, Jun;24(6):1086-94.

[103]Mackinnon, E.S., Rao, A.V., Josse, R.G., Rao, L.G. (2011). Supplementation with the antioxidant lycopene significantly decreases oxidative stress parameters and the bone resorption marker N-telopeptide of type I collagen in postmenopausal women. *Osteoporos Int*, Apr;22(4):1091-101.

8-3. PHYTONUTRIENTS: BIOFLAVONOIDS

The bioflavonoids exhibit antioxidant activity in different ways:[1]

- They directly scavenge free radicals.
- They inhibit excess nitric oxide production
- They inhibit certain enzymes responsible for free radical generation.
- They chelate trace elements, which sometimes enhance free radical generation; they help in metabolizing oxygen.

Anthocyanins

Anthocyanins are the largest group of water-soluble plant pigments. They are a group of dark-blue pigmented antioxidants found especially in dark fruit, such as blueberries, bilberries, aronia berries, and dark blue grapes. They are also present in acai fruit, cranberries, black raspberries, cherries, and black currants. In vegetables they are found in the peel of eggplant, in red cabbage, and in black rice. They are a type of flavonoid, odorless, and barely astringent. In flowers they can vary from red to purple or blue, depending on the pH of the soil in which the plant grows.

With respect to vision health, anthocyanins counter the oxidative stress in the retina,[2] reduce inflammation in the tissues of the eye,[3] and provide antiallergic, antiviral, antimicrobial, and anticarcinogenic functions.[4] They support blood circulation and the integrity of fine capillaries in the eye. Anthocyanidins inhibit growth of new blood vessels,[5] which develop in the advanced version of macular degeneration and diabetic retinopathy.

Bilberry

Bilberry is a small wild shrub growing in North America and northern Europe. Traditionally the berries have been utilized for diarrhea, urinary tract infections, and hemorrhoids. Over forty years of research establish this herb's value for vision health.[6] [7] [8] [9]

Antioxidant. Antioxidant[10] anthocyanosides are the active components of bilberry. They help improve microcirculation of tiny blood vessels[11] [12] and therefore improve the delivery of oxygen to the eyes. They accomplish this by improving rhythmic changes in the diameter of blood vessels[13] [14] in the eye's vascular system, as well as in the entire body. They help repair tissue,[15] protect retinal nerve tissue,[16] and generally support a healthy retina by supporting levels of antioxidants in the blood serum.[17]

Connective tissue. Bilberry's antioxidants strengthen collagen and promote the health of tissues.

Inflammation. Bilberry is also rich in tannins, which are astringent in nature and have anti-inflammatory properties. Bilberry was found to inhibit airway inflammation in asthma.[18]

Mitochondrial support. Bilberry is found to protect against dysfunction of mitochondria (cellular energy producers) and also against neurotoxicity.[19]

Cataract. Some studies suggest that bilberry may slow cataract formation. Bilberry, combined with vitamin E, stopped cataract formation in 48 of 50 patients with senile cortical cataracts.[20] In a later animal model, 70% of non-bilberry animals developed cataracts, while none of the animals given bilberry did so.[21]

Diabetic retinopathy. Where diabetic retinopathy is combined with wet or dry AMD, bilberry brought increased macular thickness.[22] In diabetic retinopathy, bilberry improved light sensitivity[23] and slowed onset of blood-retinal barrier disintegration.[24] Researchers reported that berry extracts and anthocyanins inhibit alpha-amylase and alpha-glucosidase in the gut, interacting with sugar transporters in the intestine, and ultimately slowing the rate of glucose entering the bloodstream. For this reason, they are important in helping to manage diabetes and diabetic retinopathy.[25]

Focusing capacity and eye fatigue. Bilberry supports focusing capacity, helps prevent eye fatigue in computer users, and supports all-over vision health.[26]

Macular degeneration. Bilberry is helpful for macular degeneration because it protects the retina against oxidative stress that results from free radicals.[27] It is an effective neuroprotector.[28]

Night vision. Bilberry helps stimulate the production of rhodopsin needed for night vision.[29] [30]

Flavanones

The flavanones are aromatic compounds best known for their presence in citrus fruits and other plants. Some of them may have therapeutic value.

Silymarin

Milk thistle contains large quantities of silymarin, for which reason it is associated with supporting the liver. As a therapy for liver cirrhosis, silymarin is found to reduce biomarkers of liver disease, and it restores levels of the antioxidant enzymes superoxide dismutase (SOD) and glutathione.[31] These enzymes are important for vision health. Silymarin is an antioxidant and anti-inflammatory agent that provides immune system protection.[32]

Milk thistle also contains a number of other components that are valuable for vision health, such as vitamin E and omega-6 fatty acids (fatty acids linoleic, oleic, and palmitic acid).[33]

Source. Milk thistle. Smaller amounts of silymarin are found in wild artichoke, turmeric, coriander seeds, and trace amounts in other foods.

Hesperetin and Hesperidin

Hesperetin and hesperidin inhibit inflammation. Hesperetin increases ocular blood flow in the iris, ciliary body, and choroid, but not the retina, and it inhibits inflammation.[34] Hesperidin is able to permeate into ocular tissues like the cornea, sclera, and retinal pigment epithelium.

Flavanols

The flavanols are aromatic, colorless compounds that occur in plants. They are found as glycosides, which means they are bound to a sugar molecule.

Quercetin

Quercetin is a flavanol that protects the eye from chronic solar radiation exposure. In addition, it may reduce inflammation, and it is being investigated for use in helping reduce eye symptoms from allergens. It functions in a synergistic manner with vitamin E and taurine. Quercetin helps protect fine capillaries in the retina from deterioration and leaking. Both quercetin and rutin are important for a healthy macula, optic nerve health, and lens support.

Glaucoma. Quercetin protects retinal ganglion cells in glaucoma models, independent of lowering intraocular pressure.[35]

Macular degeneration. Quercetin is helpful through its antioxidant capacity to protect retinal pigment from oxidative stress that is caused by solar radiation.[36] Quercetin also inhibits formation of extra blood vessels, as well as improves blood flow in the choroid layer of the retina.[37]

Source. Quercetin is highest in lingonberries. It is also found in dark red or blue fruit, such as cranberries and blueberries, as well as in black and green tea, capers, apples, red grapes, citrus, broccoli, and leafy-green vegetables. It is also in tomatoes. Interestingly, organically grown tomatoes have 79% more quercetin than chemically grown tomatoes.[38]

Caution. Supplemental quercetin may be contraindicated for quinolone antibiotics, such as fluoroquinolone, because it binds to bacteria, but researchers don't understand whether this is a problem.[39] It is also identified as having potentially interfering interactions with taxol/paclitaxel used to treat some types of cancer.[40]

Rutin

Rutin is a cousin of quercetin (part of the bonding structure of quercetin and sugar molecules). As an antioxidant, it is an excellent free-radical fighter.

Diabetic retinopathy. Rutin may reduce levels of fasting glucose and thus may protect against high levels of blood sugar.[41] In this capacity, it may prove valuable in preventing the development of diabetes into diabetic retinopathy.

Macular degeneration. Rutin combats inflammation and oxidative stress involved in the development of macular degeneration. Furthermore, research has indicated that rutin reduces leakage from tiny retina blood vessels and combats inflammation.[42]

Related disorders. Rutin slows platelet clotting[43] and blood clotting, protects from blood vessel leakage, reduces inflammation, and may be useful for other blood vessel and blood circulation issues such as varicose veins and hemorrhoids. Rutin may have a role in prevention of some chronic diseases such as diabetes, hypertension, high cholesterol, and some cancers.[44]

Source. Capers have the highest concentration of rutin, seven times as much as black olives, and nine times as much as buckwheat. It is found in large amounts in raw asparagus, black tea, and black and red raspberries. To a lesser degree, it is found in citrus fruits, mulberries, cranberries, peaches, cherries, white grapefruit, pears, grapes, red onions, onions and garlic, green cabbage, spinach, and kale.

Flavan-3-ols

Catechin

The catechins are natural antioxidant phenols. They are responsible for aromas in plants such as capsaicin, the aromatic constituent of chili peppers. They exist in most plants and plant extracts, from olive oil to rye.[45] There are a number of subgroups with valuable vision-related benefits. These include epigallocatechins and gallocatechins.

Catechins are readily absorbed in the body. They are able to cross the blood-brain barrier. They may support blood flow regulation through modulating vasodilation.[46] As a result,[47] they may be useful for glaucoma therapy. They also help improve functioning of mitochondria, the energy producers of cells.[48]

The epigallocatechin gallate subgroup of the catechins has been much researched in recent years. They have a neuroprotective effect that may be useful for glaucoma,[49] may reduce neovascularization,[50] and have an anti-clotting benefit.[51]

Source. Catechins are especially abundant in cocoa and chocolate, but you should limit the quantity. They are found in abundance in dark plums and broad beans, such as fava beans. They are also found in pecans, red wine, strawberries, apples, peaches, and black grapes.

Green Tea

Even though cocoa has more catechins per gram, green tea is more famous as a source. Through studies with lab animals, researchers have found that green tea catechins are passed from the digestive system into the tissue of the eye.[52] Green tea contains a variety of phytonutrients that support its value.

Antioxidant protection. Tea catechins protect against oxidative stress due to chemical damage; they also protect mitochondria[53] [54] and act as an antioxidant to counter the harm due to alcohol.[55]

Diabetic retinopathy. Green tea consumption appears to protect against complications of diabetes.[56] [57] [58]

Dry eye. The catechins of green tea are effective in treating dry eye and meibomian gland dysfunction.[59] These glands secrete oily meibum on top of the tear film to slow evaporation. The catechins of green tea regulate and reduce symptoms of autoimmune imbalances, as is exhibited in Sjogren's syndrome.[60] [61]

Retinal support. Green tea epigallocatechin protects lab animal retinas from the oxidative damage of hydrogen peroxide[62] and from UVB light damage. This UV light protective effect seems to have to do with the ability of cells to resist degradation when exposed to UV light.[63]

Related disorders. Green tea consumption, timed to match the high pollen counts, significantly reduces symptoms of hay fever or pollen allergy. The most effective green tea for this purpose is matured Benifuuki tea from the second crop season.[64] Other research on green tea and its effect on allergic dermatitis finds the anti-inflammatory results are helpful, without increasing skin irritation.[65]

A number of animal studies report that green tea extract combined with the amino acid l-theanine, (primarily found in green tea), is quite helpful for cognitive capacity. Researchers looked at the effect on human subjects who had mild cognitive impairment, focusing on attention and memory. They found that there were measurable improvements in memory and selective attention in a tea and l-theanine group. Brain wave research further indicated a significant increase in theta waves, known as indicators of cognitive alertness.[66]

Green tea's catechins may improve blood pressure[67] and help lower cholesterol.

Green tea catechins are effective for some conditions for which senior women are most at risk. One study concluded that through modification of estrogen metabolism, green tea might reduce breast cancer risk[68] and osteopenia, low bone density.[69] Green tea is helpful for overactive bladder,[70] regulation of glucose, LDL cholesterol,[71] and general relief of menopausal symptoms, as part of a morning and evening formula combined with other herbs.[72]

In a number of studies, researchers have found that consumption of green tea extract is associated with weight loss.[73] Others have determined that the combination of running and decaffeinated green tea extract in lab animals on a high fat diet is beneficial, reducing body mass, visceral fat mass, blood glucose, and insulin resistance.[74]

Epicatechin

Epicatechin is another flavonol of the catechin family that may improve blood flow. It is found to have three times the antioxidant value of green tea and twice the antioxidant value of red wine. It is rapidly absorbed in humans, peaking several hours after consumption.

Antioxidant. One of the primary benefits of epicatechin is that it is a powerful antioxidant, and because it can cross the blood-brain barrier it can be delivered directly to the brain (as well as reach the optic nerve and retina).[75][76]

Inflammation. Epicatechin can interact with and reduce free radicals. Many eye conditions are caused or aggravated by inflammation.[77][78]

Related conditions. Epicatechin from cocoa appears to protect the nervous system and improve cognitive functioning by enhancing blood flow and controlling vasodilation that tends to increase with aging.[79] In a mouse model it reduced atherosclerosis by 27%, compared to diet alone.

Similarly, these catechins may be helpful in preventing and healing that is associated with stroke and heart attack.[80]

Source. Cocoa contains at least twice as much epicatechin as other sources. Other good sources include prune juice, broad bean pods, apples, blackberries, peaches, and green tea.

Caution. Because hot chocolate drinks can include a lot of sugar (acidifying), either take your hot chocolate Mexican style (with little or no sugar) or favor other sources.

Stilbenoids

Stilbenoids are excellent antioxidants and antibacterial agents, and may have anticancer properties.[81] Because oxidative stress is linked to many conditions, including cancer, diabetes, cardiovascular disease,[82] and eye conditions, these compounds are of great interest to researchers. They have been well studied both as plant-derived extracts and as pure compounds; hundreds have been identified.

They are of particular interest in cancer research because they are able to inhibit a biochemical known as topoisomerase II that plays a role in DNA gene expression.[83]

Source. Foods include grapes, blueberries, and wine, as well as cocoa powder, and peanuts.

Resveratrol

Resveratrol appears to target multiple age-related issues such as mitochondrial dysfunction, inflammation, and oxidative stress.[84]

It is present in a variety of berries including blueberry, bilberry, currant, and cranberry. Heating and cooking these berries reduce the amount of available resveratrol.[85] It is concentrated in grape skin. Red wine is fermented with grape skins and therefore carries a high concentration of resveratrol.[86] Resveratrol has been derived from the skin of grapes, as well as from grapeseed extract, a common nutritional supplement.

Antioxidant. Resveratrol's antioxidant action protects the cardiovascular system, helps maintain biochemical balance, and protects neurons from injury or degeneration.[87]

Inflammation. Resveratrol's anti-inflammatory capacity helps to manage diabetic retinopathy[88] and heart disease by reducing vascular inflammation; similarly, it may help protect microcirculation in the eye.[89] By reducing inflammation, it helps maintain biochemical balance and protects the nervous system.[90]

Cataract. A large number of trials and studies report that because of its antioxidant and anti-inflammation properties, resveratrol may be a good candidate for nutritional therapy.[91] Resveratrol activates an enzyme called sirtuin type 1 (SIRT1), which protects against oxidative stress in lens epithelial cells,[92] protecting against cataract development.[93]

Diabetic retinopathy. Resveratrol has potential in the management of type 2 diabetes. The ability of resveratrol to improve blood sugar balance and lower insulin resistance in diabetes[94][95][96] may also help reduce the incidence of diabetic retinopathy,[97] a complication of diabetes. Its anti-inflammatory capacity may help prevent diabetic retinopathy.[98]

Glaucoma. Resveratrol's antioxidant capacity may also play a role in protecting retinal ganglion cells. Researchers found that when these nerve cells were exposed to intraocular pressure in a mouse model, resveratrol supplementation reduced damage in retinal thickness and protected against cell death.[99][100] Another study found that a combination of resveratrol and quercetin reduced intraocular pressure in an animal model.[101] Through improved microcirculation in the eye, it may help prevent glaucoma.[102]

Macular degeneration. Through its anti-inflammatory and antioxidant effect, resveratrol may help protect against macular degeneration.[103]

Related disorders. Resveratrol plays a role in regulating special proteins that are implicated in a number of degenerative diseases. Incorrect modulation of these proteins by the body has been linked to a number of conditions, including inflammatory and immune-related conditions and viral infections.[104] Similarly, incorrect regulation of a similar function (iron bonding to oxygen) has been linked to Parkinson's and Alzheimer's diseases.[105][106] Resveratrol appears to have the ability to reduce some problems associated with type 2 diabetes, such as restricted blood flow to the heart.[107] Finally, resveratrol is being examined with interest in its capacity to alleviate some of the symptoms of aging, such as bone mineral density loss.[108]

Another study concluded it has neuroprotective properties as well.[109]

Source. Grape skins, grapeseed extract, sprouted peanuts, and in lesser amounts cocoa powder, and dark chocolate.

Curcuminoids

Curcumin

Curcumin is a powerful anti-inflammatory and antioxidant agent with many beneficial effects. It is the primary ingredient of turmeric, a bright yellow spice used to add color and flavor to curry, mustard, and more. It is a relative of ginger.

Inflammation. Curcumin is known for its ability to fight inflammation, which is a key component of many health conditions.[110]

Neuroprotection. Curcumin has been found to reduce neuroinflammation. Researchers found that in a mouse model, curcumin suppressed neuroinflammation that in turn reduced tau/amyloid development, which results in cognitive damage.[111] Interestingly, turmeric is used to detect Alzheimer's disease, because it becomes florescent when in contact with beta-amyloid.

Diabetic retinopathy. Curcumin's anti-inflammatory effects are responsible for a number of studies that conclude it may be helpful for diabetic retinopathy.[112] [113] Researchers are examining why these nutrient therapies work. Curcumin slows blood vessel leakage by inhibiting CAMKII, a biochemical process.[114] Curcumin also slows the death of the islet cells that produce insulin in diabetics by retarding creation of islet free radicals.[115]

Eye cancer. Mitochondrial disease is a group of diseases that involve mitochondria (cellular energy producers) and are detected in dysfunction of the optic nerve, retina, and extraocular muscles. Increasingly, these conditions are being implicated in more common vision problems, such as macular degeneration, diabetic retinopathy, and glaucoma. Reviewers note that therapies which inhibit tumorous mitochondrial function and cause cell death in tumors, such as curcumin, might offer therapies for ocular neoplasms such as retinoblastoma and uveal melanoma.[116]

Glaucoma. Curcumin has a neuroprotective effect against oxidative damage to the optic nerve in vitro and in an animal model. In one study, microglia cell tissue (a kind of cell that protects nerve cells) was exposed to oxidative stress and was protected to a degree that was statistically significant. In animals, mild IOP was induced. In animals that had been given curcumin, the degree of protection was significant.[117]

Macular degeneration. Vascular endothelial growth factor (VEGF) is a protein that, among other functions, regulates cell death and has been the subject of extensive research. Anti-VEGF therapy is a common treatment for wet macular degeneration. Curcumin has been shown to inhibit VEGF and cell death and is of great interest to researchers.[118]

In other research, curcumin has been found to have a protective effect against cell damage in human retinal pigment cells caused by blue light, because it protects retinal pigment epithelial cells against oxidation, which is caused by free radicals.[119] Curcuminoids may have potential in AMD treatment.[120] This research corroborates earlier studies.[121]

Uveitis. Patients with chronic anterior uveitis were given curcumin. Compared to a control group also receiving antitubercular treatment, the patients receiving curcumin alone had a lower recurrence rate than the control in the following three years, and no side effects were reported. The researchers note that the lack of side effects for curcumin is a benefit.[122]

Related disorders. Curcumin supports the immune system's defenses against allergens,[123] [124] doing so, at least in part, by inhibiting the release of histamine from mast cells.[125] Its anti-inflammatory and antifungal capacity is a promising therapy for chronic asthma. In animal models, the herb alleviated asthma symptoms and decreased the fungal burden causing respiratory distress.[126]

Curcumin's anti-inflammatory capacity is of great value in treating and managing various forms of arthritis. Although its potential in *protecting* against osteoarthritis is recognized, its potential in *treating* osteoarthritis is less clear. Researchers evaluated whether it could treat osteoarthritis in mice. They found that curcumin suppressed expression of intermediate biochemicals in the inflammatory process at both the RNA and protein levels. Curcumin also strongly improved other biochemicals that reduce inflammation. Overall, through both avenues, it lessened inflammation, either alone,[127] or as a major component in proprietary formulations.[128]

Source. Turmeric (curcuma longa), mango ginger (curcuma amadaRoxb), and curry powder.

[1] Majumdar, S., Srirangam, R. (2015). Potential of the Bioflavonoids in the Prevention/Treatment of Ocular Disorders. *J Pharm Pharmacol,* Aug;62(8):951-965.

[2] Mykkanen, O.T., Kalesnykas, G., Adriaens, M., Evolo, C.T., Torronen, R., et al, (2012). Bilberries potentially alleviate stress-related retinal gene expression induced by a high-fat diet in mice. *Mol Vis,* 2012:18:2338-51.

[3] Miyake, S., Takahashi, N., Sasaki, M., Kobayashi, S., Tsubota, K., et al. (2012). Vision preservation during retinal inflammation by anthocyanin-rich bilberry extract: cellular and molecular mechanism. *Lab Invest,* Jan;92(1):102-9.

[4] Ghosh, D., Konishi, T. (2007). Anthocyanins and anthocyanin-rich extracts: role in diabetes and eye function. *Asia Pac J Clin Nutr,* 2007;16(2):200-8.

[5] Matsunaga, N., Tsuruma, D., Shimazawa, M., Yokota, S., Hara, H. (2010). Inhibitory actions of bilberry anthocyanidins on angiogenesis. *Phytother Res,* Jan;24 Suppl 1:S42-7.

[6] Camire M.E. (2000). *Herbs, Botanicals and Teas.* Bilberries and blueberries as functional foods and nutraceuticals; pp. 289–319. Lancaster, PA: Technomic Publishing Company.

[7] Chu, W.K., Cheung, S.C.M., Lau, R.A.W., Benzie, I.F.F. (2011). Chapter 4 Bilberry (Vaccinium myrtillus L.). *Herbal Medicine: Biomecular and Clinical Aspects. 2nd ed.* Boca Raton, FL: CRC Press/Taylor & Francis.

[8] Kemper, K.J. (1965). Bilberry (Vaccinium myrtillus). *Ann Ottalmol Clin Ocul,*1965;91:371-86.

[9] Upton, R, editor. (2001). Bilberry Fruit Vaccinium myrtillus L. Standards of Analysis, Quality Control, and Therapeutics. *American Herbal Pharmacopoeia and Therapeutic Compendium.* Santa Cruz, CA/.

[10] Zafra-Stone, S., Yasmin, T., Bagchi, M., Chatterjee, A., Vinson, J.A., et al. (2007). Berry anthocyanins as novel antioxidants in human health and disease prevention. *Mol Nutr Food Res,* Jun;51(6):675-83.

[11] Mastantuono, T., Starita, N., Sapio, D., D'Avanzo, S.A., Di Maro, M., et al. (2016). The Effects of Vaccinium myrtillus Extract on Hamster Pial Microcirculation during Hypoperfusion-Reperfusion Injury. *PLoS One,* Apr 12;11(4):e0150659.

[12] Cohen-Boulakia, F., Valensi, P.E., Boulahdour, H., Lestrade, R. Dufour-Lamarinie, J.F., et al. (2000). In vivo sequential study of skeletal muscle capillary permeability in diabetic rats: effect of anthocyanosides. *Metabolism,* Jul;49(7):880-5.

[13] Colantuoini, A., Bertuglia, S., Magistretti, M.J., Donato, L. (1991). Effects of Vaccinium Myrtillus anthocyanosides on arterial vasomotion. *Arzneimittelforschung,* Sep;41(9):905-9.

[14] Zhu, Y., Xia, M., Yang, Y., Liu, F., Li, Z., et al. (2011). Purified anthocyanin supplementation improves endothelial function via NO-cGMP activation in hypercholesterolemic individuals. *Clin Chem,* Nov;57(11):1524-33.

[15] Yamaura, K., Simada, M., Ueno, K. (2011). Anthocyanins from bilberry (Vaccinium myrtillus L.) alleviate pruritus in a mouse model of chronic allergic contact dermatitis. *Pharmacogosy Res,* Jul;3(3):173-7.

[16] Matsunaga, J., Imai, S., Inokuchi, Y., Shimazawa, M., Yokata, S., et al. (2009). Bilberry and its main constituents have neuroprotective effects against retinal neuronal damage in vitro and in vivo. *Mol Nutr Food Res,* Jul;53(7):869-77.

[17] Mazza, G., Kay, C.D., Correll, T., Holub, B.J. (2002). Absorption of anthocyanins from blueberries and serum antioxidant status in human subjects. *J Agric Food Chem,* 50:7731–7.

[18] Park, S.J., Shin, W.H., Seo, J.W., Kim, E.J. (2007). Anthocyanins inhibit airway inflammation and hyperresponsiveness in a murine asthma model. *Food Chem Toxicol,* Aug;45(8):1459-67.

[19] Yao, Y., Vieria, A. (2007). Protective activities of Vaccinium antioxidants with potential relevance to mitochondrial dysfunction and neurotoxicity. *Neurotoxicology,* Jan;28 93–100.

[20] Bravetti, G. (1989). Preventive medical treatment of senile cataract with vitamin E and anthocyanosides: clinical evaluation. *Ann Ottalmol Clin Ocul,*115:109.

[21] Fursova, A.Z., Gesarevich, O.G., Gonchar, A.M., Trofimova, N.A., Kolosova, N.G. (2005). Dietary supplementation with bilberry extract prevents macular degeneration and cataracts in senesce-accelerated OXYS rats. *Adv Gerontol,* 2005;16:76-9.

[22]Moshetova, L.K., Vorob'eva, I.V., Alekseev, I.B., Mikhaleva, L.G. (2015) Results of the use of antioxidant and angioprotective agents in type 2 diabetes patients with diabetic retinopathy and age-related macular degeneration. *Vestn Oftalmol*, May-Jun;131(3):34-44.

[23] Ibid. Moshetova. (2015).

[24]Kim, J., Kim, C.S., Lee, Y.M., Sohn, E., Jo, K., et al. (2015). Vaccinium myrtillus extract prevents or delays the onset of diabetes--induced blood-retinal barrier breakdown. *Int J Food Sci Nutr,* Mar;66(2):236-42.

[25]Castro-Acosta, M.L., Lenihan-Geels, G.N., Corpe, C.P., Hall, W.L. (2016). Berries and anthocyanins: promising functional food ingredients with postprandial glycaemia-lowering effects. *Proc Nutr Soc*, Aug;75(3):342-55.

[26] Ozawa, Y., Kawashima, M., Inoue, S., Inagaki, E., Suzuki, A., et al. (2015). Bilberry extract supplementation for preventing eye fatigue in video display terminal workers. *J Nutr Health Aging*, May;19(5):548-54.

[27] Osada, H., Okamoto, T., Kawashima, H., Toda, E., Miyake, S., et al. (2017). Neuroprotective effect of bilberry extract in a murine model of photo-stressed retina. *PLoS One*, Jun 1;12(6):e0178627.

[28]Wang, Y., Zhao, L., Lu, F., Yang, X., Deng, Q., et al. (2015). Retinoprotective Effects of Bilberry Anthocyanins via Antioxidant, Anti-Inflammatory, and Anti-Apoptotic Mechanisms in a Visible Light-Induced Retinal Degeneration Model in Pigmented Rabbits. *Molecules,* Dec 14;20(12):22395-410.

[29] Muth, E.R., Laurent, J.M., Jasper, P. (2000). The effect of bilberry nutritional supplementation on night visual acuity and contrast sensitivity. *Altern Med Rev*, 5:164-173.

[30]Ibid. Muth. (2000).

[31] Zaidi, S.N.F., Mahboob, T. (2017). Prevention of liver cirrhosis by Silymarin. *Pak J Pharm Sci*, Jul;30(4):1203-1211.

[32] Chambers, C.S., Holeckova, V., Petrakova, L., Bidermann, D., Valentova, K., et al. (2017) The silymarin composition ... and why does it matter? *Food Res Int*, Oct;100(Pt 3):339-353.

[33] Ibid. Chambers. (2017).

[34] Ibid. Majumdar. (2015).

[35] Gao, F.J., Zhang, S.H., Xu, P., Yang, B.O., Zhang, R., et al. (2017). Quercetin Declines Apoptosis, Ameliorates Mitochondrial Function and Improves Retinal Ganglion Cell Survival and Function in In Vivo Model of Glaucoma in Rat and Retinal Ganglion Cell Culture In Vitro. *Front Mol Neurosci,* Sep 7;10:285.

[36] Zhuang, P., Shen, Y., Lin, B.Q., Zhang, W.Y., Chiou, G.C. (2011). Effect of quercetin on formation of choroidal neovascularization (CNV) in age-related macular degeneration (AMD). *Eye Sci*, Mar;26(1):23-9.

[37] Ibid. Zhuang. (2011).

[38]Mitchell, A.E., Hong, Y.J., Barrett, D.M., Bryant, D.E., Denison, R.F., et al. (2007). Ten-Year Comparison of the Influence of Organic and Conventional Crop Management Practices on the Content of Flavonoids in Tomatoes. *J Agric Food Chem*, Jul 25;55(15):6154-9.

[39] Quercitin. RxList. Retrieved Sep 18 2017 from https://www.rxlist.com/quercetin-page3/supplements.htm.

[40] Samuel, T., Fadlalla, K., Turner, T., Yehualaeshet, T.E. (2010). The flavonoid quercetin transiently inhibits the activity of taxol and nocodazole through interference with the cell cycle. *Nutr Cancer*, (8):1025-35.

[41] Ghorbani, A. (2017) Mechanisms of antidiabetic effects of flavonoid rutin. *Biomed Pharmacother*, Oct 7;96:305-312.

[42] Benavente-Garcia, O., Castillo, J. (2008). Update on uses and properties of citrus flavonoids: new findings in anticancer, cardiovascular, and anti-inflammatory activity. *J Agric Food Chem*. Aug 13;56(15):6185-205.

[43]L. Navarro-Nunez, Lozano, M.L., Palomo, M., Martinex, C., Vicente, V., et al. (2008). Apigenin Inhibits Platelet Adhesion and Thrombus Formation and Synergizes with Aspirin in the Suppression of the Arachidonic Acid Pathway. *J Agric Food Chem,* May 14;56(9):2970-6.

[44] Sharma, S., Ali, A., Ali, J., Sahni, J.K., Baboota, S. (2013). Rutin: therapeutic potential and recent advances in drug delivery. *Expert Opin Investig Drugs*, Aug;22(8):1063-79.

[45] Wikipedia. Phenols. Retrieved Sep 18 2017 from https://en.wikipedia.org/wiki/Phenols.

[46]Hooper, L., Kay, C., Abdelhamid, A., Kroon, P.A., Cohn, J.S., et al. (2012). Effects of chocolate, cocoa, and flavan-3-ols on cardiovascular health: A systematic review and meta-analysis of randomized trials. *Am J Clin Nutr*, Mar;95(3):740–51.

[47] Faria, A., Pestana, D., Teixeira, D., Couraud, P.O., Romero, I., et al. (2011). Insights into the putative catechin and epicatechin transport across blood-brain barrier. *Food Funct*, Jan; 2(1):39-44.

[48] Silva Santos, L.F., Stolfo, A., Calloni, C., Salvador, M. (2017). Catechin and epicatechin reduce mitochondrial dysfunction and oxidative stress induced by amiodarone in human lung fibroblasts. *J Arrhythm*, Jun;33(3):220-225.

[49] Shen, C., Chen, L., Jiang, L., Lai, T.Y. (2015) Neuroprotective effect of epigallocatechin-3-gallate in a mouse model of chronic glaucoma. *Neurosci Lett*, Jul 23;600:132-6.

[50] Lee, H.S., Jun, J.H., Jung, E.H., Koo, B.A., Kim, Y.S. (2014) Epigalloccatechin-3-gallate inhibits ocular neovascularization and vascular permeability in human retinal pigment epithelial and human retinal microvascular endothelial cells via suppression of MMP-9 and VEGF activation. *Molecules*, Aug 13;19(8):12150-72.

[51] Joo, H.J., Park, J.Y., Hong, S.J., Kim, K.A., Lee, S.H., et al. (2018). Anti-platelet effects of epigallocatechin-3-gallate in addition to the concomitant aspirin, clopidogrel or ticagrelor treatment. *Korean J. Intern Med*, May;33(3):522-531.

[52]Chu, K.O., Chan, K.P., Wang, C.C., Chu, C.Y., Li, W.Y., et al. (2010). Green Tea Catechins and Their Oxidative Protection in the Rat Eye, *J Agric Food Chem*, 58 (3): 1523

[53] Chen, L., Yang, X., Jiao, H., Zhao, B. (2003). Tea catechins protect against lead-induced ROS formation, mitochondrial dysfunction, and calcium dysregulation in PC12 cells. *Chem Res Toxicol,* Sep;16(9):1155-61.

[54] Sinha, D., Roy, S., Roy, M. (2010). Antioxidant potential of tea reduces arsenite induced oxidative stress in Swiss albino mice. *Food Chem Toxicol*, Apr;48(4):1032-9.

[55] Skrzydlewska, E., Ostrowska, J., Stankiewicz, A., Farbiszewski, R. (2002). Green tea as a potent antioxidant in alcohol intoxication. *Addict Biol*, Jul;7(3):307-14.

[56] Ma, Q., Chen, D., Sun, H.P., Yan, N., Xu, Y., et al. (2015). Regular Chinese Green Tea Consumption is Protective for Diabetic Retinopathy: A Clinic-Based Case-Control Study. *J Diabetes Res*, 2015:231570.

[57] Landrum, J.T., Bone, R.A., Kilburn, M.D. (1997). The Macular Pigment: A Possible Role in Protection from Age-Related Macular Degeneration. *Adv Pharmacol*, 38:537-56.

[58] Silva, K.C., Rosales, M.A., Hamassaki, D.E., Saito, K.C., Faria, A.M., et al. (2013). Green tea is neuroprotective in diabetic retinopathy. *Invest Ophthalmol Vis Sci,* Feb 15;5(2):1325-36.

[59] Nejabat, M., Reza, S.A., Zadmehr, M., Yasemi, M., Sobhani, Z. (2017). Efficacy of Green Tea Extract for Treatment of Dry Eye and Meibomian Gland Dysfunction; A Double-blind Randomized Controlled Clinical Trial Study. *J Clin Diagn Res*, Feb;11(2):NC05-NC08.

[60] Dickenson, D., Yu, H., Ohno, S., Thomas, C. Derossi, S., et al. (2014). Epigallocatechin-3-gallate prevents autoimmune-associated down- regulation of p21 in salivary gland cells through a p53-independent pathway. *Inflamm Allergy Drug Targets*, Feb;13(1):15-24.

[61] Hsu, S.D., Dickinson, D.P., Qin, H., Borke, J., Ogbureke, K.U., et al. (2007). Green tea polyphenols reduce autoimmune symptoms in a murine model for human Sjogren's syndrome and protect human salivary acinar cells from TNF-alpha-induced cytotoxicity. *Autoimmunity*, Mar;40(2):138-47.

[62]Cia, D., Vergnaud-Gauduchon, J., Jacquemot, N., Doly, M. (2014) Epigallocatechin Gallate (EGCG) Prevents H2O2-Induced Oxidative Stress in Primary Rat Retinal Pigment Epithelial Cells, *Curr Eye Res*, Sep;39(9):944-52

[63] Ibid. Landrum. (1997).

[64] Maeda-yamamoto, M. (2013). Human clinical studies of tea polyphenols in allergy or life style-related diseases, *Curr Pharm Des*, 2013:19(34):6148-55.

[65]Kim, H.K., Choi, S.Y., Chang, H.K., Baek, S.Y., Chung, J.O., et al. (2012). Human skin safety test of green tea cell extracts in condition of allergic contact dermatitis. *Toxicol Res*, Jun;28(2):113-6.

[66] Park, S.K., Jung, I.C., Lee, W.K., Lee, Y.S., Park, H.K., et al. (2011). A combination of green tea extract and l-theanine improves memory and attention in subjects with mild cognitive impairment: a double-blind placebo-controlled study. *J Med Food,* April;14(4):334-43.

[67]Khalesi, S., Sun, J., Buys, N., Jamshidi, A., Nikbakht-Nasrabadi, E., et al. (2014). Green tea catechins and blood pressure: A systematic review and meta-analysis of randomised controlled trials. *Eu J Nutr*, Sep;53 (6):1299–311.

[68] Fuhrman, B.J., Pfeiffer, R.M., Wu, A.H., Xu, X., Keefer, L.K., et al. (2014). Green tea intake is associated with urinary estrogen profiles in Japanese-American women. *Nutr J*, Feb 15;12:25.

[69] Qian, G., Xue, K., Tang, L., Wang, F., Song, X., et al. (2012). Mitigation of oxidative damage by green tea polyphenols and Tai Chi exercise in postmenopausal women with osteopenia, *PLos One,*7(10):e48090.

[70]Payton, S. (2012). Green tea catechin can improve symptoms of menopause-induced overactive bladder, S. Payton, *Nat Rev Urol*, Jun 19;9(7):353.

[71] Wu, A.H., Spicer, D., Stanczyk, F.Z., Tseng, C.C., Yang, C.S., et al. (2012). Effect of 2-month controlled green tea intervention on lipoprotein cholesterol, glucose, and hormone levels in healthy postmenopausal women, *Can Prev Res*, Mar;5(3):393-402.

[72] Sun, J. (2003). Morning/evening menopausal formula relieves menopausal symptoms: a pilot study. *J Alt Complement Med*, Jun;9(3):403-9.

[73] Snoussi, C., Ducroc, R., Hamdaoui, M.H., Dhaouadi, K. Abaidi, H., et al. (2014). Green tea decoction improves glucose tolerance and reduces weight gain of rats fed normal and high-fat diet., *J Nutr Biochem*, May;25(5):557-64.

[74] Sae-tan, S., Rogers, C.J., Lambert, J.D. (2013). Voluntary exercise and green tea enhance the expression of genes related to energy utilization and attenuate metabolic syndrome in high fat fed mice, *Mol Nutr Food Res*, May;58(5):1156-9.

[75] Shay, J., Elbax, H.A., Lee, I., Sielske, S.P., Malek, M.H., et al. (2015). Molecular Mechanisms and Therapeutic Effects of (−)-Epicatechin and Other Polyphenols in Cancer, Inflammation, Diabetes, and Neurodegeneration. *Oxid Med Cell Logev*, 2015:181260.

[76] Faria, A., Pestana, D., Teixeira, D., Couraud, P.O., Romero, I., et al. (2011). Insights into the putative catechin and epicatechin transport across blood-brain barrier. *Food Funct*, Jan; 2(1):39-44.

[77] Ibid. Shay. (2015).

[78] Ibid. Shay. (2015).

[79] Nehlig, A. (2013). The neuroprotective effects of cocoa flavanol and its influence on cognitive performance. *Br J Clin Pharmacol*, Mar;75(3):716–727.

[80] Ibid. Shay. (2015).

[81] Niesen, D.B., Hessler, C., Seeram, N.P. (2013). Beyond resveratrol: A review of natural stilbenoids identified from 2009–2013. *J Berry Res*, 3:181–196.

[82] Ibid. Niesen. (2013).

[83] Ibid. Niesen. (2013).

[84] Ibid. Niesen. (2013).

[85] Ibid. Niesen. (2013).

[86] Ibid. Niesen. (2013).

[87] Abu-Amero, K.K., Kondkar, A.A., Chalam, K.V. (2016). Resveratrol and Ophthalmic diseases. *Nutrients,* Apr 5;8(4):200.

[88] Ghadiri, S. E., Arbabi-Aval, M., Rezaei, K.M, Ahmadieh, H. (2015). Anti-inflammatory properties of resveratrol in the retinas of type 2 diabetic rats. *Clin Exp Pharmacol Physiol*, Jan;42(1):63-8.

[89] Bola, C., Bartlett, H., Eperjesi, F. (2014). Resveratrol and the eye: activity and molecular mechanisms. *Graefes Arch Clin Exp Ophthalmol*, May;252(5);699-713.

[90] Ibid. Abu-Amero. (2016).

[91] Goutham, G., Manikandan, R., Beulaja, M., Thiagarajan, R., Arulvasu, C., et al. (2017). A focus on resveratrol and ocular problems, especially cataract: From chemistry to medical uses and clinical relevance. *Biomed Pharmacother*, Feb;86:232-241.

[92] Zheng, T., Lu, Y. (2016). SIRT1 Protects Human Lens Epithelial Cells Against Oxidative Stress by Inhibiting p53-Dependent Apoptosis. *Curr Eye Res,* Aug;41(8):1068-1075.

[93] Ibid. Zheng. (2016).

[94] Zhu, X., Wu, C., Qiu, S., Yuan, X., Li, L. (2017). Effects of resveratrol on glucose control and insulin sensitivity in subjects with type 2 diabetes: systematic review and meta-analysis. *Nutr Metab (Lond),* Sep 22;14:60.

[95] Anderson, G., Burkon, A., Sulzmaier, F.J., Walker, J.M., Leckband, G. (2011). High dose of dietary resveratrol enhances insulin sensitivity in healthy rats but does not lead to metabolite concentrations effective for SIRT1 expression. *Mol Nutr Food Res*, Aug;55(8):1197-206.

[96] Crandall, J.P., Oram, V., Trandadirescu, G., Reid, M. Kishore, P., et al. (2012). Pilot study of resveratrol in older adults with impaired glucose tolerance. *J Gerontol A Biol Sci Med Sci*, Dec;67(12):1307-12.

[97] Antonetti, D.A., Klein, R., Gardner, T.W. (2012). Diabetic retinopathy. *N Engl J Med*, Mar 29; 366(13):1227-39.

[98] Ibid. Bola. (2014).

[99] Seong, H., Ryu, J., Yoo, W.S., Kim, S.J., Han, Y.S., et al. (2017). Resveratrol Ameliorates Retinal Ischemia/Reperfusion Injury in C57BL/6J Mice via Downregulation of Caspase-3. *Curr Eye Res*, Dec;42(12):1650-1658.

[100]Anekonda, T.S., Adamus, G. (2008). Resveratrol prevents antibody-induced apoptotic death of retinal cells through upregulation of Sirt1 and Ku70. *BMC Res Notes*, Dec 1;1;122.

[101] Natesan, S., Pandian, S., Ponnusamy, C., Palanichamy, R., Muthusamy, S., et al. (2017) Co-encapsulated resveratrol and quercetin in chitosan and peg modified chitosan nanoparticles: For efficient intra ocular pressure reduction. *Int J Biol Macromol*, Nov;104(Pt B):1837-1845.

[102] Ibid. Bola. (2014).

[103] Ibid. Bola. (2014).

[104] Ibid. Niesen. (2013).

[105] Ibid. Niesen. (2013).

[106]Currais, A, Prior, M., Dargusch, R., Armando, A., Ehren, J., et al. (2014). Modulation of p25 and inflammatory pathways by fisetin maintains cognitive function in Alzheimer's disease transgenic mice. *Aging Cell*, Apr;13(2):379-90.

[107] Ibid. Niesen. (2013).

[108] Ibid. Niesen. (2013).

[109] Bastianetto, S., Menard, C., Quirion, R. (2015). Neuroprotective action of resveratrol. *Biochem Biophys Acta*, Jun;1852(6):1195-201.

[110]Calabrese, V., Bates, T.E., Mancuso, C., Cornelius, C., Ventimiglia, B., et al. (2008). Curcumin and the cellular stress response in free radical-related diseases. *Mol Nutr Food Res*, Sep;52(9):1062-73.

[111] Sundaram, J.R., Poore, D.P., Sulaimee, N.H.B., Pareek, T., Cheong, W.F., et al. (2017), Curcumin Ameliorates Neuroinflammation, Neurodegeneration, and Memory Deficits in p25 Transgenic Mouse Model that Bears Hallmarks of Alzheimer's Disease. *J Alzheimers Dis*, 2017;60(4):1429-1442.

[112]Aldebasi, Y.H., Aly, S.M., Rahmani, A.H. (2013). Therapeutic implications of curcumin in the prevention of diabetic retinopathy via modulation of anti-oxidant activity and genetic pathways. *Int J Physiol Pathophysiol Pharmacol*, Dec 15;5(4):194-202.

[113]Jeenger, M.K., Shrivastava, S., Yerra, V.G., Naidu, V.G., Ramakrishna, S., et al. (2015). Curcumin: a pleiotropic phytonutrient in diabetic complications. *Nutrition*, Feb;31(2):276-82.

[114] Li, J., Wang, P., Ying, J., Chen, Z., Yu, S. (2016). Curcumin Attenuates Retinal Vascular Leakage by Inhibiting Calcium/Calmodulin-Dependent Protein Kinase II Activity in Streptozotocin-Induced Diabetes. *Cell Physiol Biochem*, 2016;39(3):1196-208.

[115]Meghana, K., Sanjeev, G., Ramesh, B. (2007). Curcumin prevents streptozotocin-induced islet damage by scavenging free radicals: a prophylactic and protective role. *Eur J Pharmacol*, Dec 22;577(1-3):183-91.

[116] Schrier, S.A., Falk, M.J. (2011). Mitochondrial disorders and the eye. *Curr Opin Ophthalmol*, Sep;22(5):325-31.

[117] Yue, Y.K., Mo, B., Zhao, J., Yu, Y.J., Liu, L., et al. (2014). Neuroprotective effect of curcumin against oxidative damage in BV-2 microglia and high intraocular pressure animal model. *J Ocul Pharmacol Ther*, Oct;30(8):657-64.

[118] Saberi-Karimian, M., Katsiki, M., Caraglia, M., Boccellino, M., Majeed, M., et al. (2017). Vascular endothelial growth factor: An important molecular target of curcumin. *Crit Rev Food Sci Nutr*, Aug 30:1-14.

[119]Woo, J.M., Shin, D.Y., Lee, S.J., Joe, Y., Zheng, M., et al. (2012). Curcumin protects retinal pigment epithelial cells against oxidative stress via induction of heme oxygenase-1 expression and reduction of reactive oxygen. *Mol Vis*, 18: 901–908.

[120] Park, S.I., Lee, E.H., Kim, S.R., Jang, Y.P. (2017). Anti-apoptotic effects of Curcuma longa L. extract and its curcuminoids against blue light-induced cytotoxicity in A2E-laden human retinal pigment epithelial cells. *J Pharm Pharacol*, Mar;69(3):334-340.

[121] Zhu, W., Wu, Y., Meng, Y.F., Wang, J.Y., Xu, M., et al. (2015). Effect of curcumin on aging retinal pigment epithelial cells. *Drug Des Devel Ther*, Sep 25;9:5337-44.

[122] Lal, B., Kapoor, A.K., Asthana, O.P., Agrawal, P.K., Prasad, R., et al. (1999). Efficacy of curcumin in the management of chronic anterior uveitis. *Phytother Res*, Jun;13(4):318-22.

[123]Kurup, V.P., Barrios, C.S. (2008). Immunomodulatory effects of curcumin in allergy. *Mol Nutr Food Res*, Sep;52(9):1031-9.

[124]Oh, S.W., Cha, J.Y., Jung, J.E., Chang, B.C., Kwon, H.J., et al. (2011). Curcumin attenuates allergic airway inflammation and hyper-responsiveness in mice through NF-?B inhibition. *J Ethnopharmacol*, Jul 14;136(4):414-21.

[125]Nugroho, A.E., Ikawati, Z., Sardjiman, Maeyama, K. (2009). Effects of benzylidenecyclopentanone analogues of curcumin on histamine release from mast cells. *Biol Pharm Bull*, May;32(5):842-9.

[126]Karaman, M., Arikan, A.Z., Firinci, F., Kiray, M., Bagriyanik, A., et al. (2011). Effects of curcumin on lung histopathology and fungal burden in a mouse model of chronic asthma and oropharyngeal candidiasis. *Arch Med Res,* Feb;42(2):79-87.

[127] Sun, Y., Liu, W., Zhang, H., Li, H., Liu, J., et al. (2017). Curcumin Prevents Osteoarthritis by Inhibiting the Activation of Inflammasome NLRP3. *J Interferon Cytokine Res,* Oct;37(10):449-455

[128]Belcaro, G., Cesarone, M.R., Dugall, M., Pellegrini, L., Ledda, A., et al. (2010). Efficacy and safety of Meriva®, a curcumin-phosphatidylcholine complex, during extended administration in osteoarthritis patients. *Altern Med Rev,* Dec;15(4):337-44.

8-4. VITAMINS AND VITAMIN-LIKE

Vitamin A

Vitamin A is a group of compounds that includes retinol, retinoic acid, and retinal. In addition, certain carotenoids (beta-carotene, alpha-carotene, and beta-cryptoxanthin) are precursors. Lycopene is not itself a precursor to vitamin A but it is a precursor to beta-carotene.

Retinol is essential for cell growth and differentiation. It plays a major role in vision, immune system and brain functioning, metabolism, and tissue regeneration. Vitamin A deficiency exacerbates iodine deficient thyroid dysfunction, and it may play a role in metabolic syndrome.[1] It is needed for the reproductive system and bone growth. **Retinoic acid** apparently plays a role in structuring the fovea area of the eye.[2] The fovea is a tiny dip in the center of the macula that is responsible for high-sharpness vision. The photoreceptor cones are highly concentrated in that area, and vitamin A is required to form rhodopsin (protein + pigment found in the photoreceptor ganglion cells). **Retinal**, bound to proteins called opsins, is the chemical basis of animal vision.

Antioxidant. Vitamin A is essential for vision health. As a powerful antioxidant it is a keystone of protection against oxidative damage caused by exposure to blue, violet, and UV light.

Cataract. Researchers noted as early as 1944 that moderate levels of vitamin A in patients' diets were connected to a 40% lower risk of opaque lenses or cataracts.[3] The Nurses Health Study tracked the health of more than 50,000 female registered nurses along with their diet and levels of nutrients over 20 years. They found 39% less risk of developing a cataract in nurses with the highest 1/5th intake of vitamin A in the diet. This finding has often been replicated.[4] The risk of cataract in those taking both A and C was lowered by 45%.

More recently, researchers looked to patterns of nutrients with respect to cataracts. That is, rather than looking at vitamin A (and other nutrients) in isolation, they looked at reasonable groups. Two groups that decreased cataract risk significantly were an antioxidant group (carotenes and vitamins A and C) and an omega-3 group.[5]

Glaucoma. Giving patients vitamin A is somewhat effective in lowering IOP.[6]

Night blindness. Early research demonstrated that vitamin A supplementation could reverse the effects of night blindness. Even a small increase in vitamin A levels is helpful, and both dietary vitamin A and vitamin A supplementation are effective.[7] Successful light adaption is closely tied to blood retinol levels and markedly improves with vitamin A supplementation.[8]

Retinitis pigmentosa. In a literature review, researchers found that daily vitamin A (15,000 IU) has a small, protective effect in slowing RP progression. Also, lutein and beta-carotene (a vitamin A precursor) also show some benefit.[9] Vitamin A combined with fish oil is helpful.[10]

Source. The top source of vitamin A is beef liver. Top vegetable sources are carrots and sweet potato, followed by kale, spinach, seaweed, apricots, broccoli, butter, eggs, and winter squash.

Stargardt's warning. Stargardt's is a type of macular dystrophy similar to AMD that forms in young children. In the case of Stargardt's, vitamin A supplementation **is not recommended**. Similarly, supplementation with vitamin A precursors (alpha- and beta-carotene, and beta-cryptoxanthin) is not recommended, as they can be toxic to the photoreceptor cells in the retina. Patients with lower vitamin A intake experience better visual acuity.[11]

Caution. Mega-doses of vitamin A can be toxic, and amounts greater than 25,000 IU are not advisable unless you are deficient and under your doctor's supervision.

B Vitamins

Each of the B vitamins perform unique functions. Deficiencies in any of these B vitamins may have serious consequences for vision and/or general health. They are found in a wide variety of foods. Some, like B12, are not found in vegetables and must come from dairy, meat, or supplemental sources. Vitamin B production can be reduced by vitamin D deficiency.[12]

Vitamin B1 - Thiamine

Vitamin B1 appears in all cells, and its deficiency causes a wide-ranging set of problems. It is not synthesized in the body and must be taken in through food; the amount needed can depend on medications taken or diseases of the individual.[13] It plays an important role in nerve message transmission and maintenance of the nervous system, mucous membranes, the cardiovascular system, and the muscular-skeletal system. It affects some parts of the brain more than others.

Antioxidant. Thiamine behaves like an antioxidant,[14] especially in combination with other antioxidants. It is essential for vision and cognitive functioning. Bacteria and fungi can manufacture their own vitamin B1, but for humans, it is an essential nutrient only available through food or supplements.

Inflammation. The combination of thiamin and riboflavin (B2) inhibit cytokine production and reduce inflammation in animal models.[15]

Cataract. Long-term supplementation with vitamin E and B1 and/or B2 may slow development of cataracts.[16] Although thiamine by itself does not have statistical significance in protection against cataracts, it becomes important because deficiency impairs the function of certain metabolic pathways.[17]

Dry eye. As a result of glaucoma eye drops with preservatives, dry eye may result. A combination of forskolin, rutin, and vitamins B1 and B2 is helpful in reducing the dry eye symptoms.[18]

Glaucoma. The Rotterdam Study involving more than 3,500 participants over age 55 found that a low consumption of vitamin A-related nutrients, vitamin B1, and a high intake of magnesium were linked to an increased risk of developing open-angle glaucoma.[19]

Retinal and optic nerve edema. A known brain abnormality called Wernicke-Korsakoff syndrome results from vitamin B1 deficiency.[20] It results in eye muscle weakness, confusion, and physical coordination problems. In one case of Wernicke encephalopathy, eye doctors noted optic disc edema and retinal hemorrhage, which resolved with thiamine treatment.[21] In another case, optic nerve edema resulted from thiamine deficiency and was resolved with thiamine treatment.[22]

Related disorders. B1 supports heart muscle energy metabolism and cardiovascular functions and is therefore found in many formulas supporting heart health. Diuretics and low-dose water pills for high blood pressure can contribute to vitamin B1 deficiency.[23] After a heart attack, supplemental thiamine helps recovery and improves neurological function. In animal models, B1 improves oxygen consumption in cell mitochondria.[24] Vitamin B complex deficiencies, including vitamin B1, may contribute to cognitive decline, memory loss, and mental imbalance. It plays a role in nerve transmission in parts of the brain (called cholinergic neurons) that deteriorate in Alzheimer's disease. The activity of vitamin B1-dependent enzymes has been found to be lower in the brains of people with Alzheimer's. People with type 1 diabetes also often exhibit B1 deficiency,[25] as do alcoholics.[26]

Source. Good sources of B1 are meat, fish, whole grains, sunflower seeds, nuts, beans and peas, seaweed, asparagus, leafy-green vegetables, and eggs.

Caution. Vitamin B1 deficiency can be caused or aggravated by a diet high in raw fish and shellfish, a diet high in coffee or tea, and general malnutrition. Grains are a valuable source of B1, but removing the hulls in white rice and white flour also removes B1. In industrialized countries, B1 and other nutrients are added back to the processed flour.

Vitamin B2 - Riboflavin

Vitamin B2 (riboflavin) behaves like an antioxidant,[27] combating free radicals that cause oxidation damage to red blood cells, tissues in the eyes, and other parts of the body. Riboflavin is essential for proper functioning of many cell processes, including energy production. It bears special importance for vision, because it helps the retina receive light and is used in glutathione creation.

Immune system. Riboflavin helps regulate the immune system, and its deficiency is linked to a weak immune response. When exposed to various illness stressors, macrophages induce the immune response. Riboflavin deficiency impairs this ability.[28] [29] Macrophages are large cells created by the immune system to engulf and destroy infection-bearing cells.[30]

Cataract. B2 deficiencies may cause cataracts. Riboflavin is an indirect precursor of glutathione (essential for lens health), and as such, its deficiency can contribute to cataract development. Researchers found no link between early cataracts and a deficiency in B2, but people with mature cataract do have a B2 deficiency.[31]

Corneal health. Researchers have been investigating novel ways of using riboflavin-based eye drops in conjunction with other therapies to treat conditions such as keratoconus[32] and keratitis.[33]

Light sensitivity. Lack of B2 can contribute to migraine headaches, and it possibly contributes to a number of other conditions, including light sensitivity and sore eyes.

Related disorders. Deficiencies, or poor transport of B2, can alter biochemical pathways. Researchers found that depriving animals of B2 increased biomarkers that indicate cardiovascular problems, mitochondrial functioning, and other essential biochemical processes.[34]

Source. The best sources of riboflavin are beef liver and fish. For vegetarians, dairy products, mushrooms, almonds, eggs, quinoa, leafy-green vegetables, seeds, nuts, and tomatoes are good.

Caution. When taken in large doses, vitamin B2 may cause diarrhea and increased urine. Check with your doctor before taking extra B2 if you are taking medications for acne, depression, phenobarbital, and probenecid (or any other prescription medications). These and other medications can change the amount of B2 in your body.

Vitamin B3 - Niacin

Vision health. Vitamin B3 is one of the essential nutrients and is included in many vision health formulations. There are several forms of vitamin B3. In at least one case severe B3 deficiency, due to pellagra, reduced antioxidant capacity of the eye lens which resulted in cataracts.[35]

Related disorders. Not enough niacin in the diet may bring about problems with lesions on the skin and in the mouth, upset stomach, anemia, and headaches. Fatigue, poor concentration ability, nervousness, apathy, and depression are also associated with niacin deficiency. Chronic niacin deficiency causes a condition known as pellagra. Niacin is often prescribed to help lower cholesterol, raise HDL, and lower lipoprotein and triglycerides, while another form of B3, niacinamide (nicotinamide), does not lower cholesterol.

Source. Poultry, peanuts, mushrooms, liver, tuna, green peas, and grass-fed beef.

Caution. Too large doses of B3 can cause macular edema,[36] flushing, headaches, liver damage, and problems with diabetes, so you should always check with your health care provider. A survey of patients taking a form of niacin, nicotinic acid, for high cholesterol found that it increased the likelihood of blurred vision, eyelid swelling, and macular edema.[37]

Vitamin B5 - Pantothenic acid

Vitamin B5 (pantothenic acid) is a water-soluble essential nutrient included in many formulations supporting macular health. It is essential to energy production and synthesis of some neurotransmitters. It is generally used in combination with other B vitamins, and among many other uses, supports cardiovascular health, nerve pain, cognitive functioning, normal blood sugar levels, arthritis, protection against stress, and healing in the body.

Vision health. Vitamin B5 supports nerve health. It plays an essential role in the production of coenzyme A, which metabolizes essential omega-3 and omega-6 fatty acids.[38] It also plays an essential role in the synthesis of vitamin A.

Related conditions. Vitamin D deficiency reduces B production, and supplementing with D without also supplementing with B vitamins does not solve the problem.[39] Lack of B5 creates an inflammatory state in the immune system, which is linked to atherosclerosis and autoimmune conditions.[40] Pantothenic acid is used in synthesis of cholesterol to manufacture vitamin D along with certain steroid hormones. It may lower blood levels of cholesterol and triglycerides. Patients with rheumatoid arthritis are commonly deficient in vitamin B5.

Source. B5 is found in almost every food, but especially in egg yolks, liver, and dried mushrooms.

Caution. Patients with blood clotting disorders such as hemophilia should not take B5 without consulting their doctor. High doses of B5 can cause diarrhea and increase bleeding risk.[41]

Vitamin B6 - Pyridoxine

Most macular degeneration patients tend to be deficient in vitamin B6, and so it is generally included in vision health formulations. B6 assists in a number of enzyme activities, especially in amino acid synthesis, glucose and fat metabolism. Along with folic acid and B12, B6 is responsible for converting homocysteine to cysteine (needed for glutathione production). Low B6 levels are linked to high homocysteine levels, linked to glaucoma, diabetic retinopathy, and optic neuropathy, as well as cardiovascular and brain functioning problems.

Diabetic retinopathy. Because this condition is a complication of diabetes, the fact that B6 levels are decreased in diabetic patients makes it of interest in diabetic retinopathy.[42]

Glaucoma. A national study of 20 years of data found that B6 intake, by itself, was not associated with high rates of exfoliation glaucoma.[43] However where homocysteine levels were high, low rates of B6 were linked to glaucoma incidence. These lower levels may also be associated with deficiency of certain enzymes. The conclusion was that observed high levels of B6 in normal and open-angle glaucoma could be related to some compensatory process. But the high levels of homocysteine in the pseudo-exfoliation glaucoma are linked to low levels of vitamin B6.[44]

Macular degeneration. In people with more than three AMD risk factors or cardiovascular disease, researchers found that folic acid, B6, and B12 combined could reduce the risk of AMD.[45]

Source. Vegetables contain the most stable form of B6, pyridoxine. Good sources include avocado, wheat bran, organ meats, molasses, milk, and eggs.

Vitamin B7 - Biotin

Vitamin B7 is included in B complex formulations and supports vision health, skin and hair health, normal blood sugar levels, healthy heart functioning, nervous system support, digestive metabolism, and cell growth.

Diabetic retinopathy. Biotin supports the synthesis of fatty acids and is an important part of the metabolism of glucose. It helps with type 2 diabetes (in combination with chromium), decreases insulin resistance, and therefore may be helpful for diabetic neuropathy, a complication of diabetes. It is noted that B7 levels are low in diabetics, but the mechanics are unclear.[46]

Optic nerve atrophy. Children with B7 deficiency can experience many neurological symptoms, including optic nerve atrophy and conjunctivitis. The deficiency can be treated with biotin supplements, but symptoms such as optic nerve atrophy are usually irreversible.[47] Pregnant women have a high risk of biotin deficiency, and embryos are sensitive to a mild deficiency.[48]

Source. Although biotin is water-soluble and leaves the body quickly, it is found in many foods, but especially beef liver. It is found in eggs and salmon. It is also found in sunflower seeds, sweet potato, almonds, green vegetables such spinach and broccoli, and in dairy products.

Caution. If you take prescription drugs, check with your health practitioner before biotin supplementation. It may weaken some drugs, such as those for lowering cholesterol. Antibiotics and other drugs can lower biotin levels, as can regular consumption of raw egg whites.

Vitamin B9 - Folate, Folic Acid

Folic acid (folacin, folate) converts to vitamin B9 in the liver and is critical for many functions, such as repairing DNA and supporting healthy red blood cells. It supports cell growth and helps keep homocysteine levels low. Pregnant women need B9 to support growth of the fetus. Folic acid is water soluble, meaning that it becomes depleted rapidly and must be replenished daily.

Glaucoma. A study looked at folate intake and the risk of developing open-angle glaucoma. Twenty years of research on nearly 120,000 people in the Nurses Health Study reported higher folate intake was likely associated with a reduced risk of exfoliation glaucoma.[49]

Optic neuropathy. In a New Guinea prison system, patients with optic neuropathies were found to have folate deficiencies.[50]

Related disorders. Deficiency can contribute to inability to convert homocysteine into cysteine, causing inflammation and impacting the cardiovascular system.

Source. Good sources include legumes, asparagus, eggs, green leafy vegetables, citrus, Brussels sprouts, broccoli, nuts and seeds, beef liver, wheat germ, papaya, banana, and avocado.

Caution. Be careful when supplementing with folate. Folate, or vitamin B9, is naturally found in food. Folic acid on the other hand is synthetic and is found in many fortified foods and supplements. Folate and folic acid are often used interchangeably. Excessive folic acid intake has been linked to cancer, specifically colorectal,[51] while inadequate folate has also been linked to malignancy.[52] If you are deficient in folate, then supplementing with "5-methyltetrahydrofolate" or "5-MTHF" is safest, as opposed to the synthetic form, folic acid.

Unless your doctor recommends a higher dose, adults over 19 should not take more than 1,000mcg daily; and children should take lower doses. Consult your health provider for guidance.

Vitamin B12

The body builds up large reserves of vitamin B12 over time, and so people who lack B12 in their diets may not experience serious symptoms of deficiency for many years. It is critical to proper functioning of brain and nerve cells. Supplementation may reduce eyesight deterioration from glaucoma by supporting myelin sheath stability (the fatty layer surrounding nerve cells).

Along with folic acid and B6, B12 is responsible for converting homocysteine to cysteine. Low levels of B12 are linked to high levels of homocysteine. High homocysteine levels are associated with many vision conditions, including glaucoma, diabetic retinopathy, and optic neuropathy.

Cataract. Researchers evaluated cataract status in the more than 3,500 Blue Mountain study participants. Five years later, participants were re-evaluated. The researchers found a correlation between cataract incidence and high homocysteine levels; B12 modified that relationship.[53]

Glaucoma. A national study of 20 years of data found that low B12 intake consumption, by itself, was not associated with high rates of exfoliation glaucoma.[54]

Macular degeneration. There have been contradictory reports as to whether B12 is helpful for AMD. A review of eleven relevant studies (about 2,000 people) found that AMD is linked to high levels of homocysteine and low levels of B12.[55] Whether B12 or the other B vitamins are helpful for AMD is still under evaluation.

Optic nerve conditions. Optic neuropathy may be due to a rare vitamin B12 deficiency. In several cases, patients' vision improved after supplementation with B12.[56] The tissue layers around the retinal nerve are thinner in people with vitamin B12 deficiency.[57] There can be marked improvement of ocular neuropathic pain with B12 supplementation.[58]

Related disorders. Low B12 is linked to neurodegenerative disease and cognitive impairment. A small dementia subset is reversible with B12 therapy, but it does not improve cognition in those who are not deficient.[59]

Source. The best sources of B12 are clams and beef liver, followed by fish, milk, cheese, and eggs. Only fortified grains contain B12.

Note. Methylcobalamin, the natural form of B12 in nature, is easily absorbed and utilized by the body. In general, methylcobalamin is used mostly in your liver, brain, and nervous system. This is the only form of vitamin B12 one should supplement with. The cyanocobalamin form of B12 is completely synthetic and contains trace amounts of cyanide, which, although not considered toxic in the amounts taken in, is a toxin that has to be eliminated from the body if in excess.

Vegetarian caution. Vegetarians often have vitamin B12 deficiency, and it is a risk factor for cardiovascular disease[60] and other B12-related neurological problems. People on vegan diets must supplement with B12.

Vitamin C - Ascorbic Acid

Vitamin C is said to help support overall health in many ways, including support of the immune system and reducing the risk of cardiovascular disease. It is a necessary ingredient for many enzyme processes in the body, supporting injury healing and blood vessel integrity. It is helpful for a wide range of eye conditions, including diabetic retinopathy, glaucoma, macular degeneration, and cataracts.

Antioxidant. Vitamin C is a powerful antioxidant and helps remove oxidized waste material in the body.[61] After the adrenal glands, the second highest concentration of vitamin C is in the eye. Its power to help reduce inflammation is important for conditions like uveitis where inflammation and swelling are problematic. Vitamin C enhances the absorption of lutein, one of the most important carotenoid antioxidants in the eye.[62]

Cataract. The research is contradictory as to whether vitamin C is helpful for cataracts, with one report stating that high-dose vitamin C (sometimes used for cancer therapy) actually slightly increased the risk of cataract.[63] However, vitamin C is one of the nutrients that support glutathione production. Glutathione is essential for forming enzymes that block free radicals.[64]

Glaucoma. In its antioxidant capacity, vitamin C generally supports optic nerve health. Although blood levels of vitamin C are apparently not correlated to glaucoma incidence, supplementation with vitamin C is connected to lower risk of glaucoma.[65] One reason for this discrepancy may be the presence of genetic factors. Researchers consistently found a marked relationship between lower blood vitamin C levels and certain genetic risk factors for glaucoma.[66] It assists absorption of other nutrients such as lutein, and together they support formation of the enzyme superoxide dismutase, which in turn, has been associated with lower risk of developing glaucoma.[67]

Macular degeneration. The AREDS studies established that ascorbic acid was one of the nutrients helpful in preventing dry AMD and preventing development into wet AMD (choroidal neovascularization).[68] Best to supplement with an ascorbated vitamin C, buffered with bioflavonoids and/or minerals.

Vitreous detachment. Vitamin C supports connective tissue health because it contributes to collagen production. After a wound, blood and tissue levels of ascorbic acid are reduced, and supplementation increases them to normal levels.[69]

Related disorders. The highest concentration of vitamin C is in the adrenal glands where it is a critical component of adrenal function; there, it helps you handle stress. Vitamin C supports the health of the skin, being a necessary co-factor in collagen creation. In this regard, it is especially relevant for skin problems due to damage from the sun. It supports the immune system and is important in slowing the aging process. It helps reverse the bad effects of high levels of homocysteine, which damage the cell lining of your blood vessel walls.[70] Vitamin C protects HDL, the good cholesterol,[71] and supports the absorption of iron for those who are iron-deficient.[72] In the case of patients with bladder infections, or UTI, vitamin C restricts E. coli growth[73] and makes the urine slightly acidic, which is not a friendly environment for bacteria growth. It may be helpful, at low dosage levels, in gout treatment. In the case of diabetes, vitamin C may reduce glycosylation, lower sorbitol, and improve glucose tolerance.[74]

Source. The highest levels of vitamin C are found in rose hips, raw sweet red peppers, oranges, grapefruit, and green peppers. Other good sources are kiwi fruit, broccoli, strawberries, tomatoes, cantaloupe, and cabbage. Vitamin C is destroyed by heat and prolonged storage.

Vitamin D - Calcitriol

Fat-soluble vitamin D is actually a group of vitamins that perform a number of essential functions, including proper absorption of magnesium and calcium.[75] Vitamin D synthesis comes primarily from a process involving the sun. Our skin contains a biochemical precursor to vitamin D, a form of cholesterol called 7-dehydrocholesterol. When the skin is exposed to UV light rays, cholecalciferol is created, and a process begins that passes through the liver, then to the kidneys where it is converted into calcitriol, vitamin D.[76]

Immune system. Vitamin D is known for its support of the immune system.[77]

Diabetic retinopathy. Low levels of vitamin D are seen in patients with diabetic retinopathy.[78] Vitamin D levels are linked to artery intima-media thickness in diabetics.[79]

Dry eyes. Vitamin D deficiency is linked to dry eye according to a large study.[80] The cornea contains receptors that recognize vitamin D.[81] In dry eye patients, cornea nerve cells were less dense, shorter, thinner, and covered less total area of the cornea.[82]

Macular degeneration. Low levels of vitamin D are connected to an increase in macular degeneration, and supplementing with vitamin D may lower risk,[83] especially in women younger than age 75. It supports the health of the retinal microvascular system.[84]

Related disorders. Low levels of vitamin D contribute to weak bones and may play a role in cancer, respiratory infections, and Alzheimer's.

Food sources. Sunlight is a great source of D. Foods include fatty fish, vitamin D fortified foods, and smaller amounts of beef liver, cheese, and egg yolks.

Note. Vitamin D3 is a more readily absorbed form of D.

Caution. Get exposure to the sun in only short spurts (10-15 minutes), avoiding sunburn. Skin pigmentation and climate are factors determining when the body reaches a saturation point and stops producing vitamin D.

Vitamin E - Alpha Tocopherol

Vitamin E is made up of four tocopherols and four tocotrienols, but alpha tocopherol is the main vitamin E form in the body. It is fat-soluble and an antioxidant, and it scavenges free radicals formed from oxidation of lipids (fats).[85] Research has focused on effects of isolated chemical ingredients of vitamin E, but the isolated ingredients, while showing some good effects, do not work as well as the whole vitamin. Some researchers speculate this is because vitamin E cooperates and works in concert with other nutrients in a complex metabolic process.

The discovery of the complexity of vitamin E metabolism fostered the idea that vitamin E may be more than an antioxidant. Vitamin E is now known to affect the expression and activity of immune and inflammatory cells and to enhance dilation of blood vessels.

Cataract. The risk of both cortical and nuclear cataracts is greater when vitamin E levels are low.[86] Cortical cataracts involve the outside edge of the lens, while nuclear cataracts, the most common type of cataract, involve changes to the center of the lens. Several very large studies of over 39,000 women over ten years found that women with more vitamin E in their diet had a lower incidence of cataracts. Furthermore, women who also had greater consumption of lutein and zeaxanthin in their diet had even lower risk.[87] A meta-analysis of study through to 2014 replicates this finding.[88]

Diabetic retinopathy. Vitamin E and protein kinase C (PKC), a family of enzyme-like proteins that control other proteins, could also have a vaso-regulatory effect in the retina. In different experimental models, retinal vascular dysfunction due to hyperglycemia was reportedly prevented by vitamin E via the diacylglycerol-PKC pathway.[89]

Glaucoma. Vitamin E is known to inhibit the activity of protein kinase C (PKC). PKC inhibitors relax the trabecular meshwork and affect matrix metalloproteinase and PGF2 alpha, both of which can degrade cell structure.[90] These findings prompted researchers to evaluate vitamin E in glaucoma patients. Compared with those receiving vitamin E, non-treated subjects show statistically significant reduction in visual field at 6 and 12 months.[91]

Macular degeneration. In a study of patients and controls over 60, researchers found a marked connection between incidence of AMD and low blood plasma levels of zinc and vitamin E. In addition, they found that the lower the level of vitamin E, the greater the severity of AMD.[92] The AREDS studies of 2001, 2003, and update in 2013, confirmed the helpfulness of vitamin E.[93]

Retinitis pigmentosa. Vitamin E supplementation is not recommended. A 2014 case report mentioned that a mutation causing severely low vitamin E levels might be associated with the development of retinitis pigmentosa, as well as AMD.[94]

Related disorders. Whether vitamin E is helpful for cardiovascular problems is still controversial. It might have a protective effect against atherosclerosis.[95] Animal models suggest that E might play a role in the control of leptin (hormone regulating fat storage) status in the endothelium cells that line blood vessels.[96] Because results with respect to cardiovascular conditions are so contradictory, researchers are looking to other members of the vitamin E family.[97]

Because the brain is so vulnerable to oxidative stress, vitamin E is of great interest to researchers. Surveys have reported that memory performance is poor when blood levels of vitamin E are low, and high levels of E (and vitamin A) are found in the blood of healthy centenarians.[98] A large, long-term trial investigating the delay of Alzheimer's progression did find some benefit.[99] A review of the research reported that most studies linked high vitamin E levels with better cognitive capacity and lower Alzheimer's risk."[100]

Source. The best source of vitamin E is wheat germ. Other good sources include sunflower seeds, almonds and other nuts, spinach, and broccoli.

Retinitis pigmentosa caution. High dose vitamin E (400 IU) is not recommended for retinitis pigmentosa. A 1993 trial of 600 patients that evaluated vitamin E (and vitamin A) therapies reported that 400 IU of vitamin E tended to worsen the condition.[101] But there was no indication that dietary or small supplemental amounts have an adverse effect.[102] Since then, there has not been much research for vitamin E, although a 2014 case report mentioned that a mutation causing severely low vitamin E levels may be associated with the development of retinitis pigmentosa as well as macular degeneration.[103]

Note. Vitamin E as a supplement is most effective when taken in the mixed tocopherol form.

Alpha-lipoic Acid

Alpha-lipoic acid is not a vitamin, but we consider it vitamin-like in its vision-supporting activity. It also enhances the effectiveness of glutathione and CoQ10, and it complements the vitamin B family in generating energy through the breakdown of food into fats, proteins, and carbohydrates.

Antioxidant. Alpha-lipoic acid is a powerful antioxidant that helps prevent cell damage by neutralizing free radicals and reducing oxidative stress.[104] Because it is a water- and fat- soluble antioxidant, the brain (passes the blood-brain barrier), liver, and kidneys easily absorb it.

Cataracts. In animal models, alpha-lipoic acid prevents cataract formation.[105] [106] It accomplishes this by inhibiting cell death of the lens' epithelial cells and also activating antioxidative enzymes.[107] Administered orally, this nutrient prevents cataracts in diabetic dogs through inhibiting a sugar-related process that draws water into the lens causing opacity. The study has significance in preventing this type of condition in humans.[108]

Diabetic retinopathy. Researchers have been considering alpha-lipoic acid and other forms of alpha-lipoic acid as therapies for neuropathies that may arise from complications of either type 1 or type 2 diabetes, such as diabetic retinopathy. Their usefulness arises from their antioxidant capacity[109] and protection against cell death.[110] Several trials and reviews have demonstrated that alpha-lipoic acid is effective in treating diabetic neuropathy,[111] [112] and that this effect is more pronounced if patients control their blood sugar.[113] [114] [115]

Glaucoma. A number of studies have shown that glaucoma is associated with oxidative stress to retinal nerve cells, and that supplementing with alpha-lipoic acid helps support healthy vision for those with glaucoma.[116] [117] Researchers have found that alpha-lipoic acid is helpful in reducing oxidative stress and improving survival of nerve cells.[118] [119] [120]

Retinitis pigmentosa. This group of diseases is characterized by the death of rod cells, followed by the death of cone cells. Rod cells use a lot of oxygen, and after their death, the amount of oxygen in the retina increases, causing oxidative damage to cone cells.[121] For that reason antioxidants, including alpha-lipoic acid, are being tested as therapeutic treatments. In some cases, they did not prevent, but they did slow rod cell death.[122] [123]

Related disorders. Some of the problems that develop with aging involve dysfunction of mitochondria, the energy-producers of the cell, and loss of antioxidants. DL-alpha-lipoic acid supplementation in lab animals has been found to enhance both mitochondrial enzyme activity and antioxidant levels, and in that way, it protects mitochondria from the effects of aging.[124] [125]

Source. Spinach, cow kidney, and cow heart have the most alpha-lipoic acid. In addition, broccoli, tomato, green peas, Brussels sprouts, and other organ meats contain good levels of the nutrient.

Note. The R form of ALA (natural) is most easily absorbed versus the S-form (synthesized) form.

Co-enzyme Q10 - CoQ10

Co-enzyme Q10 is a vitamin-like antioxidant essential for its cardiovascular support. It is produced by the body and is also available in food. It supports mitochondria processes in the retina.[126] Mitochondria are the cellular energy producers that support all cellular activity. Depletion or deficiency of CoQ10 is thus a deficiency of one of the fundamental needs of the cell in every part of the body. Other nutrients such as acetyl-l-carnitine, omega-3 fatty acids, vitamin E, and alpha-lipoic acid enhance CoQ10 functioning.

Diabetic retinopathy. In combination with pine bark (pycnogenol) and vitamin E, CoQ10 helps to not only reduce free radicals but to improve the thickness of the retina.[127]

Glaucoma. CoQ10's ability to support mitochondrial function[128] and its known neuroprotective capacity makes it of interest to glaucoma researchers. In animal models, when applied topically, it is effective in reducing high intraocular pressure.[129]

Macular degeneration. CoQ10, combined with acetyl-l-carnitine or omega-3 fatty acids, supports retinal functioning more than either of those nutrients alone. In general, compounds that affect mitochondrial fat metabolism appear to improve and stabilize vision, and even improve vision in patients with early-stage AMD.[130] In combination with acetyl-l-carnitine, omega-3s, and vitamin E, it improves the retinal pigment cell tissue function[131] and reduces the drusen-covered area of the retina.[132]

Retinal disease. Not only does CoQ10 play an essential role in mitochondria processes, but it also protects fats, proteins, and DNA from oxidative stress. The reviewers note its value in treating AMD and glaucoma and propose that it could be effective for other retinal conditions.[133]

Related disorders. Use of statin drugs for cholesterol control reduces CoQ10 precursors in the body, resulting in a deficiency with symptoms that include muscle pain, cramps, and weakness.[134] Therefore, if statin drugs are prescribed, CoQ10 should also be taken. Combined with red yeast rice, CoQ10 helps reduce cholesterol levels.[135] This may be because while CoQ10 is effective in protecting against the oxidation of proteins in the body, it is especially effective against the oxidation of lipids.[136]

Research assessing the value of supplementing with CoQ10 in 109 hypertension patients found marked reduction in blood pressure.[137] [138] In eight other studies, the mean systolic decrease was 16, and the mean diastolic decrease was 10.[139] There is some evidence (from animal models only) that CoQ10 may be helpful as a neuroprotective therapy in patients with Parkinson's disease[140] or stroke (after atorvastatin), due to its anti-inflammatory and anti-cell death effects.[141]

Source. Meats and fish are among the best sources of CoQ10. Other good food sources include nuts, seeds, broccoli, cauliflower, oranges, and other fruit.

[1] Brossaud, J., Pallet, V., Corcuff, J.B., (2017). Vitamin A, endocrine tissues and hormones: interplay and interactions. *Endocr Connect*, Jul 18.i: EC-17-0101.

[2] da Silva, S., Cepko, C.L. (2017). Fgf8 Expression and Degradation of Retinoic Acid Are Required for Patterning a High-Acuity Area in the Retina. *Dev Cell*, Jul 10;42(1):68-81.e6.

[3] Mares-Perelman, J.A., Klein, B.E.K., et al. (1944). Relationship Between Lens Opacities and Vitamin and Mineral Supplement Use, *Ophthalmology*.

[4] Wang, A., Jiang, Y., Zhang, D., et al. (2014). Association of vitamin A and β-carotene with risk for age-related cataract: a meta-analysis, *Nutrition*, Oct;30(10):1113-21.

[5] Sedaghat, F., Ghanavati, M., Nezhad, Hajian, P., Hajishirazi, S., Ehteshami, M., et al. (2017). Nutrient patterns and risk of cataract: a case-control study. *Int J Ophthalmol*, Apr 18;10(4):586-592.

[6] Pescosolido, M., Malagola, R., Scarsella, G., Lenarduzzi, F., Dapoto, L., et al. (2012). Oxidative stress in the closed-eyelid test: management of glaucoma. *Eur Rev Med Pharmacol Sci, Oct*;16(10):1453-7.

[7] Haskell, M.J., Pandey, P., Graham, J.M., Peerson, J.M., Shrestha, R.K., et al. (2005). Recovery from impaired dark adaptation in night-blind pregnant Nepali women who receive small daily doses of vitamin A as amaranth leaves, carrots, goat liver, vitamin A-fortified rice, or retinyl palmitate. *Am J Clin Nutr*, Feb;81(2):461-71.

[8] Congdon, N., Dreyfuss, M., Christian, P., Navitsky, R.C., Sanchez, A.M., et al. (2000). Responsiveness of dark-adaptation threshold to vitamin A and beta-carotene supplementation in pregnant and lactating women in Nepal, *Am J Clinical Nutr*, Oct;72(4):1004-9.

[9] Brit-Garcia, N., Del Pino-Sedeno, T., Trujillo-Martin, M.M., Coco, R.M., Rodriguez de al Rua, E., et al. (2017). Effectiveness and safety of nutritional supplements in the treatment of hereditary retinal dystrophies: a systematic review. *Eye (Lond)*, Feb;31(2):273-285.

[10]Rayapudi, S., Schwartz, S.G., Wang, X., Chavis, P. (2013). Vitamin A and fish oils for retinitis pigmentosa. *Cochrane Database Syst Rev*, Dec 19;(12):CD008428.

[11] Sofi, F., Sodi, A., Franco, F., Urro, V., Biagini, D., et al. (2016). Dietary profile of patients with Stargardt's disease and Retinitis Pigmentosa: is there a role for a nutritional approach? *BMC Ophthalmol*, Jan 22;16:13.

[12] Gominak, S.C. (2016). Vitamin D deficiency changes the intestinal microbiome reducing B vitamin production in the gut. The resulting lack of pantothenic acid adversely affects the immune system, producing a "pro-inflammatory" state associated with atherosclerosis and autoimmunity. *Med Hypotheses*, Sep;94:103-7.

[13] Sica, D.A. (2007). Loop diuretic therapy, thiamine balance, and heart failure. *Congest Heart Fail*, Jul-Aug;13(4):244-7.

[14] Higashi-Okai, K., Nagino, H., Hamada, K., Okai, Y. (2006). Antioxidant and prooxidant activities of B group vitamins in lipid peroxidation. *J OUEH*, Dec 1;28(4):359-68.

[15] Menezes, R.R., Godin, A.M., Rodrigues, F.F., Coura, G.M.E., Melo, I.S.F., et al. (2017). Thiamine and riboflavin inhibit production of cytokines and increase the anti-inflammatory activity of a corticosteroid in a chronic model of inflammation induced by complete Freund's adjuvant. *Pharmacol Rep*, Oct;69(5):1036-1043.

[16] Jacques, P.R., Taylor, A., Moeller, S., Hankinson, S.E., Rogers, G., et al. (2005). Long term nutrient intake and 5-year change in nuclear lens opacities. *Arch Ophthalmol*, Apr;123(4):517-26.

[17] Mitchell, P., Cumming, R.G., Smith, W. (2001). Low thiamine intake and risk of cataract: Author's reply. *Ophthalmol*, 2001;108(7) 1167.

[18] Nebbioso, M., Rusciano, D., Pucci, B., Zicari, A.M., Grenga, R., et al. (2013). Treatment of glaucomatous patients by means of food supplement to reduce the ocular discomfort: a double blind randomized trial. *Eur Rev Med Pharmacol Sci,* Apr;17(8):1117-22.

[19] Ramdas, W.D., Wolfs, R.C., Kiefte-de Jong, J.C., Hofman, A., de Jong, P.T., et al. (2012). Nutrient intake and risk of open-angle glaucoma: the Rotterdam Study. *Eur J Epidemiol,* May;27(5):385-93.

[20] Thiamin. Wikipedia. Retrieved Nov 16 2017 from https://en.wikipedia.org/wiki/Thiamine.

[21] Serlin, T., Moisseiev, E. (2017). Fundus Findings in Wernicke Encephalopathy. *Case Rep Ophthalmol,* Jul 26;8(2):406-409.

[22] Gratton, S.M., Lam, B.L. (2014). Visual loss and optic nerve head swelling in thiamine deficiency without prolonged dietary deficiency. *Clin Ophthalmol,* May 22;8:1021–1024.

[23] Suter, P.M. (1994). Forgotten metabolic side effects of diuretics: lipids, glucose and vitamin B1 (thiamin). *Medizin Praxis,* May 12;93(20):857-63.

[24] Ikeda, K., Liu, X., Kida, K., Marutani, E., Hirai, S., et al. (2016) Thiamine as a neuroprotective agent after cardiac arrest. *Resuscitation,* Aug;105:138-44.

[25] Haugen, H.N. (1964). The blood concentration of thiamine in diabetes. *Scand J Clin Lab Invest,* 1964;16:260-6.

[26] Martin, P.R., Singleton, C.K., Hiller-Sturmhofel, S. (2003). The Role of Thiamine Deficiency in Alcoholic Brain Disease. *Alcohol Res Health,* 2003;27(2):134-42.

[27] Ashoori, M., Saedisomeolia, A. (2014). Riboflavin (vitamin B_2) and oxidative stress: a review. *Br J Nutr,* Jun 14;111(11):1985-91.

[28] Mazur-Bialy, A.I., Buchala, B., Plytycz, B. (2013). Riboflavin deprivation inhibits macrophage viability and activity - a study on the RAW 264.7 cell line. *Br J Nutr,* Aug 28;110(3):509-14.

[29] Mazur-Bialy, A.I., Buchala, B., Plytycz, B. (2015). Immunomodulatory effect of riboflavin deficiency and enrichment - reversible pathological response versus silencing of inflammatory activation. *J Physiol Pharmacol,* Dec;66(6):793-802.

[30] Mandal, A. (2014). What is a Macrophage? Retrieved Nov 18 2017 from https://www.news-medical.net/life-sciences/What-is-a-Macrophage.aspx.

[31] Skalka, H.W., Prchal, J.T. (1981). Cataracts and riboflavin deficiency. *Am J Clin Nutr,* May;34(5):861-3.

[32] Mazzotta, C., Baiocchi, S., Bagaglia, S.A., Fruschelli, M., Meduri, A., et al. (2017). Accelerated 15 mW pulsed-light crosslinking to treat progressive keratoconus: Two-year clinical results. *J Cataract Refract Surg,* Aug;43(8):1081-1088.

[33] Chan, E., Snibson, G.R., Sullivan, L. (2014). Treatment of infectious keratitis with riboflavin and ultraviolet-A irradiation. *J Cataract Refract Surg,* Nov;40(11):1919-25.

[34] Udhayabanu, T., Karthi, S., Mahesh, A., Varlakshmi, P., Manole, A., et al. (2018). Adaptive regulation of riboflavin transport in heart: effect of dietary riboflavin deficiency in cardiovascular pathogenesis. *Mol Cell Biochem,* Mar;440(1-2):147-156.

[35] Athanasiadis, I., Konstantinidis, A., Kyprianou, I., Robinson, R., Moschou, V., et al. (2007). Rapidly progressing bilateral cataracts in a patient with beta thalassemia and pellagra. *J Cataract Refract Surg,* Sep;33(9):1659-61.

[36] Makri, O.E., Georgalas, I., Georgakopoulos, C.D. (2013). Drug-induced macular edema. *Drugs,* Jun;73(8):789-802.

[37] Fraunfelder, F.W., Fraunfelder, F.T., Illingworth, D.R. (1995). Adverse ocular effects associated with niacin therapy. *Br J Ophthalmol,* Jan; 79(1): 54–56.

[38] Fidanza, A., Audisio, M. (1982). Vitamins and lipid metabolism. *Acta Vitaminol Enzymol,* 4(1-2):105-14.

[39] Ibid. Gominak. (2016).

[40] Ibid. Gominak. (2016).https://www.ncbi.nlm.nih.gov/

[41] PennState Hershey Medical Center. Vitamin B5 (Pantothenic acid). Retrieved Nov 18 2017 from http://pennstatehershey.adam.com/content.aspx?productId=107&pid=33&gid=000336.

[42] Valdes-Ramos, R., Guadarrama-Lopez, A.L., Martinez-Carrillo, B.E., Benitez-Arciniega, A.D. (2015). Vitamins and type 2 diabetes mellitus. *Endocr Metab Immune Disord Drug Targets,* 2015;15(1):54-63.

[43] Kang, J.H., Loomis, S.J., Wiggs, J.L., Willett, W.C., Pasquale, L.R. (2014). A prospective study of folate, vitamin B_6, and vitamin B_{12} intake in relation to exfoliation glaucoma or suspected exfoliation glaucoma. *JAMA Ophthalmol,* May;132(5):549-59.

[44] Turgut, B., Kaya, M., Arslan, S., Demir, T., Guler, M., et al. (2010). Levels of circulating homocysteine, vitamin B6, vitamin B12, and folate in different types of open-angle glaucoma. *Clin Interv Aging,* Apr 26;5:133–139.

[45] Christen, W.G., Glynn, R.J., Chew, E.Y., Albert, C.M., Manson, J.E. (2009). Folic Acid, Vitamin B6, and Vitamin B12 in Combination and Age-related Macular Degeneration in a Randomized Trial of Women. *Arch Intern Med*, Feb 23;169(4):335-41.

[46] Ibid. Valdes-Ramos. (2015).

[47] Gannavarapu, S., Prasad, C., DiRaimo, J., Napier, M. Goobie, S.., et al. (2015). Biotinidase deficiency: Spectrum of molecular, enzymatic and clinical information from newborn screening Ontario, Canada (2007-2014). *Mol Genet Metab,* Nov;116(3):146-51.

[48] Mock, D.M. (2009). Marginal biotin deficiency is common in normal human pregnancy and is highly teratogenic in mice. *J Nutr,* Jan;139(1):154-7.

[49] Kang, J.H., Loomis, S.J., Wiggs, J.L., Willett, W.C., Pasquale, L.R. (2014). A prospective study of folate, vitamin B6 and vitamin B12 in relation to exfoliation glaucoma or exfoliation glaucoma suspect. *JAMA Ophthalmol,* May;132(5):549–559.

[50] Tousignant, B., Brian, G., Venn, B.J., Gould, C., McKay, R., et al. (2013). Optic neuropathy in a prison population in Papual New Guinea. *Ophthalmic Epidemiol,* 2013:20(1):4-12.

[51] Mason, J.B., Dickstein, A., Jacques, P.R., Haggarty, P., Selhub, J., et al. (2007). A temporalassociation between folic acid fortification and an increase in colorectal cancer rates may be illuminating important biological principles: a hypothesis. *Cancer Epidemiol Biomarkers Prev*, Jul;16(7):1525-9.o

[52] Duthie, S.J. (1999). Folic acid deficiency and cancer: mechanisms of DNA instability. *Br Med Bull,* 199955(3):578-92.

[53] Tan, A.G., Mitchell, P., Rochtchina, E., Flood, V.M., Cumming, R.G., et al. (2014). Serum homocysteine, vitamin B12, and folate, and the prevalence and incidence of posterior subcapsular cataract. *Invest Ophthalmol Vis Sci*, Nov 18;56(1):216-20.

[54] Ibid. Kang. (2014).

[55] Huang, P., Wang, F., Sah, B.K., Jiang, J., Ni, Z., et al. (2015). Homocysteine and the risk of age-related macular degeneration: a systematic review and meta-analysis. *Sci Rep,* Jul;21;5:10585.

[56] Chavala, S.H., Kosmorsky, G.S., Lee, M.K., Lee, M.S. (2005). Optic neuropathy in vitamin B12 deficiency. *Eur J Intern Med,* Oct;16(6):447-8.

[57] Turkyilmaz, K. Oner, V., Turkyilmaz, A.K., Kirbas, A., Kirbas, S., et al. (2013). Evaluation of peripapillary retinal nerve fiber layer thickness in patients with vitamin B12 deficiency using spectral domain optical coherence tomography. *Curr Eye Res*, Jun;38(6):680-4.

[58] Shetty, R., Despande, K., Ghosh, A., Sethu, S. (2015). Management of Ocular Neuropathic Pain with Vitamin B12 Supplements: A Case Report. *Cornea*, Oct;34(10):1324-5.

[59] Moore, E., Mander, A., Ames, D., Carne, R., Sanders, K., et al. (2012). Cognitive impairment and vitamin B12: a review. *Int Psychogeriatr*, Apr;24(4):541-56.

[60] Pawlak, R. (2015). Is vitamin B12 deficiency a risk factor for cardiovascular disease in vegetarians? *Am J Prev Med*, Jun;48(6):e11-26.

[61] Cangemi, R., Angelico, F., Loffredo, L., Del Ben, M., Pignatelli, P., et al. (2007). Oxidative stress-mediated arterial dysfunction in patients with metabolic syndrome: Effect of ascorbic acid. *Free Radic Biol Med*, Sep 1;43(5):853-9.

[62] Tanumihardjo, S.K., Li, J., Dosti, M.P. (2005). Lutein absorption is facilitated with co-supplementation of ascorbic acid in young adults. *J Am Dietetic Assoc*, 105:114-18.

[63] Zheng, S.J., Rautianinen, S., Lindblad, B.E., Morgenstern, R., Wolk, A. (2013). High-dose supplements of vitamins C and E, low-dose multivitamins, and the risk of age-related cataract: a population-based prospective cohort study of men. *Am J Epidemiol*, Mar 15;177(6):548-55.

[64] Head, K.A. (2001). Natural therapies for ocular disorders, part two: cataracts and glaucoma. *Altern Med Rev*, Apr;6(2):141-66.

[65] Wang, S.Y., Singh, K., Lin, S.C. (2013). Glaucoma and vitamins A, C, and E supplement intake and serum levels in a population-based sample of the United States. *Eye (Lond)*, Apr;27(4):487-94.

[66] Zanon-Moreno, V., Ciancotti-Olivares, L., Asencio, J., Sanz, P., Ortega-Azorin, C., et al. (2011). Association between a SLC23A2 gene variation, plasma vitamin C levels, and risk of glaucoma in a Mediterranean population. *Mol Vis*,17:2997-3004.

[67] Canizales, L., Rodriguez, L., Rivera, C., Martinez, A., Mendez, F., et al. (2016). Low-level expression of SOD1 in peripheral blood samples of patients diagnosed with primary open-angle glaucoma. *Biomark Med*, Dec;10(12):1218-1223.

[68] AREDS, AREDS2: (2001, 2006, 2013) Antioxidants & Macular Degeneration. Retrieved on Oct 15 2017 from http://www.naturaleyecare.com/study.asp?s_num=105.

[69] Moores, J. (2013). Vitamin C: a wound healing perspective. *Br J Community Nurs,* Dec; Suppl:S6, S8-11.

[70] Hanashima, C., Namiki, H. (1999). Reduced viability of vascular endothelial cells by high concentration of ascorbic acid in vitreous humor. *Cell Biol Int,* 23(4):287-98.

[71] Frei B. (1991). Ascorbic acid protects lipids in human plasma and low-density lipoprotein against oxidative damage. *Am J Clin Nutr,* Dec;54(6 Suppl):1113S8S.

[72] Hunt, J.R., Gallagher, S.K., Johnson, L.K. (1994). Effect of ascorbic acid on apparent iron absorption by women with low iron stores. *Am J Clin Nutr,* Jun;59:13815.

[73] Schlager, T.A., Anderson, S., Trudell, J., Hendley, J.O. (1999). Effect of cranberry juice on bacteriuria in children with neurogenic bladder receiving intermittent catheterization. *J Pediatr,* Dec;135(6):698702.

[74] Sinclair, A.J., Lunec, J., Girling, A.J., Barnett, A.H. (1992). Modulators of free radical activity in diabetes mellitus: role of ascorbic acid. *EXS,* 1992;62:342-52.

[75] Wikipedia. Vitamin D. Retrieved Nov 2 2017 from https://en.wikipedia.org/wiki/Vitamin_D.

[76] Dietobio. Vitamin D. Retrieved Nov 2 2017 from http://www.dietobio.com/vegetarisme/en/vit_d.html

[77] Hewison, M. (2012). Vitamin D and immune function: an overview. *Proc Nutr Soc,* Feb;71(1):50-61.

[78] Aksoy H, Akçay F, Kurtul N, Baykal O, Avci B. (2000). Serum 1,25 dihydroxy vitamin D (1,25(OH)2D3), 25 hydroxy vitamin D (25(OH)D) and parathormone levels in diabetic retinopathy. *Clin Biochem,* 33:47–51.

[79] Targher, G., Bertolini, L., Padovan, R., Zenari, L., Scala, L., et al. (2006). Serum 25-hydroxyvitamin D3 concentrations and carotid artery intima-media thickness among type 2 diabetic patients. *Clin Endocrinol (Oxf),* 65:593–597.

[80] Yoon, S.Y., Bae, S.H., Shin, Y.J., Park, S.G., Hwang, S.H. et al. (2016). Low Serum 25-Hydroxyvitamin D Levels Are Associated with Dry Eye Syndrome. *PLoS One.* Jan 25;11(1):e0147847.

[81] Yildirim, P., Garip, Y., Karci, A.A., Guler, T. (2015). Dry eye in vitamin D deficiency: more than an incidental association. *Int J Rheum Dis,* Jan;19(1):49-54.

[82] Shetty, R., Sethu, S., Deshmukh, R., Deshpande, K., Ghosh, A., et al. (2016). Corneal Dendritic Cell Density Is Associated with Sub basal Nerve Plexus Features, Ocular Surface Disease Index, and Serum Vitamin D in Evaporative Dry Eye Disease. *BioMed Res Int,* 2016:4369750.

[83] Vitamin D linked to lower macular degeneration risk. (2016). Naturaleyecare. Retrieved Nov 2 2017 from http://www.naturaleyecare.com/blog/vitamin-d-linked-to-lower-macular-degeneration-risk.

[84] Mutlu, U., Ikram, M.A., Hofman, A., de Jong, P.T., Uitterlinden, A.G., et al. (2016). Vitamin D and retinal microvascular damage: The Rotterdam Study. *Medicine (Baltimore),* Dec; 95(49): e5477.

[85] Qing, J. (2014). Natural forms of vitamin E: metabolism, antioxidant and anti-inflammatory activities and the role in disease prevention and therapy. *Free Radic Biol Med,* Jul;72:76–90.

[86] Vitale, S., West, W., Hallfrisch, J., Alston, C., Wang, F., et al. (1993). Plasma antioxidants and risk of cortical and nuclear cataract. *Epidemiology,* May;4(3):195-203.

[87] Christen, W.G., Liu, S., Glynn, R.J., Gaziano, J.M., Buring, J.E. (2008). Dietary carotenoids, vitamins C and E, and risk of cataract in women: a prospective study. *Arch Ophthalmol,* Jan;126(1):102-9

[88] Zhang, Y., Jiang, W., Xie, Z, Wu, W., Zhang, D. (2015). Vitamin E and risk of age-related cataract: a meta-analysis. *Public Health Nutr,* Oct;18(15):2804-14.

[89] Lee, I.K., Koya, D., Ishi, H., Kanoh, H., King, G.L. (1999). D-alpha tocopherol prevents hyperglycemia induced activation of the diacylglycerol (DAG)-protein kinase C pathway in vascular smooth muscle cells by an increase in DAG kinase activity. *Diabetes Res Clin Pract,* Sep;45(2-3):183-90.

[90] Kunisaki, M., Bursell, S.E., Clermont, A.C., Ishii, H., Ballas, L.M., et al. (1995). Vitamin E prevents diabetes-induced abnormal retinal blood flow via the diacylglycerol-protein kinase C pathway. *Am J Physiol,* Aug;269(2 Pt 1):E239-46.

[91] Engin, K.N., Engin, G., Kucuksahin, H., Oncu, M., Engin, G., et al. (2007). Clinical evaluation of the neuroprotective effect of alpha tocopherol in glaucomatous damage. *Eur J Ophthalmol,* July-Aug;17(4):528-33.

[92] Belda, J.I., Roma, J., Vielela, C., Puertas, F.J., Diaz-Llopis, M., Bosch-Morell, F., et al. (1999). Serum vitamin E levels negatively correlate with severity of age-related macular degeneration, *Mech Ageing Dev,* Mar 1;107(2):159-64.

[93] Chew, E.Y., Clemons, T.E., Agron, E., Sperduto, R.D., Sangiovanni, J.P. (2013). Long-term effects of vitamins C and E, beta carotene, and zinc on age-related macular degeneration: AREDS report no. 35. *Ophthalmology,* Aug;120(8):1604-11.

[94] Iwasa, K., Shima, K., Komai, K., Nishida, Y., Yokota, T., et al. (2014). Retinitis pigmentosa and macular degeneration in a patient with ataxia with isolated vitamin E deficiency with a novel c.717 del C mutation in the TTPA gene. *J Neurol Sci,* Oct 15;345(1-2):228-30

[95] Wallert, M., Schmotz, L., Galli, F., Birringer, M., Lorkowski, S. (2014). Regulatory metabolites of vitamin E and their putative relevance for atherogenesis. *Redox Biol,* Feb 19;2:495-503.

[96] Krawczynska, A., Olczak, E., Rembiszewska, A., Herman, A.P., Gromadzka-Ostrowska, J. (2014). Time-dependent supplementation of vitamin E influences leptin expression in the aortic layers of rats fed atherogenic diet. *J Physiol Pharmacol,* Feb;65(1):33-9.

[97] Mathur, P., Ding, Z., Saldeen, T., Mehta, J.L. (2015). Tocopherols in the Prevention and Treatment of Atherosclerosis and Related Cardiovascular Disease. *Clin Cardiol,* Sep;38(9):570-6.

[98] La Fata, G., Weber, P., Mohajeri, M.H. (2014). Effects of Vitamin E on Cognitive Performance during Ageing and in Alzheimer's Disease. *Nutrients,* Dec;6(12):5453-5472.

[99] Dysken, M.W., Sano, M., Asthana, S., Vertrees, J.E., Pallaki, M., et al. (2014). Effect of vitamin E and memantine on functional decline in Alzheimer disease: The TEAM-AD VA cooperative randomized trial. *JAMA,* Jan 1;311(1):33–44.

[100] Ibid. La Fata. (2014).

[101] Berson, E.L., Rosner, B., Sandberg, M.A., Hayes, K.C., Nicholson, B.W. (1993). A randomized trial of vitamin A and vitamin E supplementation for retinitis pigmentosa. *Arch Ophthamol,* Jun; 111(6):761-772.

[102] Foundation Fighting Blindness. Study shows Vitamin A Slows RP. Retrieved Nov 18 2017 from http://www.blindness.org/treatments/study-shows-vitamin-slows-rp.

[103] Iwasa, K., Shima, K., Komai, K., Nishida, Y., Yokota, T., et al. (2014). Retinitis pigmentosa and macular degeneration in a patient with ataxia with isolated vitamin E deficiency with a novel c.717 del C mutation in the TTPA gene. *J Neurol Sci,* Oct 15;345(1-2):228-30

[104] Packer, L. (1998). alpha-Lipoic acid: a metabolic antioxidant which regulates NF-kappa B signal transduction and protects against oxidative injury. *Drug Metab Rev,* May;30(2):245-75.

[105] Maitra, I., Servinova, E., Trischler, H., Packer, L. (1995). Alpha-lipoic acid prevents buthionine sulfoximine-induced cataract formation in newborn rats. *Free Radic Biol Med,* Apr;18(4):823-9.

[106] Chen, Y., Yi, L., Yan, G., Fang, Y., Jang, Y. et al. (2010). Alpha-Lipoic acid alters post-translational modifications and protects the chaperone activity of lens alpha-crystallin in naphthalene-induced cataract. *Curr Eye Res,* Jul;35(7):620-30.

[107] Li, Y., Liu, Y.Z., Shi, J.M., Jia, S.B. (2013). Alpha lipoic acid protects lens from H(2)O(2)-induced cataract by inhibiting apoptosis of lens epithelial cells and inducing activation of anti-oxidative enzymes. *Asian Pac J Trop Med,* Jul;6(7):548-51.

[108] Williams, D.L. (2017). Effect of Oral Alpha Lipoic Acid in Preventing the Genesis of Canine Diabetic Cataract: A Preliminary Study. *Vet Sci,* Mar 16;4(1).

[109] Gomes, M.B., Negrato, C.A. (2014). Alpha-lipoic acid as a pleiotropic compound with potential therapeutic use in diabetes and other chronic diseases. *Diabetol Metab Syndr,* Jul 28;6(1):80.

[110] Kowluru, R.A., Odenbach, S. (2004). Effect of long-term administration of alpha-lipoic acid on retinal capillary cell death and the development of retinopathy in diabetic rats. *Diabetes,* 2004 Dec;53(12):3233-8.

[111] Lin, J., Bierhaus, A., Bugert, P., Dietrich, N., Feng, Y., et al. (2006). Effect of R-(+)-alpha-lipoic acid on experimental diabetic retinopathy. *Diabetologia,* May;49(5):1089-96.

[112] Nebbioso, M., Pranno, F., Pescosolido, N. (2013). Lipoic acid in animal models and clinical use in diabetic retinopathy. *Expert Opin Pharmacother,* Sep;14(13):1829-38.

[113] Ibrahimpasic, K. (2013). Alpha lipoic acid and glycaemic control in diabetic neuropathies at type 2 diabetes treatment. *Med Arch,* 67(1):7-9.

[114] Papanas, N., Ziegler, D. (2014). Efficacy of alpha-lipoic acid in diabetic neuropathy. *Expert Opin Pharmacother,* Dec;15(18):2721-31.

[115] Han, T., Bai, J., Liu, W., Hu, Y. (2012). A systematic review and meta-analysis of α-lipoic acid in the treatment of diabetic peripheral neuropathy. *Eur J Endocrinol,* Oct;167(4):465-71.

[116] Filina, A.A., Davydova, N.G., Endrikhovskii, S.N., Shamshinova, A.M. (1995). Lipoic acid as a means of metabolic therapy of open-angle glaucoma. *Vestn Oflalmol,* Oct-Dec;111(4):6-8.

[117] Inman, D.M., Lambert, W.S., Calkins, D.J., Homer, P.J. (2013). α-Lipoic acid antioxidant treatment limits glaucoma-related retinal ganglion cell death and dysfunction. *PLoS One*, Jun5;8(6):e65389.

[118] Ibid. Inman. (2013).

[119] Osborne, N.N. (2008). Pathogenesis of ganglion "cell death" in glaucoma and neuroprotection: focus on ganglion cell axonal mitochondria. *Prog Brain Res*, 2008;173:339-52.

[120] Filina, A.A., Davydova, N.G., Endrikovskii, S.N., Shamshinova, A.M. (1995). Lipoic acid as a means of metabolic therapy of open-angle glaucoma. *Vestn Oftalmol,* Oct-Dec;111(4):6-8.

[121] Komeima, K. Rogers, B.S., Lu, L., Campochiaro, P.A. (2006). Antioxidants reduce cone cell death in a model of retintis pigmentosa. *Proc Natl Acad Sci U S A,* Jul 25;103(30):11300-5.

[122] Sanz, M.M., Johnson, L.E., Ahuja, S., Ekstrom, P.A., Romero, J., et al. (2007). Significant photoreceptor rescue by treatment with a combination of antioxidants in an animal model for retinal degeneration. *Neuroscience*, Mar 30;145(3):1120-9.

[123] Ibid. Komeima. (2006).

[124] Arivazhagan, P., Ramanathan. K., Panneerselvam, C. (2001). Effect of DL-alpha-lipoic acid on mitochondrial enzymes in aged rats. *Chem Biol Interact,* Nov 28;138(2):189-98.

[125] Palaniappan, A.R., Dai, A. (2007). Mitochondrial ageing and the beneficial role of alpha-lipoic acid. *Neurochem Res*, 2007 Sep;32(9):1552-8.

[126] Littarru, G.P., Tiano, L. (2007). Bioenergetic and antioxidant properties of coenzyme Q10: recent developments. *Mol Biotechnol,* Sep;37(1):31-7.

[127] Domanico, D., Fragiotta, S., Cutini, A., Carnevale, C., Zompatori, L., et al. (2015). Circulating levels of reactive oxygen species in patients with nonproliferative diabetic retinopathy and the influence of antioxidant supplementation: 6-month follow-up. *Indian J Ophthalmol,* Jan;63(1):9-14.

[128] Erb, C., Koniezka, K. (2018). Mitochondrial Dysfunctions and Role of Coenzyme Q10 in patients with glaucoma. *Klin Monatsbl Augenheilkd,* 235(02):157-162.

[129] Davis, B.M., Tian, K., Pahlitzsch, M., Brenton, J., Ravindran, N. (2017). Topical Coenzyme Q10 demonstrates mitochondrial-mediated neuroprotection in a rodent model of ocular hypertension. *Mitochondrion*, Sep;36:114-123.

[130] Feher. J., Kovacs, B., Kovcs, I., schveoller, M., Papale, A., et al. (2005). Improvement of visual functions and fundus alterations in early age-related macular degeneration treated with a combination of acetyl-L-carnitine, n-3 fatty acids, and coenzyme Q10. *Ophthalmologica,* May-Jun;219(3):154-66.

[131] Feher, J., Papale, A., Mannino, G., Gualdi, Balacco, G.C., et al. (2003). Mitotropic compounds for the treatment of age-related macular degeneration. The metabolic approach and a pilot study. *Ophthalmology,* Sep-Oct;217(5):351-7.

[132] Ibid. Feher. (2003).

[133] Zhang, X., Tohari, A.M., Marcheggianai, F., Zhou, X., Reilly, J., et al. (2017). Therapeutic potential of co-enzyme Q10 in retinal diseases. *Curr Med Chem*, 2017;24(39):4329-4339.

[134] Potgieter, M., Pretorius, E., Pepper, M.S. (2013). Primary and secondary coenzyme Q10 deficiency: the role of therapeutic supplementation. *Nutr Rev,* Mar;71(3):180-8.

[135] Cicero, A.F.G., Colletti, A., Bajraktari, G., Descamps, O., Djuric, D.M., et al. (2017). Lipid lowering nutraceuticals in clinical practice: position paper from an International Lipid Expert Panel. *Arch Med Sci,* Aug; 13(5):965–1005.

[136] Littarru, G.P., Tiano, L. (2007). Bioenergetic and antioxidant properties of coenzyme Q10: recent developments. Mol *Biotechnol,* Sep;37(1):31-7.

[137] Folkers, K., Drzewoski, J., Richardson, P.C., Ellis, J., Shizukuishi, S., et al. (1981). Bioenergetics in clinical medicine. XVI. Reduction of hypertension in patients by therapy with coenzyme Q10. *Res Commun Chem Pathol Pharmacol,* Jan;31(1):129-40.

[138] Singh, R.B., Niaz, M.A., Rastogi, S.S., Shukla, P.K., Thakur, A.S. (1999). Effect of hydrosoluble coenzyme Q10 on blood pressures and insulin resistance in hypertensive patients with coronary artery disease. *J Hum Hypertens*, Mar;13(3):203-8.

[139] Rosenfeldt, F., Hilton, D., Pepe, S., Krum, H. (2003). Systematic review of effect of coenzyme Q10 in physical exercise, hypertension and heart failure. *Biofactors*, 2003;18(1-4):91-100.

[140] Attia, H.N., Maklad, Y.A. (2018). Neuroprotective effects of coenzyme Q10 on paraquat-induced Parkinson's disease in experimental animals. *Behav Pharmacol*, Feb;29(1):79-86.

[141] Nasoohi, S., Simani, L., Khodagholi, F., Nikseresht, S., Faizi, M., et al. (2017). Coenzyme Q10 supplementation improves acute outcomes of stroke in rats pretreated with atorvastatin. *Nutr Neurosci*, Sep 26:1-9.

8-5. ESSENTIAL FATTY ACIDS

Essential fatty acids are as important for chemistry balance and for good cell function as good food, vitamins, and minerals. They are an integral component of nerve cells, cell membranes, and vital hormone-like substances called prostaglandins. Prostaglandins help regulate numerous body functions, including normal immune response during inflammation.[1]

Oil	Omega-6	Omega-3
Fish	0%	100%
Flaxseed	14%	57%
Walnut	52%	10%
Canola	20%	9%
Soybean	32%	7%
Olive	9%	1%
Avocado	12%	1%
Butter	3%	1%
Safflower	75%	0%
Sunflower	65%	0%
Corn	54%	0%
Cottonseed	50%	0%
Sesame	42%	0%
Peanut	32%	0%

Fatty acids include **omega-3 fatty acids** and **omega-6 fatty acids**. The ideal ratio of omega-3 to omega-6 fatty acids in the diet is 1:2, but in the standard American diet, that ratio has shifted to almost 1:20, causing many age-related problems.[2]

Vegetable oils have a much higher omega-6 to omega-3 ratio, which can lead to health problems. Both omega-6 and 3 use the same conversion enzymes. In the body, higher levels of omega-6 from vegetable oils convert to inflammatory eicosanoids (molecules made by enzymes and used for signaling) and reduce the conversion of omega-3 to anti-inflammatory DHA/EPA.

This result is seen in Japan where the gradual change from a diet with lower omega-6 levels to a more Western diet with higher omega-6 levels corresponds to an increase in macular degeneration.[3]

Omega-3 Fatty Acids

Omega-3 fatty acids are a specific type of essential fatty acid known to reduce inflammation and lower risk of chronic diseases, such as heart disease, cancer, and arthritis. They are so essential to the retina that when omega-3 levels begin to fall, the retina begins to recycle DHA within the eye. The typical American diet is deficient in omega-3 fatty acids, whereas omega-6 fatty acids are generally plentiful due to a high intake of vegetable oils and refined grains, which include white breads, white rice, and white pasta.

There are three types of omega-3 fatty acids: **alpha-linolenic acid (ALA),** which is found in plant oils; **eicosapentaenoic acid (EPA)** used primarily in the brain and retina, and **docosahexaenoic acid (DHA)** used primarily in the heart and circulatory system; the latter two are found in fish oils.[4] EPA and DHA are not naturally present in the body; we can synthesize them from ALA, but this synthesizing ability declines with age. Therefore, it is important to get adequate EPA and DHA from other sources. Healthy oils such as flaxseed oil can provide EPA and DHA, but are not as efficient as fish oil because a two-step conversion is required to generate EPA and DHA.

Every cell in the body contains an outer layer comprised of essential fatty acids, so maintaining healthy oils in one's diet is essential for maintaining health and avoiding disease. That is why intake of poor oils, such as trans-fatty acids or commercial vegetable oils, over time, can lead to chronic inflammatory disorders. First cold pressed, extra virgin olive oil is great for salads and even cooking on low temperatures. For cooking in higher temperature, saturated fats are much better, including butter or coconut oil.

The two primary omega-3 fatty acids, DHA and EPA, may protect the retina through expression of genes, retinal cell differentiation, and survival. There has been extensive research about these two omega-3's and much less about alpha-linolenic acid (ALA). It is likely that the three have very specific and independent roles in protecting against disease.[5]

Antioxidant. A derivative of DHA protects retinal pigment epithelial cells from oxidative stress.[6] Unlike the effect of DHA in other parts of the body such as the liver, it does not appear to be subject to lipid oxidation in the retina.[7]

Inflammation. DHA reduces inflammation[8] in retinal microcapillaries[9] and in the retina, changing potent inflammatory agents to less powerful ones.[10]

Neovascularization. EPA and DHA have the capacity to regulate formation of blood vessels, which is important with respect to the advanced form of AMD, choroidal neovascularization.[11] [12] They are able to encourage immune cell movement toward the site of extraneous formations of blood vessels that distort vision. The results indicate promising potential for omega-3 as a nutritional therapy for other conditions involving inflammation and neovascularization.[13]

Computer eyestrain. In a year-long trial, 500 patients using the computer for 3 or more hours daily, received 180mg EPA and 120mg DHA. They reported improvement in dry eye symptoms.[14] In combination with bilberry and lutein, EPA improved computer eyestrain symptoms, including stiff shoulders, back pain, and dry eyes during a four-week test period.[15]

Glaucoma. Low levels of blood DHA and EPA are seen in patients with primary open-angle glaucoma along with decreased optic nerve blood flow. These omega-3s help to modulate blood circulation in the eye.[16]

Macular degeneration. While it is known that a low-fat diet that gets only 10% of its calories from fat (excluding red meat and milk products), lessens AMD risk, it has been found that omega-3 fatty acids and olive oil further reduce AMD risk.[17]

EPA and DHA, found especially in fatty fish like salmon or sardines, are important in preventing macular degeneration. Eighty-five percent of AMD patients over age 70 experienced improved vision after four weeks of supplemental omega-3s.[18] Other reports, such as a meta-analysis of more than 270 studies and papers,[19] a longitudinal study of over 1,800 people over 12 years,[20] and a large 10-year study evaluating the diets of nearly 40,000 women confirmed these findings.[21]

Photoreceptors. There is a high concentration of omega-3, especially DHA, in the retina and especially in the photoreceptors.[22] It plays an important role in the regeneration of photoreceptor cells, and its deficiency alters the rhodopsin content and photoreceptor function.[23] DHA is found to provide photoreceptor neuroprotection,[24] protecting against cell death.[25]

Retinal health. Omega-3 fatty acids are essential for nerve conduction in the retina and for reducing cholesterol; this keeps retinal blood vessels open, helping to maintain retinal nutrition levels. The omega-3s provide protection from neuroinflammation, a key component of many vision conditions.[26] Omega-3 DHA is present in large amounts in retinal epithelial cells, acting towards neuroprotection; this understanding presents possibilities for future therapies.[27]

Related disorders. Omega-3 fatty acids have a supportive effect on the circulatory system and can reduce blood cholesterol levels.[28] Alpha-linolenic acid (ALA) may inhibit inflammation, which contributes to blood vessel endothelial cells.[29] The omega-3 alpha-linolenic acid (ALA) is being investigated as a possible therapy for inflammatory bone loss in osteoporosis.[30] Omega-3 unsaturated fatty acids are necessary for healthy skin, hair, and nails.[31]

Source.

- EPA. Cold-water fish, especially mackerel, lake trout, sardines, tuna, and salmon. Also, halibut, river trout, catfish, cod, red snapper, and tuna packed in water.
- DHA. Some microalgae, anchovies, salmon, herring, mackerel, tuna, and halibut. Also, liver, fish oil, and eggs from grass fed poultry.
- ALA. Flaxseed, flaxseed oil, canola oil, pumpkin seeds, pumpkin seed oil, tofu, perilla seed oil, walnuts, walnut oil, and chia seeds.

Omega-6 fatty acids

The omega-6 fatty acids include polyunsaturated fatty acids, some of which have more negative effects and some of which have more beneficial effects. The omega-6 fatty acids include **linoleic acid (LA)** (not to be confused with the omega-3 alpha-linolenic acid), **arachidonic acid (ARA),** and **gamma-linolenic acid (GLA).** While the body does need some omega-6 fatty acids, excessive amounts interfere with the health benefits of omega-3s.[32] The body cannot synthesize omega-6 fatty acids on its own and cannot convert dietary omega-6s to omega-3s.[33]

Excessive levels of omega-6 fatty acids (except GLA) increase inflammation and autoimmune conditions. In most cancer tissues, there are higher levels of omega-6s and lower levels of omega-3s.[34] Omega-6 fatty acids support lowered LDL cholesterol, but they are not correlated with cardiovascular protection.[35]

The omega-6 GLA acids are anti-inflammatory. Both ARA (omega-6) and DHA (omega-3) are needed for brain development and function, and along with EPA (omega-3), are precursors to a wide range of biochemicals, such as endocannabinoids that play interconnected roles in controlling inflammatory response, synapse functioning, nerve growth, and neuroprotection.[36]

Source.

- LA is found in plant oils, especially safflower, evening primrose, poppy seed, grapeseed, sunflower, hemp, corn, and wheat germ.
- GLA is found in plant oils, especially blackcurrant seed oil, borage oil,[37] and hempseed oil. It is also in smaller amounts in oats and barley.
- ARA is found in meats, dairy, and egg yolks.

---

[1] Ricciotti, E., FitzGerald, G.A. (2011). Prostaglandins and Inflammation. *Arterioscler Thromb Vasc Biol*, May; 31(5):986–1000.

[2] Kain, V., Ingle, K.A., Kachman, M., Baum, H., Shanmugam, G., et al. (2018). Excess Omega-6 Fatty Acids Influx in Aging Drives Metabolic Dysregulation, Electrocardiographic Alterations and Low-grade Chronic Inflammation. *Am J Physiol Heart Circ Physiol*, Feb 1;314(2):H160-H169.

[3] Querques, G., Forte, R., Souied, E.H. (2011). Retina and Omega-3. *J Nutr Metab*, 2011:748361.

[4] Omega-3 fatty acid, Wikipedia, Retrieved Nov 18 2017 from https://en.wikipedia.org/wiki/Omega-3_fatty_acid

[5] Anderson, M.B., Ma, D.W.L. (2009). Are all n-3 polyunsaturated fatty acids created equal? *Lip Health Dis*, Aug 10;8:33.

[6] Mukherjee, P.K., Marcheselli, V.L., Serhan, C.N., Bazan, N.G. (2004). Neuroprotectin D1: a docosahexaenoic acid-derived docosatriene protects human retinal pigment epithelial cells from oxidative stress. *Proc Natl Acad Sci USA*, Jun 1;101(22):8491-6.

[7] Ibid. Querques. (2011).

[8] Calder, P.C., (2015). Marine omega-3 fatty acids and inflammatory processes: Effects, mechanisms and clinical relevance. *Biochem Biophys Acta*, Apr;1851(4):469-84.

[9] Chen, W., Esselman, W.J., Jump, D.B., Busik, J.V. (2005). Anti-inflammatory effect of docosahexaenoic acid on cytokine-induced adhesion molecule expression in human retinal vascular endothelial cells. *Invest Ophthalmol Vis Sci*, Nov;46(11):4342-7.

[10] Ibid. Querques. (2011).

[11] Ibid. Querques. (2011).

[12] SanGiovanni, J.P., Chew, E.Y. (2005). The role of omega-3 long-chain polyunsaturated fatty acids in health and disease of the retina. *Prog Retin Eye Res*, 2005;24(1): 87–138.

[13] Yanai, R., Mulki, L., Hasegawa, E., Takeuchi, K. Sweigad, H., et al. (2014). Cytochrome P450-generated metabolites derived from omega-3 fatty acids attenuate neovascularization. *Proc Natl Acad Sci U S A*, Jul 1;111(26):9603-8.

[14] Bhargava, R., Kumar, P., Phogat, H., Kaur, A., Kumar, M. (2015). Oral omega-3 fatty acids treatment in computer vision syndrome related dry eye. *Cont Lens Anterior Eye*, Jun;38(3):206-10.

[15] Kawabata, F., Tsuji, T. (2011). Effects of dietary supplementation with a combination of fish oil, bilberry extract, and lutein on subjective symptoms of asthenopia in humans. *Biomed Res*, 2011 Dec;32(6):387-93.

[16] Ren, H., Magulike, N., Ghebremeskel, K., Crawford, M. (2006). Primary open-angle glaucoma patients have reduced levels of blood docosahexaenoic and eicosapentaenoic acids. *Prostaglandins Leukol Essent Fatty Acids*, Mar;74(3):157-63.

[17] Chong, E.W., Robman, L.D., Simpson, J.A., Hodge, A.M., Aung, K.Z., et al. (2009). Fat consumption and its association with age-related macular degeneration. *Arch Ophthalmol*, May;127(5):674-80.

[18] W.E. Connor, Neuringer, M., Reisbick, S. (1992). Essential fatty acids: The importance of n-2 fatty acids in the retina and the brain. *Nutr Rev*, Apr;50(4(Pt2)):21-29.

[19] Chong, E.W., Kris, A.J., Wong, T.Y., Simpson, J.A., Guymer, R.H. (2008). Dietary omega-3 fatty acid and fish intake in the primary prevention of age-related macular degeneration: a systematic review and meta-analysis. *Arch Opthalmol*, Jun;126(6):826-33.

[20] SanGiovanni, J.P., Agron, E., Meleth, A.D., Reed, G.F., Sperduto, R.D., et al. (2009). Omega-3 Long-chain polyunsaturated fatty acid intake and 12-y incidence of neovascular age-related macular degeneration and central geographic atrophy: AREDS report 30, a prospective cohort study from the Age-Related Eye Disease Study. *Am J C Nutr*, Dec;90(6):1601-7.

[21]Christen, W.G., Schaumberg, D.A., Glynn, R.J., Buring, J.E. (2011). Dietary omega-3 fatty acid and fish intake and incident age-related macular degeneration in women. *Arch Ophthalmol,* Jul;129(7):921-9.

[22] Ibid. Querques. (2011).

[23]Bush, R.A., Malnoe, A., Reme, C.E., Williams, T.P. (1994). Dietary deficiency of N-3 fatty acids alters rhodopsin content and function in the rat retina. *Invest Ophthalmol Vis Sci.* Jan, 35(1):91-100.

[24]Bazan, N.G., Molina, M.F., Gordon, W.C. (2011). Docosahexaenoic acid signalolipidomics in nutrition: significance in aging, neuroinflammation, macular degeneration, Alzheimer's, and other neurodegenerative diseases. *Annu Rev Nutr,* Aug 21;31:321-51.

[25] Ibid. Querques. (2011).

[26] Orr, S.K., Palumbo, S., Bosetti, F., Mount, H.T., Kang, J.X., et al. (2013). Unesterified docosahexaenoic acid is protective in neuroinflammation. *J Neurochem,* Nov;127(3):378–393.

[27]Bazan, N.G. (2006). Cell survival matters: docosahexaenoic acid signaling, neuroprotection and photoreceptors. *Trends Neurosci,* May;29(5):263-71.

[28] Lecerf, J.M. (2009). Fatty acids and cardiovascular disease. *Nutr Rev,* May;67(5):273-83.

[29] Shen, Y., Chen, G., Ziao, A., Xie, Y., Liu, L., Cao, Y. (2018). In vitro effect of flaxseed oil and α-linolenic acid against the toxicity of lipopolysaccharide (LPS) to human umbilical vein endothelial cells. *Inflammopharmacology,* Spr;26(2):645-654.

[30] Song, J. Jing, Z., Hu, W., Yu, J., Cui, X. (2017). α-Linolenic Acid Inhibits Receptor Activator of NF-κB Ligand Induced (RANKL-Induced) Osteoclastogenesis and Prevents Inflammatory Bone Loss via Downregulation of Nuclear Factor-KappaB-Inducible Nitric Oxide Synthases (NF-κB-iNOS) Signaling Pathways. *Med Sci Monit,* Oct 24;23:5056-5069.

[31] Chalmers, A. (2015). Omega 3s for Healthy Hair, Nails and Skin. Usana. Retrieved Nov 22 2017 from https://whatsupusana.com/2015/06/omega-3s-healthy-hair-nails-skin.

[32] Omega-6 fatty acid. Wikipedia. Retrieved from https://en.wikipedia.org/wiki/Linoleic_acid.

[33] Zirate, R., El Jaber-Vazdekis, N., Tejera, N., Perez, J.A., Rodriguez, C. (2017). Significance of long chain polyunsaturated fatty acids in human health. *Clin Transl Med,* Dec;6(1):25.

[34] Ibid. Zirate. (2017).

[35] Ibid. Lecerf. (2009).

[36] Dyall, S.C. (2017). Interplay Between n-3 and n-6 Long-Chain Polyunsaturated Fatty Acids and the Endocannabinoid System in Brain Protection and Repair. *Lipids,* Nov;52(11):885-900

[37] Weil, A. Six Tips for Healthy Hair and Skin. DrWeil. Retrieved Nov 22 2017 from https://www.drweil.com/health-wellness/body-mind-spirit/hair-skin-nails/six-tips-for-healthy-hair-and-skin.

8-6. ENZYMES

Enzymes are one of the major classes of antioxidants. They are mostly proteins that speed up cellular processes and are essential for life and for vision. Some help break down molecules for more effective absorption; others combine molecules to form something new. Enzymes are specialized workers; each enzyme is responsible for a very specific action.[1] We produce certain enzymes naturally, but these enzymes lessen in natural production as we age.

Superoxide Dismutase

Superoxide dismutase (SOD) reduces conditions involving inflammation, infection, respiration, metabolic and cardiovascular conditions, and urinary and fertility disorders.[2] The observation that SOD levels are low in patients with a variety of vision issues has been partially responsible for the increasing understanding that oxidative stress is the cause of, or contributing factor in, many eye conditions. SOD is able to neutralize the full spectrum of free radicals in the body.

There are three types of superoxide dismutase.

- SOD1, found within the cell, interacts with copper and zinc.
- SOD2, found in mitochondria (cellular level energy producers), interacts with manganese.
- SOD3, found outside the cells, interacts with copper and zinc.[3]

Antioxidant. SOD repairs cells and reduces the damage done to them by superoxide, the most common free radical in the body. SOD is a potential therapy for oxidative-stress related conditions caused by UV light, carcinogens, cell death, and neurodegeneration.

Inflammation. Superoxide dismutase has potential for anti-inflammatory properties,[4] and has been used to help treat arthritis, inflammatory diseases, and burn injuries.[5]

Cataract. Blood levels of SOD and another enzyme, catalase, are lower in patients with both diabetic-related cataracts and age-related cataracts. In both conditions there is increased oxidative stress, damaging the lens when enzyme levels are low.[6]

Cornea. The cornea contains relatively high levels of SOD that protects it from oxidative stress. In cases of keratoconus and bullous keratopathy, it was found that extracellular levels and activity of SOD3 were half that of healthy corneas, leading researchers to speculate that these cases may arise due to low enzyme levels.[7]

Macular degeneration. Superoxide dismutase levels appear to be low in AMD patients.[8]

Glaucoma. The amount of SOD in the trabecular meshwork decreases with age, leading researchers to consider SOD's role in primary open-angle glaucoma.[9] Levels of SOD and other antioxidant enzymes increase in the aqueous humor of patients with glaucoma and may be potential stress markers for early glaucoma.[10]

Uveitis. SOD is helpful in treating uveitis; it has a greater antioxidant effect compared to the corticosteroid dexamethasone. Adding it to therapy with dexamethasone results in lower inflammation intensity and enhanced dexamethasone effect.[11]

Source. Superoxide dismutase is found in barley grass, nutritional yeast, broccoli, Brussels sprouts, cabbage, wheatgrass, and most green plants.

Nattokinase

Nattokinase (NK) is an anti-inflammatory proteolyic enzyme; that is, it breaks down proteins. It comes from boiled and fermented soybeans from which vitamin K2 is removed. While digestive enzymes are normally taken with food, anti-inflammatory enzymes such as nattokinase and serrapeptase are best taken on an empty stomach. Doing so assists with detoxification because they break down debris in the blood and tissues that may be linked to inflammatory conditions.

Inflammation. Nattokinase is often recommended to reduce inflammation, although there is not a lot of research. In the context of research on nattokinase's effectiveness in reducing or preventing blood clots, researchers do point out that there is a strong molecular link between inflammation and coagulation, and that nattokinase might be helpful for patients with inflammatory diseases.[12]

Related disorders. Nattokinase is considered to be a safe, powerful, low-cost, and all-natural supplement for the treatment of heart and cardiovascular disease.[13 14 15] NK was reported to have an effect on both oxidative injury-mediated arterial thrombosis[16 17] and inflammation-induced venal thrombosis.[18] It can be an effective thrombolytic agent.[19 20] It can be unstable however. Researchers combined it with another stable compound, polylysine dendrimer, for a more effective therapy that avoids complications.[21]

Nattokinase may be effective for high blood pressure. In an eight-week clinical study of over 70 people, both systolic and diastolic blood pressure were reduced when compared to placebo. Both men and women experienced the reduction, although it was greater for men. A subgroup had low levels of renin, which regulates blood pressure. The renin levels improved for 66% of the people after eight weeks.[22]

Caution. Use with care if you are taking blood thinners, as it can decrease blood clotting.

Serrapeptase

Also known as serratiopeptidase, serrapeptase is an anti-inflammatory proteolyic enzyme derived from silkworms. It has many of the same traits and possible benefits as nattokinase.

There has been little conclusive research on serrapeptase. Even though it is routinely used in many clinical specialties for anti-inflammatory, antiedemic, and analgesic effects, the existing scientific evidence is weak. This is because much of the research was based on poor methodology with dosage and duration missing and outcomes not clearly defined.[23]

Even so, serrapeptase appears to be an enzyme that can be useful in reducing inflammation and swelling due to arthritis and/or allergies, and consequently it may be helpful for inflammation-related symptoms of eye conditions, such as iritis, uveitis, dry eye, and Sjogren's syndrome.

Inflammation. In animal models, low doses of serrapeptase combined with other proteolyic enzymes, along with aspirin, failed individually but succeeded in combination in relieving acute inflammation. In subacute inflammation, swelling was significantly relieved, and also in combination with aspirin, inflammation was relieved.[24] It reduced inflammation-related acute or chronic ear, nose, or throat problems, and appears to act rapidly on local inflammation.[25] [26]

Related disorders. It may be effective for swelling after facial surgery to clear the sinuses.[27] It is often used for swelling, but the research-based evidence is inconclusive and more is needed.

Serrapeptase shows better ability to separate and remove insulin amyloids than nattokinase. Amyloids are clusters of proteins that are implicated in brain conditions such as Alzheimer's disease. While this research was not on beta-amyloids causing dementia, the function of serrapeptase in breaking up the clusters is similar.[28]

When compared to antibiotic use alone, serrapeptase in combination with an antibiotic, improvements resulted in an animal model of staph lung infections.[29] In another study, a variety of single enzymes, including serrapeptase, were combined with antibiotics, resulting in improved outcomes against staph infections.[30]

Caution. Because it breaks down fibrin, take care when combining with moderate blood thinners such as fish oil, and do not pair with potent blood thinner drugs.

---

[1] Castro, J. (2014). How Do Enzymes Work? LiveScience. Retrieved Nov 22 2017 from https://www.livescience.com/45145-how-do-enzymes-work.html.

[2] Carillon, J., Rouanet, J.J., Cristol, J.P., Brion, R. (2013). Superoxide dismutase administration, a potential therapy against oxidative stress related diseases: several routes of supplementation and proposal of an original mechanism of action. *Pharm Res*, Nov;30(11):2718-28.

[3] Superoxide dismutase. Retrieved Oct. 30, 2017 from https://en.wikipedia.org/wiki/Superoxide_dismutase

[4] Yasui, K., Baba, A. (2006). Therapeutic potential of superoxide dismutase (SOD) for resolution of inflammation. *Inflamm Res*, Sep;55(9):359-63.

[5] Chesnokova, N.B., Neroev, V.V., Beznos, O.V., Beyshenova, G.A., Panova, I.G., et al. (2015). Effects of dexamethasone and superoxide dismutase instillations on clinical course of uveitis and local biochemical processes (experimental study). *Vestn Oftalmol*, May-Jun;131(3):71.75.

[6] Maurya, O.P., Mohanty, L., Bhaduri, G., Chandra, A. (2006). Role of anti-oxidant enzymes superoxide dismutase and catalase in the development of cataract: study of serum levels in patients with senile and diabetic cataracts. *J Indian Med Assoc*, Jul;104(7):394, 396-7.

[7] Behndig, A., Karlsson, K., Johansson, B.O., Brannstrom, T., Marklund, S.L. (2001). Superoxide dismutase in the normal and diseased human cornea. *Invest Opthalmol Vis Sci*, Sep;42(10):2293-6.

[8] Yildirim, Z., Ucgun, N.I., Yildirim, F. (2011). The role of oxidative stress and antioxidants in the pathogenesis of age-related macular degeneration. *Clinics (Sao Paulo)*, May;66(5):743-6.

[9] De La Paz, M.A., Epstein, D.L. (1996). Effect of age on superoxide dismutase activity of human trabecular meshwork. *Invest Ophthalmol Vis Sci*, Aug;37(9):1849-53.

[10] Ferreira, S.M., Lerner, S.F., Brunzini, R., Evelson, P.A., Llesuy, S.F. (2004). Oxidative stress markers in aqueous humor of glaucoma patients. *Am J Ophthalmol*, Jan;137(1):62-9.

[11] Chesnokova, N.B., Neroev, V.V., Beznos, O.V., Beyshenova, G.A., Panova, I.G., et al. (2015). Effects of dexamethasone and superoxide dismutase instillations on clinical course of uveitis and local biochemical processes (experimental study). *Vestn Oftalmol,* May-Jun;131(3):71.75.

[12] Kurosawa, Y., Nirengi, S., Homma, T., Esaki, K., Ohta, M., et al. (2015). A single-dose of oral nattokinase potentiates thrombolysis and anti-coagulation profiles. *Sci Rep,* June 25;5:11601.

[13] Nagata, C., Wada, K., Tamura T, Konishi K, Goto Y., et. Al. (2017). Dietary soy and natto intake and cardiovascular disease mortality in Japanese adults: the Takayama study. *Am J Clin Nutr,* Feb; 105(2):426-431

[14]Dabbagh, F., Negahdaripour, M., Berenjian, A., Behfar, A., Mohammadi, F., et al. (2014). Nattokinase production and application. *Appl Microbiol Biotechnol,* Nov; 98(22):9199-206.

[15]Huang, Y., Ding, S., Liu, M., Gao, C., Yang J., et al. (2013). Ultra-small and anionic starch nanospheres: formation and vitro thrombolytic behavior study. Carbohydr Polym, Jul 25; 96(2):426-34.

[16] Suzuki, Y., Kondo, K., Matsumoto, Y., Zhao, B.Q., Otsuguro, K., et al. (2003). Dietary supplementation of fermented soybean, natto, suppresses intimal thickening and modulates the lysis of mural thrombi after endothelial injury in rat femoral artery. *Life Sci,* Jul 25; 73(10):1289-98.

[17]Jang, J.Y., Kim, T.S., Cai, J., Kim, J., Kim, Y., et al. (2013). Nattokinase improves blood flow by inhibiting platelet aggregation and thrombus formation. *Lab Anim Res,* Dec; 29(4):221-5.

[18] Xu, J., Du, M., Yang, X., Chen, Q., Chen, H., et al. (2014). Thrombolytic effects in vivo of nattokinase in a carrageenan-induced rat model of thrombosis. *Acta Haematol,* 132(2):247-53.

[19]Jang J.-Y., Kim T.-S., Cai J., Kim J., Kim Y., Shin K., Kim K.-S., Park S.K., Lee S.-P., Choi E.-K., et al. Nattokinase improves blood flow by inhibiting platelet aggregation and thrombus formation. *Lab. Anim. Res.* 2013;29:221–225.

[20]Xu J., Du M., Yang X., Chen Q., Chen H., et al. (2014). Thrombolytic effects in vivo of nattokinase in a carrageenan-induced rat model of thrombosis. *Acta Haematol.* 132:247–253.

[21] Wu, C., Gao, C., Lu, S., Xu, X., Wen, N., et al. (2018). Construction of polylysine dendrimer nanocomposites carrying nattokinase and their application in thrombolysis. *J Biomed Mter Res A,* Feb;106(2):440-449.

[22] Jensen, G.S., Lenninger, M., Ero, M.P., Benson, K.F. (2016). Consumption of nattokinase is associated with reduced blood pressure and von Willebrand factor, a cardiovascular risk marker: results from a randomized, double-blind, placebo-controlled, multicenter North American clinical trial. *Integr Blood Press Control,* Oct 13;9:95-104.

[23] Bhagat, S., Agarwal, M., Roy, V. (2013). Serratiopeptidase: A systemic review of the existing research. *Int J Surg,* Apr:11(3) 209-17.

[24] Swamy, A.H.M.V., Patil, P.A. (2008). Effect of some clinically used proteolytic enzymes on inflammation in rats. *Indian J Pharm Sci,* Jan-Feb: 70(1).

[25] Mazzone, A., Catalani, M., Costanzo, M., Drusian, A., Mandoli, A., et al. (1990). Evaluation of Serratia peptidase in acute or chronic inflammationof otorhinolaryngology pathology: a multicentre, double-blind, randomized trial versus placebo. *J Int Med Res,* Sep-Oct;18(5):379-88.

[26]Tachibana, M, Mizukoshi, O., Harada, Y., Kawamoto, K., Nakai, Y. (1984). A muti-centre, double-blind study of serrapeptase versus placebo in post-antrotomy buccal swelling. *Pharmatherapeutica,* 3(8); 526-30.

[27] Serrapeptase. WebMD. Retrieved Oct 31, 2017 from https://www.webmd.com/vitamins-supplements/ingredientmono-1115-SERRAPEPTASE.aspx.

[28] Metkar, S.K., Girigoswami, A., Murugesan, R., Girigoswami, K. (2017). In vitro and in vivo insulin amyloid degradation mediated by Serratiopeptidase. *Mater Sci Eng C Mater Biol Appl,* Jan 1;70(Pt 1):728-735.

[29] Gupta, P.V., Nirwane, A.M., Belubbi, T., Nagarsenker, M.S. (2017). Pulmonary delivery of synergistic combination of fluoroquinolone antibiotic complemented with proteolytic enzyme: A novel antimicrobial and antibiofilm strategy. *Nanomedicine,* Oct;13(7):2371-2384.

[30] Hogan, S., Zapotoczna, M., Stevens, N.T., Humphreys, H., O'Gara, J.P., et al. (2017). Potential use of targeted enzymatic agents in the treatment of Staphylococcus aureus biofilm-related infections. *J Hops Infect,* Jun;96(2):177-182.

8-7. AMINO ACIDS

Glutathione

Glutathione is essential to making tissue enzymes and crucial to stopping free-radical damage. It is involved in the control of mitochondrial membrane permeability and therefore helps protect against premature cell death.[1] It is not generally considered an essential nutrient since the body is capable of synthesizing it from a number of amino acids, including cysteine, glutamic acid, and glycine. However, cysteine is somewhat rare in foods so that the amount of cysteine in the body determines how much glutathione can be produced.

Antioxidant. Glutathione is one of the "super" antioxidants because it is capable of stabilizing the full spectrum of free radicals. It is used throughout the body and is considered one of the essential anti-aging nutrients. The amount of glutathione in blood plasma is considered an overall indicator of the body's antioxidant defense system.

Cataract. Glutathione can be helpful at preventing cataract formation.[2] It exists in unusually high concentrations in the lens, where it plays an essential free-radical scavenging function,[3] defending both the entire eye and various regions of the lens from cataracts.[4] Studies have shown that all lenses with cataracts contain a reduced amount of glutathione, about 1/15 the normal amount.[5]

Glaucoma. Glutathione is part of the optic nerve defense system against neurodegeneration.[6] Low blood levels of glutathione are observed in patients with both open-angle glaucoma and normal tension glaucoma.[7] [8] In animal testing, researchers have learned that while increased oxidative stress markers and lowered glutathione levels occur in acute glaucoma, the markers are no longer there in the chronic condition. This suggests that oxidative damage occurs early in the condition's progression.[9]

Macular degeneration. Low levels of glutathione are also observed in macular degeneration patients. Early AMD patients have high levels of oxidized glutathione (glutathione disulfide), which is a biomarker for AMD.[10] Glutathione helps protect the retina from oxidative damage.[11]

Other eye disorders. Researchers have also found that glutathione levels are low in patients with diabetic retinopathy[12] where glutathione synthesis is reduced[13] and in problems of the vitreous.[14]

Source. Since glutathione is poorly absorbed when taken directly in pill or capsule form, we recommend taking a formula that is either sublingual or submucosal and contains additional nutrients to help the liver manufacture additional glutathione.

Glutamine

Glutamine is an essential amino acid that is critical to the production of cellular energy, especially in the intestinal tract and stomach. The body produces it from glutamic acid. It represents 60% of the free amino acids in the body with the highest concentrations in blood plasma, muscles, and cerebral and spinal fluid.[15] Along with cysteine and glycine, it is one of the amino acid components of glutathione.

One of the important roles of glutamine is removing waste and toxic materials from the body. It is required in greater amounts in response to mental or physical stress.[16] Glutamine provides an energy source for the cells and for synthesizing protein. It is a popular addition to diets of athletes due to its energy boosting properties,[17] and it has been found to support immune functioning.[18]

Cataract. Glutamine residues, created as the result of deterioration of glutamine, are found in the proteins of the eye lens crystallins and in increasing amounts as we age.[19] This process, called deamidation, may be responsible for the fact that the crystallins in lenses break down, the proteins clump together, and opacity increases.[20]

Presbyopia. The stiffness of the lens, resulting in the inability to focus on near objects, occurs as a result of the same deamidation of biochemicals such as glutamine.[21]

Other eye disorders. Glutamine plays an essential role in regulating the acid-base ratio in the body, with the optimal pH of between 7.35 and 7.45 to function effectively (see the chapter on the Alkaline-Acid diet.) Glutamine separates ammonia in the kidneys and protects the brain.[22]

Source. Glutamine is especially found in poultry, meat, seafood, dairy products, seaweed, wheat, parsley, cabbage, spinach, beans, and vegetable juices.

Cysteine

Cysteine, consumed as n-acetylcysteine, helps your retina stay healthy by supporting synthesis of glutathione along with glutamine and glycine. Cysteine is the only amino acid that is not commonly found in foods. The supportive role of cysteine helps prevent primary open-angle or normal tension glaucoma and macular degeneration.

Cataract. Cysteine is essential in order to maintain a healthy lens to focus vision, to support macular health, and to prevent damage to the optic nerve. Cysteine combines with another amino acid, tryptophan, to protect the lens from UV radiation.[23] In fact, there is a special biochemical "pathway" to regulate cysteine uptake in the lens.[24]

Source. Good sources of cysteine include soybeans, sunflower seeds, legumes, kamut, oats, cheese, eggs, beef, lamb, chicken, pork, and fish.

Carnosine

Carnosine is made up of two other amino acids, beta-alanine and histidine, and is found primarily in the brain and in muscle tissue.[25] It takes several forms, including d-, l-carnosine, and n-acetylcarnosine. L-carnosine cannot be used topically in the eye though n-acetylcarnosine can; both may be taken internally as supplements.

Cataract. Researchers investigated the mechanisms behind the anti-cataract capacity of n-acetylcarnosine by evaluating both direct and indirect antioxidant properties.

In several trials, researchers investigated the possible efficacy of n-acetylcarnosine (NAC)[26] in a 1% solution for treating or reducing the risk of cataract. The study evaluated changes in lens clarity in nearly 100 subjects and controls that were given NAC, or placebo, or were untreated.[27]

Over six months, 41.5% of the treated eyes showed "marked" improvement in lens clarity; 90% of the eyes showed "gradual" improvement in lens clarity, and 88.9% of the eyes showed improvement in glare sensitivity. There was less lens density and opacity in the posterior subcapsular and cortical morphological portions of the lens. With the study extending over two years, the researchers could report that the NAC benefit continues and is sustainable.[28]

These researchers followed up with more trials identifying further conclusions: that n-acetylcarnosine reduces glare scores, that it has some antioxidant capacity, and that it breaks up lens crystallins aggregation.[29] A literature review noted that n-acetylcarnosine might be helpful in initial stages of cataract.[30]

Another form, l-carnosine, is a strong inhibitor of sugar molecules' ability to bond to proteins or fats unless an enzyme is present. This is called glycation. Glycation is implicated in cataract development (and overall aging). Other researchers have compared d- and l-carnosine, finding that both dissolved the kind of fibrils that make up cataracts.[31]

Diabetic retinopathy. Researchers concluded that because l-carnosine inhibits the ability of sugar molecules to bond to proteins without an enzyme, it could be effective in treating diabetic eye disease.[32]

Sources. Meats. The body is also able to synthesize carnosine.

Glycine

Glycine is the simplest amino acid; it is synthesized in the body and is one of three amino acids required to synthesize glutathione, the "super antioxidant" of vision.

It is an inhibitory neurotransmitter (non-stimulating) in the brainstem and spinal cord. In the retina, it plays a mediation role in neurotransmission.[33] Half of certain retinal neurons, called amacrine cells, release glycine at their synapses with a variety of other neurons. Some of these cells relay light from rods, and some modulate different types of ganglion cell responses.[34]

It is also a protein precursor in the body, where the greatest use is in collagen, which is about 35% glycine.[35]

Related disorders. Glycine modulates certain neurobiochemicals in the brain and improves sleep quality.[36] The details of why it does so are poorly understood. Researchers found that oral glycine induced non-rapid eye movement sleep, along with lowered core temperature, and they conclude that the effect may be due to dilation of peripheral blood vessels.[37]

Source. Beans, spinach, kale, cauliflower, cabbage and pumpkin are good vegetable source of glycine. It is found in fruits, including banana and kiwi, and in meat, dairy products, poultry, fish, and eggs.

Taurine

Taurine is critical for nerve health and is responsible for clearing away and regenerating old tissue. It is especially important for the health of the eye and of the inner ear.

Diabetic retinopathy. Taurine is protective against the complications of diabetes.[38] [39]

Macular degeneration. Low levels of taurine are associated with instances of AMD[40] and macular dystrophies.[41] Taurine protects against ultraviolet radiation, acts as an antioxidant to protect cells, helps move nutrients across cell membrane barriers, and helps remove debris and toxins from the system.[42]

Night vision. Taurine is found in high concentration in the retina photoreceptor rods, ten times greater than any other part of the body that is derived from the central nervous system,[43] and where there are two binding proteins specific to taurine. It plays an important role in night vision and is essential to photoreceptor integrity.[44] [45] [46]

Retinal ganglion degeneration. Taurine protects against retinal degeneration.[47] [48] Research has shown that when taurine is removed from food, animals develop retinal degeneration; when taurine is replaced, the degeneration reverses.[49] [50]

Related conditions. Patients with diabetes have an increased need for taurine; taurine levels are lower in diabetics, and research indicates that the relationship between low levels of taurine, obesity, and diabetes is a close one.[51] Taurine levels are also tied to non-alcoholic fatty liver disease[52] and cardiovascular disease.[53] [54] [55]

Food sources. Highest levels of taurine are found in shellfish, especially clams, scallops, and mussels, as well as dark poultry meat. Lower amounts of taurine are found in cheese.

L-arginine

L-arginine is important for vision because it is a nitric oxide precursor. The body needs low levels of nitric oxide for a number of functions, including keeping blood vessels dilated and flexible and supporting kidney functioning. L-arginine is used to build protein in the body. L-arginine generally supports vision indirectly, that is, through its ability to improve blood flow, improve sugar balance, and remove waste ammonia from the body.

Inflammation. L-arginine's important role in vision health is underlined by its capacity as an anti-inflammatory agent. Inflammation and resulting oxidative stress increase the risk of many eye conditions and health conditions.

Diabetic retinopathy. As a result of insufficient blood circulation to the retina, diabetic retinopathy is a common complication of type 2 diabetes. L-arginine stimulates the creation of insulin by the pancreas, improving (but not normalizing) insulin sensitivity in patients.[56]

Glaucoma. In one study, administered through an intravenous drip infusion, l-arginine reduced intraocular pressure significantly, and then the IOP increased again fairly rapidly. The test does not therefore suggest that this amino acid improves glaucoma problems, but that it lowered IOP primarily through the formation of nitric oxide.[57]

Related disorders. In the body, l-arginine is converted into nitric oxide, which expands blood vessels. So, it plays a role in supporting the heart and circulatory system, including maintenance of normal blood pressure. It may be helpful for angina and leg pain that is due to poor blood flow because it dilates blood vessels; but it, itself, does not help cardiovascular conditions.

L-arginine may be helpful in reducing high blood pressure. A review of the research indicates, overall, that it improves endothelium-derived nitric oxide production and function on endothelium cells, which line blood vessels and reduce systemic blood pressure in some models of hypertension.[58]

L-arginine helps the body get rid of waste products, such as ammonia, and supports kidney functioning. It is essential to maintain nitric oxide levels needed for proper kidney functioning. Patients with kidney failure have low levels of l-arginine in the blood. [59]

Source. Arginine is available through nuts, poultry, red meat, fish, and dairy products, as well as grains, beans, corn, and leafy-green vegetables.

Caution. People who are prone to allergies or asthma should take l-arginine with caution, as it may increase airway swelling. It may make herpes worse, should not be taken to prevent a heart attack, or by people with kidney disease. Because it can interfere with blood pressure, it should not be taken at least two weeks before surgery.[60]

L-methionine

The essential amino acid L-methionine is synthesized in the body as part of the metabolism of proteins, which is an intermediate step to the creation of cysteine, carnitine, and taurine—all critical to eye health.

Its conversion to cysteine requires adequate levels of B vitamins. As a part of certain cell functions, it contributes a molecule to the process, and is "repaid" that molecule from vitamin B12 or folic acid. However, when the body is deficient in those nutrients, this repayment (remethylation) does not occur, and homocysteine remains. Over time, high levels of homocysteine build up, which have been connected to a number of vision and health conditions.

Eye disorders. There are connections between high levels of homocysteine and advanced macular degeneration,[61] [62] other retinal conditions, and photoreceptor problems.[63] It is linked to glaucoma,[64] diabetic retinopathy,[65] and optic neuropathy.[66] Furthermore, high homocysteine levels are linked to heart disease, stroke, osteoporosis, and other health conditions.

Source. This nutrient is found in egg whites, fish, poultry, and crustaceans. In smaller quantities it is found in seaweed, sesame seed, and cottage cheese.

---

[1] Hall, A.G. (1999). The role of glutathione in the regulation of apoptosis. *Eur J Clin Invest*, Mar; 29(3):238-45.

[2] Harding, J.J. (1970). Free and protein-bound glutathione in normal and cataractous human lenses. *Biochem J,* May; 117(5):957-60.

[3] Giblin, J. (2000). Glutathione: a vital lens antioxidant. *J Ocul Pharmacol Ther,* Apr;16(2):121-35.

[4] Bhat, K.S., John, A., Reddy, P.R., Reddy, P.S., Reddy, V.N. (1991). Effect of pigmentation on glutathione redox cycle antioxidant defense in whole as well as different regions of human cataractous lens. *Exp Eye Res*, Jun; 52(6):715-21.

[5] Glutathione (2000, '02, '15, '17) & Cataract. Retrieved Oct 30 2017 from http://www.naturaleyecare.com/study.asp?s_num=426.

[6] Dringen, R. (2000). Glutathione metabolism and oxidative stress in neurodegeneration. *Eur J Biochem,* Aug; 267(16):4903.

[7] Gherghel, D., Mroczkowska, S., Qin, L. (2013). Reduction in blood glutathione levels occurs similarly in patients with primary-open angle or normal tension glaucoma. *Invest Ophthalmol Vis Sci,* May 9;54(5):3333-9.

[8] Glutathione (2005, 2013) levels low in glaucoma patients. Retrieved Oct 30 2017 from http://www.naturaleyecare.com/study.asp?s_num=57

[9] Chen, T., Gionfriddo, J.R., Tai, P.Y., Novakowski, A.N., Alyahya, K., Madl, J.E. (2015). Oxidative stress increases in retinas of dogs in acute glaucoma but not in chronic glaucoma. *Vet Ophthalmol,* Jul;18(4):261-70.

[10] Qin, L., Mroczkowska, S.A., Ekart, A., Patel, S.R., Gibson, J.M., et al. (2014). Patients with early age-related macular degeneration exhibit signs of macro- and micro-vascular disease and abnormal blood glutathione levels. *Graefes Arch Clin Exp Ophthalmol,* Jan;252(1):23-30.

[11] Sternberg, P., Davidson, P.C., Jones, D.P., Hagen, T.M., Reed, R.L., et al. (1993). Protection of retinal pigment epithelium from oxidative injury by glutathione and precursors. *Invest Ophthalmol Vis Sci, Dec*;34(13):3661-8.

[12] Kundu, D., Mandal, T., Nandi, M., Osta, M., Bandyopadhyay, U., Ray, D. (2014). Oxidative stress in diabetic patients with retinopathy. *Ann Afr Med,* Jan-Mar;13(1):41-6

[13] Sekhar, R.V., McKay, S.V., Patel, S.G., Guthikonda, A.P. Reddy, V.T., et al. (2011). Glutathione Synthesis Is Diminished in Patients With Uncontrolled Diabetes and Restored by Dietary Supplementation With Cysteine and Glycine. *Diabetes Care,* Jan; 34(1):162–167.

[14] Gherghel, D., Griffiths, H.R., Hilton, E.J., Cunliffe, I.A. (2005). Systemic Reduction in Glutathione Levels Occurs in Patients with Primary Open-Angle Glaucoma. *Invest Ophthalmol Vis Sci,* Mar;46(3):877-83.

[15] Glutamine and glutamic acid. Retrieved Oct 30, 2017 from http://www.aminoacid-studies.com/amino-acids/glutamine-and-glutamic-acid.html.

[16] Hall, J.E., Guyton, A.C. (2006). *Textbook of medical physiology* (11th ed.). St. Louis, Mo: Elsevier Saunders. 393.

[17] Yuneva, M., Zamboni, N., Oefner, P., Sachidanandam, R. Lazebnik, Y. (2007). Deficiency in glutamine but not glucose induces MYC-dependent apoptosis in human cells. *J Cell Bio,* Jul 2;178(1):93-105.

[18] Calder PC, Yaqoob P. (1999) Glutamine and the immune system. *Amino Acids*, 1999;17(3):227-41.

[19] Hooi, M.Y., Raftery, M.J., Truscott, R.J. (2012). Age-dependent deamidation of glutamine residues in human γS crystallin: deamidation and unstructured regions. *Protein Sci,* Jul;21(7):1074-9.

[20] Hains, P.G., Truscott, R.J.W. (2010). Age-Dependent Deamidation of Lifelong Proteins in the Human Lens. *Invest Ophthalmol Vis Sci,* Jun; 51(6): 3107–3114.

[21] Ibid. Hains. (2010).

[22] Ibid. Glutamine and glutamic acid. Retrieved Mar 18 2018 from http://www.Aminoacid-studies.com

[23] Schafheimer, J., Wang, Z., Schey, K., King, J. (2014). Tyrosine/cysteine cluster sensitizing human γD-crystallin to ultraviolet radiation-induced photoaggregation in vitro. *Biochemistry,* Feb 18;53(6):979-90.

[24] Lim, J.C., Lam, L., Li. B., Donaldson, P.J. (2013). Molecular identification and cellular localization of a potential transport system involved in cystine/cysteine uptake in human lenses. *Exp Eye Res*, Nov;116:219-26.

[25] Carnosine. Retrieved Oct 30, 2017 from https://en.wikipedia.org/wiki/Carnosine

[26] Confusingly, both n-acetylcysteine, and n-acetylcarnosine are commonly abbreviated as NAC. Here we refer only to the latter as NAC.

[27] Babizhayev, M.A., Deyev, A.K., Yermakova, V.N., Semiletov, Y.A., Davydova, N.G., et al. (2001). N-Acetylcarnosine, a natural histidine-containing dipeptide, as a potent ophthalmic drug in treatment of human cataracts. *Peptides*, Jun;22(6):979-94.

[28] Ibid. Babizhayev. (2001).

[29] Babizhayev, M.A., Burke, L. Micans, P., Richer, S.P. (2009). N-Acetylcarnosine sustained drug delivery eye drops to control the signs of ageless vision: glare sensitivity, cataract amelioration and quality of vision currently available treatment for the challenging 50,000-patient population. *Clin Interv Aging,* 2009;4:31-50

[30] Grover, A.K., Samson, S.E. (2014). Antioxidants and vision health: facts and fiction. *Mol Cell Biochem,* Mar;388(1-2):173-83.

[31] Attanasio, F., Cataldo, S., Fisichella, S., Nicoletti, S., Nicoletti, V.G., et al. (2009). Protective effects of L- and D-carnosine on alpha-crystallin amyloid fibril formation: implications for cataract disease. *Biochemistry*, Jul 4.

[32] Abdelkader, H., Longman, M., Alany, R.G., Pierscionek, B. (2016). On the Anticataractogenic Effects of L-Carnosine: Is It Best Described as an Antioxidant, Metal-Chelating Agent or Glycation Inhibitor? *Oxid Med Cell Longev,* 2016:3240261.

[33] Glycine. Wikipedia. Retrieved Oct 31 2017 from https://en.wikipedia.org/wiki/Glycine.

[34] Havercamp, S. (2012). Glycine Receptor Diversity in the Mammalian Retina. *Webvision,* Mar 27.

[35] Ibid. Glycine. Wikipedia.

[36] Bannai, M., Kawai, N., Ono, K., Nakahara, K., Murakami, N. (2012). The effects of glycine on subjective daytime performance in partially sleep-restricted healthy volunteers. *Font Neurol*, Apr 18;3;61.

[37] Kawai, N., Sakai, N., Okuro, M., Karakawa, S., Tsuneyoshi, Y., et al. (2015). The sleep-promoting and hypothermic effects of glycine are mediated by NMDA receptors in the suprachiasmatic nucleus. *Neuropsychopharmacology*, May;40(6):1405-16.

[38] Sarkar, P., Basak, P., Ghosh, S., Kundu, M., Sil, P.C. (2017). Prophylactic role of taurine and its derivatives against diabetes mellitus and its related complications. *Food Chem Toxicol*, Dec;110:109-121.

[39] Yu, X., Xu, Z., Mi, M., Xu, H., Zhu, J., et al. (2008). Dietary taurine supplementation ameliorates diabetic retinopathy via anti-excitotoxicity of glutamate in streptozotocin-induced Sprague-Dawley rats. Neurochem Res, 33:500–7.

[40] Birdsall, T.C. (1998). Therapeutic applications of taurine. *Altern Med Rev*, Apr;3(2):128-36.

[41] Shpak, N.I., Naritsyna, N.I., Konovalova, N.V. (1989). Taufon and emoksipin in the combined treatment of sclerotic macular dystrophies. *Oftalmol Zh*, (8):463-5.

[42] Ibid. Birdsall. (1998).

[43] Gaucher, D., Arnault, E., Husson, Z., Froger, N., Dubus, E., et al. (2012). Taurine deficiency damages retinal neurones: cone photoreceptors and retinal ganglion cells. *Amino Acids*, Nov;43(5):1979-1993.

[44] Wright, C.E. (1986). Taurine: Biological Update. *Annu Rev Biochem,*1986;55:427-53.

[45] Petrosian, A.M., Haroutounian, J.E. (1998). The role of taurine in osmotic, mechanical, and chemical protection of the retinal rod outer segments. *Adv Exp Med Biol,*1998;442:407-13.

[46] Lopez-Colome, A.M., et al. (1980). Taurine interactions with chick retinal membranes. *J Neurochem, May*;34(5):1047-52.

[47] Lombardini, J.B. (1991). Taurine: retinal function. *Brain Res Brain Res Rev*, May-Aug;16(2):151-69.

[48] Petrosian, A.M., Haroutounian, J.E. (1998). The role of taurine in osmotic, mechanical, and chemical protection of the retinal rod outer segments, *Adv Exp Med Biol*, 442:407-13.

[49] Froger, N., Cadetti, L., Lorach, H., Martins, J., Bemelmans, A.P., et al. (2012). Taurine provides neuroprotection against retinal ganglion cell degeneration. *PLoS One,*2012;7(10):342017.

[50] Imaki, H., Moretz, R., Wisniewski, H., Neuringer, M., Sturman, J. (1987). Retinal degeneration in 3-month-old rhesus monkey infants fed a taurine-free human infant formula. *J Neurosci Res,* 18(4):602-14.

[51] Franconi, F., Bennardini, F., Mattana, A., Miceli, M., Ciuti, M., et al. (1995). Plasma and platelet taurine are reduced in subjects with insulin-dependent diabetes mellitus: effects of taurine supplementation. *Am J Clin Nutr,* May;61(5):1115-9.

[52]Miyazak, T., Boucarel, B., Ikegami, T., Honda, A., Matsuzaki, Y. (2009). The protective effect of taurine against hepatic damage in a model of liver disease and hepatic stellate cells, *Adv Exp Medi Biol,* 2009;643:293-303.

[53]Murakami S., Taurine and atherosclerosis. *Amino Acids.* Jan;46(1):73-80.

[54] Ibid. Birdsall. 1998.

[55]Xu, Y.J., Arneja, A.S., Tappia, P.S., Dhalla, N.S. (2008). The potential health benefits of taurine in cardiovascular disease. *Exp Clin Cardiol,* Summer;13(2):57-65.

[56] Piatti, P.M., Monti, L.D., Valsecchi, G., Magni, F., Setola, E., et al. (2001). Long-Term Oral l-Arginine Administration Improves Peripheral and Hepatic Insulin Sensitivity in Type 2 Diabetic Patients. *Diabetes Care,* May; 24(5): 875-880.

[57] Chuman, H., Chuman, T., Nao-i, N., Sawada, A. (2000). The effect of L-arginine on intraocular pressure in the human eye. *Curr Eye Res,* Jun;20(6):511-6.

[58] Gokce, N. (2004). L-Arginine and Hypertension. *J Nutr,* Oct 1:134(10) 28075-115.

[59] Brunini, T.M., da Silva, C.D., Siqueria, M.A., Moss, M.B., Santos, S.F., et al. (2006). Uremia, atherothrombosis and malnutrition: the role of L-arginine-nitric oxide pathway. *Cardiovasc Hematol Disord Drug Targets,* Jun;6(2):133-40.

[60] L-Arginine. WebMD. Retrieved Nov 1 2017 from https://www.webmd.com/vitamins-supplements/ingredientmono-875-l-arginine.aspx.

[61] Ghosh, S., Saha, M., Das, D. (2013). A study on plasma homocysteine level in age-related macular degeneration. *Nepal J Ophthalmol,* Jul-Dec;5(2):195-200.

[62] Huang, P., Wang, F., Sah, B.K., Jiang, J., Ni, Z., et al. (2015). Homocysteine and the risk of age-related macular degeneration: a systematic review and meta-analysis. *Sci Rep,* Jul;21;5:10585.

[63] Ganapathy, P.S., Perry, R.L., Tawfik, A., Smith, R.M., Perry, E., et al. (2011). Homocysteine-mediated modulation of mitochondrial dynamics in retinal ganglion cells. *Invest Ophthalmol Vis Sci,* Jul 25;52(8):5551-8.

[64] Ghanem, A.A., Mady, S.M., El awady, H.E., Arafa, L.F. (2012). Homocysteine and hydroxyproline levels in patients with primary open-angle glaucoma. *Eye Res,* Aug;37(8):712-8.

[65] Xu, C., Wu, Y., Liu, G., Liu, X., Wang, F., Yu, J. (2014). Relationship between homocysteine level and diabetic retinopathy: a systematic review and meta-analysis. *Diagn Pathol,* Sep 26;9:167.

[66] Stanger, O., Weger, M., Obeid, R., Temmel, W., Meinitzer, A., et al. (2005). Impairment of homocysteine metabolism in patients with retinal vascular occlusion and non-arteritic ischemic optic neuropathy. *Clin Chem Lab Med,* 2005;43(10):1020-5.

8-8. MINERALS

Chromium

Chromium, in trace amounts, helps regulate blood sugar levels, the breakdown of fats, and supports healthy blood circulation.

Diabetic retinopathy. Chromium increases insulin responsiveness,[1] which might be a factor in deterring diabetic retinopathy, a complication of diabetes. Chromium supplementation might require diabetics to reduce their insulin dose with the advice of their health professional.

Eye fatigue. Low chromium levels may be associated with eyestrain, because it helps regulate glucose utilization. Poor glucose utilization is linked to the inability of ciliary muscles (in front of the eye) to bring reading materials into focus.[2]

Glaucoma. Chromium deficiency has been linked to high IOP levels, and patients with open-angle glaucoma often have low chromium blood levels.[3]

Related disorders. Supplemental chromium is linked to lower risk factors in cardiovascular disease.[4] Deficiency in chromium can lead to either hypoglycemia or hyperglycemia; in both cases, adding chromium normalizes blood sugar levels.[5] Chromium helps to keep insulin effective by assisting the transport of glucose to cells.

Source. Brewer's yeast, eggs, and potato skins.

Caution. Too much chromium can result in iron deficiency anemia.[6]

Copper

Copper is utilized in a number of enzyme functions such as with superoxide dismutase and pH balance. The balance of copper to zinc is important to healthy vision. A balance of 15 parts zinc to 1 part copper is recommended when supplementing with either zinc or copper. Copper interacts with iron to create red blood cells and enhances iron absorption.

Diabetic retinopathy. Researchers evaluated the trace mineral content of tears, which reflect the trace mineral content of the eyes. They noted that lower levels of copper were found in patients with diabetic retinopathy compared to healthy eyes.[7]

Myopia. Researchers evaluating tear trace minerals observed lowered copper levels in patients with progressive myopia, as well as a changed ratio of zinc to iron, which suggests metabolic disorders in connective tissue.[8]

Optic neuropathy. Copper deficiency can lead to nerve damage and rarely to optic neuropathy; occasionally this deficiency is acquired after gastric surgery.[9]

Related disorders. Copper deficiency can contribute to iron anemia and osteoporosis.

Source. Shellfish, whole grains, legumes, nuts, potatoes, and dark leafy-green vegetables.

Magnesium

Magnesium (Mg) is one of the most abundant elements in the body. It is critical for the metabolism of many other minerals, of nitric oxide, and of many enzymes in order to maintain equilibrium within cells. Absorption of magnesium, in turn, depends upon many other factors including magnesium in the diet, selenium, parathyroid hormone, and vitamins B6 and D. Excess fat interferes with magnesium functioning. In addition, too much alcohol, salt, sugary sodas, coffee, sweating, stress, women's menstruation issues, some drugs, and parasites decrease magnesium levels.[10]

Researcher S. Johnson writes, "It is highly regrettable that the deficiency of such an inexpensive, low-toxicity nutrient result in diseases that cause incalculable suffering and expense throughout the world. The range of pathologies associated with Mg deficiency is staggering: hypertension (cardiovascular disease, kidney and liver damage, etc.) and peroxynitrite damage (migraine, multiple sclerosis, glaucoma, Alzheimer's disease, etc.)."[11]

Blepharospasm. Treatment by magnesium often reduces facial tics such as blepharospasm,[12] which may be aggravated by imbalances of magnesium and calcium.[13]

Diabetic retinopathy. Low levels of magnesium are also detected in patients with diabetic retinopathy.[14] Magnesium deficiency is the most evident in type 2 diabetes and may heighten the risk of heart disease as well as retinopathy.[15]

Glaucoma. Magnesium has been identified as potential therapy for glaucoma, because it improves blood flow through enhancing the functioning of cells that line blood vessels (endothelial function) and nitric oxide pathways. It also protects the nervous system of the retina/optic nerve by protecting the neurons from oxidative damage.[16]

Keratoconus. Magnesium deficiency could be affecting metabolic factors that influence genetic abnormalities, causing conditions like keratoconus, Thalasselis' syndrome, type A behavior, and allergy.[17] The alterations in the molecular and cellular components of the cornea can be induced by magnesium deficiency, suggesting a possible connection.[18]

Macular degeneration. Researchers have observed that patients with macular degeneration are low in magnesium (along with lack of enough vitamin E, B6, folic acid, and zinc).[19] Poor retinal microcirculation, preventing adequate supply of nutrients, is one factor in AMD that is affected by magnesium levels.

Related disorders. Low levels of magnesium are also associated with migraines, diabetes, and osteoporosis.

Source. Dry roasted almonds, spinach, cashews, soymilk, beans, and avocado, as well as wheat germ, fish, and leafy-green vegetables.

Caution. If you are taking antibiotics, do not take magnesium because it interferes with the effectiveness of the antibiotics.

Selenium

Vision health. Selenium is an essential trace element needed to synthesize enzymes, such as the antioxidant glutathione that is essential to healthy vision.

Cataract. There appears to be a correlation between increased levels of selenium found in lens tissue and cataracts. At the same time, blood levels of selenium are low. Young diabetes patients show selenium changes in the lens. Smokers show decreased selenium levels in both lens and blood. But the reasons for these changes are still being investigated.[20]

Related disorders. Selenium is essential to the thyroid and every part of the body that relies on hormones from the thyroid. In this capacity it may inhibit Hashimoto's disease.[21] Selenium levels decrease with aging and may contribute to brain function declines, although a study finds no link between selenium deficiency and memory.[22] Low levels may also have an impact on cardiovascular disease[23] and certain types of cancer.[24]

Source. Brazil nuts, seafood, whole grains, seeds, meat, poultry, and mushrooms. Other good sources include garlic, onions, broccoli, cabbage, and sunflower seeds.

Sulfur

Sulfur, in the form of methylsulfonylmethane (MSM), also known as methyl sulfone and dimethyl sulfone, is a compound naturally occurring in humans, animal, fruits, and vegetables. It is known for its anti-inflammatory contribution to vision health, but it also has been found to relieve muscle pain and fight oxidative stress and free radicals.[25] MSM markedly slows the release of, or reduces levels of, a variety of inflammatory agents[26] with potential benefit in combating metabolic disorders.[27]

Antioxidant. MSM reduces muscle pain that is due to oxidative stress after acute exhaustive physical exercise.[28] [29]

Permeability. As a permeability enhancer, MSM is effective in combining with other substances to support absorption. For example, in this role it is effective in allowing medications to permeate the lens to reduce opacity and accumulated toxins of cataracts.[30]

Optic nerve degeneration. MSM, combined with a permeability enhancer, was effective in reducing oxidation stress to reduce both oxidative damage and inflammation in animal retinal ganglion cells and demyelination of the optic nerve.[31]

Related disorders. Patients taking MSM showed some improvement, although small, in pain relief and physical function.[32][33]

Source. Eggs, meat, poultry, fish, milk, Brussels sprouts, garlic, onions, asparagus, legumes, kale, and wheat germ.

Caution. There has been at least one case of MSM-induced acute-angle glaucoma, which resolved after intake ceased.[34]

Zinc

Zinc is not itself an antioxidant but has some antioxidant characteristics. It is part of the molecular structure of more than 100 enzymes and is involved in the synthesis of many amino acids. It has roles in RNA and DNA metabolism, cell death, gene expression, and neuron and synapse activity, but it can also be a neurotoxin in the brain.[35] It helps heal injuries, supports the immune system, and supports the functioning of many enzymes.

Zinc plays a vital role in bringing vitamin A from the liver to the retina in order to produce melanin, a protective pigment in the eyes. It helps bind the protective pigment layer of the retina to the underlying tissue. Zinc is found in high concentrations in the eye, especially the retina, its underlying tissues, and choroid (the vascular tissue layer lying under the retina).[36]

Diabetic retinopathy. Measurements of trace minerals in tear fluid suggest balance of those minerals in the health of the eye. Researchers have associated low zinc levels with diabetic retinopathy.[37]

Glaucoma. Similarly, low zinc levels have been found in the tear fluid of patients with glaucoma.[38]

Macular degeneration. The AREDS studies demonstrated that zinc is helpful for macular degeneration,[39] slowing progression of the condition and protecting retinal health.

Myopia. In myopics, the ratio of zinc to iron is abnormal, which suggests metabolic disorders in connective tissue.[40]

Related disorders. Zinc deficiency is associated with poor absorption, skin problems, liver and kidney diseases, sickle cell, diabetes, cancers, fertility, and the immune system.[41]

Source. Highest concentrations are in red meat, oysters, crab, and lobster. Vegetable sources depend on the soil quality; organic products are probably the best sources: wheat germ, wheat bran, seeds (especially sunflower and pumpkin), beans, nuts (especially almonds), whole grains, chicken, and turkey.

Caution. Zinc restricts copper, so if you are taking zinc you should also take copper as well in a 15:1 zinc to copper ratio. Consult your health care professional.

[1] Hoffman, N.J., Penque, B.A. Habegger, K.M., Sealls, W., Tackett, L. et al. (2014). Chromium enhances insulin responsiveness via AMPK. *J Nutr Biochem,* May;25(5):565-72.

[2] Essential Mineral for Treating Glaucoma. Retrieved Nov 22 2017 from https://www.healingtheeye.com/Articles/Glaucoma_chromium.html Nov 2 2017.

[3] Lane, B.C. (1980). Evaluation of intraocular pressure with daily, sustained closework stimulus to accommodation, lowered tissue chromium and dietary deficiency of ascorbic acid. *Doc Ophthalmol,* 1980;28:149-155.

[4] Anderson, R.A., (1986). Chromium metabolism and its role in disease processes in man. *Clini Physiol Biochem,* 1986;4(1):31-41.

[5] Ibid. Anderson. (1986).

[6] Nutrition and Glaucoma. Glaucoma.org. Retrieved Nov 2 2017 from https://www.glaucoma.org/treatment/nutrition-and-glaucoma.php

[7] Vinetskaia, M.I., Iomdina, E.N. (1994). Study of lacrimal fluid trace elements in several eye diseases. *Vestn Oftalmol,* Oct-Dec;110(4):24-6.

[8] Ibid. Vinetskaia. (1994).

[9] Pineles, S.L., Wilson, C.A., Balcer, L.J., Slater, R., Galetta, S.L. (2010). Combined optic neuropathy and myelopathy secondary to copper deficiency. *Surv Ophthalmol,* Jul-Aug;55(4):386-92.

[10] Johnson, S. (2001). The multifaceted and widespread pathology of magnesium deficiency. *Med Hypotheses,* Feb;56(2):163-70.

[11] Ibid. Johnson, S. (2001).

[12] Ploceniak, C. (1990). Bruxism and magnesium, my clinical experiences since 1980. *Rev Stomatol Chir Maxillofac,* 1990;91 Suppl 1:127.

[13] Alonso-Navarro, H., Jimenez-Jimenez, F. (2006). Tardive blepharospasm associated with cinnarizine use. *Clin Neuropharm,* Jul-Aug;29(4):187-9.

[14] Ibid. Vinetskaia. (1994).

[15] Tuvemo, T., Gebre-Medhin, M. (1985). The role of trace elements in juvenile diabetes mellitus. *Pediatrician,* 1983-1985;12(4):213-9.

[16] Ekici, F., Korkmaz, S., Karaca, E.E., Sul, S., Tufan, H.A., et al. (2014) The role of magnesium in the pathogenesis and treatment of glaucoma. *Int Sch Res Notices,* Oct 13;2014:745439

[17] Thalasselis, A., (1995). Thalasselis syndrome and genetic theories on keratoconus. *J Am Optom Assoc,* Aug;66(8):495-9.

[18] Thalasselis, A. (2005). The possible relationship between keratoconus and magnesium deficiency. *Ophthalmic Physiol Opt,* Jan; 25(1):7-12.

[19] Multicenter ophthalmic and nutritional age-related macular degeneration study--part 1: design, subjects and procedures. Age-related Macular Degeneration Study Group. (1996). *J Am Optom Assoc,* Jan;67(1):12-29.

[20] Dawczynski, J., Winnefeld, K., Konigsdorffer, E., Augsten, R., Blum, M., et al. (2006). Selenium and cataract--risk factor or useful dietary supplement? *Klin Monbl Augenheilkd.* Aug;223(8):675-80.

[21] Selenium. Wikipedia. Retrieved Nov 2 2017 from https://en.wikipedia.org/wiki/Selenium.

[22] Selenium. National Institutes of Health. Retrieved Nov 2 2017 from https://ods.od.nih.gov/factsheets/Selenium-Consumer.

[23] Ibid. NIH. Selenium.

[24] Ibid. Wikipedia. Selenium.

[25] Butawan, M., Benjamin, R.L., Bloomer, R.J. (2017). Methylsulfonylmethane: Applications and Safety of a Novel Dietary Supplement. *Nutrients,* Mar 16;9(3).

[26] Kim, Y.H., Kim, D.H., Lim, H., Baek, D.Y., Shin, H.K., et al. (2009). The anti-inflammatory effects of methylsulfonylmethane on lipopolysaccharide-induced inflammatory responses in murine macrophages. *Biol Pharm Bull,* Apr;32(4):651-6.

[27] Ahn, H., Kim, J., Lee, M.J., Kim, Y.J., Cho, Y.W., et al. (2015). Methylsulfonylmethane inhibits NLRP3 inflammasome activation. *Cytokine,* Feb;71(2):223-31.

[28] Nakhostin-Roohi, B., Niknam, Z., Vaezi, N., Mohammadi, S., Bohlooli, S. (2013). Effect of single dose administration of methylsulfonylmethaneon oxidative stress following acute exhaustive exercise. *Iran J Pharm Res,* Fall;12(4):845-53.

[29] Withee, E.D., Tippens, K.M., Dehen, R., Tibbitts, D., Hanes, D., et al. (2017). Effects of Methylsulfonylmethane (MSM) on exercise-induced oxidative stress, muscle damage, and pain following a half-marathon: a double-blind, randomized, placebo-controlled trial. *J Int Soc Sports Nutr,* Jul 21;14:24.

[30] Zhang, M., Shoeb, M., Liu, P., Xiao, T., Hogan, D., et al. (2011). Topical metal chelation therapy ameliorates oxidation-induced toxicity in diabetic cataract. *J Toxicol Environ Health A,* 2011;74(6):380-91.

[31] Liu, P., Zhang, M., Shoeb, M., Hogan, D., Tang, L., et al. (2014). Metal chelator combined with permeability enhancer ameliorates oxidative stress-associated neurodegeneration in rat eyes with elevated intraocular pressure. *Free Radic Biol Med,* Apr;69:289-99.

[32] Debbi, E.M., Agar, G., Fichman, G., Ziv, Y.B., Kardosh, R., et al. (2011). Efficacy of methylsulfonylmethane supplementation on osteoarthritis of the knee: a randomized controlled study. *BMC Complement Altern Med,* Jun 27;11:50.

[33] Kim, L.S., Axelrod, L.J., Howard, P., Buratovich, N., Waters, R.E. (2006). Efficacy of methylsulfonylmethane (MSM) in osteoarthritis pain of the knee: a pilot clinical trial. *Osteoarthritis Cartilage,* Mar;14(3):286-94.

[34] Hwang, J.C., Khine, K.T., Lee, J.C., Boyer, D.S., Francis, B.A. (2015). Methyl-sulfonyl-methane (MSM)-induced acute angle closure. *J Glaucoma,* Apr-May;24(4):e28-30.

[35] Zinc. Wikipedia. Retrieved Nov 2 2017 from https://en.wikipedia.org/wiki/Zinc

[36] Age-Related Eye Disease Study Research Group. (2001). A randomized, placebo-controlled, clinical trial of high-dose supplementation with vitamins C and E, beta carotene, and zinc for age-related macular degeneration and vision loss: AREDS report no. 8. *Arch Ophthalmol,* 119(10):1417–1436.

[37] Ibid. Vinetskaia. (1994).

[38] Ibid. Vinetskaia. (1994).

[39] AREDS, AREDS2: (2001, 2006, 2013) Antioxidants & Macular Degeneration. Retrieved on Oct 15 2017 from http://www.naturaleyecare.com/study.asp?s_num=105.

[40] Ibid. Vinetskaia. (1994).

[41] Ibid. Wikipedia. Zinc.

8-9. HERBS

Cineraria Maritima

Cataracts. Cineraria is useful in treating immature cataracts.[1] As an eyedrop cataract treatment, it has been listed in the Ophthalmology Physician's Desk Reference herbal section for nearly 40 years. Studies with animals find that it is effective against cataracts.[2][3] Homeopathic descriptions also mention that it is effective against conjunctivitis and eye inflammation.[4] Because it is a homeopathic remedy, the concentration of herb is so low that there are rarely any negative side effects. If side effects occur, they are minor and clear up quickly after discontinuing.

Coleus Forskohlii

Glaucoma. Coleus is used as an eyedrop to lower intraocular pressure (IOP). Its active ingredient has been used in IOP-lowering drugs,[5] sometimes combined with other known IOP-reducers, such as L-carnosine, some B vitamins, magnesium, and folic acid.[6] One such compound is forskolin, a coleus forskohlii derivative that lowers IOP by reducing flow of fluid into the center of the eye rather than increasing outflow.[7]

Note. Although coleus is not available in the United States in eyedrops form, we have found that, taken orally, it still can help lower eye pressure up to 3–5 points.

Eyebright

Euphrasia officinalis L. has been used for centuries to treat eye irritation. It is thought that the name was given to the plant because of its valuable properties as an eye medicine, which preserved eyesight and so brought gladness into the life of the sufferer.

Inflammation. In the lab, eyebright extracts were found to decrease cytokine inflammatory agent expression. Furthermore, its effectiveness depended upon the solvent used: ethanol and ethyl acetate extracts worked better than heptane extract.[8][9]

Ginkgo Biloba

Ginkgo's beneficial properties come from its flavonoid constituents. Ginkgo contains quercetin, kaempferol, and isorhamnetin, which are known as flavonoid glycosides (meaning that they include a molecule of sugar). This is important because flavonoids such as quercetin are known to be difficult to absorb, but the presence of sugar much improves the bioavailability of quercetin.[10] Even so, the bioavailability is only about 5% of intake.

Ginkgo has been used for many centuries for eye and central nervous system problems. It is a selective cerebrovascular dilator[11] and seems to increase circulation to the back of the eye, as well as increase blood flow to the eye. It is also becoming an increasingly popular adjunct in the treatment of macular degeneration and glaucoma. It has possible benefit for cancer[12] and atherosclerosis,[13] [14] due to its antioxidant capacity and ability to improve blood flow.[15]

Diabetic retinopathy. Ginkgo is associated with reduced bleeding in patients with a diabetes mellitus complication[16] and with improved color vision.[17]

Glaucoma. Ginkgo has possible therapeutic application for the treatment of glaucoma because of its ability to improve ocular blood flow and protect the optic nerve.[18]

Macular degeneration. It may help improve impaired vision due to dry age-related macular degeneration,[19] [20] by reducing oxidative stress on the retinal pigment epithelial cells.[21]

Nervous system. Ginkgo beneficially affects electrochemical, physiological, neurological, and circulatory systems without side effects.[22]

Retina. Ginkgo has a beneficial effect in reducing oxidative stress in the retina.[23]

Related disorders. Ginkgo helps reduce the accumulation of lipids associated with non-alcoholic liver disease[24] and may protect the kidneys from diabetes-related damage and oxidative stress.[25]

Grapeseed Extract

Grapeseed extract contains oligomeric flavonoid antioxidants called proanthocyanidins that are many times stronger than vitamin E and vitamin C. Proanthocyanidins have good free-radical scavenger ability, evidenced by their ability to improve antioxidant status in lab animals, in addition to improving thiol and other biomarker levels as well as memory.[26] They also strengthen capillaries, arteries, and veins, improve circulation, protect against premature cell death in diabetic retinopathy,[27] reduce capillary fragility, and reduce nerve damage in the eye. Grapeseed's flavonoids reduce inflammation and influence platelet release, giving it possible therapeutic value in cardiovascular conditions.[28]

Triphala (Chebulic, Beleric, and Emblic Myrobalans)

Vision health. Triphala is a compound of three dried and powdered fruits with both nourishing and detoxifying properties. Noted for gastrointestinal support, which in turn supports the body's ability to absorb nutrients, it contains many polyphenols, flavonoids, and vitamin C.[29] In addition it is antifungal, protects cells from harmful agents,[30] and is an anti-inflammatory antioxidant.[31]

Computer eyestrain. Triphala is effective in treating the visual problems associated with extended use of computer monitors.[32]

Diabetic retinopathy, wet macular degeneration. It has been found to be useful in reducing inflammation and growth of new blood vessels by inhibiting production of a cytokine which is implicated in diabetic retinopathy and neovascularization in the choroid and retina.[33]

Glaucoma. Triphala been used to lower intraocular pressure via parasympathetic relaxation of the body. Triphala has long been used in Ayurvedic medicine for the treatment of glaucoma.

Pycnogenol

Like grapeseed extract, pycnogenol gets its potent antioxidant capacity from proanthocyanidins. Pycnogenol is derived from French maritime pine tree bark and is known to strengthen blood vessels, improve circulation,[34] [35] [36] [37] reduce capillary fragility, reduce nerve damage in the eye, support healthy DNA function through enhanced antioxidant activity and other potential mechanisms, [38] [39] and it has potent antioxidant action. [40] [41]

Extensive research has demonstrated that these proanthocyanidins are much stronger than either vitamin C or vitamin E. Of particular note is their ability to reduce leakage into the retina by repairing capillaries in the eyes. Because of this capacity, pycnogenol is the leading prescription for diabetic retinopathy in France. Pycnogenol improves visual acuity and the functioning of the retina, especially in cases of retinal damage caused by micro bleeding of the eye capillaries, due to blood sugar imbalances.

Diabetic retinopathy. Pycnogenol was found to improve circulation of tiny capillaries in the retina, reduce swelling in the retina, and improve vision sharpness in patients with early diabetic retinopathy.[42]

Saffron

Saffron is better known as a kitchen spice that lends yellow color and a delicate flavor to many dishes. It can have wonderful results for eye problems. In a recent trial, every participant who took saffron had vision improvements, and the researchers said the aromatic herb "may hold the key to preventing the loss of sight in the elderly."

Cataract. There have also been reports of saffron significantly helping vision in the instance of cataracts.[43] [44]

Macular degeneration. Patients given saffron supplementation showed improved electroretinogram results, indicating improved flicker sensitivity in early macular degeneration, suggesting that improvements may extend beyond the benefits of antioxidant support.[45] [46] Additionally, experimental studies suggest that saffron protects the photoreceptors from oxidative stress.[47]

Vinpocetine

Vinpocetine is an extract derived from periwinkle seeds. It supports healthy circulation, and in that capacity, it is used in Europe to help prevent strokes and enhance memory.

Retinal circulation. It appears to increase retinal circulation. In one study, 100 people with atherosclerosis and eye disorders were given vinpocetine. Eighty-eight responded with increased retinal circulation and improved visual acuity. Vinpocetine enhances oxygen and glucose use in both the brain and the retina by increasing ATP concentration. ATP molecules are the energy carrying molecules located in cells.

Circulation. Vinpocetine inhibits excessive blood clotting, improves red blood cell health, and by relaxing arteries, it inhibits an enzyme that reduces blood flow.[48] Additionally, the relaxing effect normalizes blood pressure.[49] Vinpocetine improves blood supply to the brain.[50] [51]

Retinal disorders. As in the general body, retinal circulation improves, helping to protect the retina from deterioration. Vinpocetine helps protect cell death after retinal ischemia-reperfusion and improve retinal function.[52] [53]

Related disorders. It promotes optimal energy in the brain and increases the brain's use of oxygen and glucose.[54] In clinical studies, vinpocetine has been shown to benefit a wide variety of conditions, including depression, headaches, short-term memory, inner-ear conditions, tinnitus, vertigo, menopausal symptoms, and insomnia.

Also See

Chapter 5, Antioxidants

---

[1] Burdon-Cooper. (1936). Cineraria maritima and the Treatment of Cataract. *Br Med J*, Jan 11;1(3914):85.

[2] Anitha, T.S., Annadurai, T., Thomas, P.A., Geraldine, P. (2011). Prevention of selenite-induced cataractogenesis by an ethanolic extract of Cineraria maritima: an experimental evaluation of the traditional eye medication. *Biol Trace Elem Res*, Oct;143(1):425-36.

[3] Anitha, T.S., Muralidharan, A.R., Annadurai, T., Jesudasan, C.A., Thomas, P.A., et al. (2013). Putative free radical-scavenging activity of an extract of Cineraria maritima in preventing selenite-induced cataractogenesis in Wistar rat pups. *Mol Vis*, Dec 16;19:2551-60.

[4] Cineraria Maritima. Retrieved Jun 15 2018 from https://www.repldradvice.com/homoeopathic/131-cineraria-maritima.html.

[5] Wagh, V.D., Patil, P.N., Surana, S.J., Wagh, K.V. (2012). Forskolin: upcoming antiglaucoma molecule. *J Postgrad Med,* Jul-Sep;58(3):199-202.

[6] Mutolo, M.G., Albanese, G., Rusciano, D., Pescosolido, N. (2016). Oral Administration of Forskolin, Homotaurine, Carnosine, and Folic Acid in Patients with Primary Open Angle Glaucoma: Changes in Intraocular Pressure, Pattern Electroretinogram Amplitude, and Foveal Sensitivity. *J Ocul Pharmacol Ther*, Apr;32(3):178-83.

[7] Caprioli, J., Sears, M., Bausher, L., Gregory, D., Mead, A. (1984). Forskolin lowers intraocular pressure by reducing aqueous inflow. *Invest Opthalmol Vis Sci*, Mar;25(3):268-77.

[8] Paduch, R., Wozniak, A., Niedziela, P., Rejdak, R. (2014). Assessment of eyebright (euphrasia officinalis L.) extract activity in relation to human corneal cells using in vitro tests. *Balkan Med J*, Mar;31(1):29-36.

[9] Isaacs, T. Restore and Maintain Good Eye Health Naturally. Retrieved Feb 10 2018 from http://www.tbyil.com/Restored_Vision_Eye_Health.htm.

[10] Principles of herbal pharmacology. (2013). In Bone, K. and Mills, S. (Eds.), *Principles and Practice of Phytotherapy: Modern Herbal Medicine*. St. Louis, Mo: Elsevier Sanders,

[11] Mashayekh, A., Pham, D.L., Yousem, D.M., Dizon, M. Barker, P.B., et al. (2011). Effects of Ginkgo biloba on cerebral blood flow assessed by quantitative MR perfusion imaging: a pilot study. *Neuroradiology*, Mar;53(3):185-191.

[12] Feng, X., Zhang, L., Zhu, H. (2009). Comparative anticancer and antioxidant activities of different ingredients of Ginkgo biloba extract (EGb 761). *Planta Med*, Jun;75(8):792-6.

[13] Ou, H.C., Lee, W.J., Lee. I.T., Chiu, T.H., Tsai, K.L., et a;/ (2009). Ginkgo biloba extract attenuates oxLDL-induced oxidative functional damages in endothelial cells. *J Appl Physiol*, May;106:1674–85.

[14]Wu, Y.Z., Li, S.Q., Zu, X.G., Du, J., Wang, F.F. (2008). Ginkgo biloba extract improves coronary artery circulation in patients with coronary artery disease: contribution of plasma nitric oxide and endothelin-1. *Phytother Res*, Jun;22(6):734-9.

[15]Wu, Y., Li, S., Cui, W., Zu, X., Du, J., Wang, F. (2008). Ginkgo biloba extract improves coronary blood flow in healthy elderly adults: role of endothelium-dependent vasodilation. *Phytomedicine*, Mar;15(3):164-9.

[16]Huang, S.Y., Jeng, C., Kao, S.C., Yu, J.J., Liu, D.Z., (2004). Improved haemorrheological properties by Ginkgo biloba extract (Egb 761) in type 2 diabetes mellitus complicated with retinopathy. *Clin Nutr*, Aug;23(4):615-21.

[17]Lanthony, P., Cosson, J.P., (1988). Evolution of color vision in diabetic retinopathy treated by extract of Ginkgo biloba. *J Ophthalmol*, 11:671–74.

[18]Chung, H.S., Harris, A., Kristinsson, J.K., Ciulla, T.A., Kagemann, C., et al. (1999). Ginkgo biloba extract increases ocular blood flow velocity. *J Ocul Pharmacol Ther*, Jun;15:233–40.

[19]Fies, P., Dienel, A. (2002). Ginkgo extract in impaired vision--treatment with special extract EGb 761 of impaired vision due to dry senile macular degeneration. *Wien Med Wochenschr,*2002;152(15-16):423-6.

[20]Lebuisson, D.A., Leroy, L., Rigal, G. (1986). Treatment of senile macular degeneration with Ginkgo biloba extract. A preliminary double-blind drug vs. placebo study. *Presse Med*, Sep 25;15(31):1556-8.

[21]Oh, J.H., Oh, J., Togloom, A., Kim, S.W., Huh, K. (2013). Effects of Ginkgo biloba Extract on Cultured Human Retinal Pigment Epithelial Cells under Chemical Hypoxia. *Curr Eye Res*, Oct;38(10): 1072–1082.

[22]Diamond, B.J., Shiflett, S.C., Feiwel, N., Matheis, R.J., Noskin, O., et al. (2000). Ginkgo biloba extract: mechanisms and clinical indications. *Arch Phys Med Rehabil*, May;81(5):668-78.

[23]Droy-Lefaix, M.T., Cluzel, J., Menerath, J.M., Bonhomme, B., Doly, M. (1995). Antioxidant effect of a Ginkgo biloba extract (EGb 761) on the retina. *Antint J Tissue React,*1995;17(3):93-100.

[24] Wei, T., Xiong, F.F., Wang, S., Wang, K., Zhang, Y., et al. (2014). Flavonoid ingredients of *Ginkgo biloba* leaf extract regulate lipid metabolism through Sp1-mediated carnitine palmitoyltranferase 1A up-regulation. *J Biomed Sci*, Sep 3;21(1):87.

[25]Welt, K., Weiss, J., Martin, R., Hermsdorf, T., Drews, S., et al. (2007). Ginkgo biloba extract protects rat kidney from diabetic and hypoxic damage. *Phytomedicine*, Feb;14(2-3):196-203.

[26] Balu, M., Sangeetha, P., Murali, G., Panneerselvam, C. (2005). Age-related oxidative protein damages in central nervous system of rats: modulatory role of grape seed extract. *Int J Dev Neurosci*, Oct;23(6):501-7.

[27]Ren, X., Lu, H., Wang, N., Zhang, C., Ji, Y., et al. (2017). Thioredoxin is implicated in the anti apoptotic effects of grapeseed proanthocyanidin extract during hyperglycemia. *Mol Med Rep*, Nov;16(5):7731-7737.

[28]Vitseva, O., Varghese, S., Chakrabarti, S., Folts, J.D., Fredman, J.E. (2005). Grape seed and skin extracts inhibit platelet function and release of reactive oxygen intermediates. *J Cardiovasc Pharmacol*, Oct;46(4):445-51.

[29] Tarasiuk, A., Mosinska, P., Fichna, J. (2018). Triphala: current applications and new perspectives on the treatment of functional gastrointestinal disorders. *Chin Med*, Jul 18;13:39.

[30] Ibid. Tarasiuk. (2018).

[31] Peterson, C.T., Denniston, K., Chopra, D. (2017). Therapeutic Uses of Triphala in Ayurvedic Medicine. *J Altern Complement Med*, Aug:23(8):607-614.

[32] Gangamma, M.P., Poonam, Rajagopala, M. (2010). A clinical study on "Computer vision syndrome" and its management with Triphala eye drops and Saptamrita Lauha. *Ayu*, Apr;31(2):236-9.

[33] Shanmuganathan, S., Angayarkanni, N. (2018). Chebulagic acid, Chebulinic acid and Gallic acid, the active principles of Triphala, inhibit TNFalpha induced pro-angiogenic and pro-inflammatory activites in retinal capillary endothelial cells by inhibiting p38, ERK and NRkB phosphorylation. *Vascul Pharmacol*, Sep;108:23-35.

[34]Sime, S., Reeve, V.E. (2004). Protection from inflammation, immunosuppression and carcinogenesis induced by UV radiation in mice by topical Pycnogenol. *PhotochemPhotobiol*, Feb;79(2):193-8.

[35] Pneng, Y.J., Lee, C.H., Wang, C.C., Salter, D.M., Lee, H.S. (2012). Pycnogenol attenuates the inflammatory and nitrosative stress on joint inflammation induced by urate crystals. *Free Radic Biol Med*, Feb 15;52(4):765-74.

[36] Grimm, T., Chovanova, A., Muchova, J., Sumegova, K., Liptakova, A., et al. (2006). Inhibition of NF-kappaB activation and MMP-9 secretion by plasma of human volunteers after ingestion of maritime pine bark extract (Pycnogenol). *J Inflamm (Lond)*, Jan 27;3:1.

[37] Kim, Y.J., Kim, Y.A., Yokozawa, T. (2011). Pycnogenol modulates apoptosis by suppressing oxidative stress and inflammation in high glucose-treated renal tubular cells. *Food Chem Toxicol*, Sep;49(9):2196-201.

[38] D'Andrea, G. (2010). Pycnogenol: a blend of procyanidins with multifaceted therapeutic applications? Fitoterapia, Oct;81(7):724-36.

[39] Nelson, A.B., Lau, B.H., Ide, N., Rong, Y. (1998). Pycnogenol inhibits macrophage oxidative burst, lipoprotein oxidation, and hydroxyl radical-induced DNA damage. *Drug Dev Ind Pharm*, Feb;24(2):139-44.

[40] Rohdewald, P. (2002). A review of the French maritime pine bark extract (Pycnogenol) a herbal medication with a diverse clinical pharmacology. *Int J Clin Pharmacol Ther*, Apr;40(4):158-68.

[41] Ryan, J., Croft, K., Mori, T., Wesnes, K., Spong, J., et al. (2008). An examination of the effects of the antioxidant Pcynogenol on cognitive performance, serum lipid profile, endocrinological and oxidative stress biomarkets in an elderly population. *J Psychopharmacol,* Jul;22(5):553-62.

[42] Steigerwalt, R., Belcaro, G., Cesarone, M.R., Di Renzo, A., Grossi, M.G., et al. (2009). Pycnogenol improves microcirculation, retinal edema, and visual acuity in early diabetic retinopathy. *J Ocul Pharmacol Ther*, Dec;25(6):537-40.

[43] Makri, O.E., Ferlemi, A.V., Lamari, F.N., Georgakopoulos, C.D. (2013). Saffron administration prevents selenite-induced cataractogenesis. *Mol Vis,* May 30;19:1188-97.

[44] Balmani, F., Bathaie, S.Z., Aldavood, S.J., Ghahghaei, A. (2016). Inhibitory Effect of Crocin(s) on Lens alpha-Crystallin Glycation and Aggregation Results in the Decrease of the Risk of Diabetic Cataract. *Molecules,* Jan 26;21(2):143.

[45] Falsini, B., Piccardi, M., Minnella, A., Savastano, C., Capoluongo, E. et al. (2010). Influence of saffron supplementation on retinal flicker sensitivity in early age-related macular degeneration, *Invest Ophthalmol Vis Sci,* Dec;51(12):6118-24.

[46] Marangoni, D., Falsini, B., Piccardi, M., Ambrosio, L., Minnella, A.M. (2013). Functional effect of Saffron supplementation and risk genotypes in early age-related macular degeneration: a preliminary report, *J Transl Med*, Sep 25;11:228.

[47] Bisti, S., Maccarone, R., Falsini, B. (2014). Saffron and retina: neuroprotection and pharmacokinetics. *Vis Neurosci,* Sep;31(4-5):355-61.

[48] Feher, G., Koltai, K., Kesmarky, G., Horvath, B., Toth, K., et al. (2009). Effect of parenteral or oral vinpocetine on the hemorheological parameters of patients with chronic cerebrovascular diseases. *Phytomedicine*, Mar;16(2-3):111-7.

[49] Bagoly, E., Feher, G., Szapary, L. (2007). The role of vinpocetine in the treatment of cerebrovascular diseases based in human studies. *Orv Hetil,* Jul 22;148(29):1353-8.

[50] Ibid. Ryan. (2008).

[51] Horvath, S. (2001). The use of vinpocetine in chronic disorders caused by cerebral hypoperfusion. *Orv Hetil,* Feb 25;142(8):383-9.

[52] Nivison-Smith, L., O'Brien, B.J., Truong, M., Guo, C.X., Kalloniatis, M., et al. (2015). Vinpocetine modulates metabolic activity and function during retinal ischemia. *Am J Physiol Cell Physiol*, May 1;308(9):C737-49.

[53] Nivison-Smith, Khoo, P., Acosta, M.L., Kalloniatis, M. (2017). Pre-treatment with vinpocetine protects against retinal ischemia. *Exp Eye Res,* Jan;154:126-138.

[54] Hadjiev, D. (2003). Asymptomatic ischemic cerebrovascular disorders and neuroprotection with vinpocetine. *Ideggyogy Sz,* May 20;56(5-6):166-72.

9-1. TRADITIONAL CHINESE MEDICINE

The human body is a complex, organic unit. Its tissues and organs are interrelated and mutually dependent. Therefore, as the optical organ of the body, the health of the eyes can influence and be influenced by any and every other organ in the body. Traditional Chinese Medicine (TCM) has been successful in treating a wide range of visual conditions, including glaucoma, cataracts, macular degeneration, optic neuritis, and optic atrophy. The Western and Eastern medical approaches to eye health vary in a fundamental way.

Western Medicine Approach

Eye disease is defined on the basis of how "x" causes "y." Western medicine assigns a specific diagnosis to define the underlying pathology. Once this diagnosis is made, the treatment and medication given are often the same for patients with similar diagnoses, regardless of differing symptoms. This approach can be very effective for acute conditions, but often falls short for ongoing chronic conditions where the cause or causes of the symptoms are elusive.

Chinese Medicine Approach

Every individual is viewed as unique. Chinese medicine looks for patterns of disharmony to see the relationship between "x" and "y." Healing depends on how they are interrelated. Treatment is based on the pattern of symptoms and meridian imbalances. While Western medicine treats the headache symptom, Chinese medicine treats the imbalance in the body that causes the headache. Western medicine offers the same or similar treatment for a particular symptom, while TCM has many different treatments for the same symptom.

According to Traditional Chinese Medicine, all diseases involving the eye are closely related to the Liver (meridian). It is also understood that the eye is nourished by all of the internal organs in the body. An imbalance in any of the internal organs may lead to eye disease.[1]

The Modern History of Acupuncture

The first records of acupuncture were compiled in mainland China between 300 BC and 100 BC. Relatively recent archeological findings, however, suggest that acupuncture may have been around for at least the last five thousand years. Treatment methods have evolved over the last century from other cultures, including Japan, Thailand, France, and the United States.

Acupuncture and Chinese medicine have held an elite position in medicine within China for centuries. Health was so valued in China that the classical physician was only paid as long as everyone in the family maintained good health. If the head of a family became ill, it was the physician's duty to also support the family until the illness had passed. Quite a bit more responsibility than today's modern physicians and practitioners carry!

Traditional Chinese Medicine coexists equally with modern Western medicine in China; hospitals offer both modalities. The traditions of classical acupuncture in China had been maintained through centuries of political turmoil. Mao Tse-Tung found it was politically expedient to establish five TCM universities.[2] The government compiled lists of families of classical practitioners and their knowledge of Chinese medicine. Texts were written, and TCM courses of study were created. Today, 83% of Chinese patients have used TCM.[3]

In the U.S., the National Certification Commission for Acupuncture and Oriental Medicine (NCCAOM) was established in 1982 to validate entry-level competency in acupuncture. Its certification is accepted by 47 states for licensing. In addition, each state of the U.S. currently has its own licensing process.

Acupuncture Gains Popularity in the United States

Interest in acupuncture first surged in the United States after 1972, following a trip to China by President Nixon to establish political ties with Mao. James Reston, an accompanying journalist, wrote about his experiences in China. When he had a flare-up of appendicitis, Chinese doctors performed surgery using an epidural. He received acupuncture the next day for severe pain, and later he wrote extensively about acupuncture. Western media thought he'd received acupuncture in lieu of anesthesia.[4] Nonetheless, the event raised interest, not only with Western physicians, but also with the people who read about it.

More recently, Western physicians have shown increasing interest in those aspects of acupuncture that involve anesthesia, nausea relief, and pain control. There have been increasing amounts of research investigating the effects of acupuncture in treating a wide variety of human problems, ranging from infertility to eye disease. Acupuncture is becoming more widely accepted as a form of medicine; it is being utilized in hospitals and rehabilitation centers and administered by tens of thousands of independent practitioners nationwide.

Traditional Chinese Medicine

Acupuncture

Acupuncture is part of the complete and comprehensive system of Chinese medicine, which also includes Chinese herbal medicine, qigong, moxibustion, cupping, and tui na massage.

It works by adjusting and regulating "qi-energy," commonly referred to as "qi." Qi, pronounced "chee," is typically translated to mean the life force or vital-energy that flows through all things in the universe. Qi flows through the body's 20 main, but invisible, distribution channels or "meridians." There are 71 meridians altogether, though most acupuncturists focus on about 20 meridians in determining their treatment strategies. Twelve of these channels are internally connected with specific organs, such as Liver, Lungs, Heart, Kidneys, and Spleen. There are also eight "extra channels" throughout the body.

Millennia of trial and error, accompanied by meticulous observation, allowed the Chinese to accurately map out the locations of these channels. Each channel has energy nodes or neurovascular junctions called "acupoints," where the energy is concentrated and can be more easily accessed and stimulated. Additionally, the hundreds of acupuncture points (along the vessels) each have a specific regulatory function within the body.

When the qi, blood, and other fluids become blocked, and cease to flow smoothly through meridian channels, pain and degeneration manifest over time. By stimulating the blocked points, acupuncture can unblock stagnation in the meridians and regulate "flow," which helps to restore and preserve healthy function throughout the body. Acupuncture helps regulate excess and deficient organ systems and strengthen isolated weaknesses. The best way to understand the benefits of acupuncture is by thinking of each body system as an instrument in an orchestra. If one instrument is playing out of time or tune, it affects the entire performance. By adjusting flow, acupuncture helps all organ systems act together harmoniously.

Acupuncture needles are so thin that you can fit at least eight of them into the head of a hypodermic needle, which means that acupuncture treatments are generally painless. These hair-thin acupuncture needles are inserted into acupuncture points, adjusting the flow of energy through the various channels of your body. By promoting qi to flow through congested meridians involved, the body can restore its proper function and maintain a healthy, balanced state.

Acupuncture is safe and without any serious side effect. This is one of the reasons for its widespread acceptance. The very thin stainless-steel needles are pre-sterilized and disposed of after each treatment. Acupuncture has been used by millions of Americans and is recognized by the National Institutes of Health (NIH) and the Food and Drug Administration (FDA). The FDA regulates acupuncture needles as medical devices and rates them as "safe and effective." The National Institutes of Health study of acupuncture concluded:

> "While it is often thought that there is substantial research evidence to support conventional medical practices, this is frequently not the case. This does not mean that these treatments are ineffective. The data in support of acupuncture are as strong as those for many accepted Western medical therapies. One of the advantages of acupuncture is that the incidence of adverse effects is substantially lower than that of many drugs, surgeries, or other accepted medical procedures used for the same conditions."[5]

Moxibustion

Moxibustion is an acupuncture technique of heat therapy using tiny pieces of processed dried mugwort that are burned on top of a thin layer of cream on the skin. The heat from the moxa brings blood, qi, and warmth to the area being treated.

Cupping

Cupping involves putting a small glass or plastic cup on the skin with suction. This is done in order to increase the flow of qi, blood, and fluids in the treated area and is used for many conditions such as pain reduction, migraines, and nervous system imbalances.

Herbal Medicine

Herbal medicine is based on restoring balance to energy flow through the body, by means of traditional herbal decoctions.

Qigong

Qigong is a series of body postures and movement, breathing, and meditation for health, healing, and increased vitality. It is over 3,000 years old and is the basis for both acupuncture and martial arts. Qi is vital life force. Gong (pronounced "gung") means accomplishment, or skill, that is cultivated through steady practice. Together, qigong (chi kung) means cultivating energy.

Tui Na

Tui na is a therapeutic form of massage over 2,000 years old that uses a rocking motion to help balance out meridian imbalances. Rhythmic compression techniques along different meridians help to establish harmonious flow of qi throughout the body and bring the body back into balance.

---

[1] The English-Chinese Encyclopedia of Practical Traditional Chinese Medicine, Volume 17, Ophthalmology, p. 8-10. Beijing, China: Higher Education Press.

[2] Wikipedia. Traditional Chinese Medicine. Retrieved Jun 8 2018 from https://en.wikipedia.org/wiki/Traditional_Chinese_medicine.

[3] McQuade, J.L., Meng, Z., Chen, Z., Wei, Q., Zhang, Y., et al. (2012). Utilization of and Attitudes towards Traditional Chinese MedicineTherapies in a Chinese Cancer Hospital: A Survey of Patientsand Physicians.*Evid Based Complement Alternat Med,* 2012:504507.

[4] ScienceBasedMedicine. James Reston's Appendectomy. Retrieved Jun 8 2018 from https://sciencebasedmedicine.org/acupuncture-anesthesia-a-proclamation-of-chairman-mao-part-i/.

[5] National Institutes of Health. (1997). Acupuncture. Retrieved Jun 7 2018 from https://consensus.nih.gov/1997/1997acupuncture107html.htm.

9-2. TCM: DISEASE AND FOOD

Life according to Chinese philosophy is all about balance: the perfect balance of yin and yang. It is believed that everything in life is subject to this philosophy that you will see exhibited in nature, often in the form of opposite forces.

Yin energy, for example, is cooling energy; it relates to sunset and nighttime, to rest and repair, and to building blood and fluids. It has "descending" energy (yin energy flows inward and downward), dominates the left side of the body, and embodies qualities of the Mother. As far as foods go, yin is the realm of salty, bitter, and sour. **Yang**, on the other hand, is warming energy; it relates to morning energy, the sunrise, and daytime activity. Yang has "ascending" energy (energy that rises outward and upward), dominates the right side of the body, and embodies qualities of the Father. In terms of foods, yang is associated with both sweet and pungent foods.

All of Traditional Chinese Medicine (TCM) naturally works to balance yin and yang. Whether the purpose is to maintain proper body temperature, correct acid (yang) and alkaline (yin) levels in the tissue and blood, or overall harmony in the body, yin and yang are always at work. When either yin or yang becomes imbalanced, discomfort occurs. If steps are not then taken to address the underlying cause of the imbalance, pain and disease will occur. The type of disease that occurs, and where it occurs in the body, depends on any number of factors in addition to the underlying condition or imbalance, such as genetics and lifestyle choices.

Source of Disease

For example, excess yin reduces the heat in the body, while excess yang increases it. People with excess yin tend toward diseases with a quality of dampness, such as high cholesterol and obesity. People with excess yang can be prone to conditions like arthritis, hypertension, and headaches.

Furthermore, timing of the development of a disease is unknown. It may take weeks, months, several years, and even decades for a disorder to appear. But one thing is certain: it will appear! Acute conditions like stings and accidents may be an exception, but even in the case of sport injuries, an underlying imbalance (sometimes called a "weakness") could very well be in place long before a larger injury occurs. This is why complementary therapies like TCM, diet, exercise, and lifestyle choices, are so crucial. Collectively, they work toward maintaining balance.

The Western medical paradigm is concerned with reducing or eradicating symptoms after a disease has manifested; it relies on pharmacology and surgery to do so. Neither of these therapies addresses the root, or underlying cause, of a disorder. Worse, sometimes both surgery and pharmaceuticals create added imbalances. Although they may be temporary, often there are long-term side effects; this is particularly true of pharmaceutical use over time. Without a strong and comprehensive preventive plan to maintain balance in the body, the underlying imbalances not only remain but also may accumulate over time, resulting in further breakdown. This is especially true when drugs mask the underlying problem and push it deeper into the body.

TCM looks at all issues related to the health of the body from the perspective of a balanced yin and yang. From a dietary standpoint, the key is to balance warming (yang) and cooling (yin) foods. Some foods warm the body, some cool it, some create moisture, some cause dryness, etc. The key is to eat foods that have properties that balance the body and its systems.

Cooling versus Heating Foods

When people are healthy, their body temperature can adjust to temperature changes in their environment with relative ease. But some people are always too hot; they dislike heat and crave cool food and drinks. Others dislike cold and crave warmth, hot drinks, and hot food. In TCM, these people can balance their body's temperature with the help of acupuncture, herbs, and food.

Foods that Increase Heat

In terms of Chinese medicine, foods that cause more heat in the body include the following:

- Red meat and chicken
- Coffee and alcohol
- Spicy food

Foods that Decrease Heat

Cooling foods include the following:

- Vegetables such as cucumber, celery, spinach, bok choy, broccoli, sweet corn, zucchini, radish, lettuce, and eggplant
- Fruits such as apple, cantaloupe, watermelon, tomato, pear, and banana

Consequences of Excess

Here are examples of eating excessive types of foods:

- Excessive eating of cold foods, raw food, salads, and fruit can weaken the Spleen (and Stomach), the meridian affecting digestion and nutrient distribution.
- Excessive consumption of hot-energy and spicy foods (lamb, beef, curry, chili, and hot sauce) causes heat, especially of Stomach and Liver.
- Excessive consumption of greasy/fried foods (deep fried foods, fatty meats, nuts, milk, cheese, cream, and butter) causes phlegm or dampness, which can obstruct Spleen function of transformation and transportation (poor distribution of essential nutrients from food).

Patterns of Imbalance

What we eat affects how we feel, supports heath and balance in the body, and reduces the risk of disease onset. In Chinese medicine, balanced meridians are key; western medicine refers to it as homeostasis. Basically, when we are in balance, we can avoid disease. Being chronically out of balance eventually results in pain and disease.

Meridian balances and imbalances in TCM are related to patterns with names like Liver Yang Rising, Yin Deficiency, and Spleen Dampness. The patterns may be described as follows:

- Too much or too little yin or yang
- Too much or too little functioning of one or more meridians
- Too warm or too cold
- Too moist or too dry
- Not enough qi, the flow of energy
- Movement upward or downward

All of the TCM meridian systems (organs) have patterns that pertain to ocular functioning. Some imbalances stand on their own and are not "types" of yin or yang. Others are too much or too little yin or yang. Following are a few examples along with food considerations.

Deficient Yin

Deficient Liver and Kidney Yin

Major ocular symptoms include cataracts, AMD, Stargardt's, open-angle glaucoma, retinitis pigmentosa, Usher syndrome, dry eye, optic neuritis, and retinal bleeding. Retinal bleeding may be considered more of a Spleen deficiency, heat, or stasis.

Blood Deficiency

Major ocular symptoms include Stargardt disease, floaters, dry eye, retinal vein or artery occlusion, and night blindness. Occlusion may be considered to be more Blood Stasis.

Foods that help build blood include the following:

- **Vegetables**. Alfalfa sprouts, artichoke, avocado, beetroot, cabbage, celery, dandelion leaf, chlorophyll-rich foods, kelp, dark leafy-green vegetables, garlic, fresh ginger, leeks, shiitake mushroom, button mushroom, onions, spinach, watercress, wheatgrass, winter squash and pumpkin, parsnips, black sesame, and spirulina
- **Meats**. Beef, liver (both pork and sheep), bone stock/soup, chicken, oysters, and eggs
- **Grains**. Molasses, barley, corn, bran, rice, oats, sweet rice, and wheat
- **Fruit**. Apple, apricot, avocado, date, fig, grape, and goji berries

Deficient Yang

Deficient Yang (Heat)

Major ocular symptoms include diabetic retinopathy, retinitis pigmentosa, Usher syndrome, choroidal dystrophy, and optic nerve atrophy.

Foods that help tonify yang include the following:

- **Fruits**. Cherries, persimmon, coconut, lemons, raspberries, blackberry, mulberry
- **Vegetables**. Cauliflower, mustard greens, beets, string beans, onion, cabbage, kale, garlic, fresh ginger, chestnuts, soups with onions, garlic, ginger, and leeks
- **Meats**. Chicken and turkey
- **Dairy.** Yogurt and butter
- **Grains.** Barley, wheat, rice, quinoa, amaranth, and sweet brown rice
- **Seeds and nuts**. Pumpkin seeds, walnuts, and millet
- **Legumes.** Tofu, kidney beans, black beans, mung beans, and mung bean sprouts
- **Other**. Seaweeds and micro-algae (especially chlorella and spirulina), coffee

Deficient Kidney Yang

Major ocular symptoms include diabetic retinopathy, Usher syndrome, choroidal dystrophy, optic nerve atrophy, and retinitis pigmentosa. Retinitis pigmentosa may be considered more Lung Deficiency, but may also be Kidney Yang Deficiency.

Excessive Yang

Excessive Yang (Heat)

Major ocular symptoms include wet macular degeneration, diabetic retinopathy, ocular (and regular) migraines, dry eyes, glaucoma, eyestrain, and blurry vision.

Common disorders that may show up in other areas of the body include dry skin, excessive thirst, heat intolerance, nosebleeds, high blood pressure, a rapid pulse, temple headaches, tremors, tinnitus, hearing impairment, rashes, swelling, restlessness, skin eruptions, local inflammation, inflammation in any part of the body, constipation, blood in the urine, and thick yellow or green phlegm, as with a cold or bronchitis.

Foods to help reduce excess yang include the following:

Cooling foods. Simultaneously, decrease your consumption of heating foods down to 10%-15% of the diet for 3-6 months, and check with your TCM practitioner. Increase cooling foods to 85%-90% of the diet. Cooling foods include the following:

- **Vegetables**: cucumber, celery, spinach, bok choy, broccoli, sweet corn, zucchini, radish, lettuce, and eggplant
- **Fruit**: apple, cantaloupe, watermelon, tomato, pear, banana, and apples
- **Fluids.** These should also be cooling, such as vegetable or fruit juices, broths, and herbal teas; room temperature green tea is also permitted. Ideally, beverages should be consumed at room temperature, rather than when cold, as cold foods and beverages disrupt stomach acid, and can further weaken the body.
- **Reduce meat**. Reduce red meat, chicken, coffee, alcohol, and spicy foods, in particular.

Excessive Yin

Excessive Yin (Cool)

Major ocular symptoms include myopia, astigmatism, blurry vision, cataracts, macular degeneration, retinitis pigmentosa, diabetic retinopathy, photophobia, and/or poor night vision.

Other conditions signaling excessive yin are cold intolerance, chill sensations, body pain from cold weather conditions, copious excretions of clear body fluids such as with the onset of cold symptoms, afternoon headaches, dry stools, restlessness, poor sleep, dizziness, diabetes, tuberculosis, hypoglycemia, chronic inflammation, and infection (from viruses, parasites, bacteria, and fungi).

Excessive yin can be caused by overconsumption of rich or denatured foods, which includes all fast food, processed food, and those foods high in fat and sugar. In addition, the consumption of alcohol and coffee contribute, as does smoking, taking synthetic drugs (pharmaceuticals), being overly competitive, and not managing chronic stress.

Blood and tissue also may be lacking in calcium, as well as other cooling minerals and even essential fatty acids (particularly omega-3 fatty acids), which help keep the arteries clean, prevent inflammation, and therefore prevent the buildup of heat.

Recommended foods include the following:

- **Fruits.** Watermelon, blackberry, raspberry, grapes, banana, melons, pear, and persimmon
- **Vegetables.** Beets, string beans, spinach, leafy-green vegetables, asparagus, kuzu, and daily soups
- **Grains.** Quinoa, millet, barley, and amaranth
- **Legumes.** Black beans, mung beans, and kidney beans
- **Seafood.** Crab, anchovies, and sardines
- **Other.** Pine nuts, sprouts, microalgae, tofu, seaweed, chlorella, and spirulina
- **Avoid spicy** and overly warm foods, alcohol, coffee, and black tea

Liver (Sour) Wind

Major ocular symptoms include acute-angle closure glaucoma, open-angle glaucoma (usually not so much unless it is sudden), sudden retinal bleeding, optic neuritis, cataracts (more fluid deficiency and Liver Kidney Yin deficiency), NAION, retinal detachment, occlusions, sudden eye pain, stye, and nystagmus.

Foods that help reduce or extinguish Liver Wind include:

- **Vegetables.** Celery, cucumber, lettuce, watercress, basil, sage, fennel, ginger, anise, oats, black soybean, black sesame seed, mung beans and their sprouts, pine nuts, coconut, tofu, fresh cold-pressed flax oil, lemon, plum, rhubarb root, radish, and chamomile

Foods that worsen Liver Wind:

- Eggs, crabmeat, and buckwheat
- Excessive meat in the diet can also be toxic to the Liver

Deficient Qi

Major ocular symptoms include retinitis pigmentosa, macular degeneration (wet and dry), Usher syndrome, and presbyopia.

Foods that help build "qi" include the following:

- **Grains**. All grains including quinoa, oats, pearl barley, and brown rice
- **Meats**. Chicken and lamb
- **Legumes**. All lentils and legumes, soybeans and tofu
- **Eggs**
- **Fish**
- **Vegetables**. Green beans, leeks, onion, root vegetables, mushrooms, pumpkin, and squash
- **Fruits**. Goji berries, cherries, dates, figs, loganberry, and coconut
- **Other**. Fox nut, ginseng, nutmeg, green tea, jasmine tea, and raspberry leaf tea

Excessive Dampness

Major ocular symptoms include macular degeneration (wet and dry), diabetic retinopathy, macular edema, cystoid macula edema, and central serous retinopathy.

Foods to help reduce excess dampness include the following:

- **Vegetables**. Organic lightly cooked vegetables, corn, celery, watercress, lettuce, turnip, pumpkin, alfalfa sprouts, button mushrooms, radish, turnip, and scallion
- **Grains**. Rye, amaranth, brown rice, barley, and oats
- **Legumes**. Adzuki beans, kidney beans, and lentils
- **Meat**. Small amount of lean organic meat, poultry, and fish
- **Fruit**. Small amount of whole fruits and lemon
- **Other**. Raw honey, all bitter herbs, sesame seeds, pumpkin seeds, sunflower seeds, wild blue-green algae, seaweed, and kelp

Avoid dairy, cold raw foods, cold drinks, wheat (and refined wheat flour) for those that are gluten sensitive, peanuts and peanut butter, avocado, coffee, and alcohol. Avoid overeating.

9-3. THE CHINESE FIVE ELEMENTS

In Chinese medicine, the five-element or five-phase theory can help explain both the basis of disease and specific acupuncture and herbal treatment strategies. The five elements are wood, fire, earth, metal, and water. Each element has a range of traits and foods associated with it. Yin and yang theory is an essential part of all Chinese medicine and the five-element theory, but the five-element theory gives us another approach to look at health, disease, and treatment strategies.

Wood (Sour)

The Wood element is connected to the Liver and Gallbladder meridian systems. The sense organs associated with Wood are the eyes, and you will often read throughout this book that the Liver "opens to the eyes." It is also related to tendon health; its color is green; its developmental stage is birth, and its season is spring. When emotions related to wood are out of balance, the result is often anger and resentment, irritability and depression, or pronounced mood swings.

Wood governs sour foods, and they are recommended when Wood conditions are out of balance.

- Foods include raw and sprouted foods, as well as rye, oats, wheat, avocado, zucchini, string beans, lettuce, green peppers, pickles, lemons, limes, sour apples and plums, rose hips, sauerkraut, mung and lima bean, garbanzo bean, green lentils, and vinegar.

Sour foods have astringent properties and cause contraction of body tissues. As such, they can be helpful for preventing or slowing abnormal leakage of fluids and energy such as retinal bleeding, edema anywhere in the body, ease of bruising, and for drying and firming up tissues.

In Your Diet

If the Liver is out of balance, one should avoid soft dairy and salty foods.

Fire (Bitter)

Fire is connected to the Heart and Small Intestine meridian systems. The Heart meridian "opens to the tongue;" its color is red, and its season is summer. The developmental stage associated with Fire is growth, and when emotions related to fire are out of balance, a person can either experience excessive joy or sadness. The sense organ linked to Fire is the tongue, and the taste is bitter foods.

- From a dietary perspective, bitter foods include alfalfa sprouts, rye, romaine lettuce, and bitter melon. Bitter foods have a cooling effect; they can lower fevers, dry up fluids, reduce dampness, and induce bowel movements. They can also help to clear heat, clean the arteries, and lower blood pressure.
- Other balancing foods include red pepper, beets, tomato, scallion, salads, okra, dandelion, persimmon, cherries, lemon and lime, red lentil, apples, watermelon, sunflower seed, pistachio, corn, and amaranth.

In Your Diet

Helpful herbs include fresh ginger, horseradish, cayenne red pepper, and black pepper.

Limit or avoid chocolate and sugar, as well as iced drinks and ice cream as these hold in heat, contract the stomach, and stop digestion. Limit heavy foods on hot days including meats, eggs, and excess nuts, seeds, and grains.

Earth (Sweet)

The Earth element is connected to the Spleen and Stomach meridian systems. Its color is yellow; its season is late summer, and the developmental stage associated with earth is growth and transformation (both in the physical form and emotionally). The Earth element is also connected to the muscles, and when emotions related to Earth are out of balance, it can be due to over-thinking or pensiveness and excessive worry. The sense organ is the mouth, and its associated taste is for sweet foods.

Sweet foods help expand energy upward and outward in the body, and they have a calming and relaxing effect. Earth energy can help retard acute disease symptoms, soothe aggressive behavior such as anger and impatience, moisten dry conditions of the lungs, and slow down an interactive heart and mind (particularly for those prone to worry and overthinking or pensiveness).

- From a dietary perspective, Earth foods include sweet rice, sweet potato, spinach, squash, carrot, parsnip, cabbage, rutabaga, millet, barley, garbanzo beans, amaranth, molasses, sunflower seeds, pine nuts, chestnuts, pumpkin, yam, tofu, walnuts, rice syrup, cherries, pineapple, strawberries, fig, papaya, orange, apricots, and cantaloupe.

In Your Diet

Limit or avoid meat. Food should be moderately cooked and well chewed. Avoid late night and overeating. Butter is the only recommended dairy product.

Metal (Pungent)

Metal is connected to the Lung and Large Intestine meridian systems. In terms of organ connections, Metal "opens to the Lungs." Its color is white; its season is autumn, and its developmental stage is harvest. When emotions related to Metal are out of balance, the experience is sadness and/or grief. Metal is also connected with skin and hair, and its associated sense organ is the nose; its taste is for pungent foods.

Pungent and salty foods strongly move energy inward and downward and help with cleansing and protection against colds. Health conditions include heat congestion in the lungs; symptoms include dry cough, painful sore throat, shortness of breath, as well as yellow-green sputum with pus, and yellow nasal discharge.

- From a dietary perspective, pungent foods to eat include sourdough bread, cucumber, broccoli, celery, onion, mustard greens, bok choy, seaweeds, cauliflower, cabbage, radish, asparagus, adzuki beans, navy and soybeans, cheese, sauerkraut, almonds, grapefruit, papaya, grapes, pear, peach, persimmon, pumpkin, apricot, plums, rose hip teas, watercress, and cantaloupe.

In Your Diet

Useful herbs for cooking include kuzu root, chickweed, and horehound leaf. From a dietary perspective, the diet should include primarily cooked foods, and limit cooling or mucous forming foods such as citrus fruits, milk, salt, and other dairy products. Limit or avoid eggs. In general, cook with less water, and cook at a lower heat for longer periods of time. Crockpots work well.

Water (Salty)

Water is connected to the Kidney and Bladder meridians. Water "opens to the ears." Its color is blue/black; its season is winter, and its developmental stage is storing (as in building reserves). When emotions related to Water are out of balance, a person has high amounts of fear. The taste is for salty food.

Common symptoms of Kidney imbalance include any urinary, sexual, and reproductive imbalances, hearing loss, bone problems (especially related to knee and lower back), teeth problems, premature aging, hair loss, and premature graying of hair.

Salty and bitter foods are appropriate for winter, as they promote "sinking in," and centering; they also cool the exterior of the body, deepening body heat.

- Salty foods include soy sauce, miso, millet, barley, and seaweeds. Other related foods include buckwheat, kale, mushrooms, string beans, water chestnut, black sesame seeds, walnut, raspberry, mulberry, pomegranate, watermelon and other melons, beans (kidney, adzuki, pinto and black), tofu, almonds, clarified butter (ghee), royal jelly and bee pollen, chlorella, sardines, crab, and eggs.

In Your Diet

Helpful herbs include marshmallow root, asparagus root, rehmannia root, and aloe vera gel. Use salt with moderation as it can cause coldness and weaken the kidneys, bladder, and heart. Also, limit or avoid cheese.

General Note

If a meridian is in excess, then you should avoid the foods associated with that meridian until the meridian is back in balance. This would be best discussed with your acupuncturist/herbalist.

9-4. ACUPUNCTURE

From a Western medical standpoint, acupuncture increases blood flow to the eyes. We know this because research using ocular Doppler imaging and ultrasound have shown that certain acupuncture points directly increase blood flow to the eye.[1]

Many ophthalmic conditions progress because of impaired blood and energy flow, which results in reducing the flow of oxygen and vital nutrients to the eyes. Impaired circulation to the eyes also results in toxic accumulation of metabolic ocular waste products, which are waste products produced by the eye in its normal day-to-day functioning.

Another way acupuncture improves vision is by stimulating the ocular nerve cells (retina,[2] ganglia, optic nerve[3], etc.). Nerve cells need ongoing nourishment to function optimally, including B vitamins, vitamins C, E, zinc, copper, selenium, trace minerals, and essential fatty acids.[4]

Acupuncture can arouse dormant nerve cells that often result in visual acuity improvement. The amount of improvement in vision that patients will see is directly related to the ratio of dormant-to-dead ocular nerve cells. The more dormant cells a person has, the greater the improvement. A small or no gain may indicate that there is relatively little or no cell dormancy. Acupuncture can also help improve vision related to nearsightedness and farsightedness by strengthening overall circulation and the flow of energy to the muscles of the eyes.

This concept has been critical in terms of explaining and demystifying the improvement that people have with acupuncture treatment. Until recently, it was believed that non-functional ocular nerve cells were dead, and that no improvement in vision was possible simply because dead nerve tissue is permanently inactive. Now that we know that these cells can lie dormant,[5] it has become easy to explain how some vision can be restored.

Five Elements and Eye Symptoms

Wood	Fire	Earth	Metal	Water
Liver / Gallbladder	Heart/ Small Intestine	Spleen/ Stomach	Lung/ Large Intestine	Kidney/ Bladder
Sudden, rapid onset, common in acute eye diseases	Swelling, inflammation, redness, common in acute eye diseases	Mucus, edema, secretions, slow onset	Dryness, itching, redness	Slow onset, sharp pain, chronic degenerative vision loss

The TCM five element theory organizes health and overall system balance into five elements: Wood, Fire, Earth, Metal, and Water. Each element corresponds to major TCM meridian systems, or organs: the Liver, Heart, Spleen, Lung, and Kidneys.

Each organ has a series of sensory and functional relationships in the body that are specifically related to our overall health; imbalances help the practitioner determine treatment strategies.

Function	Liver	Heart	Spleen	Lung	Kidney
System	Vision	Tongue/Circulation	Mouth/Digestion	Nose/Immune	Ears/Endocrine
Tissue	Tendons	Vessels	Muscles	Skin	Bones
Color	Green	Red	Yellow	White	Blue/Black
Season	Spring	Summer	Late Sumer	Autumn	Winter
Emotion	Anger	Joy	Worry/Pensiveness	Grief/ Sadness	Fear
Taste	Sour	Bitter	Sweet	Pungent	Bitter
Direction	East	South	Center	West	North
Odor	Rancid	Scorched	Fragrant	Rotten	Putrid

Element	TCM Organs	Color	Eye Structure	Excess Emotion	Balanced Emotion
Wood	Liver/ Gallbladder	Blue-Green	Iris, eye muscles and cornea	Anger/ Resentment	Compassion/ Tranquility
Fire	Heart/ Small Intestine	Red	Inner Canthus	Chaos/ Overexcitement/ Overstimulation	Ritual/ Proprietary
Earth	Spleen/ Pancreas/ Stomach	Yellow	Spleen-top eyelid Stomach-lower eyelid Aqueous Fluid	Worry/ Obsession	Faith/ Comfort
Metal	Lung/ Large Intestine	White	Sclera and cornea	Grief/ Melancholy/ Depression	Rectify/ Resolve
Water	Kidney/ Bladder	Black	Pupil, lens, macula, retina	Terror/ Flight	Resolution/ Calm

Using Pattern Discrimination

TCM bases treatment protocols on pattern discrimination, rather than on symptoms or test results only. For example, for glaucoma patients there are specific eyedrops to lower eye pressure, even though many people with glaucoma may have normal and even low IOP, yet they may be treated the same way as patients with elevated tension.

Chinese medicine practitioners view each person as an individual. While the symptoms may be the same, the treatment protocol may vary significantly, based on a number of factors deemed important to the diagnosis, which include the following:

- Taking the patient's pulse
- Viewing his/her tongue
- Looking at the patient (shape, smell, temperament, and other visible indicators)
- Asking the patient about their symptoms

Glaucoma is a good example. Liver Yang Rising is the most common imbalance pattern. But because all meridians can affect eye health, the actual TCM treatment for glaucoma can vary dramatically based on which meridians are out of balance.

TCM Patterns

Liver Patterns

Liver Yin Deficiency. The liver in Chinese medicine "opens to the eyes," and imbalances to the Liver meridian often result in eye issues.

> **Major ocular symptoms** include myopia, astigmatism, AMD, retinitis pigmentosa, presbyopia, dry eyes, floaters, glaucoma, Stargardt's, cataracts, red and dry eyes, bloodshot eyes, poor night vision, and other symptoms such as dry skin and dry stool.

> **Treatment principles**. Nourish Liver Yin and Blood. Liver Yin deficiency can result in the blockage of nourishment and blood to the eyes.

Liver Yin Deficiency with Heat. The yin (cooling) should be in balance with the yang (heat) in the body. When the yin is deficient and cannot hold the yang down, this results in heat rising.

> **Major ocular symptoms** include glaucoma, myopia, AMD, astigmatism, retinitis pigmentosa, Stargardt disease, photophobia, red and dry eyes, bloodshot eyes, poor night vision, blurry vision, headaches, as well as other symptoms such as dry stool, scanty urine, night sweats, malar flush and afternoon hot flashes, restlessness, and poor sleep.

> **Treatment principles**. Nourish Liver Yin and Blood

Liver Qi Congestion. This pattern is the blockage of the free flow of energy and blood.

Major ocular symptoms include eyestrain headaches, glaucoma (early stage, open-angle), and myopia, as well as other symptoms such as irritability, sighing, flank pain/distention, depression/mood swings, belching, and abdominal distention.

Treatment principles. Regulate Liver Qi.

Liver Wind/Liver Yang Rising. This pattern results when the yin energy of the liver and the kidney becomes extremely depleted, the Liver Yang energy becomes erratic, undernourished, and imbalanced. This can also result in heat rising.

Major ocular symptoms include glaucoma, wet or dry AMD, eyestrain or temple headaches, blurry vision, as well as other symptoms such as tinnitus, hearing impairment, tremors, tics, hypertension, and restlessness.

Treatment principles. Nourish the Liver and Kidney Yin to help control the rise of the heat due to Liver Yang rising, and unblock the Liver Qi congestion to allow the free flow of energy and blood.

Liver Blood Deficiency. This pattern reflects the lack of proper amount of blood and essential fluids in the body.

Major ocular symptoms include floaters, red and dry eyes, cataracts, presbyopia, photophobia, poor night vision, blurry vision, as well as other symptoms such as dizziness, soft or brittle nails, dry skin, and muscle twitches.

Treatment principles. Nourish Liver Blood, and nourish Kidney and Liver Yin

Liver Qi and Blood Stagnation with Lung Qi Stagnation. This pattern is the blockage of the free flow of qi and blood in the body, the stagnation of the ease of flow of blood, and a reduction in the free flow of Liver energy as well as a lack of Lung energy.

Major ocular symptoms include AMD, retinitis pigmentosa, glaucoma, myopia, peri-orbital edema, as well as other symptoms such as headaches, irritability, sighing, flank pain/distension, depression/mood swings, belching, abdominal distention, prone to catch colds, and quiet voice or "soft spoken."

Treatment principles. Regulate the liver, move Qi and Blood, nourish the Lungs, and strengthen the Lung Qi.

Gallbladder Patterns

Disharmony between the Gallbladder and Stomach with Phlegm-Heat. This pattern draws on the fact that the gallbladder secretes bile fluids required to digest and metabolize fats and oils. It also provides energy for muscular strength and vitality. Imbalances in the gallbladder reduce the body's ability to digest food and can create excess heat in the body due to the build-up of phlegm.

Major ocular symptoms include glaucoma, diabetic retinopathy, as well as other symptoms such as lack of initiative, timidity, edema in the extremities, tight chest, palpitations, and anxiety.

Treatment principles. Warm the Gallbladder and transform dampness, clear heat.

Kidney Patterns

Kidney Yin Deficiency. This pattern arises from the reduction of essential fluids in the body, which keeps the body moist and balances yang (heat).

Major ocular symptoms include dry AMD, myopia, astigmatism, cataracts, dry eyes, floaters, photophobia, as well as other symptoms such as dry mouth with thirst (especially at night), scanty urine, dizziness, and tinnitus.

Treatment principles. Nourish Kidney and Liver Yin

Kidney Yin Deficiency with Heat. Heat rising results from deficient essential fluids in the body.

Major ocular symptoms include open-angle glaucoma, dry AMD, myopia, astigmatism, cataracts, photophobia, dry eyes, itchy eyes, and other symptoms such as night sweats, dry mouth with thirst (especially at night), scanty urine, dizziness, and tinnitus.

Treatment principles. Nourish Kidney and Liver Yin, clear heat, and moisten dryness.

Kidney Yin, Liver Blood, and Heart Yin Deficiency. This pattern is a deficiency in the essential fluids and blood in the body.

Major ocular symptoms include myopia, astigmatism, as well as symptoms such as restlessness, palpitations, poor memory, night sweats, dry mouth with thirst (especially at night), scanty urine, dizziness, and tinnitus.

Treatment principles. Nourish Kidney and Heart Yin, nourish Liver Blood, calm spirit.

Kidney Yang Weakness. This is a deficiency in the heat and daytime energy in the Kidney meridian.

Major ocular symptoms include retinitis pigmentosa, AMD, diabetic retinopathy, glaucoma, poor night vision, and other symptoms such as cold and sore knees, lower back pain, frequent and clear urination, decreased sexual function, and cold extremities.

Treatment principles. Strengthen the Kidney Qi and warm yang.

Spleen and Stomach Patterns

Spleen and Stomach Weakness with Damp Accumulation. This pattern results in a lessening of the body's ability to digest and breakdown food effectively due to qi weakness and build-up of phlegm in the body.

Major ocular symptoms include wet AMD, diabetic retinopathy, night blindness, other symptoms such as fatigue (especially after eating), reduced appetite, pale complexion, loose stools, heavy limbs, dizziness, abdominal distention/fullness, and edema.

Treatment principles. Strengthen the Spleen and Stomach, transform damp accumulation, and regulate qi.

Central (Spleen) Qi Weakness. This results in a lessening of the body's ability to digest and breakdown food effectively due to qi weakness.

Major ocular symptoms include retinitis pigmentosa, choroidal dystrophy, night blindness, diabetic retinopathy, AMD, Usher syndrome, and other symptoms such as fatigue (especially after eating), reduced appetite, pale complexion, loose stools, heavy limbs, dizziness, and abdominal distention/fullness.

Treatment principles. Raise the central qi, and strengthen the Spleen Qi.

Spleen Qi Weakness and Heart Blood Deficiency. This pattern affects the body's ability to digest food and poor circulation of blood in the body.

Major ocular symptoms include wet AMD, diabetic retinopathy, and other symptoms such as bleeding under the skin (purpura), uterine bleeding, bruising easily, anxiety, poor sleep, and fatigue.

Treatment principles. Strengthen the Spleen Qi, nourish the Heart Yin and Blood, and calm the mind.

Heart and Liver Blood Stagnation Patterns

Blood Stagnation. This pattern affects the free flow of blood throughout the body, resulting in reduced nourishment to the organs and tissues.

Major ocular symptoms include glaucoma, dry AMD, and other symptoms such as sharp localized pain, angina, palpitations, insomnia, and nightmares.

Treatment principles. Move qi and blood in the chest and head areas.

Chinese Herbal Patent Formulas

Chinese herbal patent formulas are based on the pattern differentiation (as well as the acupuncture point strategy). Here are common patent formulas by eye condition:

Wet Macular Degeneration

- Yunnan paiyao or sanqi powder (dissolve 2g in water, two times per day)
- Ming mu di huang tang (bright eye tea)
- Xiao yao san

Dry Macular Degeneration

- Ming mu di huang tang (bright eye tea)
- Xiao yao san

Retinitis Pigmentosa

- Ming mu di huang wan

Diabetic Retinopathy

- You gui wan (restore the right decoction) helps strengthen the Kidney Yang
- Er chan tang drains mucus and dampness and opens/clears yang passage to the eyes
- Wen dan tang (warm the gallbladder decoction) to nourish Kidney and Liver Yin and to brighten the eyes

Retinal Vein and Artery Occlusion

- Ming mu di huang wan
- Qi ju di huang wan
- Preserve vistas pill
- Xiao yao san
- Shu gan tang + er chen tang
- Wen dan tang
- Modified xuefu zhuyu tang
- Gui pi tan

Open-Angle Glaucoma

- Wen dan tang (warm the gallbladder decoction) to nourish Kidney and Liver Yin, and to brighten the eyes
- Qi ju di huang wan (rehmania 6 plus chrysanthemum and lycii) to nourish kidney and Liver Blood and yin
- Xiao yao san
- Shu gan tang

Cataracts

- Shi hy ye guang wan
- Ming mu di huang wan (to brighten the eyes) nourishes the liver, enriches the kidneys, and improves vision.
- Shi hu ye guang wan
- Qi ju di huang wan

Myopia, Farsightedness, and Presbyopia

- Ba zhen tang to strengthen qi and nourish blood

Herbal recommendations will vary, based on your acupuncturist intake evaluation.

Acupuncture Methods

Repeated experience in using certain acupuncture points on specific areas of the body in similar cases provides the practitioner with many tried and proven acupuncture treatment protocols. The modern-day creation of TCM was geared toward establishing these protocols, wherein selected acupuncture points are used to treat specific conditions. Research studies have helped confirm efficacy that can result in improved blood flow to the retina, stimulate dormant ocular nerve cells, and activate the visual cortex of the brain.

In TCM, once the pattern(s) of imbalances related to the meridians are determined from the acupuncturist's intake and evaluation, herbal formula(s) may be given based on the imbalance. Acupuncture points are often predetermined once the herbal formula is identified, though many acupuncturists will adjust their treatment strategy for best results. Many practitioners are trained in multiple acupuncture models to choose from.

Traditional Acupuncture

Traditional acupuncture is the insertion of fine needles at specific acupuncture points in order to regulate circulation of qi and blood. Today, practitioners use pre-sterilized, disposable needles. They are used once and discarded in accordance with OSHA medical biohazard regulations and guidelines. Acupuncture is typically painless, with a gentle insertion of very thin, sterile needles that can be gently manipulated to stimulate the acupuncture point.

Electro-Acupuncture

Low-level electricity is attached to the needles (through wires) to get stronger stimulation. This method uses very low (and gentle) electrical impulses through the acupuncture needles. This technique is generally used for analgesia (pain relief or prevention). The amount of power is only a few microamperes, but the frequency of the current can vary from 5 to 2,000 Hz.

Laser Acupuncture

Laser acupuncture uses a low-level laser (LLLT) to stimulate acupuncture points without penetrating the skin. In practice, we find laser acupuncture most effective for children. Adults don't seem to respond as well, perhaps because, in general, children have more clear responses. It is a very safe, painless, and effective method.

Furthermore, we have recently observed that laser acupuncture on specific acupoints can be tremendously beneficial for retinal bleeding and retinal or macular edema. LLLT can help reduce the need for ongoing anti-VEGF injections due to retinal bleeding and/or edema. It can also help in cases where a resistance to these medications has developed, and they are no longer effective.

Acupressure

Acupressure is a manual technique in which pressure is applied to specific acupuncture points. Pressure can be applied with the fingers, hands, or devices. Acupressure is often combined with "trigger-point" therapy to alleviate pain and muscle spasms. Acupressure and massage are most often the treatment of choice for pediatric cases. See Chapter 10-4 for more information on acupressure.

Essential Acupuncture

Essential acupuncture is where essential oils are placed on specific acupuncture points. The oils are absorbed into these points and/or activate the acupuncture points. Essential acupuncture is one of the easiest home therapies you can do. See Appendix 9 on essential oils.

Auricular (Ear) Acupuncture

Auricular acupuncture is one of the most important components of traditional Chinese acupuncture. In Chinese medical theory there are more than 120 points on each ear related to specific parts of the body. Modern practitioners can simulate ear acupoints using needles, laser, and electrical stimulants.

Auricular acupuncture theory suggests that the ear represents an inverted fetus, with stimulation points affecting the corresponding parts of the body. All major energy channels of the body are thought to cross through the ear. Recently developed protocols related to auricular acupuncture are being introduced throughout the U.S. and Europe and are being shown to have great results with many eye conditions. Based on the auricular acupuncture model, specific points on the auricle of the ear have been identified to benefit vision.

There are eight suggested points documented to help vision loss. An acupuncture "point locator" device is often used to determine which of these "active" points are to be treated (usually 2–5 points in each ear). The locator detects areas of reduced electrical resistance on the surface of the skin. Once these points have been identified they may be stimulated with microcurrent stimulation (MENS), needles, acupuncture press tacks, and/or pellets. Pellets and press-tacks are usually left in for a number of days to promote ongoing stimulation. Stimulating these specific points has been shown to have remarkable clinical results for vision loss patients. From our clinical experience, this is a promising system of acupuncture for degenerative vision loss.

Traditional Japanese Acupuncture (TJM)

Chinese medicine arrived in Japan through Korea in the 6th century and has been practiced for over 14 centuries. Its theoretical foundation is derived from the Chinese medical classics. Japan has developed its own version of acupuncture, still based on theories related to TCM. Chinese acupuncturists use the patient's pulse, tongue, and face to make their diagnosis. Japanese acupuncturists rely more on palpatory findings of the pulse, abdomen, back, and meridians. While Chinese acupuncture today is closely allied with herbal medicine, Japanese acupuncture has developed in close proximity to massage and moxibustion. Great importance is placed on palpation, careful location, and stimulation of reactive points in Japanese acupuncture. The needles used in meridian therapy tend to be much thinner, and do not go as deep as traditional Chinese medicine, so therefore it is a much gentler technique.

Scalp Acupuncture

Scalp acupuncture is a relatively modern specialized acupuncture technique. Treatment zones have been mapped onto the scalp, which are associated with body functions and broad body regions. The zones include a few standard acupuncture points, but the treatment principle for point selection is usually not based on the traditional indication for the point or associated meridian. Scalp acupuncture can be of particular benefit for eye stroke (retinal occlusions) and optic nerve atrophy.[6][7][8]

Micro Acupuncture 48 System

This modern hybrid system involves forty-eight acupuncture points located only in the hands and feet, and is not associated with any other acupuncture system. The system was developed by Freddy Dahlgren in Denmark in the 1980s, and was further developed by Dr. Andy Rosenfarb.

Dalhgren had originally used the micro acupuncture system to treat arthritis and noticed patients reporting improved vision. Dalhgren showed his friend Per Otte this acupuncture point-protocol, and the two treated eye patients using the new protocol in a barn in Denmark with reported excellent results. Otte brought the system to the U.S., treated patients, and showed a few acupuncturist the protocol he used.

Dr. Rosenfarb learned the acupoint protocol from Per Otte and further developed it into the complete Micro Acupuncture 48 system. After 15 years of developing and refining the MA48 system in clinic, Dr. Rosenfarb felt that he had enough experience and understanding with the MA48 system to begin to teach these methods. Until the publication of Rosenfarb's, *The Black Book of Micro Acupuncture 48,* only a handful of acupuncturists knew the secret micro acupuncture protocol. Otte and Dalhgren had treated thousands of individuals using the micro acupuncture protocol with mostly degenerative eye diseases like macular degeneration, glaucoma, eye stroke, retinitis pigmentosa, diabetic retinopathy, and dry eye.

None of the MA48 treatment methods are intended to be curative in nature. Clinical results have shown to recover lost vision in some patients and slow (and in some cases arrest) progressive vision loss in most cases. Not everyone responds to MA48 acupuncture (approximately 85% respond). The developers have found it to be among the most powerful and effective acupuncture methods for recovering and preserving vision. As we know, for many of these degenerative eye diseases there is no conventional treatment.

Theory and Point Map

The results are, at this point, clinically based, although a recent pilot study suggests that acupuncture can be effective for patients with retinitis pigmentosa.

The MA48 system combines elements from three other systems: traditional meridian-based acupuncture, reflexology, and ECIWO acupuncture (a system based on the understanding that the whole organism is found projected on part of the body such as the hands or feet.)

The following diagrams show the 12 MA48 acupoints on each hand and foot.

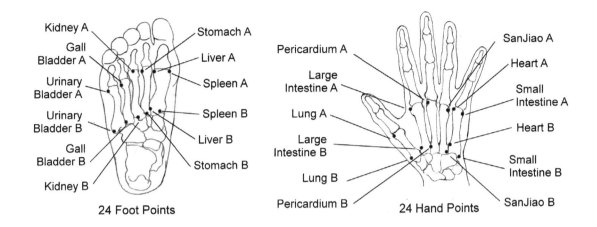

Kidney A
Gall Bladder A
Urinary Bladder A
Urinary Bladder B
Gall Bladder B
Kidney B

Stomach A
Liver A
Spleen A
Spleen B
Liver B
Stomach B

24 Foot Points

Pericardium A
Large Intestine A
Lung A
Large Intestine B
Lung B
Pericardium B

SanJiao A
Heart A
Small Intestine A
Heart B
Small Intestine B
SanJiao B

24 Hand Points

Chinese Moxibustion

Chinese moxibustion (moxa) is the process of burning a dried herb (mug wort) on, over, or near acupuncture points, in order to increase circulation and function. Moxa can be applied locally or distally (points below the elbows and knees) to various acupuncture points. Moxibustion herbal heat therapy remains one of the best means of dispersing cold-stagnation of qi and blood in the eyes. A few methods of applying moxa follow:

- Direct moxa applied to the skin
- Moxa stick (indirect)
- Needle-moxa
- Moxa-shells for the eyes

In one method, walnut shells are soaked in a ginger and clove tea, dried, and then rested on the eyelids as half-shells. Moxa is ignited over the shells to warm them. This brings about rapid, penetrating warmth to the eyes, dispersing the cold. This method is still widely practiced in TCM hospitals throughout China and is highly effective for helping various degenerative vision conditions.

The basic idea of how moxa therapy works for retinal bleeding and edema is similar to the mechanism of a pipe freezing and bursting in your house during the winter. The old pipes get cold and brittle and then crack, allowing the fluid to leak out. Laser surgery is similar to "soldering" the old brittle pipes, and injections are like "caulking" the leaks. In most cases, this is just patchwork and the pipes can easily burst again. The moxa therapy warms the vessels and increases the mending, flexibility, and strengthening of the weak blood vessels and reduces obstructions in blood vessels. It also helps the body effectively reabsorb the fluids. Taking herbs and foods to warm the body internally will help expedite this process.

Though there is good research using moxa for a wide range of health problems,[9] the results on its use for retinal bleeding and edema are based on clinical experience at this point. Moxa can be done at home by just about anyone, using certain precautions. Only a trained practitioner who has had experience in treating degenerative eye conditions should apply the specific methods of using moxa for retinal bleeding.

In Summary

In summary, there are many tools available for acupuncturists to maximize the benefits of treatments, and these will vary, based on the acupuncturist's training and background. Along with these treatments should go the fundamentals of good vision health: pure water, nourishing food, UV and blue light protection, eye and whole-body exercise, and nourishing sleep.

About the Author

Andy Rosenfarb, N.D., L.Ac. is an acupuncturist and naturopathic doctor who has practiced in Westfield, New Jersey since 1997. He has been leading the field in integrated treatment methods that combine Traditional Chinese Medicine, Naturopathic Medicine, and new cutting-edge therapies to help sufferers of debilitating eye disease improve and maintain their eyesight.

See Also

Chapter 10-4, Eye Exercises and Acupressure

---

[1] Bittner, A.K. (2016). Improvement in Ocular Blood Flow and Vision following Electro Stimulation Therapies for Retinal Disease. *Florida International University, Biomedical Engineering, Wallace H. Coulter Foundation Lecture Series, Feb 5, 2016.*

[2] Bittner, A.K., Gould, J.M., Rosenfarb, A., Rozanski, C., Dagnelie, G. (2014). A pilot study of an acupuncture protocol to improve visual function in retinitis pigmentosa patients. *Clin Exp Opt,* May;97(3):240-7.

[3] Qin, Y., Yuan, W., Deng, H., Ziang, Z., Yang, C., et al. (2015). Clinical Efficacy Observation of Acupuncture Treatment for Nonarteritic Anterior Ischemic Optic Neuropathy. *Evid Based Complement Alternat Med,* 2015:713218.

[4] Gibson, G.E., Blass, J.P. (1999). Nutrition and Functional Neurochemistry In Siegel, G.J., Agranoff, B.W., Albers, R.W., et al. (Eds.), Basic *Neurochemistry: Molecuar, Cellular and Medical Aspects. (6th Ed.).* Philadelphia, PA: Lippincott-Raven.

[5] Li, H.J., Sun, Z.L., Yang, X.T., Zhu, L. Feng, D.F. (2017). Exploring Optic Nerve Axon Regeneration. *Curr Neuropharmacol,* Aug;15(6):861-873.

[6] Li, C., Sun, L. (2014). Research on Treating Stroke by Head Acupuncture Therapy. *Clin J Chin Med,* 6.1.

[7] Zheng, G.Q. (2009). Methodological standards for experimental research on stroke using scalp acupuncture. *Acupunct Electrother Res,* 34(1-2):1-13.

[8] Zheng, G.Q., Wang, Y., Wang, X.T. (2006). Literature foundation of scalp-acupuncture treatment of cerebral hemorrhage and its recent progress in clinical research. *Acupunct Res,* 31:181–184.

[9] Deng, H., Shen, X. (2013). The Mechanism of Moxibustion: Ancient Theory and Modern Research. *Evid Based Compl Alt Med,* 2013:379291.

10-1. SELF-HELP SUGGESTIONS

Here are basic self-help suggestions that apply to every vision condition and to all good health.

Diet

Limit Sugar

Reduce or eliminate all types of refined sugars. White sugar in particular should be avoided, but also fructose, sucrose, fruit juice concentrates, maltose, dextrose, glucose, and refined carbohydrates. This includes "natural" drinks that contain a lot of sugar, including all fruit juices. Another sugar, galactose ("milk sugar"), may have an impact for people who are lactose intolerant, putting them at higher risk for cataracts.[1]

Favor an Alkaline Diet

Eat an alkaline-based diet. The standard Western diet is high in acid, due to the increase in grains eaten, particularly refined carbohydrates and processed foods, also meat, sugars, and poor-quality oils (for cooking). Acidic balanced diets versus an alkaline diet high in fruits and vegetables contribute to inflammation in the body and overall chronic illness, and may, in many cases, be the ultimate cause of chronic health conditions, such as autoimmune disease.

Drink Pure Water

Drink eight glasses of water daily, in small doses. You will have heard many wholistic health practitioners tell you to sip water throughout the day. This is optimally taken as a four-ounce glass of water every half-hour to equal 16 four-ounce glasses. Our bloodstream can only effectively handle about four ounces at any one time.

When you drink more than four ounces at a time, the kidneys must work more to filter this water that hasn't had a chance to travel through the lymph system and clean body tissues. Adequate water intake helps maintain the flow of nutrients to the eyes and to release wastes and toxins from tissues. Favor purified water.

Increase Antioxidants

Eat foods high in antioxidants. Antioxidants come from enzymes, phytonutrients such as carotenoids and bioflavonoids, and some vitamins and vitamin-like biochemicals. Most of the important nutritional components of vision-disease prevention and reversal are related to boosting antioxidant levels. Antioxidants are one of the most important combatants against free radicals, a major cause of inflammation. A good diet that is supplemented with antioxidant vitamins and minerals can help prevent the damage due to oxidation.

Lifestyle

Wear Sunglasses

Wear 100% ultraviolet-blocking wrap-around sunglasses (polarized) and a hat, since ultraviolet light from the sun can cause damage to the lens of the eye. Amber colored lenses are best for neutralizing blue light. Brown lenses are second best. Ongoing exposure to sunlight increases the risk of macular degeneration, cataracts, and more.

Note: Cheaper glasses may have a coating to block out UV light that, over time, can rub off. Many people think it is the tint that helps protect the eyes, but it is actually the UV filter on, or in, the lens that is helpful. A dark lens without UV protection increases pupil dilation, allowing more light to enter the eyes.

Avoid Microwaves

Radiation leakage from microwave ovens is a direct cause of some conditions like cataracts; so, avoid constant peeking into the door window while you cook. The severity depends upon the duration and power.[2] Steaming and slow cooking is the best option for retaining the maximum amount of nutrients in food. High temperature cooking and microwaving both cause greater nutritional deterioration. We feel that if you are going to use a microwave, then warming up foods in the microwave is preferable to cooking in the microwave.

Avoid Chemical Toxins

Many synthetic chemicals and pharmaceuticals can cause vision problems. Steroids, for example, taken internally or applied to the skin, are a typical cause of cataracts, because they block the normal metabolism of the connective tissue, one of the components of the lens. In addition, the steroid "estrogen," which is prescribed for menopause and breast cancer, impacts eye function.[3] Steroids such as glucocorticoids are photosensitizing, and they make you more susceptible to cataracts[4] and glaucoma.[5][6] See Chapter 12 for more information on harmful drugs.

Stop Smoking

Cigarette smoking causes about 20% of all cataracts. Men who smoke more than 15 cigarettes a day increase their risk for cataracts by 42%.[7] For female smokers, the risk of getting cataracts is also high. Quitting without supplementing the diet with additional vitamins and minerals doesn't seem to eliminate the increased risk for almost ten years.[8] This is likely due to how smoking depletes antioxidant levels in the body and the eyes. Numerous studies have shown smoking to be associated with the development of cataracts.[9][10][11]

Get Exercise and Take Breaks

Exercise regularly several times a week. Researchers find that exercise improves almost all health conditions, including vision conditions.

Take breaks. Most importantly, take time away from your electronic devices, as computer use is directly linked to many eye conditions, including glaucoma[12] [13] and dry eye syndrome.[14] Your eyes and your body need regular breaks from computers, phones, and televisions. Rest periods of at least a couple of minutes every hour will do wonders for your eyes and your body.

Make sure your "rest" activities are the opposite of your current preoccupation; the point is to engage your eyes and body in different ways. For example, if you have been sitting, doing close-up work, stand up and stretch, while looking out a window into nature. Better yet, take a walk around the block. If, on the other hand, you've been engaged in broader visual work, a rest might include checking your emails on your phone. Doing eye exercises during your rest period is also recommended.

Meditation

Find time for meditation each day. Walking in nature, without electronic devices, can be extremely meditative; it is very relaxing to both our psyche and our physical body. That is, if we are successful at focusing our awareness on the activity of walking itself.

Also See

Chapter 7, Vision Diet

Chapter 8, Nutrients

Chapter 10-4, Eye Exercises

Appendix 7, Additional Therapies

[1] Birlouez-Aragon, I., Ravelontseheno, L., Villate-Cathelineau, B., Cathelineau, G., Abitbol, G. (1993). Disturbed galactose metabolism in elderly and diabetic humans is associated with cataract formation, *J Nutr,* Aug;123(8):1370-6.

[2] Lipman, R.M., Tripathi, B.J., Tripathi, R.C. (1988). Cataracts induced by microwave and ionizing radiation. *Surv Ophthalmol,* Nov-Dec;33(3):200-10.

[3] Hutchinson, C.V., Walker, J.A., Davidson, C. (2014). Oestrogen, ocular function and low-level vision: a review. *J Endocrinol,* Nov;223(2):R9-18.

[4] Leuschen, J., Mortensen, E.M., Frei, C.R., Mansi, E.A., Panday, V., et al. (2013). Association of statin use with cataracts: a propensity score-matched analysis. *JAMA Ophthalmol,* Nov;131(11):1427-34.

[5] Jeppesen, P., Krag, S. (2015). Steroid treatment and risk of glaucoma. *Ugeskr Laeger,* Aug 17;177(34):1620-3.

[6] Rufer, F., Uthoff, D. (2013). Symptoms and therapy for steroid glaucoma. *Klin Monbl Augenheilkd,* July;230(7):692-6.

[7] Lindblad, B.E., Hakansson, N., Wolk, A. (2014). Smoking cessation and the risk of cataract: a prospective cohort study of cataract extraction among men. *JAMA Ophthalmol,* Mar;132(3):253-7.

[8] Wintraub, J.M., Willett, W.C., Rosner, B., Golditz, G.A., Seddon, J.M., et al. (2002). Smoking cessation and risk of cataract extraction among US women and men. *Am J Epidemiol,* Jan 1;155(1):72-9).

[9] Kelly, S.P., Thornton, J., Edwards, R., Sahu, A., Harrison, R. (2005). Smoking and cataract: review of causal association. *J Cataract Refract Surg,* Dec; 31(12):2395-404.

[10] Nirmalan, P.K., Robin, A.L., Katz, J., Tielsch, J.M., Thulasiraj, R.D., et al. (2004). Risk factors for age related cataract in a rural population of southern India: the Aravind Comprehensive Eye Study. *Br J Ophthalmol,* Aug; 88(8):989-94.

[11] Shalini, V.K., Luthra, M., Srinivas, L., Rao, S.H., Basti, S., et al. (1994). Oxidative damage to the eye lens caused by cigarette smoke and fuel smoke condensates. *Indian J Biochem Biophys,* Aug; 31(4):261-6.

[12] Tatemichi, M, Nakano T, Tanaka K, Hayashi, T., Nawa, T. et al. (2004). Possible association between heavy computer users and glaucomatous visual field abnormalities: a cross sectional study in Japanese workers. *J Epidemiol Community Health,* Dec;58(12):1021-7.

[13] Nakano, T., Hayaski, T., Nakagawa, T., Honda, T., Owada, S., et al. (2017). Increased Incidence of Visual Field Abnormalities as Determined by Frequency Doubling Technology Perimetry in High Computer Users Among Japanese Workers: A Retrospective Cohort Study. *J Epidemiol,* Nov 25.

[14] Rosenfeld, M. (2011). Computer vision syndrome: a review of ocular causes and potential treatments. *Ophthalmic Physiol Opt,* Sep;31(5):502-15.

10-2. ABOUT JUICING

Food for Your Eyes

Juicing provides a concentrated source of nutrients and antioxidants. It is particularly important for those people with health conditions, or even healthy people on the go who do not have the time to consistently eat a healthy diet. We recommend using only organic foods for juicing.

Juicing versus Smoothies and Green Drinks

Some of us don't juice. We don't have time, we don't have a juicer, we don't like the cleanup, or we just are not wild about juice. Although juicing allows us to have maximum usable nutrients, instead, we can make smoothies using the same recipes. If you have a blender that turns raw fruits and vegetables to a smooth puree or near liquid consistency, then you can make great smoothies and green drinks.

Making freshly juiced drinks of mostly organic fruit and vegetables is a critical part of the process of healing your eyes and body. The health of your eyes is tied to the health of your body. Juicing is a great way to get the freshest, purest nutrients into your body in an easily digested manner. Once consumed, they are carried everywhere through the blood stream and to your eyes.

Benefits of Juicing

Enzyme Protection

Juicing is a way to consume maximum enzymes, the catalysts for your body's essential and effective functioning. They increase the rate of most chemical reactions in every cell. A variety of glands and organs produce these enzymes while regulating metabolism, circulation, respiration, reproduction, and functioning of the brain. Within your digestive system, specific enzymes help digest food. They break down food into smaller building blocks so that the body can absorb them rapidly. They are found in your saliva, stomach, intestinal tract, gall bladder, and pancreas.

Enzymes convert proteins into peptides and amino acids that are the building blocks for muscles and hormone production. They convert fat into fatty acids and glycerol. They convert starches and sugars into glucose. Enzymes help in the breakdown of those foods by your body. But enzymes become sluggish when they reach temperatures above 118 degrees F, and they deteriorate completely above 130 degrees F.[1]

Some juicers or blenders operate at such high speed that the temperature rises over 130 degrees or even to 188 degrees, and this high heat destroys some of the vitamins and enzymes in the juice.

Faster Digestion. When you consume solid foods, it takes several hours for your body to break it down into usable components. Although fiber is important for good health, the juicing process removes fiber, making digestion faster, approximately 20–30 minutes.[2][3]

Concentrated Nutrients. Juicing concentrates the nutrients. By juicing the various recipes that we recommend, you quickly introduce ample amounts of nutrients into your system, more than you could take in comfortably if you ate all of those fruits and vegetables whole.

Living Juice. Many people feel that to nourish your own life, it is important to consume foods that are "alive." Juicing preserves this quality of life that is destroyed through cooking.

Vegetable Protein

Vegetables contain more protein than you may think. Vegetables such as green beans, corn, artichoke, watercress, and the cabbage family (broccoli, cauliflower, brussels sprouts, etc.) have the most protein of vegetables. And juicing is an easy way to include additional protein to your ingredients, such as brewer's yeast, wheat germ, or whole grains.

Phytochemicals

Juicing is a wonderful way to get large quantities of phytochemicals, like carotenoids, readily absorbed into the body.

These chemical compounds are responsible, among other things, for the color and smell of each plant. The colors and smells attract pollinators, and more importantly, the colors protect the plants from damaging UV radiation from the sun. Likewise, when you consume them, they help protect your health and vision. For example, lutein is found in yellow fruits and vegetables; it is also in the macula of the eye where it acts as a potent antioxidant and internal sunscreen, protecting the most sensitive part of the eye from blue, violet, and UV light.

Other Nutrients

Incorporating dark leafy-green vegetables in your juices or smoothies also provides nutrients such as B vitamins (like folate), which are methyl donors. The addition of methyl groups (CH3) to molecules (called methylation) helps many processes in our body, such as producing neurotransmitters for brain function, repairing DNA, turning genes on and off, and improving immunity and detoxification.

Juicing Tips

Follow your comfort. You may consume as much fresh juice as you wish, as long as you don't force it. Follow your comfort level. At least ½–1 pint daily is great. For therapeutic purposes, your healthcare professional may recommend larger amounts, daily.

Limit sweet juices. Don't use too much fruit, or many carrots because of their high natural sugar content. We suggest one carrot per 12–16 oz. juice.

Note about weak digestion. If you have weak digestion, then juices or smoothies may not be the best for you. If you experience pain, gas, bloating, or diarrhea, then reduce the amount and number of juices you drink. Do not add ice or frozen vegetables or fruit. Allow fresh fruits and vegetables to warm to room temperature before juicing. If symptoms persist, you can switch to warm cooked vegetable soups or purees.

Freshness. You should drink your fresh juice promptly and not store it for later. Many enzymes and vitamins break down quickly once they are exposed to the air or sunlight.

Organic. Non-organic products usually contain pesticides, and not only on the surface of their skin. If you juice non-organic foods, you are likely consuming concentrated amounts of those pesticides. Some feel pesticides reside mostly in fiber, which is removed, but it is better to be safe.

Equipment

There are many excellent juicers. We recommend those that operate at a slow 80RPM, slow enough to not create heat. Most types of juicing equipment operate at 3600RPM or higher. "Masticating juicers" chew up fruits and vegetables slowly, preserving nutrients and enzymes. The downside of these is simply a slightly slower operating time and slightly longer cleanup. There are now a number of slow juicers available, which are increasingly affordable. Omega has several in various configurations, as does Hurom (43RPM), Hamilton Beach, Super Angel, Fagor, and Tribest. Vitamix has a reputation for being an excellent machine; Nutribullet and Ninja, at a lower cost, are also good. Note: These machines are not low speed and generate heat; some nutrients and enzymes are lost. However, they are better than not making a refreshing nourishing drink at all. The Vidia vacuum blender removes air to prevent oxidation. It has a maximum speed of 20,000 RPM, not low speed. Other juicers are available on the market, so read reviews to determine the best one for you.

Also See

Chapter 7, Nutrients

Appendix 1, Juicing Recipes

---

[1] CalorieBee. (2017). At What Temperature are Enzymes in Raw Food Destroyed. Retrieved Jun 5 2018 from https://caloriebee.com/diets/Food-Enzyme-Facts.

[2] Digestion Times by Food Groups (2015). Retrieved Jun 5 2018 from http://www.9tofine.net/en/diet/digestion-time-of-different-foods/.

[3] Suzuki, S. (1987). Experimental studies on the presumption of the time after food intake from stomach contents. *Forensic Sci Int*, Oct-Nov;35(2-3):83-117.

10-3. MICROCURRENT STIMULATION

An Overview

Microcurrent stimulation (MCS) is recommended by vision doctors for its effect in helping protect vision by stimulating ocular circulation, removing waste, and potentially repairing damage.

Who Uses MCS?

There are a number of circumstances in which this technology is currently used in Western allopathic medicine.[1] In orthopedics it is used to promote bone healing, but not all orthopedic doctors use it. Sports medicine is the biggest user.[2][3] MCS is used in veterinary medicine (with racehorses as a safe alternative to doping) and in Olympic training centers. Some plastic surgeons use it to reduce scar formation after elective surgery. Neurologists use it to promote healing in the central nervous system, especially following brain or spinal cord injury and after a stroke. Wholistic eye doctors use it in degenerative retinal diseases to support the health of the retina.

Development of MCS

Reinhold Voll

In the 1950s, the German physician Dr. Reinhold Voll began to study the electrical qualities of acupuncture points as a tool for diagnosis because many of these points correspond with the classical acupuncture points. Voll was looking at changes in the resistance of these points that occurred in different states of disease and how the resistance changed as the disease progressed or as it improved with treatment. Dr. Voll's work is now referred to as Electro Acupuncture of Voll, or EAV. In the U.S., it remains a tool, mainly for measuring electrical balance and imbalance in the body and how the body reacts to different agents and substances. Other technologies that have arisen from his work are now referred to broadly as Electro-Dermal Screening or EDS.

Voll's work with the electrical qualities of acupuncture points did much to allow the modern MCS treatment of tissues, deep in the body, without the need for surgical placement of electrodes. Understanding the acupuncture meridians helps to predict how the application of current to a particular point might affect tissues at a distance from that point. Understanding these qualities of the points helps the practitioner decide where to apply microcurrent stimulation.

S.D. Smith

S. D. Smith worked with salamanders and certain species of frogs which will spontaneously regenerate a limb if it is lost or damaged. There are certain species of frogs that don't regenerate a missing limb on their own, and Smith investigated the regeneration possibilities in these animals. He found that by implanting a device made of silver and platinum wires along the bone remnant in the amputated limb, he could stimulate regeneration by means of a weak current.

Robert Becker

In the 1960s, Robert Becker, M.D., an orthopedic surgeon,[4] [5] [6] developed a technique[7] [8] to regenerate amputated legs on animals. His research was built on the work of S. D. Smith. It was, for the time, an incredible concept that begins the evolution of today's microcurrent stimulation technology. Dr. Becker took Smith's work further when he started working with rats. He tried to apply Dr. Smith's work to mammals and succeeded.

Becker's book, *The Body Electric*,[9] documents his early studies with the regeneration of animal limbs. Becker had observed that there were subtle electrical signatures around the stump of the amputated legs in frogs, and the same weak electrical signals were found around injured limbs in rats. He developed a theory that these electrical signals weren't accidental but were there for a reason. Perhaps these signals were part of an attempt by the body to regenerate. But when regeneration did not occur, it could have been because there was not enough current created. To test out his theory, he brought more of the proper electrical activity to the end of the amputated limb by surgically moving the subscapular nerve and implanting it at the point of amputation. Just as he predicted, the limb did start to regrow, but when the newly regenerating limb grew away from the implanted nerve, the leg quit growing.

Dr. Becker was convinced that there was a connection between the electrical activity he had observed around areas of injury, and the body's attempts to repair and regenerate it. He analyzed the nature of these electrical signals produced naturally in the body, and he developed electronic equipment that could duplicate those signals. When he used that equipment, and when he applied the current directly at the point of injury, in this case the end of the amputated limb, the leg began to regrow, and he was able to almost completely regrow a perfect leg. His findings were nothing short of miraculous. The equipment he invented is the basis for the modern microcurrent stimulators we now use.

Cynthia Illingworth

Becker was also aware of, and was inspired by, the work of a surgeon, Cynthia Illingworth, M.D. who had observed the apparently spontaneous regeneration of a child's cut-off fingertip. She went on to document hundreds of cases in children where doing nothing led to perfect healing of an amputated finger. For this regrowth to work, the cut needed to be clean, beyond the last joint of the finger, and the child needed to be 11 years old or younger.

How Does This Relate to Vision?

We are spending time on Becker's work in orthopedics with limb regrowth and bone healing, because the techniques that these doctors developed to promote regeneration are some of the very techniques we now use to support the health of your eyes. We simply do not know what the body is capable of when it comes to regenerating tissues that have been damaged by trauma or chronic degenerative disease. Prior to Dr. Illingworth's papers, doctors laughed at the idea that a finger could regenerate itself. She showed that, at least in children, there was a vestige of limb regeneration that occurred spontaneously and naturally, if allowed.

Dr. Becker took this further and developed therapies allowing almost complete regeneration of the leg in animals. Researchers are going back for a new look at Becker's work.[10]

Bjorn Nordenström

The doctor and scientist Bjorn Nordenström, M.D. was a prominent physician and researcher in Sweden, head of the Karolinska Institute, and for a time, head of the Nobel Prize committee. A diagnostic radiologist by training, Dr. Nordenström noticed some odd patterns of calcification in the tissues around, not in, certain tumors that he could see on radiographs. His investigation found that the same patterns of electrical activity that Dr. Becker had noted around areas of trauma and injury also existed around tumors and areas of inflammation. Dr. Becker had named the electrical activity that he observed "currents of injury." Dr. Nordenström showed that this type of electrical activity was found around many types of injury and disease in the body, and his patterns of electrical flow were actually another type of circulation in the body.

Nordenström developed his work into a system that he named "Biologically Closed Electrical Circuits" (BCEC). It's a mouthful, but it's descriptive. His work was published in the book *Biologically Closed Electrical Circuits.*[11] Prior to Nordenström's work, the conventional wisdom was that the body was simply a large sack of saltwater, and that it would be impossible to generate or maintain any sort of meaningful current outside of the myelinated (insulated) nerves. Any current that was generated would simply dissipate immediately.

Intracellular-Extracellular Membrane Potential

Nordenström demonstrated that blood vessels and different spaces of the body separated by tissue planes create a perfect environment for generating and maintaining electrical currents, at the level of the cell. There is an electrical gradient between the inside and the outside of every cell in every living thing. This is now named the "intracellular-extracellular membrane potential," and it is maintained by machinery in the membrane of every cell that can selectively move charged ions in and out of the cell to maintain the electrical gradient.[12]

This phenomenon helps us understand one of the primary mechanisms behind the effects we see with microcurrent stimulation therapy. When properly designed and properly applied, very low-level currents act as a sort of battery charger for the cell and can quickly restore a healthy electrical potential in the body's cells.

In a healthy cell, the membrane potential has a value of about 0.9 mV, which is actually quite a large potential. When the health of the cell or the health of tissues is compromised, this membrane potential can fall to 0.1 mV or less. Why is this important? Almost all of the significant metabolic activity in any cell takes place near the cell membrane. In part, the cells rely upon this membrane potential to power all of the functions of the cell. If the battery runs low because the cell is not healthy, the cell may not die but it certainly ceases to function and becomes unable to repair itself if damaged. Put simply, one function of microcurrent stimulation therapy is to restore cell health, enabling normal function, proper healing, and repair.

How long can a tissue maintain current once the electrical potential is created? Fallen autumn leaves look dead. But, Kirilian photos of "dead" leaves show continued electrical activity generated by the leaf. More relevant to our discussion is that studies have shown that, following the application of microcurrent stimulation to challenged tissues, the normal intracellular-extracellular membrane potential is quickly restored, and the normal potential can be maintained for days with no additional treatment.

Parallel Technologies

Stem Cells

Much of the current thinking on the mechanisms of regeneration, center on an understanding of our endogenous stem cells, also called our adult stem cells.[13] [14] [15] [16] [17] [18] The adult stem cell system is the system we were born with that allows us to fix anything that is broken, injured, or damaged, and make it new again. There is not a single cell in the body that is not capable of regenerating. If you cut yourself shaving, the skin regrows to look like new, and if you damage your spinal cord in an accident, we now know that significant regeneration and repair is possible with the proper support. In both of these examples, your adult stem cells are responsible for the body's ability to regenerate itself.

Stem Cells Repair Damage

Adult stem cells spend most of their time in the bone marrow, but when there is a need for repair somewhere in the body, chemical signals are released from the damaged tissues that signal for adult stem cells to enter the blood stream and travel to the area needing healing. Under a microscope, the adult stem cells look like simple white blood cells, but they can be identified with special testing that can recognize unique proteins present in their cell membranes. When these adult stem cells reach the damaged tissue, they merge with the tissue in need of repair, determine the nature of the tissue, and then initiate the process of regeneration. Once regeneration has begun, it becomes impossible to identify the unique adult stem cell that began the process.

Our Eyes Have the Potential to Heal

This means your eyes are at least capable of healing. Doctors don't know how to heal your eyes, but your body does, and if we support the systems responsible for regeneration, then regeneration is possible. We don't know the limits of the body's ability to regenerate itself. We do know that regeneration happens.

When Dr. Becker was re-growing legs on animals, he knew that there was some sort of stem cell-like activity responsible for the regeneration he was observing. Little was known about adult stem cells during his research in the 1970s. The theories at the time centered on cells that were present at the site of the injury. In amphibians, like frogs and salamanders, the red blood cells still have a nucleus. Adult stem cells are understood to be "pluripotent," meaning they are capable of producing any type of cell. When Becker was doing his research, the popular idea was that the red blood cells in salamanders and frogs were somehow becoming less specialized (de-differentiating), and in doing so, became capable of participating in the regeneration of bone, muscle, nerve, and skin. Since mammals have red blood cells that lose their nuclear material before they enter circulation, Dr. Becker thought that perhaps it was fibroblasts or other cells participating in healing and scar formation that contributed to the regeneration of normal tissues. The current thinking is that regeneration involves populations of adult stem cells; often bone-marrow derived stem cells.

Empirical Evidence for MCS

The role of adult stem cells in the regeneration of tissues is now better understood, but the role that microcurrent stimulation therapy has in promoting the function of adult stem cells is not. Making that connection, drawing a straight line between the external application of electrical stimulation and an effect on adult stem cells, is hard to do. The proof is mainly empirical, meaning that in experiments where something is done to promote and accelerate the healing of injured or damaged tissue, that tissue heals quickly with the application of MCS.

Adult stem cells are released from the bone marrow in response to chemical signals produced by injured tissues. The products of inflammation that accompany injury not only serve to trigger the release of adult stem cells but also serve to guide the circulating adult stem cells to the area of injury. One theory is that in chronic diseases like macular degeneration, retinitis pigmentosa, and Stargardt disease there is often very little or no inflammation present, and therefore there is nothing to signal to the adult stem cells to let them know where the damaged cells are that need to be repaired. Perhaps the microcurrent stimulation serves as a signal to circulating adult stem cells, and it attracts them to the area that is being treated. Currently, this is just a theory.

MCS Research

The research on microcurrent stimulation suggests that it improves small vessel circulation in the areas treated, restores the normal intracellular-extracellular membrane potential that we discussed earlier, appears to improve lymphatic flow, and it improves something called nerve conduction velocity. All of these effects essentially make the tissues that are treated more normal and healthier, and much of the positive effect we see with MCS may be due to the many things it does to restore normal functioning. Healthy tissue is better able to repair itself, and repair and regeneration are always an "inside job."

Grace Halloran

Grace Halloran pioneered the treatment of severe degenerative retinal diseases using a program that includes microcurrent stimulation, an off-label use. Her work is being continued in restoring vision for those with macular degeneration, retinitis pigmentosa, and Stargardt disease. Understanding the process Dr. Halloran went through to decide which microcurrent equipment to use and how to apply it will help inform doctors' decisions.

Halloran gave a talk at the Fourth International Symposium on Biologically Closed Electric Circuits in 1997. Along with another talk by John Jarding, O.D. research they had been doing with treatment programs for macular degeneration and other degenerative eye conditions was discussed. John Jarding has been continuing work begun by his mentor, Leland Michael (O.D.), and Leland Michael had been trained in these techniques by Grace Halloran. Both were using the microcurrent unit developed by the company MicroStim Technologies, Incorporated. Damon Miller (M.D. and author of this chapter), who worked with Grace Halloran, furthered this knowledge until her death in 2005.

Grace Halloran came from a family with a history of retinitis pigmentosa (RP). It was a particularly troublesome variant of RP that included both peripheral and central vision loss. She, her mother, sisters, and brother all had compromised vision, and when she gave birth to a son, with signs of RP in the first months of life; he would be legally blind by the time he was a teenager. Ophthalmologists said nothing could be done. But Dr. Halloran found a way to stop the progression of her son's retinitis pigmentosa and she was able to restore her own vision as well.

Her initial program involved multiple self-administered therapies based on diet, nutrition, exercises, self-administered acupressure, visualization, and stress management resulting in significant vision improvement. This early program did not yet include microcurrent stimulation. She had met Dr. Joel Rossen, and her first experience with MCS came when her young son suffered a serious arm injury expected to result in arm deformation. A high-quality microcurrent stimulation device was used to apply treatment close to the site of the injury. The arm healed perfectly, contrary to doctors' expectations.

This experience, treating her son's injured arm, was Dr. Halloran's initiation into the world of microcurrent stimulation therapy. She learned of the work of Dr. Robert Becker, and she had the thought that if this technology could help regrow an amputated limb on a mammal, then what else could it help regenerate? With the help of Dr. Joel Rossen, she developed a protocol that applied stimulation at acupuncture points as a way of using microcurrent stimulation to support the health and functioning of the eyes. At the time, Dr. Rossen was working with the Electro-Acuscope Company and even in the 1980s, their treatment units cost about $30,000. Grace was working with some people who were willing to pay this kind of money, if there was any hope at all that it might help their vision. Dr. Halloran had seen great success with restoring vision, and with the addition of microcurrent stimulation therapy to her program, people saw even greater improvement, and the improvements came more quickly.

Dr. Joel Rossen went on to develop and patent a portable unit that incorporated the same sophisticated and high quality microcurrent generation found in the Electro-Acuscope unit, but for a price closer to $1000. In the early 1990s, Dr. Halloran partnered with a neuro-ophthalmologist in San Francisco, and together they researched, not only patients with macular degeneration, retinitis pigmentosa, and Stargardt disease, but also people with diabetic retinopathy, AIDS-related retinopathy, and severe glaucoma. The combination of simple therapies that Dr. Halloran had developed was combined with an affordable microcurrent stimulation unit, and with the combination of all of these modalities, almost 90% of the people in their study showed significant improvement in just six weeks. Dr. Halloran presented the results from this study at the 1997 conference (Fourth International Symposium on Biologically Closed

Electric Circuits). You can learn more from her book, *Amazing Grace: Autobiography of a Survivor*. The book is a story of hope that any person with a degenerative eye disease would appreciate.

About the MCS Device

Any discussion of the use of microcurrent stimulation by someone who has a degenerative eye disease involves the use of this technology outside the uses for which the Food and Drug Administration (FDA) originally approved the device. This is called an "off-label" use and is legal when the clinician who recommends it believes that it is likely to be a safe and effective therapy for their patient. The off-label use of drugs and medical devices is common in the modern practice of medicine. When an orthopedic surgeon recommends the use of MCS to help with a non-healing bone fracture, they are also recommending an off-label use of a medical device.

There are many microcurrent stimulation machines on the market, and much confusion about their differences, partly because of how the FDA classifies them. The FDA calls all devices of this type TENS (Transcutaneous Electrical Nerve Stimulation) units. A TENS unit is a Class II medical device intended to treat pain. Any device that has a battery and wires coming out of it to allow the application of electrical currents to the skin is classified by the FDA as a TENS unit. A device with a battery and a couple of capacitors that can be found on eBay for $29 is classified as a TENS unit. A device with a sophisticated microprocessor with an output that involves complex waveforms and precise control of the current that is delivered and that costs $30,000 is classified as a TENS unit. You can understand how this might be confusing for both doctors and patients.

The off-label use of microcurrent stimulation devices to support the health and functioning of eyes has become more common. There are, however, many units that are marketed as MCS devices that are not suitable for the treatment of eye disease. In general, MCS is a very safe modality. The risk is in using an inadequate machine.

MCS treatment protocols are designed to help people with retinal disease. They work by supporting the body to allow the healing and regeneration that only the body can provide. Retinal tissue is easily the most complex tissue in the entire body, and we tell people that they need to commit to regular treatment for a year, because it may take a year before they first see results.

There are a few parameters that are important when choosing a microcurrent stimulation device where the intent is to promote tissue regeneration. The most critical parameter is how tightly the unit "controls" the current output. Tight control of current can only be accomplished with a microprocessor. Inexpensive TENS units without a microprocessor are considered voltage control devices and are inappropriate. Controlling current is a trivial matter if you are passing current through a copper wire, but when you start passing current through biological tissues, keeping the current constant is very difficult. The path that the current follows as it moves through the body can change moment to moment, and this can cause the resistance in the path to change moment to moment. Also, the very act of passing microcurrents through biological tissues changes the electrical qualities of those tissues. Diseased or inflamed tissue has high electrical resistance, and as you treat, the resistance falls, and as the resistance falls, the current that is flowing changes.

Resistance and Current Density

This relationship between resistance and current density is important to understand. In physics, the general law that describes the relationship between current, voltage, and resistance is Ohm's Law, but Ohm's law only applies if the material you are working with has a constant resistance. The electrical resistance in tissue can vary, so we will refer to a reformulation of Ohm's law by the physicist Gustav Kirchoff. His reformulation is expressed as $J = \sigma E$, where J is the current density at a given location in a resistive material, E is the electric field at that location, and σ (Sigma) is a material-dependent parameter called the conductivity. (Conductivity is basically the inverse of resistance.) Since the voltage in a current controlled microcurrent unit is held constant, if the conductivity changes, the current density will change. In order to maintain a constant current density, needed for the treatment to be effective, a microcurrent unit must continuously measure the conductivity in the circuit being treated and adjust the current as needed.

The original device used by Dr. Halloran did this task well. The later portable device invented and patented by Dr. Rossen is capable of adjusting the current output over 1000 times a second and provides excellent current control. The MicroStim 100ile device (was Microstim 100) from Dr. Rossen was used to gather most of the earliest data that reports the effectiveness of therapies in helping people with macular degeneration, retinitis pigmentosa, and Stargardt Disease.

Carrier Wave Technology

The next parameter that is critical in the design of an effective microcurrent stimulation unit is the addition of carrier wave technology. The earliest devices required that the treating current be applied directly at the site where it was needed. If an orthopedic surgeon wanted to utilize microcurrent stimulation to help with the union of a non-healing bone fracture, she needed to surgically implant electrodes directly at the site of the fracture. The addition of a carrier wave is a later refinement. Very high frequency signals penetrate deeply into the body, but the frequencies that are needed for the treatment itself are much lower frequencies. The combination of a higher frequency as a carrier wave with the lower frequency treating waves superimposed allows the treating frequencies to be delivered deeply into the body when the treatment is at the level of the skin. With an understanding of how acupuncture points on the surface of the body relate to structures within the body, we can design treatment protocols where treatment be applied at some distance from the area treated. The addition of carrier waves creates a more complex waveform capable of penetrating the body to the level needed. Again, part of the patent that Dr. Rossen was granted on his MicroStim 100ile unit was for this carrier wave enhancement. To this day, no one has found a better way to deliver the treating current.

Frequency

Much thought and research has evaluated which frequencies to use. There are several classes of frequencies that are important. Higher frequencies of around 300Hz and intermediate frequencies of around 30Hz, when used as the first frequencies in a treatment, help to depolarize tissues, making the remainder of the treatment more effective. The body has an innate frequency of health at which most of tissues resonate, and this is somewhere between 9Hz and 10Hz. This is the main frequency used, and is the most effective at restoring intracellular-extracellular membrane potential in compromised cells. Finally, a very low frequency of about 0.5Hz helps normalize blood flow in the small vessels, and usually this is the last frequency used in a treatment. The MCS 100ile home unit uses the frequency settings that were used in the main research studies. It is preset to automatically run through 4 frequencies in a preset 5-minute cycle before turning off. The four frequencies are: 292Hz for 30 seconds, 30Hz for 30 seconds, 9.1Hz for 2 minutes, then finally .3Hz for 2 minutes. Voltage is up to 22, and amps range 700 microAmps. This unit checks the current 1,000 times a second to maintain consistency through the retinal tissue.

Waveform and Current Type

The final parameters are the shape of the waveform and whether the current is applied as direct current or alternating current. The MicroStim 100ile unit allows treatment with both square wave and slope wave. Square wave is best at restoring healthy electrical activity and healthy circulation to tissues. Slope wave is used in more acute problems, such as treating trauma and injury, for example a sprained ankle. In general, better results are obtained using alternating current.

Safety

Finally, a word on safety: These are very safe machines. They are battery powered and designed so that they cannot generate enough current to damage tissue. They are shielded. The amount of current a unit can deliver is considered physiologic, meaning that the currents generated are currents on a level that the body would produce naturally. We generate more current in our body when we sneeze than this machine is capable of producing. If your doctors didn't warn you about sneezing, then we would say, go ahead and use microcurrent stimulation therapy.

Implanted Devices

Caution. If you have an implanted defibrillator or neuro-stimulator, then you should not use microcurrent stimulation therapy. If you have a simple pacemaker, and it was implanted after 1986, then there should be no problems using microcurrent stimulation therapy. It's always good to check with your cardiologist first.

Sub-Threshold

To get the best results, the amount of current delivered is adjusted. The most effective treatment is considered a "sub-threshold" treatment, meaning that you are treating current that you cannot feel: less than the sense of tingling. People like to feel something when being treated. Even the current is adjusted to feel only a slight tingling, it doesn't hurt and there is no danger, but the treatment loses much of its effectiveness. If a sensation is felt, reflexes are brought into play, mediated through the brain stem and the spinal cord that start to decrease circulation of blood and energy and, in many ways, undo what you're trying to achieve. It doesn't provide any risk, it doesn't cause any harm, but it can really undercut what you're trying to do with the therapy.

Disclaimer

This discussion includes off-label uses of microcurrent stimulation (MCS). We describe some of the findings from research, as well as case studies, but there are no promises that what is described here will work for you as an individual. An "off-label use" occurs when a clinician recommends a drug or medical device for use "different" than the use for which it was originally approved by the Food and Drug Administration (FDA). This very commonly occurs in medicine, and it is perfectly legal when the clinician believes that the use or practice they are recommending is safe and likely to be effective.

---

[1] Fu, X., Han, B., Cai, S., Lei, Y., Sun, T. and Sheng, Z. (2009). Migration of bone marrow-derived mesenchymal stem cells induced by tumor necrosis factor-α and its possible role in wound healing. *Wound Repair Regen*, 17:185-191.

[2] Lambert, M.I., Marcus, P., Burgess, T., Noakes, T.D. (2002). Electro-membrane microcurrent therapy reduces signs and symptoms of muscle damage. *Med Sci Sports Exerc,* Apr;23(4):602-7.

[3] Curtis, D., Fallows, S., Morris, M., McMakin, C. (2010). The efficacy of frequency specific microcurrent therapy on delayed onset muscle soreness. *J Bodyw Mov Ther,* Jul;14(3):272-9.

[4] Becker RA, Marino AA. (1982). *Electromagnetism and Life*. State University of New York Press, Albany.

[5] Becker, R.O., Selden, G. (1985). The *Body Electric: Electromagnetism and the Foundation of Life*. Morrow, New York.

[6] Becker, R.O. (1990). *Cross Currents. The Promise of Electromedicine*, the Perils of Electropollution. Torcher, Los Angeles.

[7] Becker, R.O. (1972). Stimulation of partial limb regeneration in rats. *Nature, Jan;235(5333):109-11.*

[8] Becker, R.O. (1961). Search for Evidence of Axial Current Flow in Peripheral Nerves of Salamander. *Science,* Jul 14;134(3472):101-2.

[9] Ibid. Becker. (1985).

[10] Leppik, L.P., Froemel, D., Slavici, A., Ovadia, Z.N., Hudak, L., et al. (2015). Effects of electrical stimulation on rat limb regeneration, a new look at an old model. *Sci Rep,* Dec 17;5:18353.

[11] Nordenstrom, B. (1983). Biologically Closed Electrical Circuits – Clinical, Experimental And Theoretical Evidence For A Third Circulatory System, Nordic Medical Publications. Note: Excerpts of this book can be found on organicmd.com.

[12] McCaig, C.D., Rajnicek, A.M., Song, B., Zhao, M. (2005). Controlling cell behavior electrically: current views and future potential. *Physiol Rev,* Jul;85(3):943-78.

[13] Takahashi, K., Tanabe, K., Ohnuki, M., Narita, M., Ichisaka, T., et.al. (2007). Induction of Pluripotent Stem Cells from Adult Human Fibroblasts by Defined Factors. *Manuscript-1 Department of Stem Cell Biology*, Institute for Frontier Medical Sciences, Kyoto University, Kyoto 606-8507, Japan: 67.

[14] Jiang, Y., Jahagirdar, B.N., Reinhardt, R.L., Shwartz, R.E., Keen, C.D., et.al. (2002). Pluripotency of mesenchymal stem cells derived from adult marrow. *Nature,* Jul;418:41-49.

[15] Kicic, A., Shen, W.Y., Wilson, A.S., Constable, I.J., Robertson, T., et.al. (2003). Differentiation of Marrow Stromal Cells into Photoreceptors in the Rat Eye. *J Neurosci,* Aug 27;23(21):7742–7749.

[16] Tomita, M., Adachi, Y., Yamada, H., Takahashi, K., Kiuchi, K., et.al. (2002). Bone Marrow-Derived Stem Cells Can Differentiate into Retinal Cells in Injured Rat Retina. *Stem Cells,* 2002(20): 279-283.

[17] Tropepe, V., Coles, B.L., Chiassoh, B.J., Horsford, D.J., Elia, A.J., et.al. (2000). Retinal Stem Cells in the Adult Mammalian Eye. *Science,* Mar 17;287(5460): 2032-2036.

[18] Borlongan, C., Glover, L.E., Tajiri, N., Kaneko, Y., Freeman, T.B. (2011). The great migration of bone marrow-derived stem cells toward the ischemic brain: Therapeutic implications for stroke and other neurological disorders. Prog Neurobiol, 95(2): 213-228.

10-4. EYE EXERCISES AND ACUPRESSURE

The muscles in the eyes are no different than other muscles. If we exercise them, they become stronger. The ciliary muscles flex the lens of the eyes to adjust from near to far and far to near focusing. The intraocular and extraocular muscles enable us to move our eyes around.

The Chinese have been doing eye exercises for ages, but it was Dr. William Horatio Bates who popularized eye exercises in the 1990s. The Bates Method taught people to support their eyesight naturally through a series of daily eye exercises to reduce strain that affects vision. Though still an excellent stand-alone system, vision therapy has evolved a long way since then, incorporating Bates' methods with other visionary approaches. For basic eye exercises and acupressure massage, we recommend 10-12 minutes per day.

The Research

The research as to whether eye exercises are effective is mixed. Eye exercises which rely on self-massage of acupoints appear to be more effective in reducing myopia[1] than improving near vision. Eye exercises appear to enhance accuracy and letter recognition, but not the speed with which one is able to discern letters.[2] In one study there was no general reduction in myopia risk in school children, but those who performed "high quality" eye exercises experienced a slightly lower myopia progression.[3] Eye exercises may have a role in improving muscle weakness of facial nerves. In a study of patients where the facial nerve impairment cause was unknown 68% of patients experienced improvement compared to those who did not do eye exercises.[4] Controlled trials suggest that eye exercises may be helpful for convergence insufficiency, and possibly for 3D vision and visual field after brain damage.[5] Generally, because of small sample sizes and other factors more research is needed.

Nonetheless, we feel that eye exercises are a valuable part of a healthy vision protocol because they improve microcirculation, stimulate acupressure points, and are generally relaxing.

Tips for Success

The following are essential components of a vision improvement program.

Breathe. As in yoga, the importance of good breathing is essential to getting the most out of your exercises. As you look around your world, become aware of when you are holding your breath. Breathing regularly brings more oxygen to your eyes and reduces stress.

Blink. Remembering to blink will help keep you from staring and working too hard on exercises. It will also soothe and moisturize your eyes.

Smile. Adding a smile to your exercises may help reduce any tension you may be holding in your eyes. So, smile as you go through life.

Have fun. Consider these exercises as something you enjoy rather than a task.

Commit. As in anything you really want in life, success requires that you commit to the goal. If you don't think this is the proper time for you to commit to improving your vision, then you may have to put off an eye exercise program until another time.

Believe. Check in with your belief systems about improving your eyes. Improvement is possible.

The Exercises

The following exercises are to be practiced for three to five minutes. Unless otherwise noted with instructions for a specific exercise, try to practice these exercises without glasses or contact lenses.

1. Breathing

How you breathe is an integral part of your health and your vision improvement. Smooth, even, deep, and rhythmic breathing helps to center our attention on our inner selves. We concentrate on the steady intake and exhalation of breath. Most of us breathe very shallowly. We extend our lungs, pull our stomach in, and lift our shoulders while we inhale, and do the opposite while we exhale. This is backward!

Instead, take in air all the way down to the bottom of the lungs. As air fills the lungs, they expand, and our stomach pushes outward. As we exhale, pushing air up slowly from the bottom of the lungs, our stomach contracts. This breathing exercise is very soothing. It can be done anytime, anywhere. It may be difficult at first, so practice it patiently.

Instructions

- Sit comfortably in a quiet room, or stand with knees slightly bent, and close your eyes.
- Notice the rhythm of your breathing.
- Inhale deeply through your nose. Try to let your shoulders remain down and loose. Lungs are like balloons, so let them expand. As they fill, imagine that they go all the way down to your pelvic seat (a full intake of breath should expand both the lungs and the stomach, starting first with the lungs).
- Exhale slowly and evenly through your mouth, pushing the air out from the bottom of your lungs. Feel your stomach and chest flatten but do not squeeze the air out. Let your lungs rest at the end of your exhalation, and simply allow your body to begin its next inhalation. Try not to force the inhalation, but wait for the natural impulse to breathe.
- Repeat the inhalation and exhalation, letting a natural rhythm flow continuously. Do not over-breathe.
- Gently direct your attention to the intake and exhalation of air. Let thoughts simply evaporate.
- Let your eyelids hang heavy until they gently close. Your eyes should be unfocused and the eye muscles relaxed. Let your jaw go slack. Your mouth should be slightly opened. Say the word "Duuuh" in order to help your jaw drop.
- Let your body move slightly to prevent muscles from becoming locked.

- Continue breathing for three minutes. When you open your eyes, don't look at anything in particular; just let your eyes open without refocusing, so that they can momentarily receive light in the most natural and relaxed way.

Practice this breathing technique as often as you wish, with and without your glasses or contacts.

2. Vision Statements

Your attitudes and belief systems are extremely important to improving your vision. Anatomy and physiology show that the eyes are tools for the mind; therefore, your positive intention is essential for improving your vision. You should begin your program by declaring your intentions about your vision. The following are some possible statements you may use.

- I can improve my vision.
- My eyesight can get better.
- I don't have to depend on my glasses to survive.
- I am ready to see the world.
- I can see without glasses.

You can create your own vision statements or adjust these to your particular vision condition.

3. Palming

This exercise is practiced without glasses or contact lenses. Palming reduces stress around the eyes. By placing your palms around your eyes, you are stimulating powerful acupuncture points to calm the mind, relax the muscles around the eyes, and bring healing energy to the eyes (through increased circulation and energy flow). Palming allows you to relax mind and eyes.

Instructions

- Remember to breathe. Take two deep breaths.
- Sit at a table, lean forward, place your elbows on the table, and close your eyes gently.
- Now, place the palm of your left hand over your left eye, your fingers on your forehead. The hollow of your palm is directly over the eye, but not touching it (there is still room to blink), and the heel of your hand is resting on your cheekbones.
- Place your right hand over the right eye with the fingers crossing over the fingers of the left hand. The palm should be over the eye and the heel of the hand resting on your cheekbones.
- Make sure your elbows are low enough so that your face and the weight of your head are resting in your palms. This avoids stress on the neck.

In Daily Life

Even though we recommend that you do this for only three minutes, palming can be done as few or as many times as you like throughout the day. Palming is a way to relax your eyes and calm down from tensions of daily life. It is a great tool for relaxing after long hours on the computer.

4. Figure Eights

This exercise increases the flexibility of your eye muscles in a relaxed way.

Instructions

- Remember to breathe. Take two deep breaths.
- Either stand or sit with your feet shoulder-width apart and your hands at your sides. Do not cross your hands. Let your knees bend slightly.
- Imagine a figure eight positioned horizontally, approximately ten feet away from you.
- Without moving your head, let your eyes trace the figure eight, first in one direction, then in the opposite. Always remember to continue to breathe and to blink as your eyes move effortlessly along the figure eight. Check for tension in your jaw, and let it release.

In Daily Life

This is another exercise you can easily do while at work, even in a busy office, to relax the muscles around your eyes.

5. The Hot Dog

This exercise is practiced to improve the flexibility of the inside muscles of your eyes (the ciliary muscles).

Instructions

- Remember to breathe. Take two deep breaths.
- Either stand or sit with your feet shoulder-width apart. If you are standing, make sure your knees are slightly bent.
- Aim your eyes on any target in the distance.
- While looking at your distant target, bring both your index fingers into your line of sight, horizontally, tips touching, about eight inches in front of your eyes.
- Still aiming your eyes at the distant target, notice that a mini hot dog has appeared between the tips of your fingers. Remember to continue to breathe easily and deeply. Continue to aim your eyes towards the distant target.
- Pull the tips of your fingers apart slightly and observe the hot dog floating in the air.
- Now keep the hot dog within your sight for two breaths; then look directly at your fingers. The hot dog will disappear. Do not retrieve the hot dog for two breaths; then look again in the distance and find it once again. Switch back and forth for two minutes.

In Daily Life

After a long stint of near work, this is a great way to relax the ciliary muscles that have been holding near vision in focus.

6. Scanning

Staring is bad for your eyes because it freezes the energy and muscles, restricting blood flow. Scanning is the opposite of staring. Scanning keeps you alive and energetic.

Instructions

- Remember to breathe. Take two deep breaths.
- You can stand, sit, or move around your environment.
- As you look at objects, let your eyes glide over them as if you were outlining them. Continue to breathe deeply and easily.
- As your eyes shift from object to object, allow them to move easily without staring, and continue breathing and blinking. Your eyes should move in a relaxed manner, without tension. Make sure to release any tension in the mouth or the jaw.

In Daily Life

This is another exercise that you can do inconspicuously in the office.

7. Effortless Focus

This exercise is practiced to increase awareness of the object on which you are focusing and what surrounds it. This way of effortless seeing should permeate your everyday sight.

Instructions

- Remember to breathe. Take two deep breaths.
- Choose a point on which to focus your attention.
- Apply great effort towards the point, then relax your focus, and look at it effortlessly.
- Be aware of the difference in how you look with effort and without effort.
- Notice how your peripheral vision expands when you look with ease.

In Daily Life

Notice that if you are having difficulty reading something at a distance, relaxing your gaze makes it easier to see.

8. Near and Far Focus

This exercise improves the flexibility of the eyes changing from far viewing to near visual focus.

Instructions

- Remember to breathe. Take two deep breaths.
- Either sit or stand with feet shoulder-width apart. If standing, bend your knees slightly.
- Hold your thumb six inches away from your eyes and directly in front of your nose.
- Gaze easily at the thumb and take a deep breath.
- Then focus on a distant object at least ten feet away and take a deep breath. Change this focus every breath. Feel the muscles in your eyes change as you shift your focus.

In Daily Life

This exercise is exceptionally effective in soothing tired eyes when you have been focused on the computer or other near work for a long time.

9. Eye Massage

Throughout China, eye exercises are practiced in schools, offices, and factories. Regular breaks for eye exercises allow many people to prevent the need for glasses. These massage exercises are primarily concerned with relaxing the eye muscles. You will be using finger massage to stimulate what are known as "acupressure points."

Instructions

- Remember to breathe. Take two deep breaths.
- Sit quietly and relax, feet shoulder-width apart, knees slightly bent.
- Close the eyes gently.

When you press or massage each point, be gentle. Don't use too much force, and avoid putting pressure on the eyeballs.

- Put your thumbs below your eyebrows and above the inside corners of your eyes (not on your eyes), and place the other four fingers of each hand on your forehead. Press your thumbs into the point for four breaths.
- Use the thumb and index finger of either hand to massage the bridge of your nose. Press and then squeeze with an upward motion. Press and squeeze four times, four breaths.
- Place your middle fingers on your cheekbones, directly below the center of each eye. Massage the center part of your cheek for four breaths.
- Massage a point, starting at your temples right below the eyebrows and level with the outside end of your eyes.
- Next, place your thumbs on the inside end of the eyebrows and massage.
- Move to the middle of the eyebrow and massage.
- Then massage the end of the eyebrow.
- Finally, massage right below the middle of your eye.

In Daily Life

These can be done at a specified time in the given order or incorporated into your daily activities.

10. Zooming

This exercise is designed to improve the flexibility of your eye muscles.

Instructions

- Remember to breathe. Take two deep breaths.
- Place your thumb at arm's distance straight out in front of your eyes.
- While you breathe in, move your thumb slowly towards you as you focus your eyes on it.
- When your thumb is three inches from your face, move your arm away, and begin again.

In Daily Life

This is a good relaxation technique when stuck at the computer for a long time.

11. Sunning

This exercise is practiced without any glasses or contact lenses. The eyes are light-sensing organs. They are designed to receive and interpret light energy. Eyes need good, natural light in order to stay healthy and vibrant. Even though we have heard about the reduction in the ozone layer and the need to protect ourselves from ultraviolet radiation, the eyes should still receive natural sunlight for at least 20 minutes per day. (Full spectrum lights can be used if it is not possible to experience natural light).

Instructions

- Remember to breathe. Take two deep breaths.
- Sit or stand in a sunny place or under a full spectrum light source.
- Close your eyes gently.
- Move your head slowly from side to side so that you go from an area of shade into an area of light falling on your closed eyelids. Remember to continue to breathe easily and deeply. Feel the light on your eyelids; visualize accepting the light energy.

In Daily Life

Alternate between five breaths of sunning and two breaths of palming (exercise 3).

12. Visualization for Nearsighted People

Instructions

- Find a quiet relaxed environment.
- Remember to breathe. Take two deep breaths.
- Close your eyes and imagine gently sitting on the top of a mountain. Feel the warm breeze on your face and body, and let the sun fall on your face. You see an eagle flying in front of you. It flies within 20 feet of you; then it flies farther and farther away until it lands on the next mountaintop about one mile away.
- Next, you look up to the sky and watch the clouds as they move slowly away from you in many changing shapes. A plane emerges through the clouds. It moves farther and farther away until it disappears from your sight.
- Now open your eyes slowly and blink, remembering to breathe gently.

In Daily Life

Visualization helps connect your visual cortex to your visual system, and it enhances your ability to reduce stress and relax.

13. Visualization for Farsighted People

This exercise is designed to help integrate the mind and the eye as a synchronized unit.

Instructions

- Find a quiet relaxed environment
- Remember to breathe.

- Close your eyes gently, and imagine sitting at a large table in a conference room.
- At the other end of the table, about ten feet away, is a white sign with black letters that spell the word "You." Scan each letter.
- At eight feet away is another sign that says the word "Can." Scan each letter.
- Shift to the next sign at four feet away that says "Improve" and scan each letter.
- Shift now to a sign two feet away that says "Your" and scan each letter.
- There is a sign at one foot that says "Eye" in small print. Scan each letter.
- Now shift to a sign six inches away with tiny letters that say "Sight" and scan each letter.
- Finally take a deep breath, and gently open your eyes.

In Daily Life

This exercise is designed to help integrate the mind and eye as a synchronized unit.

14. Hop Scotch

This exercise is designed to strengthen the focusing ability of the eyes for near visual tasks.

Instructions

- Remember to breathe. Take two deep breaths.
- Sit or stand with your feet shoulder-width apart, knees slightly bent.
- Hold your thumb out at arm's length. Look directly at your thumb, and take a deep breath.
- Move the thumb three inches closer. Again, look directly at it, and take a deep breath.
- Continue to move your thumb closer by three inches at a time, focusing on it each time and breathing. Once the thumb is three inches from your eyes, begin again.

In Daily Life

This is another exercise that is quite soothing for tired eyes.

15. Line Counting, Filling in Os, Tracing

These exercises are designed for the eye to learn to focus on detail at near distance.

Instructions

- Remember to breathe. Take two deep breaths.
- Sit comfortably at a table, feet shoulder-width apart.
- In real time, draw five sets of vertical lines with at least five to eight lines in each set. Now count the number of lines in each set and write the number you've counted underneath.
- Draw ten small o's on a piece of paper, and fill in the o's with a pen.
- Draw three curvy lines and trace over them with your pen.

In Daily Life

Have fun with this and improve your doodling!

Acupressure Points

Acupuncture/acupressure is an ancient system of healing, developed over thousands of years as part of the traditional medicine of China, Japan, and other Eastern countries. The practice of acupuncture is thought to have begun with the discovery that the stimulation of specific areas on the skin affects the functioning of certain organs of the body, and that there exist currents of energy that flow in distinct patterns throughout the body called "meridians." Theory holds (and experience confirms) that when these currents of energy are flowing smoothly, there is health. When any of these currents are blocked, there is pain and disease.

There are a number of acupuncture/acupressure points around the eyes, basically around the orbits of the eyes, which are the bones that surround the eyeballs. The points provided here are some of the major local eye points.

Jingming. (Bl-1) urinary bladder channel lies where the inner corner of the eye meets the nose. Bladder 1 and 2 (Bl-1 and Bl-2) are perhaps the best two points for eye problems of all kinds from early-stage cataracts or glaucoma to hysteria with vision loss. They are also used for problems with conjunctivitis and blurred vision in the elderly.

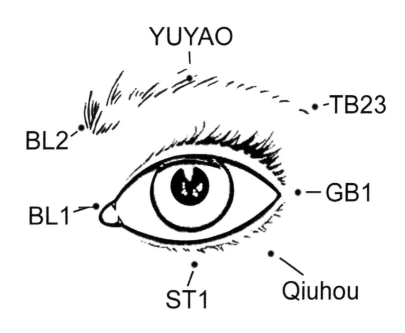

Zanzhu. (Bl-2) urinary bladder channel lies in the depressions at the inner ends of the eyebrows. See Bl-1.

Yuyao. This is located midpoint of the eyebrow in the hollow and is good for eye problems related to worry, excessive study, and mental strain.

Sizhukong. (TB-23) sanjiao or triple burner channel is in the depression at the outside end of the eyebrow. This is a local point that is good for eye and facial problems.

Tongziliao. (GB-1) gall bladder channel lies in the cavities on the outside corners of the eye sockets. Good for eye problems including conjunctivitis, red sore eyes, photophobia, dry and itchy eyes, early-stage cataracts, blurred vision, and lateral headaches.

Chengqi (St-1). This is located directly below the pupil on the infraorbital ridge bone and is the main point for all eye problems.

Qiuhou. This lies midway between St-1 and GB-1 along the orbit of the eyes.

Self-Acupressure Instructions

Gently massage each acupuncture point around the eye, starting with B1-1, and massaging each point as you go up and outward. Each point should be massaged for approximately 5–10 seconds. You can massage both eyes at the same time. You can do this massage as often as you like over the course of the day. You may find that each point feels different in terms of sensitivity. Keep breathing as you massage. Deep breathing helps the cells of your eyes receive the oxygen they need for healing. Practice long and slow abdominal breathing while massaging the points.

Caution. If you are pregnant, consult a trained acupuncturist before treating yourself. Do not massage on an area if it has a scar, burn, or infection.

Magic Eye

Magic Eye 3D images are created by using computer generated images comprised of randomly placed dots to study depth perception.

- Makes the eyes more flexible in focusing, and seeing peripheral and distance vision.
- Reduces strain related to high volume computer use.
- Increases one's ability to recall printed information
- Improves depth perception
- Helps relieve overall stress.
- Helps integrate the physical, mental and spiritual energies

See Appendix 8 for more information.

---

[1] Lin, Z, Vasudevan, B., Fang, S.J., Jhapji, V., Mao, G.Y., et al. (2016). Eye exercises of acupoints: their impact on myopia and visual symptoms in Chinese rural children. *BMC Complement Altern Med,* Sep 6;16:349.

[2] Di Noto, P., Uta, S., DeSouza, J.F. (2013). Eye exercises enhance accuracy and letter recognition, but not reaction time, in a modified rapid serial visual presentation task. *PLoS One,* 2013;8(3):359244.

[3] Kang, M.T., Li, S.M., Peng, X., Li., L., Ran, A., et al. (2016). Chinese Eye Exercises and Myopia Development in School Age Children: A Nested Case-control Study. *Sci Rep,* Jun 22;6:28531.

[4] Rodriguez, S.L., Hopman, W.M., ten Hove, M.W. (2012). Eye exercises for treatment of idiopathic cranial nerve VII paresis: pilot study. *Can J Neurol Sci,* Mar;39(2):196-201.

[5] Rawstron, J.A., Burley, C.D., Elder, M.J. (2005). A systematic review of the applicability and efficacy of eye exercises. *J Pediartr Ophthalmol Strabismus,* Mar-Apr;42(2):82-8.

10-5. VISION AND PERSONALITY

"Seeing within changes one's outer vision."
--Joseph Chilton Pearce--

The Basic Personality Types

Dr. Grossman practiced as a behavioral optometrist for over a decade before he began his study of Oriental Medicine in order to acquire a better context for understanding his patients and their vision conditions. He continued creating individualized healing protocols. The expansive application of TCM enabled him to help his patients start to heal, no matter their vision ailment.

Often, in order to help his patients make the deep changes within themselves for the healing of a visual impairment, he found it valuable to work on the level of persona. And here Chinese medicine is useful. TCM divides humanity into five types, based on the five elements of Nature. He learned to adapt these five types, not only according to vision issues but to their underlying causes, and he began to see how beneficial these applications were.

Understanding Personality

As people begin to identify their personality type, they attain a new understanding of patterns in their lives and how these patterns influence them and those around them. They better recognize their own strengths and weaknesses and can set a pathway of reasonable goals, based on a more complete understanding of their own nature. The five basic types as they pertain to persona is not only a tool for self-examination but is also a tool for building bridges toward others.

Patients discover that both their vision and their well-being depend upon living in increasing harmony with the natural world. As a result, they learn tolerance and compassion for others and gain a deeper appreciation for the various components that determine their basic nature. Importantly, patients learn who they are and how to be true to themselves. So many of our problems—physical, emotional, and spiritual—come from trying to be someone or something that we are not. When we live in situations and relationships where we are constantly struggling to fit in, we develop illnesses of all sorts.

For this reason, we include information on the five personality types, based on the five elements of TCM. The categories have been developed over many years from a synthesis of observations made in Dr. Grossman's clinical experience in behavioral optometry.

The Peacemaker (Earth)

This type might also be called the worrier, although we don't want to identify any type by just one emotion, positive or negative, as we all feel a wide range of emotions each day. And yet, The Peacemaker is a powerful worrier. In their eyes, no matter their color, no matter their gender or age, you will see a look of deep concern.

First Impressions

What is most interesting about Peacemakers when you first meet them is the message that they are sending with their eyes. And, make no mistake about it, they send forth a good deal of energy with their eyes. The eyes say, "You are safe with me. You can trust me." And they hold you in contact, without shifting, without turning away.

As we examine Peacemakers, their answers to questions quickly identify them. They worry that they will not give the right answers, as if there are right or wrong answers. During an exam, Peacemakers tend to ask many very analytical questions. And they really want responses. They always seek information. They also want an assurance that it is all right for them to ask questions, and that they themselves are providing good answers to their own questions.

Creating Harmony

When asking a Peacemaker how they best describe themselves, they will say they are sympathetic and caring. And indeed, they are. Peacemakers are among the most supportive of people. They universally have trouble shaping the word "No" with their lips. They tend to be very patient and very willing to listen to others and their troubles. Peacemakers (and not without reason) consider themselves to be wonderful friends, loving parents, and in general, spokespersons for peace, harmony, and cooperation for the peoples of the earth.

What Peacemakers tend not to say about themselves, or even not to know about themselves, is that underneath the harmony is a good deal of insecurity and sometimes, a good deal of anxiety. If you ask the object of the Peacemaker's affection how he or she feels about the Peacemaker, they may report that they feel a bit smothered by their love, that he or she cares a bit too much. They may say that the energy coming out of the Peacemaker's eyes is like that of a mother to her child.

The Peacemaker's desire for harmony can be thrown off balance easily when it is lacking, and Peacemakers have a real knack for getting involved in situations in which positive emotions are lacking. These situations drain Peacemakers of their energy. Negative situations bring out the mother in Peacemakers who will seek to create harmony for others and loved ones and not to take care of themselves. For the Peacemaker, this pattern leads to disharmony and illness.

Peacemakers tend to be trapped in the present moment. They lack fluidity with time. The present surrounds them, envelops them, and chokes them. They cannot look beyond the details around them. They get lost in details, the details of their own lives, and the details of the lives of others. They lose the ability to put details into context and see the big picture. Just as they cannot see the patterns formed by the details of life, they lack the ability to put those details into the timeline of life. This leaves the Peacemaker stuck, frozen in space and time, and very worried.

Prone to Myopia

Peacemakers have a unique visual style. Just as they question things verbally, so too, they question visually. They take in a great deal of information with their eyes, but they are likely to over-focus on it with both mind and eyes. This leads to a condition that an eye care professional would term "exophoria." This means that, while their eyes tend to drift out, they over-converge in a manner that locks them in. This visual pattern leads to eyestrain, fatigue, and nearsightedness. Peacemakers particularly are prone to myopia, and they use more energy to be able to see than they actually need. In short, they try too hard to see, just as emotionally, they are trying too hard to create harmony.

Symptoms

- Heaviness in their arms and legs, trouble moving around physically
- General lack of energy and/or endurance
- Tendency to have headaches, especially during times of conflict or excessive worrying
- Tendency to be obsessive in their emotional ties; may show obsessive/compulsive behaviors
- Need for constant love and affection
- Need to be needed, to be included, to be important to the lives of others
- Hypersensitive to criticism and conflict and an inability to handle rude or abrupt behavior
- Find times of change or transition difficult

Physical Description

Physically, Peacemakers have dark complexions and are somewhat overweight. Their systems retain water easily. They often have a large head and/or a large stomach, with small hands and feet. They carry their strength in their thighs. They have wide jaws. Peacemakers are likely to have an excessive flow of saliva and swollen and tender gums that bleed easily. The mucus in their mouth, nose, and throat tends to be thick but clear, like raw egg white.

You can often spot them by the way they walk, as they move without lifting their feet off the ground. Peacemakers lack energy and endurance. They have a slow and sluggish metabolism. Also, Peacemakers have weak joints, especially ankles and hips. They have functional disorders like chronic fatigue and hypoglycemia.

Example of a Peacemaker

Jeanette was a 45-year-old teacher of learning-disabled children. Dr. Grossman asked why she had come and she said, "I can see, but my eyes hurt all the time. I can't go on like this." Before she came to his office, Jeanette had visited three other eye doctors within a six-month period, all of whom told her the same thing: her eyes were healthy and her eyeglass prescription was correct.

Jeanette had two children in college and a husband who worked full time for the telephone company. On the surface, everything about her seemed solid and middle class. And yet, Jeanette had been on medication for chronic pain in her stomach, and she suffered from migraine headaches. Her neck, shoulder, and back muscles were very tight. She had visited a chiropractor but had received only temporary improvement in her symptoms. She also reported that she liked sweets and tended to put on weight easily if she was not careful.

It was important to Jeanette that Dr. Grossman take his time to really examine and listen to her. It was important to her that he answer all her questions. When it became apparent to her that her needs would be met, she began to relax. She said that she was worried, that she was always worried about her health, her students, her children, and her husband. Jeanette reported that she felt irritable and frustrated, often over small matters.

Jeanette's visual pattern included the onset of nearsightedness at about age 14. Her eyes also tended to over-converge. When asked to target her eyes on a specific object, she would over focus on the target. She said that often she felt she would lock in on something and could not look away. In doing so, she failed to see the big picture. All of this was causing a great deal of stress to her visual system, leaving her with chronic eye and body pain.

As they talked, it occurred to Dr. Grossman that perhaps Jeanette was too practical, too grounded, and that perhaps she would benefit by having her head in the clouds. And Dr. Grossman gave her a very simple first exercise. Any time Jeanette began to feel stressed and over-burdened she was to look up at the sky and the clouds and observe their shapelessness and graceful motion. If she could not go outside, she was to close her eyes and visualize a bright blue sky filled with beautiful white clouds. She was to spend some time with her head in the clouds.

After a six-month period of vision therapy, during which Jeanette was encouraged to relax both her mind and her eyes, Jeanette was nearly pain-free. She reported that her headaches had all but disappeared, along with her neck pain, shoulder pain, and eyestrain. She was able to use her glasses without any form of discomfort. Her husband had recently expressed his amazement with the changes in her character, as she had, according to him, become a much more relaxed and happier person. By allowing herself the practice of building skyscrapers in the sky, Jeanette had released her old and damaging patterns and created healthy instincts toward harmony.

Peacemaker Overview

What Peacemakers have in common is that their primary focus in life is being helpful to others. They gather their feelings of self-worth through their love and concern for others. They take on the role of the "good mother" for all those around them. They are likely to enter the helping professions, such as teaching, social work, therapy, nursing, and the clergy. The message they present to the world is "Let me take care of you," or "Don't worry about that, I'll worry for you."

The Performer (Fire)

Performers are warm-hearted people who fill their lives and the lives of those around them with excitement and emotion. They love to be with others and connect emotionally and very easily. They love being the center of attention and enjoy art forms such as singing, dancing, and acting.

First Impressions

When Dr. Grossman walks in to meet a Performer in the waiting room, their eyes are darting all over the room, never resting in one place. Even when in the exam chair, they do not make sustained eye contact, as if their eyes are thinking, "I am not comfortable here. I have to move."

In both children and adults of this type, there is a distinct tendency to talk and talk and talk. In an exam, one simple question during the exam returns a lengthy answer, giving far more information than was requested. Yet, they never make eye contact. Their answers are inconsistent and often contradictory, requiring simple questions with simple yes or no answers. This is difficult for Performers, as are the most basic eye tests. If asked to look at the tip of a pen, they do so for a second before their eyes begin moving around the room once more.

In Life

Performers are highly intuitive. They seem to know how others are feeling before the others know themselves. They are given to emotional highs and lows. They feel especially low when physically separated from people they love. Performers often have difficulty concentrating and paying attention. With their highly developed artistic and performance sensibilities, they might lack analytical skills. Their thinking process tends to be chaotic and unfocused and they lose direction easily, both emotionally and physically. They often feel that the circumstances of their lives are outside their control.

The eyes of a Performer are in constant turmoil. They are not able to find and sustain a target. They tend to be highly verbal and to enjoy storytelling and performing, but they have trouble matching what they are saying to what they are seeing.

Chaotic forms of communication and forms of energy output can confuse the other, making learning especially difficult. Poor focusing, poor eye teaming, and poor eye movement skills further hamper their learning skills. Visually, nothing comes easy for them. Because of their verbal and visual difficulties, and because of their desire to move, both physically and emotionally, children of this type are often diagnosed with Attention Deficit Disorder.

Under the performance and under the constant motion, Performers fear losing control and being trapped or controlled in any way. They cannot bear boredom or inactivity, but feel the need, at all times, to be emotionally and physically active. They often have very fragile personal boundaries. They are therefore easily overwhelmed by other people's intense feelings and easily exhausted by the people around them.

Symptoms

- Flushed complexion
- Tendency toward excessive perspiration and a tendency to overheat
- Chronic sleep disturbances: insomnia, nightmares, and restless sleep
- Restless, agitated, and explosive energy
- Tendency to speak in a manner that is both inappropriate and overly loud
- Tendency toward free-floating anxiety and emotional and physical restlessness
- Inability to concentrate easily, irrational thinking processes, lack of analytical skills
- Intense mood swings

Physical Description

Performers have strong, slim bodies, with sinewy hands and feet. They often have long necks, arms, and legs. Their skin is soft, warm, and moist. Many of their symptoms are related to the skin. Performers are prone to rashes, to skin irritations, including sores of the mouth, tongue, and lips. Their skin easily colors. In Caucasians, the skin often takes on a rosy or bright red hue.

Although Performers are highly verbal, they commonly have speech disorders, with stuttering or strained speech. They often must work hard on their concentration in order to speak clearly.

Example of a Performer

George was a 14-year-old having trouble in school in learning and in being disruptive in his class because of his need to constantly talk and move away from his desk. George tested with an IQ that was well above average, but he had been diagnosed with ADD. His teachers were at their wits end as to how to help him live up to his potential without sacrificing the needs of the other members of his class.

Just giving George a vision exam proved to be a major undertaking. He seemed to be everywhere in the room at once, touching every piece of equipment, exploring every corner. In the exam chair, he squirmed constantly. He repeated over and over again to his mother, as if chanting, "Can we go now? Can we go now?" The exam confirmed that George was seeing with 20/20 acuity in both eyes, and that his eyes were healthy. However, it was not possible to get a true reading of his eye teaming skills because he could not focus long enough on any visual target.

Dr. Grossman explained to George's mother all that he knew about the Performer and recommended a home-based course in vision therapy. Over the next few months, George's mother managed to corral his energy daily into the therapy program. After a year, George was far more capable of targeting with his eyes and sustaining a target. His eye teaming ability now proved to be excellent. Following this year of hard work, George was again tested by his school district. This time they found no sign of ADD.

Performer Overview

What all the members of this category have in common is an amazing amount of enthusiasm for whatever they do in life, and many of them channel it, one way or another, into show business. Life for them is an adventure, a game in which they are always looking forward to whatever is coming next. They have a creative outlook, a quick mind, and a great sense of humor. The messages they bring into the world scream "I don't think that I am ever going to grow up!" and "I want to do everything today."

The Critic (Metal)

Precise, Polite, Direct

Critics are precise people. These are the new patients who become upset when the doctor is behind schedule, as usual. They are polite and speak with clear and courteous speech. After they announce the fact that they have arrived for their appointment, they sit up straight in a chair with their hands folded in their laps. These are people of direct and strong eye contact, whose eyes send the message, "Why is this world so out of order?" Their eyes miss nothing and judge everything. They are the natural critics of world order.

When asked about their lives, they will tell the doctor that nothing is more important than philosophy. Different critics have different philosophies. Some are very religious, others very esoteric, but all adhere to a central philosophy that they enjoy sharing with others. They also tend to love classical music. They say that they need order in their lives. And they spend energy every day creating and maintaining that order. They will make a list every morning of the things they need to do that day, and they become frustrated when they cannot accomplish everything on their list by the day's end.

Looking for Perfection

On a perfect day, an adult Critic will get up and shower, take time to read the newspaper while eating breakfast, and then take time to work in the garden before lunch. In the afternoon, they go to a lecture or to a museum, meet some friends for dinner, and attend a classical music concert in the evening. Time here is the key. Critics dream of having time enough for all the things they enjoy. Usually, the Critic feels that time is the enemy and there is never enough time to get everything done. Their dream is to wake in the morning without an alarm clock and have enough time for their beloved garden.

Relationships work for them in the same manner. Critics say that they have to stress quality of time versus quantity in their relationships, as they have trouble taking time away from work for relationships.

Prone to Nearsightedness

Critics have eyes with patterns every bit as rigid as their personality. Because of a lack of flexibility in both their being and their visual system, Critics are almost universally nearsighted. They also tend to be overly convergent, with their eye muscles locked and tight.

Critics can be very difficult to work with. They are stuck in their visual pattern and have little interest in trying different ways of looking at their world. They want to stay locked in their own perspective. In fact, if they could have their way, they would see to it that the rest of us see things from their perspective. That the world does not follow their rhythm and organization is a constant source of frustration.

In Life

Naturally, Critics experience a good deal of stress. First is the stress they create in holding themselves up to almost impossible standards. Second is the stress they create in their relationships when they try to hold others up to their own, often invisible and incomprehensible standards. Underneath this stress is a deep pool of anxiety.

Critics may often become so absorbed in organizational details that they lose sight of core issues. They can forget why something is so important to them and cling only to the fact that it is important. As they become more and more stuck, they become vulnerable to spontaneous behavior. Anything that does not fall into their personal pattern of order can become confusing, frustrating, and ultimately frightening.

Of course, Critics like to be in control. They can be overbearing. They are judgmental and critical of others. In short, they are addicted to being right. Their greatest fear is losing control and falling apart. Their second greatest fear is that their holy cause of bringing order to the world will somehow be corrupted.

Symptoms

- Chronically stiff and tight muscles
- Unnaturally rigid posture, inflexible spine, especially the neck
- Sensitivity to odors
- Tendency to be emotionally distant
- Difficulty with conflict and disorder
- Overly critical and judgmental attitude, intolerant of the viewpoints of others
- Strict disciplinarian
- Emphasis on order, love of routine and of lists

Physical Description

Physically, Critics tend to be erect, and their physiques tend to be symmetrical. They are likely to have light toned, clear and dry skin, hair, and lips; their skin tends to have a low level of perspiration. Critics have delicate features with small bones and compact muscles.

Breathing problems of all sorts are common to the type. They have chronic sinus conditions and a distinct sensitivity to any number of odors. They tend to develop environmental sensitivities, especially to mold, chemicals, and animals.

Example of a Critic

Upon entering Dr. Grossman's office, Vincent told him politely that his office was too stuffy. He was dressed in a suit and tie and had shiny black shoes and perfectly combed hair. He brought with him all his records from previous doctors' offices, carefully filed, dating back ten years. Vincent was 57 years old. He worked as an art dealer and was a self-described perfectionist. He said that he loved order in his environment, his garden, his kitchen, and particularly his music collection. His need for organization was apparent in his body as well. His tall and lean body was held taut. His jaw was set and determined. His eyes were rigidly held.

Vincent said that his vision, when seeing very near and very far, was not as clear as he thought it should be. He said that he frequently cleaned his glasses with a special lens cleaner in the hope of having a little clearer image. His current prescription corrected his vision to 20/20, although Vincent felt it was not strong enough. He had an astigmatism which required one of his lenses to be slightly stronger than the other and that bothered him.

As is so often the case, Vincent's greatest strength was also his greatest weakness. His amazing visual ability to discriminate, which had brought him to the top of his profession as an art dealer, was crippling his ability to live a full and happy life. His hope for greater clarity and the slight difference between his lenses haunted and tormented him.

As the torment had begun in the previous few months, Dr. Grossman asked whether there were changes in the last year and particularly if he had started to play any musical instrument. Vincent's face broke into a broad smile as he answered that, just nine months before, he had joined a group that met weekly to play classical music. He played violin and practiced daily. Dr. Grossman explained that the practice was likely the cause of his visual disorientation. As violinists tilt their heads to play, their eyes tilt as well, and when Vincent tilted his eyes, he could not help but notice the difference in the prescriptions of his two eyes. Over time, the tilt itself could be responsible for a change in his astigmatism.

Dr. Grossman gave Vincent a slight change in his prescription and recommended that he explore the Alexander Technique as a means of relaxation, that he practice some basic vision therapy exercises at home every day, and that he have a weekly massage. By the end of just three months, all Vincent's symptoms had disappeared.

Critic Overview

Critics carry the common theme of letting the rest of us know how to live properly. They have definite opinions, and each also has a distinct philosophy of how the world should act, look, and be. They live their lives in a very idealistic manner. They each, in different ways, tend to be rather rigid. Order, cleanliness, and a sense of aesthetics help to structure their lives. The messages they bring into the world are "There is a right way and a wrong way of doing things," and "The world needs more order."

The Controller (Wood)

First Impressions

Energy pours from the eyes of The Controller. Their eyes are penetrating and almost aggressive in their glance. They walk into a room with a true entrance, never slipping in unnoticed. After that entrance, they demand total attention. The Controller has a firm handshake and a forceful voice. The Controller has a hard time containing his/her energy and sitting still. Controllers tend to talk with their hands and to tap their feet while sitting.

Eye Exam

The Controller typically has little interest in giving a case history. History is dead and gone and doesn't matter. What matters is what's ahead. Controllers want to know what the doctor can do for them right now. They have a fierce determination about getting things done, lacking both patience and compassion for those who cannot get things done as quickly. The Controller seems to be moving through life at 70mph in a 50mph zone. This is revealed in the manner in which they speak and in which they accomplish things, that is, by "pushing themselves to the limit."

The Controller is by nature independent and self-reliant. "Slow and steady" go against their nature. They don't mind taking risks and love new challenges. Unfortunately, they seem to lack an internal braking system. They don't know when to stop, only how to keep pushing. In many situations, this life strategy leaves Controllers feeling frustrated, angry, and emotionally unstable.

Prone to Over-Convergence

In terms of vision, Controllers tend to display over-convergence and a turn in one or both eyes. This creates a tension in their eye muscles and in the muscles of their neck and back. The Controller, like The Critic, displays a tense and rigid visual pattern that manifests in their body structure and their persona.

As their life and visual stress patterns build, Controllers tend to cling stubbornly to their adaptations. They push themselves and others. The muscles of their eyes, face, neck, shoulders, and back become tighter. This typically results in myopia.

Hiding Fear

Beneath their surface strength and stubbornness, The Controller is deeply afraid. Controllers are afraid of becoming helpless and losing their sense of control. They tend to rush about in many directions at once, addressing the problems this creates by slamming against them. As they get older, they naturally lose some of the overwhelming energy of youth and begin to panic. They fear illness and weakness. They hate and fear any situation—including relationships—that makes them feel confined or trapped. They love to compete and to win. Often, they go into competitions, such as for control of the left lane of the highway, in which the opponents are not even aware of being in a competition. And when they compete, they need to win.

Symptoms

- An overly serious attitude to life, lack of a sense of humor
- Difficulty relaxing
- Direct and penetrating eye contact
- Overpowering need to win, some win at any cost
- Fear of confinement or restraint, fear of losing, fear of illness or helplessness
- Tension in the neck, shoulders, and back
- Rigidity and lack of smoothness
- Tendency to walk forcefully, demand center stage

Physical Description

Physically, Controllers tend to have strong, square-shaped musculatures. They often are sports enthusiasts who thrive on watching and taking part in competitive games and vigorous exercise. Regular exercise is of vital importance to them. Controllers are likely to have coarse, thick, and oily skin that is predisposed to acne. Look for their skin to have cysts, and lumps of all kinds.

Controllers are prone to muscular tightness and pain. Muscular cramps and spasms are common throughout their body, especially in their necks and shoulders and in their digestive tract. They tend to get many headaches, especially migraines, that typically are accompanied by visual disturbances, eyestrain, and sharp eye pain. They might also have ringing in their ears, dizziness, and nausea with their headaches. Females of this type are likely to have menstrual irregularities, including heavy bleeding and abnormally frequent periods. They also suffer from excessive symptoms of PMS, such as cramping, abdominal distension, and severe mood swings. Controllers are susceptible to high blood pressure. Of all the types, they are the most vulnerable to stress.

Example of a Controller

Elizabeth always had perfect vision. But at age 24, things were starting to look a little blurry. A doctor had given her glasses for distance seeing. Even now, at age 36, she was still bothered that her vision was not perfect. She was an executive, exercised an hour a day and had a marriage and two young children. She handled all these responsibilities beautifully. She was an example of all that success implied: good looks, good marriage, large income, and a super-mom to boot.

As she walked into Dr. Grossman's office, he noticed that her stride was long, strong, and secure. She walked in like she owned the place. She gave a firm handshake and made direct eye contact. She immediately said she had made the appointment because she wanted her vision to improve, and she did not want stronger glasses. But also, as her glasses had gotten stronger, she was increasingly suffering from neck pain. A friend whose neck pain had been eased by vision therapy recommended she try it. Elizabeth's neck pain was so great that she was on medication to allow her to function. She said, in trying to solve the problem, she had already had massage, but massage only helped for a little while, and besides, who had time to have a massage every day?

After listening to all that Elizabeth had to tell, and after examining her eyes, Dr. Grossman discussed her lifestyle with her. Her life strategy had served her well, as it had brought her a functioning marriage, a high paying job, and two children; but, he pointed out, it had caused the tension in her body and her strong PMS symptoms. It also quite possibly affected other aspects of her life that she was not even aware of.

Dr. Grossman created a vision therapy program for Elizabeth that would allow her to explore her own nature and the nature of her relationships with others. This program would also let her discover the difference between "reacting" to obstacles in her life and "responding" to them. The therapy was, at its core, a program that would let Elizabeth discover and define for herself the true nature of "success." Due to her schedule, Elizabeth was able to come to the office only once a month. But she did follow through with her homework with true Controller zeal. Within nine months, she was able to live and work without her glasses, except for night driving.

As she worked through her program, Elizabeth added twice-weekly yoga sessions and a weekly massage into the mix. After a few more months, she reported that her neck pain had all but vanished, and that when it did occur, she used it as a sign that she needed to relax. She now saw those small tweaks of pain as a blessing.

Controller Overview

Controllers often achieve a high degree of success in their lives and do so by their own hand and in their own way. In their professions, they work hard to be recognized as the best. They give little time to doubting themselves and are always ready for new challenges. They are highly competitive by nature. Their messages to the world are "Nothing can stop me if I work hard enough," and "I have the ability and desire to be the best at whatever I choose to do."

The Thinker (Water)

No other type has as much going on in the eyes as The Thinker. From birth, their eyes connect with the world. They learn and communicate with their eyes. There is a certain softness and thoughtfulness to their gaze, as if they were seeing each thing, especially you, for the very first time each time they see you. The message in the eyes of a Thinker is "I am here to learn the truth." Thus, there is great power in their eyes.

First Impressions

Yet, after the initial communion, Thinkers have difficulty maintaining eye contact. Even if eye contact remains, their minds will seem to have moved off to something or somewhere else. Thinkers tend to be patient, introspective, and even shy. In the waiting room, they are usually sitting in the corner reading a magazine.

When Thinkers report their case histories, they speak in terms of what happened in the past that led them into their present state of being. They show themselves to be analytical and logical thinkers who are interested in knowing just how and why things work the way they do. Thinkers are interested in anything new; for example, they are curious about the new equipment in the eye doctor's office. Thinkers are interested in their present health problems. More than any other type, they have come to the doctor, not just for information, but for an explanation. They want to know how their vision got the way it is. This is an important step in their healing.

Thinkers' introspection is their survival strategy. When they deal with a situation that cannot be understood, they tend to retreat. They move to a pattern of solitude until an answer can be found.

Lack of Focus

Thinkers' most common vision issue has to do with a lack of ability to focus. When they feel interested, their focus is strong. But when they are in a state of confusion, their eyes have the same lack of focus that frustrates their mind. Processing visual information can drain energy and they lose perspective on what else is going on around them. They have to work and work hard, not only to see what is in front of them, but also to understand what they are seeing.

Thinkers often have a weakness in their ability to converge their eyes and in focusing. This means that they have trouble seeing and understanding the details of life. The energy they need to both converge and focus can drain them, leading to a sense of fatigue, not just in their eye muscles, but in their whole bodies and minds. The Thinker's search for truth covers an underlying deep-seated lack of trust. They tend not to trust the world, just as they cannot trust the information their eyes are taking in. Therefore, they always need to verify and test what they have seen through the use of their other senses.

Thinkers do not want to be intruded upon or controlled, however, they also do not like to be alone. It creates tension within their system. They want contact with others, yet they feel the need to withdraw. Thinkers cannot have faith in something that can't be proven to them, and yet they yearn for spiritual enlightenment. Thus, the Thinker tries to reconcile the rational with the irrational, the visible with the invisible, as he or she struggles through life.

Symptoms

- Dark blue-black circles around the eyes
- Headaches in the occiput, where the back of the neck meets the skull
- Emotional inaccessibility and tendency to withdraw, deep feelings of insecurity
- Preoccupation with inner dialogue
- Tendency to procrastinate, lack of will power and motivation to solve problems
- Lack of trust in others

Physical Description

Thinkers have long, narrow heads and faces, large, long bones, and long fingers and toes. They tend toward narrow shoulders, large hips, and deep-set eyes. They are often hypersensitive to light. Thinkers are prone to deterioration of their gums and teeth. They are also likely to have chronic low back pain and knee problems. Men of this type tend to have prostate troubles, and men and women alike have ailments of the bladder, most commonly urinating difficulty.

Example of a Thinker

Janice, 46, was a divorced woman who supported herself by writing freelance magazine articles. She lived in a large house, by herself. She was referred to Dr. Grossman by her chiropractor, after having complained to him that she never felt secure in crowded places. Janice told Dr. Grossman that she did not like closed doors, and she always slept with her windows and the door to her room open. She felt claustrophobic in small rooms or among crowds. She added that it was hard for her to make eye contact with people. In short, she often felt that the world was closing in around her, and that made her nervous.

Before coming to see Dr. Grossman, Janice had eye exams every two years and was given reading glasses in mid-life. She had been told that, except for slight presbyopia, her eyes were fine.

After examining her, Dr. Grossman disagreed.

Janice's visual patterning showed Dr. Grossman that she had very little ability to converge her eyes and focus on a target. She all but lacked the ability to focus her full attention on whatever she was looking at. When she tried to focus centrally on what was right in front of her, she was unable to sustain awareness of what was going on around her. If she paid attention to what was going on in her periphery, she was unable to focus on what was in front of her. This inability to be aware simultaneously of her central and her peripheral vision was what left her constantly confused and disorganized.

Dr. Grossman told Janice that he understood that to her, the world seemed too big to process all at the same time. She now had to become aware that, as she became more and more adept at taking in information visually in small pieces, she would feel happier and safer. He set to work with Janice doing a six-month, home-based program of vision therapy. After that time, her eyes were much more fluid at focusing near and far, centrally and peripherally. Her eyes also worked more smoothly as a team. She was better able to record and process information without strain, and she was free to shop in crowded areas as much as she wanted.

Thinker Overview

Thinkers are intrigued by the idea of discovery or finding out why things are as they are. They want to understand how everything works. They continue to search, asking questions, taking things apart. They love to research all the aspects of a situation. Thinkers prefer to observe the world in order to understand it. Because of this, they tend to stand back a bit, to be aloof. Others of this type are drawn into technical subjects like engineering, computers, and science. The messages they send to the world are "I need to understand what is going on," or "I am going to solve this problem."

Summary

If a behavioral optometrist can, in addition to diagnosing specific eye and eye/brain disorders, properly identify a patients' personality type, he is in a better position to select the proper form of treatment. Such treatment reaches all aspects of a patient's being, allowing for a process of transformation.

10-6. VISUAL HYGIENE

Headaches, squinting, and eyes that burn, ache, water, or tire easily are indications that the visual system needs help. Most people are born with the potential for good eyesight. Vision, however, is learned. And the way you use and care for your vision directly affects your success at school or work and enjoyment of play. Your visual system can undergo tremendous stress.

Changing Vision Needs

Students now read three times the number of textbooks their grandparents did. Though book reading can lead to eyestrain, textbooks are becoming anachronistic as we shift to digital texts and other digital learning software, which has its own problems in vision.[1] Children and teens are increasingly relying on digital materials at school and are obsessing with digital games, social media, and more, which is leading to additional serious consequences in vision health. Some children start looking at electronic screens from infancy.

Although parents may be familiar with vision damage from UVA and UVB light from the sun, few are aware of the damage to the retina from blue light, which is emitted by the digital screens of electronic devices and fluorescent and LED lighting.

The most common visual problems reported among college-aged computer users were headache (53.3%), burning sensation in the eyes (54.8%), and tired eyes (48%).[2] While studies on the effects of computer eyestrain are not yet prevalent, taking a look at data related to repetitive strain injuries (RSIs) can help put this problem in perspective.

Adults constantly use near vision at work and play. The shift to computers has engaged a growing number of workers in prolonged, near-vision tasks. Eye discomfort, headaches, blurred vision, lowered visual performance, and a wide array of vision-linked problems are related to this heavy, near-point vision overload, not to mention increased risk of glaucoma,[3] [4] dry eye,[5] advanced macular degeneration, damage to rods and cones[6] and to the retinal pigmented layer of macula,[7] and eye cancer.[8]

In addition to the direct physical damage from blue light emitted from electronic screens, the slumped physical position that the body adopts causes indirect damage to the eyes and body. Prolonged hunching over a computer terminal increases neck-muscle tightness, which causes neuro-vascular compression, reduces available oxygen and nutrients, and impinges on nerve conduction to and from the body and the head. Additionally, this position compresses the lung cavities, preventing full, nourishing breathing.

Hunter-Soldier Eyes

The problem is that human beings were not designed to do constant viewing within an arm's length. We evolved hunter-soldier eyes for survival and for spotting game and enemies at a distance. Only in the last half-century have so many people been forced to deal with sustained, near-visual tasks. The result has been a constant stress on the visual system that we were not designed to endure, producing eye symptoms and related problems. Many vision and eye problems are the direct result of a failure to adapt to these relatively new, near-centered visual tasks. It's no wonder that ignoring good visual hygiene, the impact of long-term visual stress, or the failure to heed symptoms of vision problems can have a significant effect on the quality and enjoyment of a person's life.

More than 20/20

The standard eye test uses the Snellen chart, which was designed around 1860 to test students' ability to read a chalkboard from the back of a schoolroom; it indicates distance visual acuity.

The Snellen chart does not, however, test the ability of a person to handle near-visual work such as reading, writing, or prolonged close-up activities—"near-point vision." Near-point visual stress, despite 20/20 distance clarity, has been shown to lead to the development of visual problems and eye conditions, including dry eyes[9] (often the result of a reduced blinking rate), increased myopia,[10] and glaucoma.[11] Blurred vision, dry eyes, burning sensation, redness of eyes, and headache are the main symptoms resulting from improper use of computers,[12] as well as visual fatigue symptoms such as sore eyes and increased glare sensitivity.[13]

Myopia (nearsightedness) is one of these eye conditions. Between 1999 and 2004, approximately 41.6% of the population of the United States was diagnosed as nearsighted, compared to 25% measured and assessed between the years 1971–1972; that is a 16.6% increase in three decades. Myopia now appears at earlier ages, and usually the earlier it appears, the deeper the person advances into nearsightedness. Increasingly strong lenses for distance vision are required as myopia progresses.

A good treatment option is to work with a vision therapist to help maintain your prescription and possibly reduce it. Daily exercising and taking regular breaks from reading and computer use to do these eye exercises can help maintain strong, healthy vision.

The most common result of visual stress is lowered achievement.[14] When chronic stress is present, people usually do one of several things:

- Avoid the task by doing as little as they can to get by
- Experience pain or other symptoms (such as aches, visual or body fatigue, and falling asleep when reading)
- Suppress the sight of one eye at the cost of reduced efficiency and understanding
- Develop myopia or astigmatism
- Get frustrated because of difficulty concentrating
- Strain harder to get the work or reading done
- Any combination of the above

How to Take Better Care of Your Vision

Here are some basic guidelines for reducing visual stress.

Looking up. Both children and adults need to look up and away from near tasks to distant objects regularly. From a Chinese medicine perspective, electronic devices give off Fire energy. When looking at computer or cell phone screens, it would help to look far away, every 30 minutes, to something green, like trees, which helps to reduce Fire energy.

Lighting. The illumination on your work should be three times brighter than the rest of the room. Don't read under a single lamp in a dark room. Eliminating glare is especially important for close-up work. Don't use fluorescent or LED lights as they have an imbalanced color spectrum, too strong in the blue range, which can contribute to impaired sleep in the short term and to retinal damage in the long run. Additionally, fluorescent lights flicker at a rate that is undetectable to the human eye and can cause eyestrain and dizziness. Incandescent lighting is the better choice. Try to avoid exposure to bright lights, computer screens, and cell phones for 3–4 hours before sleep.

Sitting straight. Have chest up, shoulders back, and weight over the seat so both eyes are at the eye task level and at an equal distance from what is being seen.

Best distance. Reading, writing, or close-up work is best done at an eye-to-activity distance equal to the length between middle knuckle and elbow (14–16 inches for adults).

Posture. Sit upright while reading or watching TV in bed, not lying on your back or stomach.

Writing. Hold your pencil or pen an inch or so from the tip so you can see and guide it without tilting your head or body to the side.

Television. Watch TV from a distance equal to seven times the width of the screen (about eight to ten feet), and sit upright. Have indirect lamps on in the room but placed to eliminate glare on the screen. Watching television involves and develops very few visual skills and should be limited to a few hours or less daily, especially for children.

Participating. Perform outdoor activities that require seeing at a distance. Become aware of what and where things are on all sides. When walking, keep your head up, eyes wide open, and look toward objects but avoid staring at them.

Nutrition. A good diet, high in fruits and vegetables along with supplementation of lutein, zeaxanthin, bilberry, and Vitamin A, is beneficial for keeping the eyes healthy. Additional nutrients may be required for specific eye conditions.

Nourishing Your Eyes

Medical science doesn't really know why or how most poor eyesight develops. It wrongly believes that once eyesight starts to go, nothing can be done, and that all we can do is stand by idly and watch it deteriorate. The good news is that we don't have to be passive victims of deteriorating eyesight. The following information from a variety of approaches can help preserve your gift of sight. Good nutrition, physical exercise, and recommended eye exercises all support your vision. See chapter 10-4 for eye exercises and acupuncture points that are good for all eye conditions and overall eye health. Other health modalities, including acupuncture, spinal adjustments, massage, and craniosacral work, can also help your vision.

Nutrition

When Mom and Dad told you to eat your carrots because they were good for your eyes, they were on the right track. Researchers are continually documenting that we really are what we eat. The role of nutrition in the health of our eyes is undoubtedly a key factor.

Consider this. It is believed that more than 25% of the nutrients we absorb from our food goes to nourish our "visual system," which includes our eyes, nerves, blood vessels, and the tissues that support our vision. The concentration of Vitamin C in healthy eyes is higher than almost anywhere else in the body.

Inflammation

Chronic inflammation causes increased production of free radicals in the body and oxidative stress. Antioxidants reduce oxidative stress, neutralize free radicals, and many reduce inflammation. See our chapters on diet and inflammation for natural ways to help reduce and manage chronic inflammation.

Exercise

Aerobic exercise not only benefits your heart, but it is good for your eyes. Exercise helps prevent your eyes from worsening. It raises oxygen levels in the cells and increases lymph and blood circulation. Healthy circulation is a prerequisite for good vision. We recommend that you gently build up to aerobic exercise for a minimum of 20 minutes per day, four days per week. You don't have to join a health club, run five miles a day, or bench press 300 pounds to have good vision. The following are some great ways of staying in shape and helping to maintain healthy eyes:

Walking or jogging. Get a good, comfortable, supportive pair of walking or jogging shoes and select a route that won't have you pounding concrete (which is bad for your joints).

Rebounding. A rebounder is a mini-trampoline. Gentle jumping on a rebounder keeps blood flowing and improves circulation, particularly in the legs and head. Rebounding is also a great way to stimulate the lymphatic system, which removes toxins from the body.

Jumping rope. This childhood activity is actually a wonderful way to stay in shape and only requires a jump rope and 5–10 minutes per day.

Eye exercises. Everyone knows that you have to exercise muscles in order to keep them fit. This applies not only to heart, leg, and arm muscles, but to eye muscles as well. To improve visual fitness, you need to regularly exercise your eye muscles.

Earthing / grounding. In the behavior of electricity, earthing means that a circuit is directly connected to the ground, and grounding means that although there is no direct connection, there is zero electrical potential. As a therapy, grounding may be an inexpensive and easy way to reduce inflammation in the eyes and body. By simply walking barefoot on grass or sand, you will absorb negative electrons from the earth. Additionally, grounding can be achieved by purchasing grounding bedsheets to be used during sleep and mats to be used while on the computer or while watching TV. See Appendix 7 for more information grounding.

Also See

Chapter 7, Vision Diet

Chapter 8, Nutrients

Chapter 10-4, Eye Exercises

Chapter 12, Drugs

Chapter 15-4, Computer Vision Syndrome

[1] T.F. Ross (2015). The Death of Textbooks? The Atlantic, Mar 6.

[2] Shantakumari, N., Eldeeb, R., Sreedharan, J., Gopal, K. (2014). Computer Use and Vision-Related Problems Among University Students In Ajman, United Arab Emirate. *Med Health Sci Res*,.4 Mar-Apr; 4(2): 258–263.

[3] Tatemichi M, Nakano T, Tanaka K, Hayashi, T., Nawa, T. et al. (2004). Possible association between heavy computer users and glaucomatous visual field abnormalities: a cross sectional study in Japanese workers. *J Epidemiol Community Health*, Dec;58(12):1021-7.

[4] Nakano, T., Hayaski, T., Nakagawa, T., Honda, T., Owada, S., et al. (2017). Increased Incidence of Visual Field Abnormalities as Determined by Frequency Doubling Technology Perimetry in High Computer Users Among Japanese Workers: A Retrospective Cohort Study. *J Epidemiol*, Nov 25.

[5] Uchino, Y., Uchino, M., Yokoi, N. (2014). Alteration of Tear Mucin 5AC in Office Workers Using Visual Display Terminals: The Osaka Study. *JAMA Ophthalmol*,132(8):985-992.

[6] Hunter, J.J., Morgan, J.I., Merigan, W.H., Sliney, D.H., Sparrow, J.R., et al. (2012). The susceptibility of the retina to photochemical damage from visible light. *Prog Ret Eye Res*, Jan;31(1):28-42.

[7] Narimatsu, Tl, Negishi, K., Miyake, S., Hirasawa, M., Osada, H., et al. (2015). Blue light-induced inflammatory marker expression in the retinal pigment epithelium-choroid of mice and the protective effect of a yellow intraocular lens material in vivo. *Exp Eye Res*, Mar;132:48-51.

[8] Logan, P., Bernabeu, M., Ferreira, A., Burner, M.N. (2015). Evidence for the Role of Blue Light in the Development of Uveal Melanoma. *J Ophthalmol*, 2015:386986.

[9] Wimalasundera, S. (2009). Computer vision syndrome. *Galle Med J*, 11(1):25–9.

[10] Fernandez-Montero, A., Olmo-Jimenez, J.M., Olmo, N., Bes-Rastroll, M., Moreno-Galarraga, L., et al. (2015). The impact of computer use in myopia progression: a cohort study in Spain. *Prev Med*, Feb;71:67-71.

[11] Ibid. Tatemichi. (2004).

[12] Bergqvist, U.O., Knave, B.G. (1994). Eye discomfort and work with visual display terminals. *Scand J Work Environ Health*, Feb; 20(1):27-33.

[13] Abdelaziz, M.M., Fahim, S.A., Mousa, D.B., Gaya, B.I. (2009). Effects of computer use on visual acuity and colour vision. *Eur J Sci Res*, 2009;35:99–105.

[14] Charpe, N.A., Kaushik, V. (2009). Computer vision syndrome (CVS): Recognition and control in software professionals. *J Hum Ecol*, 2009;28:67–9

10-7. YOGA AND VISION IMPROVEMENT

Use the light that is within you to regain your natural clearness of sight.
Seeing into the darkness is clarity. Knowing how to yield is strength.
Use your own life and return to the source of life. This is called practicing the eternal.
—Lao-Tzu—

Yoga means unity, connection, wholeness. It is an ancient Indian system that contains exercises, which improve strength and flexibility and enhance awareness by supporting unity of body and mind. In a nutshell, as we relax and open the body through yoga, we simultaneously relax and open the mind. As we relax the mind, our vision both inside and outside is enhanced. What does vision inside mean? It means our sense of self, our identity, our purpose, our "beingness" in the world. And outside? This includes not only our sight and appreciation of color and form, but also the ability to perceive the beauty that surrounds us with clarity and vividness.

Breaking it Down

Basically, yoga works on three facets of the human being. These are the physical body, the energy body or spirit, and the mental body or mind. The yoga practitioner seeks to harmonize these three dimensions of the human being, and through this, achieve optimal health, happiness, and self-understanding. This includes optimal inner and outer vision. The yogic techniques developed for working on each of these "bodies" support the overall health and vision[1] of the individual.

Physical Body

The physical poses of yoga known as asanas are designed to increase both strength and flexibility of the body, improve balance, enhance circulation and energy flow, and cleanse the organs and other systems. These poses also open the Chinese energy pathways called meridians.

Inversions

The poses that most benefit the eyes are inversions, which increase blood flow to the head. These include the headstand, shoulder stand, forearm balance, and other poses where the head is lower than the heart. Consult your doctor before doing inversions if you have a history of glaucoma or retinal bleeding; they may be contraindicated.

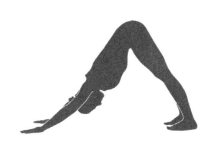

Adho mukha svanasana, Downward-facing dog.

This is one of the most widely recognized yoga poses, an all-over, rejuvenating stretch, which enhances blood flow to the brain.

Salamba sirsasana

Supported head stand

Standing on your head in proper alignment increases blood flow to the head, calms the brain, and strengthens the body.

Salamba sarvangasana

Supported shoulder stand

This version of the shoulder stand is performed with blanket support under the shoulders.

Viparita karani

Legs-up-the-wall pose.

Said to reverse the normal downward flow of a precious subtle fluid called amrita (immortal) or soma (extract) in the hatha yoga pradipika, modern yogis agree that viparita karani may have the power to cure whatever ails you.

Chinese Meridians and Yoga

In Chinese medicine, there are twelve fundamental organ meridians and eight extraordinary meridians or pathways that circulate the energy of heaven and earth in the body, bringing nourishment and vitality to the organs. Many yoga asanas have been identified with specific meridians. The following poses, through the meridian system, most directly benefit the eye health. There are many more poses for meridians, but these are great basic ones to start with.

Kidney Meridian: Cataracts and Presbyopia

Baddha konasana

Bound angle pose

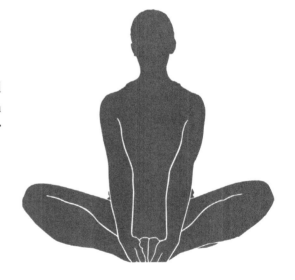

Also called the cobbler's pose after the typical sitting position of Indian cobblers, badda konasana is an excellent groin- and hip-opener and stretches the Kidney meridian.

Liver and Gallbladder Meridians:

Glaucoma, Myopia, Macular Degeneration

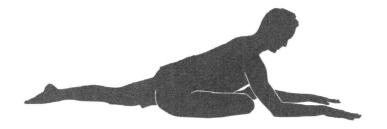

Eka pada rajakapotasana

One-legged king-pigeon pose

This is a hip opener and deep backbend that puffs the chest, making a yogi resemble a pigeon. It opens the Gallbladder meridian.

Parighasana

Gate pose

In this pose, the torso is curved to the side over the straightened leg, so that the underside of the torso is compressed, and the topside is fully stretched, opening the Liver meridian.

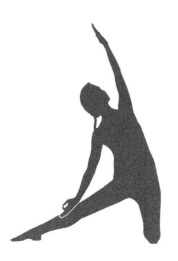

Spleen and Stomach Meridians: Macular Degeneration

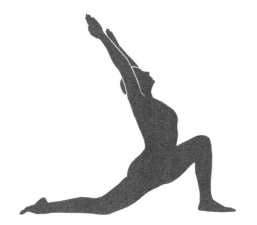

Anjaneyasana

Low lunge pose

This pose opens the Stomach meridian. It is a basic lunge that is found in many yoga classes and routines, and is known to stretch the hips, gluteus muscles, and quadriceps while improving balance, concentration, and core awareness.

Prasarita padottanasana

Wide-legged forward bend.

This pose not only stretches the back of the legs, but the inner legs as well.

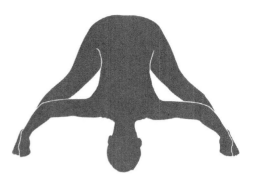

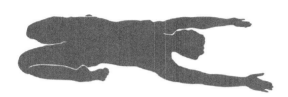

Supta virasana

Reclining hero or heroine pose

Reclining hero or heroine pose stretches the front groins, the psoas muscles, and the deep hip flexors, opening the Stomach meridian.

Upavistha konasana

Wide-angle seated forward bend

Upavistha konasana is a good preparation for most of the seated forward bends and twists, as well as the wide-leg standing poses.

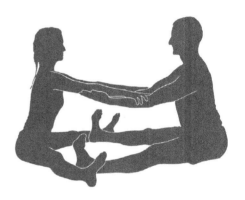

Governing and Conception Vessels: Glaucoma

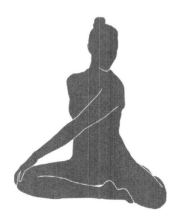

Bharadvajasana

Bharadvaja's twist

This gentle twist is a tonic for the spine and the abdominal organs.

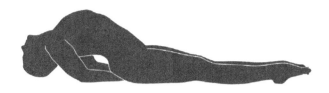

Matsyasana

Fish pose

This is a gentle reclined backbend; it can be done as a restorative pose with a bolster.

Setu bandha sarvangasana

Bridge pose

This active version of bridge pose calms the brain and rejuvenates tired legs.

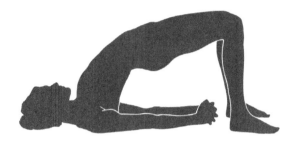

For All Meridians

Savasana

Corpse pose

Savasana is a pose of total relaxation, making it one of the most challenging of asanas.

Energy Body (Spirit)

All the breathing exercises in yoga are designed to enhance energy, oxygenate the blood, and improve circulation while removing stress. The "inhale" brings in life force, or prana, and the "exhale" cleanses the body of toxins. Through these various breathing exercises, the yoga practitioner increases circulation and brings oxygen to all parts of the body, including the eyes.

When doing yoga poses, inhale in the opening position, then exhale when closing or compressing the body. If the breath is suspended after inhalation, don't move. Only move during breath suspension if it is following an exhalation. Breathe in a relaxed and effortless manner.

Mental Body: Meditation

The goal of yoga is union with the "divine," which can also be called reality, or the Tao, the Creative Infinite, nature, "that which is," or the Universal. In yoga philosophy, the Universal is said to exist in the non-thinking space between thoughts, which is non-thinking; in this infinite space, the Truth of Being is said to reside.

Many advanced practitioners of yoga and meditation who are able to enter the "space between thoughts" report improved vision afterwards. To quote Michael Hutchison from *The Book of*

Floating, "As I went out into the world (after going into the state of no mind) my senses were extremely—almost unbelievably—sharp and keen. Everything I saw seemed beautiful and miraculous, and the colors of everything were extraordinarily rich and beautiful. I saw everything clearly, as if objects had sharp edges around…Everything has become much sharper and clearer than it normally was."

The takeaway here is that external vision can improve as you raise your level of consciousness. In other words, meditation and deepening your meditation practice (inner vision) can be a doorway to improving your eyesight (outer vision).

There are many meditation methods, but all aim to quiet the mind and bring it to focus and concentration, to the place of "no mind."

One yoga meditation technique works directly with the eyes. It is named trataka, and according to the *Hatha Yoga Pradipika*, one of the earliest texts on hatha yoga, trataka is said to eradicate all eye diseases, fatigue, and sloth, and to close the doorway creating these problems. In addition to improving concentration and memory, trataka cleanses both the eyes and the cerebral cortex, balances the nervous system, and relieves depression, anxiety, and insomnia. Another yogic text, the *Gheranda Samhita*, states that the practice cultivates clairvoyance and inner vision.

Trataka has to do with gazing on one point, either on an object or often on a candle flame. In a study performed at Svyasa University, Bengaluru, India, and published in 2014, one month of trataka intervention improved cognition when compared to a control group.[2]

Stress is often a big factor in contributing to poorer vision and even eye disease. Meditation and relaxation techniques are increasingly recognized for their value in reducing stress.[3] [4] There are several main types of meditation, and each provide comfort and value,[5] depending on your own style of functioning, how much time you can make for your practice, and whether the practice requires a quiet place.

Focused attention (FA). Trataka is an example of a focused meditation in which you focus your attention on one single object. If you live a very relaxed life, then this technique may help sharpen your attention.[6] Trataka requires sitting cross-legged, with a straight back and a candle at the level of your eyes. This form has been found to support improved vision.[7]

Open monitoring (OM). Buddhist mindfulness techniques are good examples in which you contemplate breath or thoughts in order to detach from being controlled by them. OM techniques have been found to produce beneficial mental and physical health outcomes. In experienced practitioners, measured brain patterns in the frontal lobe are found to powerfully change during this practice.[8]

Automatic self-transcending (AST). Transcendental meditation (TM) and vedic meditation are examples in which no concentration/contemplation is used, but which yield qualitatively different end results. These are good techniques even if you live a demanding, stressful life. They have been found to produce good physical outcomes, especially reducing anxiety, addiction, hypertension, sleeplessness, and migraines. As in OM techniques, frontal lobe activity changes; in addition, alpha functioning improves across the brain.[9]

Conclusion

A synthesis of practices of yoga and the Chinese meridian system for the improvement of vision, inside and out, is worthy of application for those individuals desiring to see more clearly without the aid of corrective lenses, or, at least, with milder corrective lenses. From the physical body, to the energetic and mental bodies, all the bases are covered for greater health, wellness, and clearer eyesight.

[1] Gosewade, N.B., Shende, V.S., Kashalikar, S.J. (2013). Effect of Various Eye Exercise Techniques along with Pranayama on Visual Reaction Time: A Case Control Study. *J Clin Diagn Resv*, 7(9); 2013 Sep.

[2] Talwadkar, S., Jagannathan, A., Raghuram, N. (2014). Effect of trataka on cognitive functions in the elderly. *Int J Yoga*, Jul-Dec;7(2):96-103.

[3] Sabal, B.A., Wang, J., Cardenas-Morales, L., Faiq, M., Heim, C. (2018). Mental stress as consequence and cause of vision loss: the dawn of psychosomatic ophthalmology for preventative and personalized medicine. *EPMA J*, May 9;9(2):133-160.

[4] Cahn, B. R., Goodman, M.S., Peterson, C.T., Maturi, R., Mills, P.J. (2017). Yoga, Meditation and Mind-Body Health: Increased BDNF, Cortisol Awakening Response, and Altered Inflammatory Marker Expression after a 3-Month Yoga and Meditation Retreat. *Front Hum Neurosci*, 2017:11:315.

[5] Angelina, J. How Meditation Practices Help in Improving Eyesight. Retrieved Jul 9 2018 from https://www.mindbodygreen.com/0-15506/how-to-choose-the-right-meditation-technique-for-you.html.

[6] Williams, W. (2014). How to Choose the Right Meditation Technique for You. Retrieved Jul 9 2018 from https://www.mindbodygreen.com/0-15506/how-to-choose-the-right-meditation-technique-for-you.html

[7] Ibid. Talwadkar. (2014).

[8] Ibid. Williams. (2014).

[9] Ibid. Williams. (2014).

10-8. AGING AND VISION

With aging come changes to digestion, poorer nutrient absorption, and circulation as well as hormonal changes that impact our vision and overall health. By being more attentive to eating habits, getting regular exercise, and taking targeted supplements, we can make this transition smoother and help maintain overall health and vision. Life expectancy is increasing, and the concept of what we can accomplish at any age is changing as well.

Digestion

As we age past 40 years, our ability to produce the necessary digestive enzymes decreases; our body may not receive all the nutrients it needs for good vision.

Recommended. Supplementing with a good digestive enzyme such as a formula containing amylase, protease, lipase, and cellulose, about 10 to 15 minutes before each meal or during the meal (depending on label instructions) is recommended. Another option is to take with meals one tablespoon of apple cider vinegar, the juice of half a lemon diluted in a cup of water, or Swiss bitter herbs taken after meals. These all support healthy digestion.

For those with high cholesterol or circulatory problems, there are specific enzymes that should be taken on an empty stomach. These enzymes help break down debris and waste materials in tissue and blood that can contribute to chronic inflammation and clogged blood vessels.

Recommended. Talk with your wholistic health provider about including enzymes such serrapeptase and/or nattokinase, follow the Vision diet, and get regular exercise.

Protein Digestion

Proteins are digested in a "fast" or "slow" manner; researchers have reported that whey protein digests quickly, and casein (milk) protein digests slowly. Whey protein stimulates amino acid production and protein synthesis without changing protein breakdown. Casein protein, on the other hand, has a lesser amino acid producing effect than other proteins, and it breaks down more slowly. In one study for young men, the "slow" protein was more effective; **for older men, the "fast" protein source, whey, was more effective** in limiting protein loss.[1] Adding fats and carbohydrates to these whey or casein protein sources lessened the differences.

Most commercial whey protein is a mixture of whey and casein, which is a common immunogen. Native whey protein (by counter-flow technique) is the cleanest, most easily digested and assimilated whey protein. Whey protein has high amounts of the amino acid cysteine, which is important to help our bodies make glutathione, the most important antioxidant.

Recommended. Talk with your health provider about whether you should pay attention to these differences; an issue will be whether you are lactose-sensitive. Look for a "native whey protein by counter-flow" label.

Bioavailability and Cooking Methods

Another issue is how the cooking method impacts nutrients. Here's an important example. Lutein and zeaxanthin are important nutrients to maintain healthy vision. These nutrients can be obtained through supplements, but also through foods. Let's take eggs as an example: the lutein and zeaxanthin in scrambled eggs are less bioavailable than in boiled eggs.[2]

Lightly steamed vegetables are an effective way to help preserve the nutrients while making them easier to digest. Adding a little fat such as olive oil to the steamed vegetables will increase the absorption of fat-soluble vitamins, such as lutein, zeaxanthin, CoQ10, and vitamins A, E, D, K.

Recommended. If you get your vision nutrients only through foods and not through supplements, consult your nutritionist (and do some research) regarding the impact of various cooking methods on the specific nutrients you are targeting.

Circulatory system

Poor Circulation

Another consideration as we age is poor circulation. If tissues of the eye do not receive adequate blood flow, delivering oxygen, essential nutrients, and the ability to efficiently discard waste products, then a variety of vision conditions can result, including glaucoma,[3] macular degeneration,[4] cataracts,[5] and diabetic retinopathy.[6]

Another factor is that impaired blood flow appears to be linked to gender. It is thought that the hormones estrogen, progesterone, and testosterone are important blood flow regulators in the choroid and retina.[7]

Supplementing with targeted nutrients such as ginkgo biloba or vinpocetine, resveratrol, cayenne, ginger, garlic, hawthorn, olive leaf extract, bilberry, or butcher's broom, to name a few, will help keep blood moving in the system and will support the integrity of blood vessels. There are good formulas that contain a combination of a number of these nutrients (see the product list in Appendix 5).

Other factors that can reduce blood flow to the eyes and brain are stress-related muscular compression (particularly neck and shoulder) and even tight neckties.[8]

Recommended. Get regular exercise, follow the Vision diet, and talk to your wholistic health provider about these targeted nutrients.

Vascular Resistance

In the case of macular degeneration, not only does the structure of blood vessels in the retina change, as well as the growth of new fragile blood vessels (particularly in wet AMD) to try to make up for inadequate oxygen supply, but the way blood circulates also changes. The blood flow velocity decreases, and the relationship of peak systolic and minimum diastolic blood flow velocity (pulsatility) changes.[9] These add up to increased vascular resistance—a decrease in the force needed to push blood through the circulatory system.[10]

- Foods that support circulation include oranges, dark chocolate, garlic, goji berries, salmon, avocados, watermelon, ginger root, sunflower seeds, and cayenne pepper.

Recommended. Get regular exercise, follow the Vision diet, and talk with your wholistic health provider about these targeted nutrients.

High Blood Pressure

High blood pressure can result in a range of eye conditions, including hypertensive choroidopathy or hypertensive retinopathy, hypertensive optic neuropathy,[11] [12] macula edema, glaucoma (both high- and low-blood pressure),[13] wet macular degeneration,[14] retinal vein occlusion,[15] diabetic retinopathy,[16] eye stroke[17] or nerve fiber layer ischemia, or damage to the nerve fibers.[18] It may also contribute to color-vision loss.[19] To make things more complicated, patients being treated with antihypertensive medications are more likely to have glaucoma or become glaucoma suspects.[20]

- Foods and common herbs that lower blood pressure naturally, include basil,[21] celery[22] and celery seed,[23] garlic,[24] [25] [26] flaxseed,[27] tomato,[28] pomegranate,[29] dietary fiber,[30] [31] wheat bran,[32] sesame and sesame oil,[33] green or oolong tea,[34] and dark chocolate.[35]
- Nutrients include coleus forskohlii,[36] taurine (shown to help heart disease in a number of ways including atherosclerosis),[37] [38] [39] omega-3 fatty acids,[40] and maritime pine (pycnogenol).[41] Less known foods and herbs include prickly custard apple,[42] bread fruit,[43] radish seed extract,[44] kudzu,[45] agathosma betulina,[46] psyllium (plantago species),[47] rauwolfia (considered one of the most potent anti-hypertensive plants),[48] Chinese hawthorne,[49] and cat's claw herb.[50]

Recommended. Get regular exercise, follow the Vision diet, and talk to your wholistic health provider about these targeted nutrients.

Exercise

It is well known that exercise is a critical tool in reducing age-related eye disease.[51] Aerobic exercise protects the retina from deterioration[52] (and in lab animals, protects even in cases of genetically-based retinal degeneration[53]). Exercise reduces intraocular pressure, central retinal vein occlusion, and age-related macular degeneration, as well as hypertension and diabetes.[54]

Recommended. At a minimum, take a brisk 15–20-minute walk per day. Jogging and running are not essential but are helpful if you enjoy them. The point is to get outside everyday and move around. If you are working at a desk job, full or part time, then be sure to get up and move around for a few minutes every hour or two.

Breathing

Additionally, if you work at a desk, at a computer, or if you have poor, slouched posture, the ability to obtain deep, full, cleansing breaths is more difficult, which not only affects eye health but also directly affects energy, vitality, and general health.

Recommended. Consider seeing a Buteyko breath instructor to learn how to breathe properly.

Vision Conditions

Dry Eyes

Seventy-five percent of those over age 65 experience dryness of eyes, due to a decrease in the production of tears and often due to a tear-drainage dysfunction. The resulting ocular tear-film reduction impacts visual function and comfort, even though it may not directly reduce vision clarity.[55] For men, there is a weak relationship between low androgen levels and dry eye.[56] One of the causes of dry eye in the aging population is meibomian gland dysfunction with consequent reduction of meibum, which protects the tear film from evaporation. Note that retinoids used in cosmetics promote this type of dysfunction.[57] In the aging population, dry eyes can become a particularly annoying problem, and if it is severe enough and not treated, it can cause damage to the cornea. From a Chinese medical perspective, internal dryness becomes more common with age, resulting in less tear production (a common Chinese medicine pattern called Kidney yin deficiency, although other meridian imbalances can contribute to dry eyes as well).

Recommended. Drinking coffee, overuse of sugar, excessive protein consumption, or dehydration can worsen dry eyes. Limit coffee to a few times a week, avoid sodas and sugary drinks, and drink plenty of fresh pure water. Homeopathic dry-eye drops can be very helpful.

Cataract

Cataracts are so frequent among seniors that some doctors consider them to be normal. Cataract risk is greater in people who have spent a lifetime out-of-doors due to solar radiation exposure.[58]

Recommended. Wear 100% UV resistant sunglasses whenever outdoors. Amber colored glasses will give you the best protection against blue light—which does not contribute directly to cataract, but damages the retina and is a risk factor for other conditions.

Macular Degeneration

Although macular degeneration can develop at any age, it is especially prominent in the aging population. Like cataracts, it is greater in those who've been exposed to higher levels of UV radiation.[59] Blue light is a big risk factor for AMD. Therefore, wearing blue-blocking lenses or putting a blue-blocking program on the computer and cell phones is of paramount importance, especially for younger people and people who have had cataract surgery with clear implants.

Recommended. Wear 100% UV resistant sunglasses when outdoors. Talk to your health provider about targeted nutrients that support retinal health.

Glaucoma

Another condition common to aging populations is glaucoma. With the increasing popularity of computer use, glaucoma risk is even higher in as new computer-savvy generations age.

Recommended. If you use a computer or mobile device frequently, don't forget to have your eyes tested for glaucoma regularly.

Vitreous/Retinal Tears and Detachments

As one ages past 50, the vitreous which maintains the shape of the back of the eyes starts to liquify and/or clump, causing more pulling on the attachments to the retina. The most common effects are vitreous tears and detachments (no medical intervention typically required) or retinal tears and detachments (medical intervention is required).

Floaters

Changes to the vitreous can also cause floaters (generally benign) as tiny pieces of connective tissue float free, resulting in eye floaters "floating" in the vitreous. In Chinese medicine, floaters are often caused by kidney and liver/gallbladder imbalance. Floaters have been associated with the presence of candida.

Also See

Chapter 7, Vision Diet

Chapter 8, Nutrients

Chapter 10-4, Eye Exercises

Chapter 12, Drugs

Chapter 15-1, Cataracts

Chapter 15-7, Dry Eyes

Chapter 15-9, Floaters

Chapter 15-11, Glaucoma

Chapter 15-18, Macular Degeneration

Chapter 15-25, Retinal Detachment

Chapter 15-32, Vitreous Detachment

[1] Dangin, M., Boirie, Y., Guillet, C., Beaufrere, B. (2002). Influence of the protein digestion rate on protein turnover in young and elderly subjects. *J Nutr,* Oct;132(10):3228S-33S.

[2] Nimalaratne, C., Savard, P., Gauthier, S.F., Schieber, A., Wu, J. (2015). Bioaccessibility and digestive stability of carotenoids in cooked eggs studied using a dynamic in vitro gastrointestinal model. *J Agric Food Chem,* Mar 25;63(11):2956-62.

[3] Fan, N., Wang, P., Tang, L., Liu, X. (2015). Ocular Blood Flow and Normal Tension Glaucoma. *Biomed Res Int,* 2015:308505.

[4] Friedman, E., Krupsky, S., Lane, A.M., Oak, S.S., Friedman, E.S., et al. (1995). Ocular blood flow velocity in age-related macular degeneration. *Ophthalmology,* Apr;102(4):640-6.

[5] Michael, R., Bron, A.J. (2011). The ageing lens and cataract: a model of normal and pathological ageing. *Philos Trans R Soc Lond B Biol Sci,* Apr 27;366(1568):1278-1292.

[6] Gilmore, E.D., Hudson, C., Nrusimhadevara, R.K., Harvey, P.T., Mandelcorn, M. (2007). Retinal arteriolar diameter, blood velocity, and blood flowresponse to an isocapnic hyperoxic provocation in early sight-threatening diabetic retinopathy. *Invest Ophthalmol Vis Sci,* Apr;48(4):1744-50.

[7] Schmidl, D., Schmetterer, L., Garhofer, G., Popa-Cherecheanu, A. (2015). Gender differences in ocular blood flow. *Curr Eye Res,* Feb;40(2):201-12.

[8] Bozic, M., Hentova, S.P., Brankovic, A., Marjanovic, I., Dordevic, J.J., et al. (2012). Effect of a tight necktie on intraocular pressure. *Med Pregl,* Jan-Feb;65(1-2):13-7.

[9] Ibid. Friedman. (1995).

[10] Wikipedia. Vascular resistance. Retrieved from https://en.wikipedia.org/wiki/ Vascular_resistance.

[11] Tos, M.O., Jampl, L.M. (1982). Pathophysiology of hypertensive retinopathy. *Ophthalmology,* Oct;89(10):1132-45.

[12] Chatterjee, S., Chattopadhyay, S., Hope-Ross, M., Lip, P.L. (2002). Hypertension and the eye: changing perspectives. *J Hum Hypertens,* Oct;16(10):667-75.

[13] He, Z., Vingrys, A.J., Armitage, J.A., Bui, B.V. (2011). The role of blood pressure in glaucoma. *Clin Exp Optom,* Mar;94(2):133-49.

[14] Hyman, L., Schachat, A.P., He, Q., Leske, M.C. (2000). Hypertension, cardiovascular disease, and age-related macular degeneration. Age-Related Macular Degeneration Risk Factors Study Group. *Arch Ophthalmol,* Mar;118(3):351-8.

[15] Barnett, E.M., Fantin, A., Wilson, B.S., Kass, M.A., Gordon, M.O., et al. (2010). The incidence of retinal vein occlusion in the ocular hypertension treatment study. *Ophthalmology,* Mar;117(3):484-8.

[16] Hendrick, A.M., Gibson, M.V., Kulshreshtha, A. (2015). Diabetic Retinopathy. *Prim Care,* Sep;42(3):451-64.

[17] Henderson, A.D., Bruce, B.B., Newman, N.J., Biousse, V. (2012). Hypertension-related eye abnormalities and the risk of stroke. *Rev Neurol Dis, 2011;8(1-2):1-9.*

[18] Shen, J., Yang, Q., Yu, D., Wu, J., Zhu, Y., et al. (2017). Vulnerability study of myelinated and unmyelinated nerve fibers in acute ocular hypertension in rabbit. *Mol Med Rep,* Nov;16(5):6794-6802.

[19] Shoji, T., Sato, H., Chihara, E., Sakurai, Y. (2015). Are middle-age blood pressure levels related to color visionimpairment? The Okubo Color Study. *Am J Hypertens,* Jan;28(1):98-105.

[20] Deb, A.K., Kaliaperumal, S., Rao, V.A., Sengupta, S. (2014). Relationship between systemic hypertension, perfusion pressure and glaucoma: A comparative study in an adult Indian population. *Indian J Ophthlmol,* Sep;62(9):917-922.

[21] Azhar, I., Aftab, K., Usmanghani, K. (1995). Naturally occurring calcium channel blockers. *Hamdard Medicus,* 1995;38:5–16

[22] Somanadhan, B., Varughese, G., Palpu, P., Sreedharan, R., Gudiksen, L., et al. (1999). An ethnopharmacological survey for potential angiotensin converting enzyme inhibitors from Indian medicinal plants. *J Ethnopharmacol,* May;65(2):103-12.

[23] Simpson, D. (1998). Buchu--South Africa's amazing herbal remedy. *Scott Med J,* Dec; 43(6):189-91. Scott Med J. 1998 Dec; 43(6):189-91.

[24] Reinhart, K.M., Coleman, C.I., Teevan, C., Vachhani, P., White, C.M. (2008). Effects of garlic on blood pressure in patients with and without systolic hypertension: a meta-analysis. *Ann Pharmacother,* Dec;42(12):1766-71.

[25] Ried, K., Frank, O.R., Stocks, N.P., Fakler, P., Sullivan, T. (2008). Effect of garlic on blood pressure: a systematic review and meta-analysis. *BMC Cardiovasc Disord,* Jun16;8():13.

[26] Dhawan, V., Jain, S. (2005). Garlic supplementation prevents oxidative DNA damage in essential hypertension. *Mol Cell Biochem,* Jul; 275(1-2):85-94.

[27] Bloedon, L.T., Szapary, P.O. (2004). Flaxseed and cardiovascular risk. *Nutr Rev,* Jan; 62(1):18-27.

[28] Paran, E., Novack, V., Engelhard, Y.N., Hazan-Halevy, I. (2009). The effects of natural antioxidants from tomato extract in treated but uncontrolled hypertensive patients. *Cardiovasc Drugs Ther,* Apr; 23(2):145-51.

[29] Aviram, M., Dornfeld, L. (2001). Pomegranate juice consumption inhibits serum angiotensin converting enzyme activity and reduces systolic blood pressure. *Atherosclerosis*, Sep; 158(1):195-8.

[30] Burke, V., Hodgson, J.M., Beilin, L.J., Giangiulioi, N., Rogers, P., et al. (2001). Dietary protein and soluble fiber reduce ambulatory blood pressure in treated hypertensives. *Hypertension,* Oct; 38(4):821-6.

[31] Keenan, J.M., Pins, J.J., Frazel, C., Moran, A., Turnquist, L. (2002). Oat ingestion reduces systolic and diastolic blood pressure in patients with mild or borderline hypertension: a pilot trial. *J Fam Pract,* Apr; 51(4):369.

[32] Behall, K.M., Scholfield, D.J., Hallfrisch, J. (2006). Whole-grain diets reduce blood pressure in mildly hypercholesterolemic men and women. *J Am Diet Assoc,* Sep; 106(9):1445-9.

[33] Nakano, D., Itoh, C., Takaoka, M., Kiso, Y., Tanaka, T., et al. (2002). Antihypertensive effect of sesamin. IV. Inhibition of vascular superoxide production by sesamin. *Biol Pharm Bull,* Sep; 25(9):1247-9.

[34] Yang, Y.C., Lu, F.H., Wu, J.S., Wu, C.H., Chang, C.J. (2004). The protective effect of habitual tea consumption on hypertension. *Arch Intern Med*, Jul 26; 164(14):1534-40.

[35] Ludovici, V., Barthelmes, J., Nagele, M.P., Enseleit, F., Ferri, C., et al. (2017). Cocoa, Blood Pressure, and Vascular Function. *Front Nutr,* 2017;Aug 2.

[36] Dubey, M.P., Srimal, R.C., Nityanand, S., Dhawan, B.N. (1981). Pharmacological studies on coleonol, a hypotensive diterpene from Coleus forskohlii. *J Ethnopharmacol,* Jan; 3(1):1-13.

[37] Murakami, S. (2014). Taurine and atherosclerosis. *Amino Acids*, Jan;46(1):73-80.

[38] Xu, Y.J., Arneja, A.S., Tappia, P.S., Dhalla, N.S. (2008). The potential health benefits of taurine in cardiovascular disease. *Exp Clin Cardiol*, Summer;13(2):57-65.

[39] Yamori, Y., Taguchi, T., Hamada, A., Kunimasa, K., Mori, H., et al. (2010). Taurine in health and diseases: consistent evidence from experimental and epidemiological studies. *J Biomed Sci,* Aug 24;17 Suppl 1:S6.

[40] Alasil, T., Lee, N., Keane, P., Sadda, S. (2009). Central retinal vein occlusion: a case report and review of the literature. *Cases J, 2009;2:7170.*

[41] Liu, X., Wei, J., Tan, F., Zhou, S., Würthwein, G., et al. (2004). Pycnogenol, French maritime pine bark extract, improves endothelial function of hypertensive patients. *Life Sci,* Jan 2; 74(7):855-62.

[42] Hasrat, J.A., Pieters, L., Vlietinck, A.J. (2004). Medicinal plants in Suriname. *J Pharm Pharmacol*, 2004;56(3):381–7.

[43] Ibid. Hasrat. 2004.

[44] Ghayur, M.N., Gilani, A.H. (2006). Radish seed extract mediates its cardiovascular inhibitory effects via muscarinic receptor activation. *Fundam Clin Pharmacol*, Feb; 20(1):57-63.

[45] Fan, L.L., Zeng, G.Y., Zhou, Y.P., Zhang, L.Y., Cheng, Y.S. (1982). Pharmacologic studies on Radix puerariae: effects of puerariae flavones on coronary circulation, cardiac hemodynamics and myocardial metabolism in dogs. *Chin Med J (Engl),* Feb; 95(2):145-50.

[46] Ibid. Simpson. (1998).

[47] Burke, V., Hodgson, J.M., Beilin, L.J., Giangiulioi, N., Rogers, P., et al. (2001). Dietary protein and soluble fiber reduce ambulatory blood pressure in treated hypertensives. *Hypertension,* Oct; 38(4):821-6.

[48] Jerie, P. (2007). Milestones of cardiovascular therapy. IV. Reserpine. *Cas Lek Cesk,* 2007; 146(7):573-7.

[49] Brixius, K., Willms, S., Napp, A., Tossios, P., Ladage, D., et al. (2006). Crataegus special extract WS 1442 induces an endothelium-dependent, NO-mediated vasorelaxation via eNOS-phosphorylation at serine 1177. *Cardiovasc Drugs Ther,* Jun; 20(3):177-84.

[50] Horie, S., Yano, S., Aimi, N., Sakai, S., Watanabe, K. (1992). Effects of hirsutine, an antihypertensive indole alkaloid from Uncaria rhynchophylla, on intracellular calcium in rat thoracic aorta. *Life Sci,* 1992;50(7):491-8.

[51] Pardue, M.T., Chrenek, M.A., Schmidt, R.H., Nickerson, J.M., Boatright, J.H. (2015). Potential Role of Exercise in Retinal Health. *Prog Mol Biol Transl Sci,* 134:491-502.

[52] Lawson, E.C., Han, M.K., Sellers, J.T., Chrenek, M.A., Hanif, A. (2014). Aerobic exercise protects retinal function and structure from light-induced retinal degeneration. *J Neurosci,* Feb 12;34(7):2406-12.

[53] Hanif, A.M., Lawson, E.C., Prunty, M., Gogniat, M., Aung, M.H., et al. (2015). Neuroprotective Effects of Voluntary Exercise in an Inherited Retinal Degeneration Mouse Model. *Invest Ophthalmol Vis Sci,* Oct;56(11):6839-46.

[54] Gale, J., Wells, A.P., Wilson, G. (2009). Effects of exercise on ocular physiology and disease. *Surv Ophthalmol,* May-Jun;54(3):349-55.

[55] Sharma, A., Hindman, H.B. (2014). Aging: a predisposition to dry eyes. *J Ophthalmol,* 2014:781683.

[56] Azcarate, P.M., Venincasa, V.D., Feuer, W., Stanczyk, F., Shally, A.V., Galor, A. (2014). Androgen deficiency and dry eye syndrome in the aging male. *Invest Ophthalmol Vis Sci*, Jul 3;55(8):5046-53.

[57] Ding, J., Sullivan, D.A., (2012). Aging and dry eye disease. *Exp Gerontol,* Jul;47(7):483-90.

[58] Roberts, J.E. (2011). Ultraviolet radiation as a risk factor for cataract and macular degeneration. *Eye Contact Lens,* Jul;37(4):246-9.

[59] Ibid. Roberts. (2011).

11. NATURAL EYE CARE FOR PETS

Pets often respond well to herbs and nutrients for maintaining health. With a balanced diet, appropriate exercise, and your attention to their silent (and vocal!) messages, there is no reason your pet, your dog or cat, cannot live a long, full, and happy life.

These recommendations are not meant to replace medical advice by your veterinarian.

Cataracts

Cataracts are common in older dogs and occur rarely in older cats. A healthy lens is transparent. You might notice a milkiness in your pet's eyes as they age. The growing opacity is due to changes in the lens fibers of the eye that are found behind the iris and pupil. Cataracts in dogs or cats often occur if they have diabetes. They are found in older pets that have immune disorders, chronic diseases, chronic skin problems, hip dysplasia, and ear problems.

Senile cataracts are most common and tend to occur simultaneously in both eyes. The following breed of dogs are more at risk: Afghans, cockers, Chesapeake Bay retrievers, German shepherds, golden retrievers, Labradors, Schnauzers, old English sheepdogs, huskies, poodles, westies, and springers.

Causes

Although the exact cause of cataracts in dogs or cats is not known, chemical changes within the lens may contribute to cataract development. Other factors such as genetics, congenital defects, eye infection, trauma to the eye, nutritional deficiencies, exposure to heat or radiation, toxins, eye disorders, or diabetes may also be associated with cataracts.

Regarding diabetes, cataract formation is very common due to the increased levels of sugar in the blood and fluids of the body, causing damage in the lens and body overall, and possibly systemic inflammation.

Conventional Treatment

If the cataract worsens to the point that it affects your pet's mobility, then surgery is often recommended. There is a new eyedrop called "lanosterol" that has shown promise in reducing certain types of cataracts in pets.[1]

Complementary Approach

There is very little research in nutrients for pets' eye conditions, but it has been our experience that natural remedies for cataracts in dogs and cats have been extremely useful. Wholistic veterinarians have found that many of the nutrients studied for people also apply to pets, though the dosages obviously are much lower. The recommendations below are based on veterinarian clinical experience.

Cineraria is the traditional homeopathic remedy and is the most common eyedrop recommended by wholistic veterinarians for cataracts in pets.[2]

Vitamin C with bioflavonoids is recommended as a general supplement, as well as vitamins A and E that have antioxidant properties, which fight free radicals that can damage the lens of the eye.

Eyebright and bilberry are two herbs integral to wholistic cataract treatment and helpful for pets.

N-acetylcarnosine (Can-C), according to researchers, is also beneficial for dogs with 96% success.[3]

Mixed carotenoids contain antioxidants found in carotenoid-rich food, that is, fresh produce items that are rich in color. Two specific carotenoids, **lutein** and **zeaxanthin**, provide antioxidant protection in the macula region of the eye and have been found to reduce the incidence of cataracts.

Diabetic Retinopathy

Diabetic retinopathy is a weakening of the blood vessels in the retina due to chronic blood-sugar imbalances caused by diabetes. This can lead to leaking of blood and other liquid into the retina from the blood vessels, causing vision loss, and possibly eventually blindness, if not controlled.

Blindness is a frequent occurrence in diabetic dogs and less frequent in diabetic cats. Although diabetes in dogs and cats can occur at any age, it is more common in dogs 4–14 years of age, and most are diagnosed at roughly 7–10 years of age. Most diabetic cats are older than 6 years of age. Diabetes occurs in female dogs twice as often as male dogs. Certain breeds of dogs may be predisposed to diabetes.[4]

Symptoms

Early signs of diabetes include symptoms such as sudden weight loss or gain, accompanied by excessive drinking and urination. The pets' appetite may become ravenous or absent. In dogs, the next symptom may be vision problems, including cataracts. Cats more commonly suffer from peripheral neuropathy. You will see a weakening of the hind legs, and the cat's gait may become stilted or wobbly.

Owners should watch for noticeable thinning of the skin and apparent fragility.

Complementary Approach

Fatty acids are important. Get a blend that is rich in the omega-3 constituents EPA and DHA.

Add **general supplements**, including ones that include plenty of vitamin C and bioflavonoids. Supplements should include important antioxidants and herbs that support healthy vision and strengthen blood vessels, such as eyebright, grapeseed extract, taurine, and bilberry.

CoQ10 supports heart functioning and may help animal patients with retinal damage.

Glaucoma

Glaucoma is typically linked to increased pressure within the eye, and it affects animals in the same way that it affects humans. Cells inside the eye produce a clear fluid called "aqueous humor" that maintains the shape of the eye and nourishes the tissues inside the eye. The eye is constantly producing more aqueous humor and drains the excess to maintain the proper balance and eye pressure. Most cases of glaucoma occur when the drain becomes clogged, resulting in an increase in eye pressure. This can result in the stretching and enlarging of the eye, as well as eventual blindness if not treated.

A sudden rise in pressure can damage the retina (which acts like the film in a camera) and the optic nerve, which sends information from the eye to the brain. Unfortunately, the damage is permanent and irreversible, resulting in partial or total vision loss.

Types of Glaucoma in Pets

Glaucoma is classified as either primary or secondary in animals, and also as open- or closed-angle glaucoma.

Determining whether your pet has primary or secondary glaucoma is important, because the treatment needed and the prognosis for vision is different for each type. Veterinary ophthalmologists use slit-lamp biomicroscopy, indirect ophthalmoscopy, and gonioscopy to determine the type and cause of glaucoma. Gonioscopy helps determine how predisposed the remaining visual eye is to developing glaucoma when primary glaucoma is suspected. This test involves placing a special contact lens on the eye, which allows examination of the drainage angle. Gonioscopy is usually performed under sedation or anesthesia.

Primary glaucoma is an inherited condition and is the most common cause of glaucoma in dogs, particularly American cocker spaniels, basset hounds, chow chows, shar peis, Labrador retrievers, and arctic circle breed dogs (huskies, elkhounds, etc.). Primary glaucoma is rare in cats.

Secondary glaucoma occurs when other eye diseases cause decreased fluid drainage. Common causes of secondary glaucoma are inflammation inside the eye (uveitis), advanced cataracts, cancer in the eye, lens subluxation or luxation, and chronic retinal detachment. Glaucoma in cats is usually secondary to chronic uveitis.

Narrow-angle (closed) glaucoma is the most common in dogs. It occurs as a result of other diseases within the eye, such as inflammation, eye tumor, trauma, or a displaced lens that blocks drainage.

Open-angle glaucoma occurs as a result of being an inherited disease, often associated with a mutation in the ADAMTS10 gene. Beagles have a high incidence of the open form of glaucoma.

Symptoms
- Enlarged pupil that doesn't constrict normally in bright light
- Red, teary, and cloudy eyes (the problem is mistaken for conjunctivitis or an eye allergy)

- Dilated pupil
- Cloudiness in the cornea
- Pain, which may be exhibited by squinting, holding the eye closed, keeping the third eyelid up over the eye, crying out if eye is bumped, rubbing at eye with paw, or rubbing face against furniture and carpets, possibly fluttering of eyelids or squinting
- Personality changes, such as depression, lethargy, and sleepiness

Diagnosis

Although many veterinarians have the equipment needed to check for glaucoma, an animal ophthalmologist will be able to give a more accurate diagnosis, using a small device called a tonometer that tests the eye pressure. If the test indicates that glaucoma is present, a second test may be done called a gonioscopy, which determines if the glaucoma is the wide-angle or narrow-angle type. The doctor will also examine the shape and color of the optic nerve and the drainage channels. If the ophthalmologist finds that the pressure is elevated or if the optic nerve looks unusual, he will examine the drainage channels to determine what type of glaucoma is present.

Conventional Treatment

The treatment your doctor recommends will depend on the type of glaucoma your pet has. It may include eye drops or pills to reduce the fluid pressure, surgery treatments that range from laser treatment to removal of a blinded eye, or a combination of treatments. Interestingly, often the same medication is given to pets as those given to humans for glaucoma.

The important thing to remember is that immediate medical attention is needed in order to preserve your pet's eyesight if you suspect that it has glaucoma. At the same time, however, you can support your pet's vision by giving it nutritional support.

Complementary Approach

CoQ10 30 is a supplement available for pets. CoQ10-30 is composed of 30mg, pure pharmaceutical grade Coenzyme Q10.

Fatty acid blends from high-grade marine lipid concentrate, rich in the omega-3 constituents EPA and DHA is recommended.

Whole food concentrate for nutritional support.

Eyebright and bilberry are two herbs that help eye health and microcirculation. Bilberry extract is derived from a fruit similar to the blueberry and contains active ingredients for eye health and proper vision. The berries are rich in the antioxidant anthocyanosides, the red pigments that are beneficial in ophthalmology and vascular diseases.

Zinc is a mineral linked to good vision and may protect eye tissue from damaging light and inflammation. Zinc is naturally found in healthy retinal tissue.

Taurine is an amino acid found to be "neuroprotective," meaning it helps protect nerves of the body from damage such as the optic nerve.

Quercetin is a natural antioxidant bioflavonoid that protects cells from damage by free radicals.

Alpha-lipoic acid is the "universal antioxidant" because it works in both water and fatty tissues, providing antioxidant protection to all your pet's cells. It restores numerous biological functions that become diminished with aging and helps support the optic nerve.

> **Warning**. Supplementing with alpha-lipoic acid for cats can be toxic in high dosages and should be limited to 25mg per day.

Grape seed extract has a high content of compounds called OPCs (oligomeric proanthocyanidins), which are potent antioxidants, supporting healthy skin, providing cardiovascular support, and improving blood circulation.

Retinal Degeneration

Retinal degeneration refers to a number of progressive eye diseases that lead to blindness. When the disease comes on slowly, it is referred to as progressive retinal atrophy (PRA). Sudden acquired retinal degeneration (SARD) can also develop spontaneously, without any previously perceptible signs.

Retinal degeneration is not always easy to spot, but be aware if your pet displays any of these signs or behaviors:

- Dilated pupils and more visible eye shine from the back of the eye
- Walking into objects
- Unwillingness to jump up onto objects
- Reluctance to go outside
- Poor vision in dim light or darkness

Cause

Retinal degeneration is commonly believed to be an incurable genetic condition. Some studies relate the condition to inadequate nutrition in both dogs and cats and specifically taurine deficiency in cats.[5]

Because it is an inherited disease, retinal degeneration is more likely to appear in certain breeds that have a genetic predisposition for this eye problem; both parents must carry an abnormal gene. Two parents who do not have the condition themselves may still pass on the disease to their offspring.

The sudden onset version of retinal degeneration (SARD) is not believed to be inherited, and is not usually explained by previous history of exposure to toxins or signs of other diseases. It is idiopathic (meaning no underlying cause can be determined), but the disease possibly involves autoimmune disease, toxins, elevations in adrenal sex hormones,[6] or Cushing's disease.[7]

Complementary Approach

Because retinal degeneration is considered a genetic disorder, neither afflicted animals nor their littermates should be bred.

Since this condition so often results in blindness, it is important to be aware of your pet's needs as the condition progresses. Cats generally adapt fairly well to life with diminished sight since they rely so heavily on their senses of smell and hearing. Dogs can cope with a loss of sight as well, but you should ensure that the home environment stays consistent and uncluttered; your dog can walk into furniture that has been moved or trip on unaccustomed objects left on the floor. Scent the areas at the top and bottom of household stairs with air freshener or other natural fragrances so that your dog can orient himself. Be sure that your dog still gets enough exercise, as s/he may be more timid when outdoors than s/he once was and may be more prone to obesity due to inactivity.

The studies that cite other potential causes of retinal degeneration, besides genetic factors, reference the following nutrients for improvement:

Taurine, which is a required supplement for cats.[8]

Fatty acids are important for good health. Add a highly potent fatty acid blend, rich in the omega-3 constituents EPA and DHA, to your pet's diet. Studies indicate that afflicted pets benefit from the EPA and DHA compounds in omega-3 fatty acids.[9]

General nutritional supplement. An aging pet's digestive system may not be absorbing what is needed. Consult your vet to learn what's needed.

CoQ10 exists in abundance in people and pets, is a potent antioxidant, and facilitates energy production within the heart, brain, and eyes.

Retinal Tear or Detachment

The retina is a layer of special light-sensitive cells that lines the back of the eye and functions like the film in a camera. Upon capturing the light and images, it then sends these visual images to the brain via the optic nerve.

A retinal detachment occurs if the layer of light-sensitive cells is pulled away from the back of the eye. When the retina becomes separated from the support tissue underneath (the choroid, which supplies the retina with blood and oxygen), it can no longer function and is termed "detached." If not treated promptly and properly, the affected animal will become blind, sometimes within a matter of days.

In animals, this problem tends to present late in the illness, and may be difficult to identify at first, as a dog or cat cannot let us know that some of their vision is impaired. Retinal detachments tend to be picked up only when there is significant visual loss, often affecting both eyes.

Causes

Causes of retinal detachment include an injury to the eye or head, an inherited tendency, tumor, or health condition such as diabetes, high blood pressure, lupus, kidney disease, and sickle cell anemia. Other causes include congenital defects, such as retinal dysplasia (seen in Labradors), infection, mature cataracts, any eye surgery, poisoning, or hyperviscosity (thickness) syndromes.

Success of treatment depends on how bad the damage is, and how long it has been there. In some cases, surgery is just not feasible.

Symptoms

Retinal detachments can occur slowly or quickly. If it is occurring slowly and only in one eye, you may not notice any difference in your pet's behavior. You may notice that the pupil of the affected eye dilates and remains dilated as the pet's vision decreases.

Conventional Treatment

Modern surgery involves the use of extreme cold or laser to place parts of the retina back in position by producing scar tissue. This then allows the blood supply to re-establish. It is essential that a vet examine any animal with a suspected retinal detachment, urgently. Any additional treatment to your vet's recommendation should be complementary rather than alternative.

Complementary Approach

Eyebright and **bilberry**, two herbs integral to wholistic eye treatment, are primary nutrients that may support healing.

Essential fatty acids are important for retinal (and heart) health. We recommend a product featuring a high-grade marine lipid concentrate, rich in the omega-3 constituents EPA and DHA.

---

[1] Zhao, L., Chen, X.J., Zhu, J., Xi, Y.B., Yang, X. et al. (2015). Lanosterol reverses protein aggregation in cataracts. *Nature*, Jul 30;(523):607-611.

[2] Excerpts from a 1982 Clinical Study: The Effects of Three Topical Agents on Posterior Subcapsular Cataract Progression in Royal College of Surgeons (R.S.C.) Rats. Retrieved Jul 11 2018 from http://www.natoph.com/pdf-files/article-study-cataracts.pdf.

[3] Babizhayev, M.A. (2004). Lipid peroxidation and cataracts: N-acetylecarnosine as a therapeutic tool to manage cataracts in human and canine eyes. *Drugs R D*, 2004;5(3):136-39.

[4] Diabetes in Pets. Retrieved Jul 11 2018 from https://www.avma.org/public/PetCare/Pages/Diabetes-in-Pets.aspx.

[5] Hayes, K.C. (1982). Nutritional Problems in Cats: Taurine Deficiency and Vitamin A Excess. *Can Vet J*, Jan;23(1):2-5.

[6] Carter, R.T., Oliver, J.W., Stepien, R.L., Bentley, E. (2009). Elevations in sex hormones in dogs with sudden acquired retinal degeneration syndrome (SARDS). *J Am Anim Hosp Assoc*, Sep-Oct;45(5):207-14.

[7] Gelatt, Kirk N. (ed.) (1999). *Veterinary Ophthalmology (3rd ed.)*. Philadelphia, PA: Lippincott, Williams & Wilkins.

[8] Ibid. Hayes. (1982).

[9] Bauer, J.E. (2011). Therapeutic use of fish oils in companion animals. *J Am Vet Med Assoc*, Dec 1; 239(11):1441-51.

12. DRUGS

The human body is an organic unit with tissues and organs that are interrelated and mutually dependent. The health of the eyes, as the body's optical organ, can influence, and be influenced by, any and every other organ in the body. When medications are taken for conditions anywhere in the body, they frequently have visual side effects. All drugs have side effects. Even herbs, foods, and vitamins may have side effects, though they tend more to nourish the body. Prescription drugs are not completely safe.

Drug reactions are not always noticed immediately. Some medications produce gradual symptoms that require a visit to the doctor. Sometimes a return visit is to a doctor other than the doctor who prescribed the drug. This second doctor may unknowingly prescribe one or more drugs to treat symptoms that are actually the side effects of the originally prescribed medication.

Thomas Moore, author of *Prescription for Disaster: The Hidden Dangers in Your Medicine Cabinet*,[1] points out that every year, drugs kill more people than guns, cigarettes, auto accidents, or plane crashes. The lifetime risk for the general population of developing lung cancer is one-third that of being harmed by a prescription drug. Modern drugs are rapidly integrated throughout our bodies and can throw our systems out of balance.

With that said, drugs when prescribed properly, can help manage difficult health problems and even save vision, so one has to weigh the pros and cons with the physician, before taking any medication. To research the effects of drugs and their interactions, a few excellent website sources include www.drugs.com, www.rxlist.com, and medscape.com

The following is a review of the most common medications taken in the United States that have a range of effects on the eyes.

Common Drugs with Visual Side Effects

Acne

Isotretinoin (Accutane) is a photosensitizing drug prescribed for acne that can cause blurred vision, other changes in vision, excessive tears, and possibly eye discharge. An ocular side effect may be eye abnormalities, including microphthalmia.[2]

Minocycline may result in a pigmentation of the sclera, typically a blue-grey color, worse in sunlight, which goes away with discontinued use of the drug. If not stopped, ocular side effects may include blurry vision due to aqueous-tear deficiency and bilateral-vision loss due to the effect on the back of the brain.[3]

Other related drugs can lead to sensations of dust in the eye, redness, burning eyes, temporary vision distortion, dry eye syndrome, and night blindness.

Alzheimer's

Cholinesterase hemorrhaging inhibitors, often prescribed to those suffering from Alzheimer's disease, can contribute to hemorrhaging in the eye. An example of one drug used is Donepezil. Common ocular side effects include cataracts, eye irritation, and blurred vision. Less common side effects are dry eyes, glaucoma, blepharitis, retinal or conjunctival bleeding, spots before eyes, and periorbital edema.[4]

Antibiotics

Important. Whenever taking antibiotics, also take probiotics such as acidophilus or bifidus between antibiotic doses. Vitamin C can significantly increase the effectiveness of antibiotics. Vitamin C and antibiotics could be up to 100 times more effective than drugs at killing cancer cells and without the side effects.[5]

When antibiotics are given topically for eye problems, they may have side effects that include dermatological side effects, such as skin irritation, itching or rash, burning eyes, redness/pain or swelling in or around the eyes, and vision problems.

Systemic antibiotics taken orally, intramuscularly, or intravenously to treat bacterial infections may cause some visual symptoms, including a higher risk of retinal disorders such as retinal detachments, often resulting in trips to the emergency room.[6] Known eye problems include sensitivity to bright lights, dry eye syndrome, allergic conjunctivitis, temporary vision distortion (which can even progress to night blindness), and increased risk of glaucoma (especially in patients who have diabetes).[7]

Synthetic penicillin (amoxicillin and ampicillin) may cause puffiness or swelling of the eyelids or around the eyes, face, lips, or tongue, red irritated eyes or yellow eyes or skin.[8]

Tetracyclines can cause increased sensitivity of skin to sunlight[9] or yellowing eyes or skin.[10]

Sulfonamides or "sulfa drugs" may cause allergies. These may also cause a decrease in visual acuity, pupil dilation, increase in intraocular pressure, visual field defects, and retinal toxicity disturbances on color vision. Optic neuritis and retrobulbar neuritis may result from the use of **chloramphenicol**.[11]

Amphotericin B can lead to blurred vision or other vision change.[12]

Nalidixic acid is associated with light sensitivity/photophobia, change in color perception, difficulty in focusing, decrease in visual acuity, and double vision. The antibiotic **linezolid** can contribute to optic nerve damage.[13]

Antidepressants

Antidepressants, and other drugs that act on the nervous system, change how information is processed in the nerves of the brain. Any medication that affects neurological function can affect vision and can cause changes in the cornea, optic nerve, lens, macula, and retina. Many antidepressants are drugs that increase your sensitivity to the sun and can make you more susceptible to cataracts and macular degeneration.

Cymbalta has been found to cause blurred vision, decreased vision, and eye pain.[14]

Mirtazapine, in unusual cases, can cause eye pain, abnormality of accommodation, conjunctivitis, keratoconjunctivitis, tear duct disorder, and angle-closure glaucoma.[15]

Prozac (fluoxetine hydrochloride), a commonly prescribed SSRI (selective serotonin reuptake inhibitor), may cause changes in vision, including blepharitis, double vision, exophthalmos (eye bulging), glaucoma, scleritis, strabismus, visual field defects, as well as cataracts, oculogyric crises (upward-turned eyes), and optic neuritis.[16]

Tricyclic antidepressants (amitriptyline, desipramine, imipramine, and nortriptyline) might have visual effects such as accommodation disorder, mydriasis, and more uncommonly, intraocular pressure increase.[17]

Valium (diazepam), an anti-anxiety drug, may cause double vision upon initial usage, which usually clears up after continued use. Less commonly, it can cause blurred vision, diplopia (double vision), conjunctivitis, or nystagmus (repetitive uncontrolled movements).[18]

Venlafaxine, which is prescribed for depression, has common side effects that include abnormal vision, abnormality of accommodation (ability to focus), and mydriasis (pupil dilation). Less common side effects include cataracts, conjunctivitis, corneal lesion, diplopia, dry eyes, eye pain, photophobia, or visual field defects. In rare cases, eye problems can include blepharitis, chromatopsia (abnormal color vision), conjunctival edema, exophthalmos (bulging eye), angle-closure glaucoma, retinal hemorrhage, subconjunctival hemorrhage, keratitis, pupil constriction, papilledema (optic nerve swelling), decreased pupillary reflex, scleritis, or uveitis.[19] [20]

Zoloft (sertraline hydrochloride), another popular SSRI, can cause abnormal vision and visual disturbance/impairment. Less common side effects include eye pain, mydriasis, periorbital edema, and rarely, diplopia, glaucoma, hyphema (blood pooling), lacrimal disorder, photophobia, scotoma, visual field defect, blindness, cataract, or optic neuritis.[21]

Other antidepressants (including **fluvoxamine** (Luvox) and **paraxetine** (Paxil) raise the risk of cataracts by 23–39%.[22]

Antihistamines

Just as antihistamines have a drying effect on your nose, they can affect your eyes and contribute to cataracts, increased light sensitivity,[23] burning/stinging/irritation, and dry eye syndrome.[24] In rare instances, they may make your pupils dilate or become unequal in size, decrease accommodation, increase blurred vision,[25] and worsen narrow angles, which may induce angle-closure glaucoma.[26] If you experience any unusual symptoms, report them to your doctor.

Note. Any medication with the side effect of dilated pupils increases your susceptibility to narrow-angle glaucoma.

Antimalarial Drugs

Chloroquinecan causes irreversible maculopathy and macular degeneration. Irreversible retinal damage has been reported in patients receiving long-term or high-dose **4-aminoquinoline** therapy. Less commonly reported eye issues include retinopathy, which is dose-related, visual disturbances (blurred vision, focusing, or accommodation difficulty), decreased visual acuity, and color-vision defects. Other visual field defects may include difficulty in reading, with words tending to disappear, seeing half an object, misty vision, and fog before the eyes. Damage may include pigment changes in the retina, pigmentary retinopathy, corneal deposits (which are typically reversible after discontinuing drug use), keratopathy, decreased corneal sensitivity, corneal edema, and reversible corneal opacities.[27]

Hydroxychloroquine can cause vision blurriness, which tends to be dose-dependent and reversible, and less commonly, it can cause retinopathy (with changes in pigmentation and visual field defects), corneal changes, haloes, photophobia, or nystagmus.[28]

Quinacrine used in low doses for malaria prophylaxis, can be associated with a delayed, severe maculopathy, indistinguishable from chloroquine maculopathy in certain patients.[29]

Plaquenil (hydroxchloroquine sulfate) commonly causes blurred vision. Less common side effects include retinopathy (with changes in pigmentation and visual field defects), corneal changes, haloes, or photophobia. Rare side effects include maculopathies, macular degeneration (may be irreversible), extra-ocular muscle palsies (reversible), and nystagmus.[30]

Asthma

Long-term use of nasal steroids, commonly inhaled for asthma, is connected to open-angle glaucoma, as they can increase intraocular pressure. Newer intranasal steroids are thought to have a minimal effect on IOP because of their low bioavailability.[31]

Birth Control Pills

Women taking birth control pills have a higher incidence of migraine headaches, problems with contact lenses due to dry eyes, color vision disturbances, retinal vascular problems, corneal edema, lens opacities, and retinal neuro-ophthalmologic or vascular complications.[32]

Blood Thinners

Hesparin, warfarin, coumadin, anisindione, and other oral anti-coagulants prescribed to prevent blood clotting can cause blurred vision, and rarely, swelling of the eyes or eyelids, yellow eyes and skin, and unusual bleeding or bruising.[33]

Bone Support

Fosamax is a common drug recommended to build bone. Possible ocular side effects include orbital inflammation, uveitis, and scleritis.[34]

Benign prostatic hyperplasia

Tamsulosin hydrochloride (Flomax) is an uroselective alpha-blocker, the most commonly prescribed drug for enlarged prostate and lower urinary tract symptoms. Most of the patients who develop inoperative floppy iris syndrome (IFIS) are taking tamsulosin. Tamsulosin impedes pupil dilation and can lead to IFIS and associated complications during cataract surgery.[35]

Cancer Drugs

Common cancer drugs include **tamoxifen, busulphan, methotrexate, toremifene, cyclophosphamide, 5-fluorouracil, cyclophosphamide**, and **interferon**.

Ocular side effects of cancer drugs can include blepharitis and eyelid dermatitis, excessive tearing, ocular irritation (occurs in 5.8% of users), conjunctivitis (3.8%), keratitis (3.8%), tearing (26.9%), and blurred vision (11.5%). Also, corneal opacity changes with **tamoxifen**, posterior subcapsular cataracts, ocular pruritus, and or burning sensation, ocular pain, foreign body sensation, blurred vision, and bilateral conjunctival hyperemia.

Combination chemotherapy for acute lymphoblastic leukemia with standard doses of **vincristine, cyclophosphamide** or **teniposide, cytarabine**, and **asparaginase** have been associated with corneal toxicity, especially when cytarabine is used.

Visual loss secondary to retinopathy occurs with the use of **cisplatin**, as well as retinal ischemia and neovascularization in a patient on combination chemotherapy (**bleomycin, etoposide and cisplatin**). Retinopathy also occurs with **mitotane** and **tamoxifen**; tamoxifen can cause bilateral pigmentary retinopathy, severe enough to warrant discontinuation of therapy.

Interferon associated retinopathy is typically characterized by retinal hemorrhages and cotton wool spots in the posterior fundus, but visual function is usually maintained. Other ocular reactions to interferon include ischemic retinopathy and macula edema.[36]

Important. Make sure your ophthalmologist carefully monitors your eyes when under cancer treatment.

Dermatology

The use of many drugs in dermatologic diseases may cause ocular side effects, including **anti-malarial medicines, glucocorticoids, retinoids,** and **psoralens.** Retinoid-induced ocular side effects include ocular surface disease as well as retinal dysfunction.[37] Also see steroid discussion.

Diabetes

Oral anti-diabetes drugs are photosensitizing. They absorb light energy and undergo a photochemical reaction resulting in chemical modification of tissue. They can make you more vulnerable to cataracts and macular degeneration.

Patients taking diabetes drugs known as **thiazolidinediones, pioglitazone,** and **rosiglitazone** have 3–6 times increased risk of developing diabetic macular edema.[38] [39] Actos (piogliazone) is also potentially linked to increased risk of bladder cancer.[40]

Rarely, diabetic medications such as **chlorpropamide** are connected to optic nerve degeneration,[41] and can cause blurred vision, and red, irritated eyes.[42]

Erectile dysfunction

Erectile dysfunction drugs tadalafil, vardenafil hydrocholoride, and **sildenafil citrate** (Viagra) may lead to nonarteritic anterior ischemic optic neuropathy (sudden vision loss), especially if the patient has had a past heart attack.[43]

Viagra can commonly cause abnormal vision (11% of users), including retinal hemorrhage, blurred vision, photophobia, eye irritation, and ocular hyperemia. Uncommon reactions include conjunctival disorders, eye pain, reduced visual acuity, diplopia, abnormal sensation in eye, photopsia, visual brightness, abnormal vision (mild to moderate and transient), light sensitivity, or visual color changes (chloropsia, chromatopsia, cyanopsia, erythropsia, and xanthopsia), and/or lacrimation disorders resulting in dry eyes. Rare (less than 0.1%) side effects include arteriosclerotic retinopathy, retinal disorder, glaucoma, myopia, asthenopia, floaters, iris disorder, mydriasis, halo vision, eye and eyelid swelling, scleral discoloration, nonarteritic anterior ischemic optic neuropathy, retinal vascular occlusion, or cataracts.[44]

Headaches

See Pain Relief.

Heart Disorders

Digitalis (Lanoxin), used to treat heart failure, can cause vision changes, such as blurred or yellow/green vision.[45]

Digoxin (a form of digitalis) is used for heart failure or heart irregularity. Common ocular effects are blurred vision or visual disturbances.[46]

Amiodarone is commonly associated with irreversible corneal microdeposits (up to 90% or more), visual disturbance, and less commonly, optic neuropathy/neuritis.[47] [48]

High Blood Pressure

The visual side effects of hypertension medications will reverse when you stop taking the drugs, but do not stop your medication without talking to your doctor. The optic nerve can suffer a type of stroke if it doesn't receive enough blood at night. Research has proven that taking blood pressure medications before bed can lower blood flow to the optic nerve and may cause an optic nerve stroke, resulting in permanent vision loss. The primary symptom of an optic nerve stroke is blurred vision upon awakening. There may be blackness or grayness in a portion of vision. If you are on this type of drug and awake with blurred vision, immediately seek medical attention, as early intervention can minimize vision loss.

Blood pressure drugs cause your body to excrete excess fluid and ease the blood vessels. But in the eyes, less fluid means dry eyes, light sensitivity, possible blurred and/or double vision. Analysis of data from the 2-year Beaver Dam study showed that use of vasodilator and hypertension medications increases the risk of developing macular degeneration by 72%. This research continued through 2013 with almost 5,000 patients with the same results.

Lasix, used as a component of therapy for high blood pressure, removes body fluids. Uncommon side effects can include visual disturbance, and rarely, myopia-aggravated-blurred vision.[49]

Beta-blockers are sometimes used to reduce high blood pressure by slowing the kidneys' production of a protein called renin. Renin normally causes the release of a powerful blood vessel constrictor called angiotensin II, which makes it harder for blood to flow through the arteries (thus raising blood pressure), and it also causes secretion of hormones that cause water retention, which increases the amount of fluid in the blood.

The most significant side effects of systemic beta-blocker and diuretic use are dry eye, conjunctivitis, corneal epithelial damage, and corneal irritation, secondary to decreased tear production. Furthermore, patients on beta-blockers and diuretics may experience difficulty wearing contact lenses due to significant ocular-surface dryness.[50]

Additional symptoms are dilated pupils and light sensitivity. Less common side effects include blurred vision or other change in vision, different size pupils of the eyes, discoloration of the eyeball, droopy upper eyelid, eye pain, seeing double, swelling, irritation or inflammation of eye or eyelid,[51] and a 71% increased risk of wet macular degeneration, the more severe and advanced form of AMD. Beta-blockers may also cause double vision in some people.

ACE inhibitors (angiotension converting enzymes) are also often prescribed for high blood pressure. Ocular side effects of ACE inhibitors include decreased vision, photophobia, and conjunctivitis. Further, the anemia associated with ACE inhibitors can cause retinal hemorrhaging.[52]

Alpha-1 blockers, used to lower blood pressure, can cause a condition (that doesn't affect vision) called "floppy iris syndrome." If you are going to have eye surgery, you should let your doctor know that you've been taking this type of medication, especially tamsulosin,[53] which is prescribed for benign prostatic hyperplasia and lower urinary tract symptoms.

Clonidin (Catapres), if used on an ongoing basis, can contribute to damage of the retina and cause damage to the lacrimal gland (causing dry eyes),[54] and lead to accommodation disorder, blurred vision, burning of the eyes, decreased lacrimation, and dry eyes.[55]

High Cholesterol

Cholesterol lowering drugs also can accelerate cataracts and produce fatigue. If you have high cholesterol, we suggest you include the following in your diet:

- Olive oil, omega-3 fatty acids
- Oatmeal
- Soy, garlic, onions, and shitake mushrooms
- Vitamin C, vitamin E, and niacin
- Red rice yeast

Simvastatin (Zocor) may lead to ptosis (droopy upper eyelid), diplopia, and ophthalmoplegia (paralysis of eye muscles), which tend to resolve after cessation of taking this drug.[56] In rare cases, cataracts develop. Unexplained visual blur and non-specific eye irritation have been reported in patients who use **lovastatin.**[57]

Also see steroid discussion.

Hormone Replacement

Estrogen or androgen replacement with synthetic hormones can cause blood clotting and reduction of blood circulation in the eyes. The ocular side effects of **stradiol** hormone replacement therapy include visual disturbances, contact lens intolerance,[58] and steepening of corneal curvature.[59] Estrogen hormone replacement may cause blepharospasm or eye twitching.

Insomnia

Benzodiazepines prescribed for insomnia may cause blepharospasm (eye twitch). Benzodiazepines also lead to weaknesses in concentration and memory. These include Midazolam, Trazolam, Temazepam, Oxazepam, Lorazepam, Alprazolam, Clonazepam, Diazepam, Florazepam, Clorazepam, Zolpidem, Zopiclone, and Zaleplon. For example, ocular side effects of Midazolam can include nystagmus, blurred vision, diplopia, pinpoint pupils, visual disturbance, difficulty focusing eyes, or cyclic movement of the eyelids.[60]

Muscle spasms

Gastric antispasmodics, prescribed to stop muscle spasms, can lead to optic nerve damage and/or glaucoma.

Benzodiazepines prescribed for muscle spasms or seizures can cause blepharospasm. For example, an ocular side effect of **diazepam** (Valium) is double vision, which occurs at the start of treatment, but usually disappears with continued use. Less common ocular reactions include blurred vision, conjunctivitis, diplopia, nystagmus, and visual disturbances.[61]

Pain Relief

Aspirin may exaggerate bleeding of the eye, though research is mixed.

NSAIDS are popular drugs, available over-the-counter and in prescription strength. Examples of these nonsteroidal anti-inflammatory drugs include **aspirin, ibuprofen** (e.g., Motrin or Advil), and **naproxen** (e.g., Aleve, Anaprox). Side effects can include cataracts and dry eyes. Retinal hemorrhages might result from long-term use of these drugs. Blurry vision, for example, is a common side effect of naproxen. Less common side effects include ptosis, amblyopia, scleritis, cataract, conjunctivitis, keratoconjunctivitis, lacrimation disorder, eye pain, diplopia, and optic nerve problems such as retrobulbar optic neuritis, corneal opacity, papillitis, or papilledema.[62]

Vicodin (hydrocodone/acetaminophen) along with **OxyContin** (oxycodone) are the most prescribed pain medications in the United States. Unexplained diplopia and blurred vision mandate a detailed history of prescription painkiller use. Ocular side effects can infrequently include nonspecific visual distortions, minor hallucinations, and conjunctival yellowing.[63] Double vision and transient blur are commonly reported in patients using **gabapentin**.[64]

Parkinson's Drugs

Drugs such as **levodopa**, may aggravate or cause blepharospasm. It can cause blurred vision, dilated (large) pupils, double vision, inability to move the eyes, and muscle twitching.[65]

Amantadine is often prescribed for patients with Parkinson's. Ocular side effects include dry eye, cataract, or blurred vision. Less common ocular side effects include visual disturbance, corneal opacity, corneal swelling, decreased visual acuity, sensitivity to light, or optic nerve palsy.[66] Extra care is recommended in monitoring cornea edema in such patients, as well as patients who have had cataract surgery or who have glaucoma, uveitis, or Fuch's dystrophy.

Photosensitizing Drugs

Photosensitizing drugs increase sensitivity to the sun. These drugs absorb light energy and undergo a photochemical reaction, resulting in chemical modification of tissue. They increase susceptibility to cataracts and macular degeneration. Anytime you take a drug that makes you more sensitive to light, wear sunglasses that block out 100% of the ultraviolet rays, and take antioxidants such as vitamin C, vitamin E, vitamin A, selenium, alpha-lipoic acid, lutein, zeaxanthin, mesozeaxanthin, and astaxanthin.

Drugs in the following categories are photosensitizing:

- Antihistamines
- Birth control pills
- Tranquilizers
- Sulfa drugs
- Oral antidiabetic drugs
- Antibiotics
- Antidepressants
- NSAIDS such as aspirin, ibuprofen, and naproxen
- Cholesterol lowering drugs

Recreational Drugs

Cocaine has been shown to lead to retinal artery occlusion and rapid and often irreversible loss of vision. The snorting of cocaine can result in corneal damage, decreased tear production, prolonged interblink time, and potentially corneal lesions resulting in vision impairment.[67]

Methamphetamines can cause ocular problems such as decreased visual acuity, as well as possibly retinal vasculitis, episcleritis, panophthalmitis, endophthalmitis, scleritis, retinopathy, corneal ulceration, and transient visual losses.[68] Also see weight loss discussion.

Smoking tobacco significantly increases the risk of cataract and age-related macular degeneration, diabetic retinopathy, open-angle glaucoma, retinal ischemia, anterior ischemic optic neuropathy, and Graves ophthalmopathy. It is highly irritating to the conjunctiva[69] and affects the eyes of nonsmokers through secondhand exposure. For pregnant women, cigarette smoke passes through the placenta, and the offspring of smoking mothers are prone to develop strabismus.[70]

Many recreational drugs make you more light sensitive, cause photochemical tissue changes, and may make you more vulnerable to cataracts and macular degeneration.

Psychiatric medications

The most common ocular side effects of psychogenic drugs are blurred vision, photophobia, and nonspecific visual complaints.[71] Dry eyes are a common complaint.

Psychiatric medications, such as the **phenothiazines** (thorazine and thioridazine), in large doses, can lead to pigmentation of the conjunctiva, cornea, and eyelids.

Chlorpromazine (thorazine) commonly causes blurred vision, photophobia, corneal/eye deposits, and pupil dilation or constriction. Uncommon eye disorders include optic atrophy, lens opacities, pigmentary retinopathy, precipitation/aggravation of narrow-angle glaucoma, and an accommodation disorder, which is related to the anticholinergic effects of this drug. Eye deposits occur in the front of the eye from drug accumulation; but usually do not have impact on sight.

Thioridazine (for schizophrenia) can cause blurred vision, pupil constriction, oculogyric crises, progressive conjunctival pigmentation, discoloration of exposed sclera and cornea, and stellate/irregular-shaped opacities of anterior lens and cornea.[72]

Thioridazine and chlorpromazine are both associated with night blindness, a browning of vision, cataract development, and a salt-and-pepper pigmentation of the fundus.

Selective serotonin reuptake inhibitors (SSRI), including **citalopram** and **escitalopram**, have been implicated in angle-closure glaucoma, with attacks typically occurring within six months of beginning the therapy.[73]

Antipsychotic medications, such as **Haldol,** can commonly cause oculogyric crisis (eyes turned upwards), visual disturbance, and less commonly, blurred vision, cataracts, and/or retinopathy.[74]

Benzodiazepines prescribed for alcohol withdrawal or anxiety can cause blepharospasm.

Seasickness

Stimulants such as **ephedrine,** sometimes prescribed for seasickness, give rise to dilation of the pupils and may increase risk of angle-closure glaucoma.

Steroids

- Drugs ending in **-one** (prednisone, hydrocortisone, clocortolone, etc.)[75]
- Drugs ending in **-ide** (fluocinonide, budesonide, desonide, etc.)[76]
- Drugs with **pred** in the name (prednisolone, loteprednol, prednicarbate, etc.)[77]
- Drugs with **cort** in the name (fluocortin, Cyclocort, Entocort)[78]

Steroids are commonly prescribed for inflammatory conditions such as rheumatoid arthritis, lupus, Sjögren's syndrome, shingles, systemic poison ivy or poison oak, gout, Crohn's disease, or lupus.

The most important ocular manifestations of steroid management are irreversible optic nerve damage in "steroid responders" (steroid glaucoma) and cataracts. Steroid use also can damage the eyes indirectly by causing an increase in blood sugar, leading to diabetes, and can cause ptosis, red eye, corneal deposits, and changes in color vision and the optic nerve.

Steroids, such as **prednisone** can cause blurred vision, cataracts (including posterior subcapsular cataracts), central serous chorioretinopathy, secondary bacterial infections (also fungal and viral), exophthalmos, glaucoma, and increased intraocular pressure.[79] Subcapsular cataracts will develop in up to 50% of people taking 10–15mg of prednisone daily for one to two years. These cataracts are very dense and can cause a rapid loss of vision. They will not go away, even after you stop the medication, and will have to be surgically removed.

Important. If you must take steroids, make sure you take high doses of antioxidants such as alpha-lipoic acid, vitamin C, vitamin E, and lutein to help prevent cataract formation.

Thyroid medications

There are rare reports of thyroid medication causing eye fatigue, blurred vision, or other eye disorders or impairment. **Levothyroxine, armour, unimazole (methimazole),** and **cortef** have been reported to cause blurred vision and/or dry eyes. Levothyroxine, for example, can cause swelling of the eyes, blurred or double vision, and eye pain.[80]

Synthroid, especially in women with hypertension, has been reported to cause eye fatigue. Although ocular side effects associated with levothyroxine are extremely rare, ptosis, diplopia, and ophthalmoplegia (eye muscle paralysis) have been reported.[81]

Tuberculosis

Ethambutol and **isoniazid**, used for tuberculosis, can lead to optic nerve degeneration, though rarely. The ocular side effects, for example, of ethambutol can include visual field defects, and less commonly, numbness/tingling of extremities, peripheral neuritis, and peripheral neuropathy.[82] With isoniazid, there have been reports of optic nerve atrophy.[83]

Ulcers

Proton pump medications can cause hypersensitivity, especially **omeprazole**. Irreversible visual impairment has been reported in critically ill patients who received high doses of IV omeprazole;

however, no causal relationship has been established. On rare occasions, it may cause blurred vision, and possibly optic atrophy, anterior ischemic optic neuropathy, optic neuritis, dry eye syndrome, ocular irritation, or double vision.[84]

Vitamins

Vitamin A megadoses can increase the pressure of fluid around the brain, which in turn can cause swelling of the optic nerve, headache, and visual distortions. The maximum we recommend is 15,000 IU per day of vitamin A palmitate (unless pregnant). 15,000 IU is only for people with retinal disorders such as retinitis pigmentosa. For higher dosage, consult your doctor.

Weight Loss

Appetite suppressants (**amphetamines, dextroamphetamines, methamphetamines,** and **phenmetrazine** compounds) may contribute to the following visual side effects: dry eyes, dilated pupils, difficulty focusing the eyes, and difficulty converging the eyes when reading.

Amphetamines can contribute to optic nerve damage and/or glaucoma and lead to a reduced focusing capacity and a risk for acute angle-closure glaucoma, a serious eye emergency. Some are prescribed for conditions such as attention deficit hyperactivity disorder (ADHD) and narcolepsy (where a person has an uncontrollable urge to sleep). Many are mind-stimulating drugs taken illegally such as crystal methamphetamine (ice).

Drugs for Specific Visual Disorders

Important. Patients must be told to evaluate how they feel after beginning any medication or herbal formula and to report any changes. These changes will give the practitioner information on how to adjust the medication or formula, if necessary.

Antibiotics for Ocular Surface Infections

Topical antibiotics may be prescribed for conditions such as conjunctivitis and blepharitis. Topical antibiotics often cause itching, reddening, and edema of the conjunctiva and eyelid.[85]

First Line Drugs

The following three first line drugs treat most ocular bacterial infections. They fight most common ocular pathogens. They come as eyedrops and ointments, but should be used first as drops.

Tobramycin has broad-spectrum activity. It is the drug of choice for its effectiveness and minimal side effects. Tobramycin is available in generic form, further reducing its expense. Ocular side effects include red eye or eyelid itching/swelling.[86]

Polytrim is a combination product that is relatively inexpensive. It is the pediatric drug of choice unless the infection is severe. Polytrim is excellent for treating bacterial conjunctivitis in children and adults. It is very effective against streptococcus and haemophilus, the most common causes of bacterial eye infections in children. It combines trimethoprim (good against gram-positive and gram-negative organisms) and polymyxin B. Dosage is one drop every two hours while awake for two days, then one drop every four hours while awake for five more days. Ocular side effects are the most common, and they include local irritation, increased redness, burning, stinging, and/or itching. This may occur initially, within 48 hours, or at any time with extended use.[87]

Fluoroquinolones are used primarily to treat moderate to severe conjunctival and corneal bacterial infections, such as corneal bacterial ulcers. The fluoroquinolones include ciloxan ophthalmic solution and ointment (Alcon), ocuflox ophthalmic solution (Allergan), and chibroxin ophthalmic solution (Merck). The unique chemical structure and mechanism of this category of antibiotics make them the most effective of the currently available eye medications.

These drugs work by inhibiting a bacterial DNA gyrase, an enzyme necessary for bacterial replication. Fluoroquinolones are highly bactericidal, even in very low concentrations. However, they are also very expensive. Generally safe when used for ocular conditions, ocular toxicity appears to be dose-dependent. Phototoxicity and neurotoxicity have been reported, and toxic effects on ocular collagen may be associated with Achilles tendinopathy.[88]

Other Topical Antibiotics

Other drugs used to treat eye infections include polysporin, which has a broad spectrum of activity and little surface toxicity, and erythromycin, which is virtually nontoxic to the corneal surface and has a good range of antibacterial activity.

Erythromycin is available as an ointment and is the drug of choice for using an eye patch in the case of corneal abrasions and for nighttime use. It is gentle on the cornea and provides good antibacterial protection. It is available generically and is used extensively for primary care of the external eye tissues. It works by inhibiting protein synthesis and is effective against most gram-negative and gram-positive organisms. Staphylococcal resistance may develop however, when erythromycin is used over several days. It is not a drug of choice for active therapy since it is available only in ointment form (not as eyedrops) but is a good supportive antibiotic. It is used in newborns as a second line treatment for prevention of possible chlamydial infection.

Gentamycin and neomycin are also available as topical antibiotics for use in the eyes and work by inhibiting protein synthesis. They are most effective against gram-negative bacteria, especially pseudomonas, but are also effective against gram-positive bacteria. They are relatively inexpensive and effective for most cases of bacterial conjunctivitis. **Tobramycin** (discussed above), however, is slightly more effective and slightly less toxic than gentamycin.

Bacitracin is the drug of choice to treat bacterial blepharitis. It breaks down cell walls and works well against staphylococcal bacteria, the main bacterial cause of blepharitis. If there is also a lot of lid margin inflammation, then a one-week course of **tobradex** is used also.

Polymyxin B Combinations

Many drugs are relatively broad spectrum yet do not work well against pseudomonas and other gram-negative species. Polymyxin B is a potent killer of gram-negative bacteria and pseudomonas. It works by destroying the cell membrane's structural and functional integrity, resulting in cell death. Polymyxin B is found in a number of products, including Polytrim (Allergan), polysporin, and neosporin.

Polytrim is a first-line drug of choice for eye infections. **Polysporin** is a combination of polymyxin B and bacitracin. It works well against gram-negative and gram-positive pathogens and is relatively nontoxic to the epithelial tissues.

Neosporin is a combination of bacitracin, polymyxin B, and neomycin. **Gramacidin** can replace the bacitracin of this combination since it is more water-soluble. Neosporin is effective but used infrequently because neomycin can have side effects such as edema of the eyelids.

Sulfa drugs

The sulfa drugs include **sodium sulfacetamide** and **sulfisoxazole**. Although sulfa drugs are broad spectrum, about 60–70% of staphyloccocal organisms (staph) are resistant to them, as are most pseudomonas species. Many people are allergic to sulfa drugs. For these reasons sulfa drugs are now considered poor choices. Polytrim, tobramycin, or a fluoroquinolone are more effective.

The one exception is in childhood bacterial infection, when the child will not cooperate with eyedrop therapy. Most childhood bacterial infections are caused by streptococcus pneumoniae ("strep") or haemophilus influenza. Ten percent sodium sulfacetamide ointment is effective against these. But staphylococcus also can cause infection, and sodium sulfacetamide may not be effective against staph. Polytrim is the best choice for children who will take eyedrops. Unfortunately, the eyedrops sting when putting them in.

Note. More relevant, even than selecting the right drug, is determining the optimal frequency of instillation. These medications should not be used for more than one week.

Corticosteroids Used for Eye Inflammation

Topical corticosteroids are the main medications for ocular anti-inflammatory therapy. The risks associated with short-term use are minimal.

Steroids with Maximal Clinical Action

Prednisolone acetate 1% (Pred Forte) is the most commonly prescribed and clinically proven topical steroid. It has the greatest anti-inflammatory efficacy of all topical ophthalmic steroids. Pred Forte is used for moderate to severe ocular inflammation such as episcleritis, iritis, keratitis, chemical or thermal burns of the cornea, and a host of other ocular inflammatory conditions. As with other steroids, frequent instillation is given until the inflammation is under control.

Possible ocular side effects, over time, may include increased intraocular pressure, glaucoma, optic nerve damage, posterior subcapsular cataract formation, acute anterior uveitis, perforation of globe, keratitis, conjunctivitis, corneal ulcer, mydriasis, conjunctival hyperemia, ptosis, loss of accommodation, secondary ocular infection, visual acuity or field defect, transient discomfort, oscleral/corneal perforation, foreign body sensation, burning, stinging, irritation, blurred vision, and corneal calcification. In rare cases, a side effect may be a filtering bleb, which is when the aqueous flows into the subconjunctival space, usually leading to an elevation of the conjunctiva.[89]

Other maximal action steroids are:

- Prednisone sodium phosphate (Inflamase Forte)
- Rimexolone (Vexol)
- Loteprednol etabonate (Lotemax)

Steroids with Moderate Strength

Fluorometholone alcohol (FML or Flur-Op) is a well-known moderate-strength steroid used to treat a host of mild to moderate ocular surface inflammatory conditions. It is also useful in treatment of chronic inflammation that lasts beyond three to four weeks. The most common side effect may be minimal tendency to raise intraocular pressure. Other possible, but less likely side effects include corneal calcification, eye irritation, conjunctival/ocular hyperemia, eye pain, visual disturbance, foreign body sensation in eyes, eyelid edema, blurred vision, eye discharge, eye pruritus, increased lacrimation, mydriasis, cataract (including subcapsular), ulcerative keratitis, ocular infection (bacterial, fungal, and viral), visual field defect, punctate keratitis, acute anterior uveitis, perforation of the globe, conjunctivitis, corneal ulcers, and loss of accommodation.[90]

Fluorometholone acetate (Flarex, Eflone) is another moderate-strength steroid used in treatment of eye disorders.

Steroid-Antibiotic Combinations

Steroid-antibiotic combination drugs are widely used in the ophthalmic community. The main use of these drugs is inflammation control when an antibacterial agent is also needed. Such combination drugs include:

- TobraDex. A combination of dexamethasone alcohol with tobramycin.
- Vasocidin, Blephamide, Isopto-Cetapred. Combinations of prednisolone with sodium sulfacetamide (a sulfa drug).
- Pred-G. A combination of prednisolone with gentamycin.
- Maxitrol, Dexacidin. Combinations of prednisolone, neomycin, and polymyxin B.

Dry Eye Products

The most commonly used drugs in eye doctors' offices are "artificial tear" type products. There are a wide variety of artificial tear products currently available. There are typically no negative effects of taking preservative-free over-the-counter eyedrops.

Low Viscosity Artificial Tears

Preservative-free or nontoxic preserved artificial tears are used with corneal abrasion and other types of non-specific ocular surface conditions.

There are a number of low viscosity, preservative-free tears that work well to treat mild to moderate dry-eye-syndrome symptoms. These include Gen Teal, HypoTears, Moisture Eyes, Refresh Plus, Refresh Tears, Tears Naturale, and Thera Tears. See the Dry Eye Chapter for more information and recommendations.

For advanced ocular surface disease Bion Tears and Ocu Coat are used.

Glaucoma Medications

Patients with glaucoma represent some of the most poorly cared for people in the United States and probably the world.

Dr. Grossman saw a patient who was using beta-blocker eyedrops for her eye pressure. She had a very hoarse, phlegmy voice that had developed since she had begun the drops. After switching to alternative therapies and stopping the beta-blockers, her hoarseness got better and the phlegm disappeared. Any changes in medications should be coordinated with your eye doctor, and not without medical supervision.

An extensive discussion of glaucoma medications appears in Chapter 15-11, Glaucoma.

Retinal Bleeding

Lucentis, Avestin, and **EyLea** are the most common drugs used as an injection in the eyes to help stop bleeding in the retina and reduce inflammation.

Ocular side effects from injections, such as Lucentis injections, include conjunctival hemorrhage (up to 74% of users experience this side effect), eye pain (up to 35%), vitreous floaters (up to 27%), increased intraocular pressure (up to 24%), vitreous detachment (up to 21%), intraocular inflammation (up to 18%), vision disturbance/blurred vision (up to 18%), cataract (up to 17%), foreign body sensation in eyes (up to 16%), eye irritation (up to 15%), increased lacrimation (up to 14%), blepharitis (up to 12%), dry eye (up to 12%), eye pruritus (up to 12%), ocular hyperemia (up to 11%), maculopathy (up to 11%), retinal disorder (10%), vitritis, and retinal hemorrhage.

Common (1–10%) side effects are retinal degeneration, retinal detachment or tear, retinal pigment epithelium break with or without detachment, reduced visual acuity, vitreous hemorrhage, vitreous disorder, uveitis, iritis, subcapsular cataract, punctuate keratitis, corneal abrasion, anterior chamber flare, eye hemorrhage, conjunctivitis, allergic conjunctivitis, eye discharge, photopsia (light flashes), photophobia (light sensitivity), ocular discomfort, eyelid edema, eyelid pain, conjunctival hyperemia, posterior capsule opacification, endophthalmitis, and injection site hemorrhage.

Uncommon (0.1–1%) side effects include blindness, hypopyon, hyphema, keratopathy, iris adhesion, corneal deposits, corneal edema, corneal striae, injection site pain, injection site irritation, abnormal sensation in eye, and eyelid irritation.[91]

Environmental Toxins

Although these are not drugs that your doctor might prescribe, you should remember that many "safe" chemicals used in the home and yard are toxic and can affect your vision directly, or affect your general health and thus indirectly damage your vision. Many herbicides and pesticides (and drugs that damage the retina[92] [93] [94] [95] [96]) can harm your eyes and your vision.

Recommended. Avoid the use of home chemicals, herbicides, and pesticides. If you have a food-producing garden, this is especially important.

A Few Terms

accommodation (ability to focus)
chromatopsia (abnormal color vision)
chloropsia (green-tinted vision)
cyanopsia (blue-tinted vision)
diplopia (double vision)
erythropsia (red-tinted vision)
exophthalmos (bulging eye)
hyperemia (excess blood)
hypopyon (inflammation in front of eye)
hyphema (blood pooling inside front chamber of eye)
lacrimal disorder (tear duct disorder)
mydriasis (pupil dilation)
nystagmus (repetitive uncontrolled movements)
oculogyric crises (upward-turned eyes)
ophthalmoplegia (paralysis of eye muscles)
papilledema (optic nerve swelling)
papillitis (optic nerve inflammation)
photopsia (flashes of light)
pruritus (itching)
ptosis (droopy upper eyelid)
retrobulbar (behind the eyeball)
xanthopsia (yellow-tinted vision)

---

[1]Moore, T. (1998). Prescription for Disaster: The Hidden Dangers in Your Medicine Cabinet. Simon & Schuster, New York.

[2] RXList. Acutane. Retrieved Jun 2018 from https://www.rxlist.com/accutane-drug.htm.

[3]Stephenson, M. (2011). Systemic Drugs with Ocular Side Effects. *Rev Opthalmol*, Oct 4.

[4] Drugs. Donepezil Side Effects. Retrieved Jun 10 2018 from https://www.drugs.com/sfx/donepezil-side-effects.html.

[5]Whiteman, H. (2017). Combining vitamin C with antibiotics destroys cancer cells. *Medical News Today, Jun 13*.

[6] Etminan, M., Forooghian, F., Brophy, J.M. (2012). Oral Fluoroquinolones and the Risk of Retinal Detachment. *JAMA*, 307(13):1414-1419.

[7]SWEye. How Antibiotics Can Damage Eyes and Vision. Retrieved Jun 14 2018 from https://www.sweye.com/blog/general/how-antibiotics-can-damage-eyes-and-vision/

[8] Drugs. Amoxicillin Side Effects. Retrieved Jun 8 2018 from https://www.drugs.com/sfx/amoxicillin-side-effects.html.

[9] Drugs. Tetracycline Side Effects. Retrieved Jun 8 2018 from https://www.drugs.com/sfx/tetracycline-side-effects.html.

[10] RXList. Tetracycline. Retrieved Jun 8 2018 from https://www.rxlist.com/consumer_tetracycline_sumycin_actisite/drugs-condition.html.

[11] Jaanus, S.D. (1992). Ocular side effects of selected systemic drugs. *Optom Clin,* 2(4):73-96.

[12] Drugs. Amphotericin B Side Effects. Retrieved Jun 8 2018 from https://www.drugs.com/sfx/amphotericin-b-side-effects.html.

[13] Gonzalez, S.N., Galvis, T., Borbolla, P., Mondragon, P., Juarz, O. (2017). Linezolid-associated optic neuropathy in a pediatric patient with mycobacterium nonchromogenicum: A case report. *Medicine (Baltimore),* Dec;96(50):e9200.

[14] Drugs. Cymbalta Side Effects. Retrieved Jun 8 2018 from https://www.drugs.com/sfx/cymbalta-side-effects.html.

[15] Drugs. Mirtazapine Side Effects. Retrieved Jun 8 2018 from https://www.drugs.com/sfx/mirtazapine-side-effects.html

[16] Drugs. Prozac Side Effects. Retrieved Jun 8 2018 from https://www.drugs.com/sfx/prozac-side-effects.html.

[17] Drugs. Amitriptyline Side Effects. Retrieved Jun 8 2018 from https://www.drugs.com/sfx/amitriptyline-side-effects.html.

[18] Drugs. Valium Side Effects. Retrieved Jun 8 2018 from https://www.drugs.com/sfx/valium-side-effects.html.

[19] Drugs. Venlafaxine Side Effects. Retrieved Jun 8 2018 from https://www.drugs.com/sfx/venlafaxine-side-effects.html.

[20] Etminan, M., Mikelberg, F.S., Brophy, J.M. (2010). Selective serotonin reuptake inhibitors and the risk of cataracts; a nested case control study. *Ophthalmology, Jun;117(6):1251-5.*

[21] Drugs. Zoloft Side Effects. Retrieved Jun 8 2018 from https://www.drugs.com/sfx/zoloft-side-effects.html.

[22] Ibid. Etminan. (2010).

[23] WebMD. Antihistamine Eye Drops. Retrieved Jun 8 2018 from https://www.webmd.com/drugs/2/drug-164414/antihistamine-eye-drops/details.

[24] Ibid. Jaanus. (1992).

[25] Wren, V.Q. (2000). Ocular & Visual Side Effects of Systemic Drugs. *J Behav Optom,* 11;(6):149.

[26] Caceres, V. (2016). Dermatology drugs, ocular side effects. *Eye World,* Sep.

[27] Drugs. Chloroquine Side Effects. Retrieved Jun 8 2018 from https://www.drugs.com/sfx/chloroquine-side-effects.html#refs.

[28] Drugs. Hydroxychloroquine Side Effects. Retrieved Jun 8 2018 from https://www.drugs.com/sfx/hydroxychloroquine-side-effects.html.

[29] Browning, D.J. (2004). Bull's-eye maculopathy associated with quinacrine therapy for malaria. *Am J Ophthalmol,* Mar;137(3):577-9.

[30] Drugs. Plaquenil Side Effects. Retrieved Jun 8 2018 from https://www.drugs.com/sfx/plaquenil-side-effects.html.

[31] Simsek, A., Bayraktar, C., Dogan, S., Karatas, M., Sarikaya, Y. (2016). The effect of long-term use of intranasal steroids on intraocular pressure. *Clin Ophthalmol,* 10:1079–1082.

[32] Moschos, M.M., Nitoda, E. (2017). The impact of combined oral contraceptives on ocular tissues: a review of ocular effects. *Int J Ophthalmol,* 10(10): 1604–1610.

[33] Drugs. Coumadin Side Effects. Retrieved Jun 8 2018 from https://www.drugs.com/sfx/coumadin-side-effects.html.

[34] Ibid. Stephenson. (2011).

[35] Zaman, F., Bach, C., Junaid, I., Papatsoris, A.G., Pati, J., et al. (2012). The Floppy Iris Syndrome – What Urologists and Ophthalmologists Need to Know. *Current Urol,* May;6(1):1-7.

[36] Omoti, A.E., Omoti, C.E. (2006). Ocular toxicity of systemic anticancer chemotherapy. *Pharm Pract (Granada),* Apr-Jun;4(2):55-59.

[37] Turno-Krecicka, A., Grzybowski, A., Misiuk-Hojto, M., Patryn, E., Czajor, K., et al. (2016). Ocular changes induced by drugs commonly used in dermatology. *Clin Dermatol,* Mar-Apr;34(2):129-37.

[38] Lamb, T. (2011). Actos And Avandia Use Associated With Diabetic Macular Edema, Which Can Lead To Blindness. Retrieved Jun 7 2018 from http://www.drug-injury.com/druginjurycom/2011/06/avandia-actos-side-effect-eye-disease-diabetic-macular-edema-dme-blindness.html.

[39] Simo, R., Hernandez, C. (2017). GLP-1R as a Target for the Treatment of Diabetic Retinopathy: Friend or Foe? *Diabetes,* Jun;66(6):1453-1460.

[40] Ibid. Lamb. (2011).

[41] Miller, N.R. (2007). Optic Neuropathies. Retrieved June 8 2018 from https://www.sciencedirect.com/topics/neuroscience/optic-neuropathy.

[42] Drugs. Chlorpropamide Side Effects. Retrieved June 9 2018 from https://www.drugs.com/sfx/chlorpropamide-side-effects.html.

[43] Fraunfelder, F.W., Shults, T. (2006). Non-arteritic anterior ischemic optic neuropathy, erectile dysfunction drugs, and amiodarone: is there a relationship? *J Neurophthalmol,* Mar;26(1):1-3.

[44] Drugs. Viagra Side Effects. Retrieved June 9 2018 from https://www.drugs.com/sfx/viagra-side-effects.html.

[45] RXList. Lanoxin Side Effects. Retrieved June 9 2018 from https://www.rxlist.com/lanoxin-tablets-side-effects-drug-center.htm.

[46] Drugs. Digoxin Side Effects. Retrieved June 9 2018 from https://www.drugs.com/sfx/digoxin-side-effects.html.

[47] Drugs. Amiodarone Side Effects. Retrieved June 9 2018 from https://www.drugs.com/sfx/amiodarone-side-effects.html#refs.

[48] Kaplan, L.J., Cappaert, W.E. (1984). Amiodarone-induced corneal deposits. *Ann Ophthalmol,* Aug;16(8):762-66.

[49] Drugs. Lasix Side Effects. Retrieved June 9 2018 from https://www.drugs.com/sfx/lasix-side-effects.html.

[50] Muchnick, B.G. (2013). Which Side Effects of Lurking in the Shadows? *Rev Optom,* Feb 15.

[51] MayoClinic. Beta-Adrenergic Blocker (Ophthalmic Route). Retrieved Jun 9 2018 from https://www.mayoclinic.org/drugs-supplements/beta-adrenergic-blocker-ophthalmic-route/side-effects/drg-20069403.

[52] Petrounis AD, Akritopoulos P. (1989). Influence of topical and systemic beta-blockers on tear production. *Int Ophthalmol,* Jan;13(1-2):75-80.

[53] Handzel, D.M., Briesen, S., Rausch, S., Kalble, T. (2012). Cataract Surgery in Patients Taking Alpha-1 Antagonists. *Dtsch Arztebl Int,* May;109(21):379-384.

[54] Drugs. Clonidine Side Effects. Retrieved June 9 2018 from https://www.drugs.com/sfx/clonidine-side-effects.html.

[55] Drugs. Catapres Side Effects. Retrieved June 9 2018 from https://www.rxlist.com/catapres-drug.htm#side_effects_interactions.

[56] Fraunfelder FW, Fraunfelder FT. (2012). Drug-related adverse effects of clinical importance to the ophthalmologist. Course presented at the American Academy of Ophthalmology Annual Meeting, Chicago. November 10-13.

[57] Mills, E.J., Wu, P., Chong, G., Ghement, I., Singh, S., et al. (2011). Efficacy and safety of statin treatment for cardiovascular disease: a network meta-analysis of 170,255 patients from 76 randomized trials. *QJM,* Feb;104(2):109-24.

[58] Drugs. Estradiol Side Effects. Retrieved June 9 2018 from https://www.drugs.com/sfx/estradiol-side-effects.html.

[59] RXList. Esclim Drug. Retrieved June 9 2018 from https://www.rxlist.com/esclim-drug.htm.

[60] Drugs. Midazolam Side Effects. Retrieved June 9 2018 from https://www.drugs.com/sfx/midazolam-side-effects.html.

[61] Drugs. Diazepam Side Effects. Retrieved June 9 2018 from https://www.drugs.com/sfx/diazepam-side-effects.html.

[62] Drugs. Naproxen Side Effects. Retrieved June 9 2018 from https://www.drugs.com/sfx/naproxen-side-effects.html.

[63] Richa S, Yazbek J. (2010). Ocular adverse effects of common psychotropic agents: a review. *CNS drugs,* Jun;24(6):501-26.

[64] Bookwalter T, Gitlin M. (2005). Gabapentin-induced neurologic toxicities. *Pharmacotherapy,* Dec;25(12):1817-9.

[65] Drugs. Levodopa. Retrieved June 9 2018 from https://www.drugs.com/cons/levodopa.html.

[66] Drugs. Amantadine Side Effects. Retrieved June 9 2018 from https://www.drugs.com/sfx/amantadine-side-effects.html.

[67] Mantelli, F., Lambiase, A., Sacchetti, M., Orlandi, V., Rosa, A., et al. (2015). Cocaine snorting may induce ocular surface damage through corneal sensitivity impairment. *Graefes Arch Clin Exp Ophthalmol,* May;253(5):765-72.

[68] Hazin, R., Cadet, J.L., Kahook, M.Y., Saed, D. (2009). Ocular manifestations of crystal methamphetamine use. *Neurotox Res,* Feb;15(2):187-91.

[69] Klein, B.E., Klein, R. (2007). Lifestyle exposures and eye diseases in adults. *Am J Ophthalmol,* Dec; 144(6):961-969.

[70] Solberg, Y., Rosner, M., Belkin, M. (1998). The association between cigarette smoking and ocular disease. *Surv Ophthalmol,* May-Jun;42(6):535-47.

[71] Costagiola C, Parmeggiani F, Sebastiani A. (2004). SSRIs and intraocular pressure modifications, evidence, therapeutic implications and possible mechanisms. *CNS Drugs,* Aug;18(8):475-84.

[72] Drugs. Thioridazine Side Effects. Retrieved Jun 10 2018 from https://www.drugs.com/sfx/thioridazine-side-effects.html.

[73] Ibid. Costagiola. (2004).

[74] Drugs. Haldol Side Effects. Retrieved Jun 10 2018 from https://www.drugs.com/sfx/haldol-side-effects.html.

[75] Oto, B. (2011). Drug Families: Steroids and Antibiotics. Retrieved Jun 7 2018 from http://emsbasics.com/2011/04/04/drug-families-steroids-and-antibiotics/.

[76] Ibid. Oto. (2011).

[77] Ibid. Oto. (2011).

[78] Ibid. Oto. (2011).

[79] Drugs. Prednisone Side Effects. Retrieved Jun 10 2018 from https://www.drugs.com/sfx/prednisone-side-effects.html.

[80] Drugs. Levothyroxine Side Effects. Retrieved Jun 10 2018 from https://www.drugs.com/sfx/levothyroxine-side-effects.html.

[81] Crilly, M. (2003). Thyroid function tests and hypothyroidism: reducing concentrations further would be harmful. *BMJ,* May 17;326(7398):1086.

[82] Drugs. Ethambutol Side Effects. Retrieved Jun 10 2018 from https://www.drugs.com/sfx/ethambutol-side-effects.html.

[83] Drugs. Isoniazid Side Effects. Retrieved Jun 10 2018 from https://www.drugs.com/sfx/isoniazid-side-effects.html.

[84] Drugs. Omeprazole Side Effects. Retrieved Jun 10 2018 from https://www.drugs.com/sfx/omeprazole-side-effects.html.

[85] RXList. Neosporin Ophthalmic Ointment. Retrieved Jun 10 2018 from https://www.rxlist.com/neosporin-ophthalmic-ointment-drug.htm.

[86] WebMD. Tobramycin Ophthalmic Drops. Retrieved Jun 10 2018 from https://www.webmd.com/drugs/2/drug-14396-396/tobramycin-ophthalmic-eye/tobramycin-ophthalmic-drops/details.

[87] Drugs. Polytrim Side Effects. Retrieved Jun 10 2018 from https://www.drugs.com/sfx/polytrim-side-effects.html.

[88] Thompson, A.M. (2007). Ocular toxicity of fluoroquinolones. *Clin Exp Ophthalmol,* Aug;35(6):566-77.

[89] Drugs. Prednisone Forte Side Effects. Retrieved Jun 10 2018 from https://www.drugs.com/sfx/pred-forte-side-effects.html.

[90] Drugs. Fluorometholone Ophthalmic Side Effects. Retrieved Jun 10 2018 from https://www.drugs.com/sfx/fluorometholone-ophthalmic-side-effects.html.

[91] Drugs. Lucentis Side Effects. Retrieved Jun 10 2018 from https://www.drugs.com/sfx/lucentis-side-effects.html.

[92] Seoane, A., Espejo, M., Pallas, M., Rodriguez-Farre, E., Ambrosio, S., et al. (1999). Degeneration and gliosis in rat retina and central nervous system from 3,3'-iminodipropionitrile exposure. *Brain Res,* Jul 3:833(2):258-71.

[93] Roy, N.M., Carneiro, B., Ochs, J. (2016). Glyphosate induces neurotoxicity in zebrafish. *Environ Toxicol Pharmacol,* Mar;42:45-54.

[94] Timchaulk, C., Dryzga, M.D., Johnson, K.A., Eddy, S.L., Freshour, N.L. (1997). Comparative pharmacokinetics of [14C]metosulam (N-[2,6-dichloro-3-methylphenyl]-5,7-dimethoxy-1,2,4- triazolo[1,5a]-pyrimidine-2-sulfonamide) in rats, mice and dogs. *J Appl Toxicol,* Jan-Feb; 17(1):9-21.

[95] Kamal, M.A., Al-jafari, A.A. (1999). Kinetic constants for the inhibition of camel retinal acetylcholinesterase by the carbamate insecticide Ianate. *J Biochem Mol Toxicol,* 1999;13(1):41-6.

[96] Paganelli, A., Gnazzo, V., Acosta, H., Lopez, S.L., Garrasco, A.E. (2010). Glyphosate-based herbicides promote teratogenic effects on vertebrates by impairing retinoic acid signaling. *Chem Res Toxicol,* Oct 18;23(10):1586-95.

PART THREE

VISION CONDITIONS

13-1. ASTIGMATISM

An astigmatism is usually due to an imperfection in the curvature of the cornea, resulting in perception of objects as oblong and blurred. Sometimes an astigmatism can result from an irregular shaped lens inside the eye. Astigmatism is quite common and frequently occurs along with nearsightedness and farsightedness. It is usually in both eyes but may be found just in one eye. Between 30% and 60% of adults in Europe and Asia have astigmatism.[1]

Like other visual conditions, astigmatism is not necessarily a fixed entity. In a study on musicians around symphony season, researchers noted that the musicians held their eyes and head in a tilted posture for long periods of time. Corneal changes occurred seasonally in a high percentage of the musicians, resulting in astigmatism. The researchers attributed these changes to the fact that the musicians' eyes tilted to adapt to their body distortion to try to maintain balance, causing the chronic straining of some eye muscles and relaxing of others. There was a near 100% correlation between the instruments played, the corresponding posture necessary to play the instruments, and the predicted astigmatism.[2] This is an example of "function affecting structure."

Anatomy of Astigmatism

The cornea is a transparent dome-shaped cover of the front part of the eye. It is normally round-shaped. When a cornea is astigmatic, it is shaped more like a football (egg-shaped), with a steeper, more-curved portion, and a flatter, less-curved portion. This does not allow light to be focused evenly on the retina.[3]

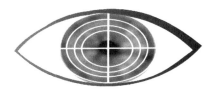

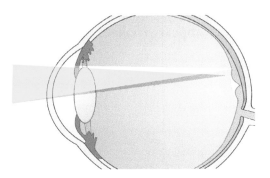

The steeper portion of the cornea focuses light more than the flatter portion, causing two different focal points within the eye. Depending on which side of the cornea is steeper, the focus may be on the retina, but also in front of the retina, behind the retina, or the two focus points may straddle the retina.

Types of Astigmatism

Astigmatisms are described relative to the shape of the cornea.

Regular. The midlines (meridians) are perpendicular.

With-the-rule. The vertical meridian is the steepest, like a football on its side.

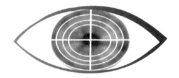

With-the-rule

Against-the-rule. The horizontal meridian is the steepest.

Oblique. The steepest curve is between 120 and 150 degrees and 30 and 60 degrees.

Against-the-rule

Irregular. The principal meridians are not perpendicular.

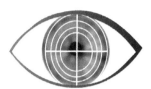

Astigmatisms are also described in terms of where the focus falls on the retina.

Simple astigmatism can cause hyperopic vision (farsighted) or myopic vision (nearsighted) with one focus point on the retina, and the other either behind or in front of the retina, respectively.

Oblique

Compound astigmatism. Both focus points are either behind (hyperopic) or in front of (myopic) the retina.

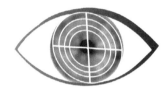

Mixed astigmatism. One focus point is in front of the retina, and the other is behind it.

Signs and Symptoms

- **Blurred vision** or distorted vision at near, distant, or both.
- **Eyestrain**, such as headaches, blurred vision, eye redness, eye fatigue, and/or twitching.
- **Distorted line perception**, such as when straight lines appear crooked, or lines appear clearer in one direction than the other.
- **Monocular double vision**[4] is double vision when only one eye is open.
- **Migraine headaches**[5] may be experienced.

Causes and Risk Factors

Genetics. The cause may be inherited, which may include other related eye conditions, such as keratoconus.[6]

Environment. Temporary or seasonal astigmatism may result from working for long hours with one's head at an angle. This can often be corrected naturally.

Corneal conditions. In less common cases, astigmatism can be due to corneal conditions, such as keratoconus. Scarring or thinning of the cornea creates a risk for astigmatism.[7]

IVR injection. Intravitreal injection of ranibizumab for wet AMD may cause astigmatism.[8]

Intraocular lens implant. Astigmatism may become more severe after cataract surgery when a standard monofocal IOL is implanted.[9]

Pterygium. Corneal tissue growth may cause astigmatism; it may eventually cover the cornea.[10]

Excessive near- or far-sightedness.[11]

Conventional Treatment

Glasses and contacts. If astigmatism interferes with vision, or causes eyestrain, glasses are the safest method of correction. Contact lenses are an option, but they are not always appropriate.[12]

LASIK surgery is also another option. A technique known as topography-guided excimer laser surgery has been found to be effective for those with irregular astigmatism by making it possible to fine-tune LASIK surgery for meridian irregularities.[13]

Toric lens. During cataract surgery, toric intraocular lenses, instead of traditional spherical lenses, may be implanted to correct astigmatism. Toric lenses are a relatively new option. In the past, intraocular lenses could not correct astigmatism, although corneal incisions during cataract surgery (limbal relaxing incisions) could sometimes help. Toric lenses take into account meridian steepness, and accordingly, apply very precise corrections. These lenses have to be placed quite precisely during installation. In addition, both monofocal and multifocal toric lenses are available for those with low levels of astigmatism who wish to improve their reading vision.[14]

Complementary Approach

Vision is not static and changes over time. Even without any pathology, vision tends to weaken as we age, as our eye muscles weaken. The eye lens becomes less flexible, and our ability to break down nutrients and deliver them to our eyes becomes compromised. Much can be done to maintain healthy vision, however, through diet, regular exercise (including daily eye exercises), and targeted supplementation. These can significantly help reduce the risk of future eye disease.

Nutrients

Nutritional supplements especially may be of value, if the astigmatism is combined with retinal weakness involving macular pigment, photoreceptors, or other eye conditions.

Helpful

Lutein. 10mg per day. This carotenoid is well researched for retinal support and essential for supporting macular pigment density.[15] Since excessive near- or far-sightedness is a risk factor for astigmatism, the ability of carotenoids to improve macular density becomes relevant. A Chinese study investigating axial length found that macular pigment density is inversely correlated with axial length.[16] Taking lutein along with zeaxanthin and astaxanthin results in significant improvement in visual acuity (vision sharpness).[17]

Whole-food, organic multivitamin. Take daily, follow the directions.

Vitamin D3. 2,000 IU–5,000 IU per day. Lower levels of vitamin D are associated with retinal microvascular damage, suggesting that the link with cardiovascular risk may partly run through changes in the microvasculature. A study of more than 900 subjects found that nearsighted people had significantly lower levels of vitamin D3 concentration.[18]

Astaxanthin. 6mg per day. Researchers concluded that astaxanthin is effective in protecting against damage from light, due to its antioxidant effect.[19] Because oxidative stress is a factor in many eye conditions,[20] astaxanthin's antioxidant capacity is critical for eye support.

Diet

Juicing. We recommend the following vegetables and fruits for general vision health and astigmatism. Choose at least 4–6 items to combine.

- Ginger, broccoli, cabbage, carrots, celery, leafy-green vegetables, and berries (preferably all organic)
- You can add your favorite fruits and vegetables as well. Do not use too many carrots due to its high natural sugar content.

Follow the Vision diet described in Chapter 7.

Lifestyle

Eye exercises. We recommend the following exercises for general vision support.

- Palming
- Eye massage of acupressure points around the eyes
- Near and far
- Figure eights
- Hot dog
- Zooming

See Chapter 10 for eye exercises and acupuncture points that are good for all eye conditions and overall eye health.

Natural daylight. Some research suggests that natural light exposure may counter-balance too much indoor/close up work causing strain on the eyes. Even on an overcast day, exposure to natural light for 2–3 hours may be helpful.

Manage chronic stress. Research has shown that long-term tension contributes to serious disease, which factors in to the causes of eye conditions.

Exercise. Develop a regular exercise routine. A minimum of 20–30 minutes of vigorous walking, swimming, etc. five days a week, for example, is excellent for eye and overall health.

Computer users. If you are a computer user, review our chapter on computer eye syndrome to learn how to minimize eyestrain.

Other Modalities

Chinese Medicine

The Liver is the main meridian in Chinese medicine responsible for health vision, as this meridian "opens to the eyes." The Kidney meridian helps nourish the retina and support lens health.

Common Chinese Medical Patterns for General Eye Health

Ming mu di juang wan is a classic formula used in Chinese medicine for eye health that helps nourish the Kidneys and Liver. It is also known to help with blurriness of vision, tearing against wind, conjunctival congestion with pain, and swelling of the eye.

Xiao yao san is a classic Liver tonic used in Chinese medicine. The Liver "opens to the eyes" and is the primary meridian (flow energy) that supports healthy circulation and the free flow of energy in the eyes, as well as throughout the body.

Herbal formula and treatment strategies can vary significantly, based on the Chinese medicine practitioner's evaluation and intake.

On the Horizon

Optical systems, such as cameras, have features like automatic focus and zooming. Ultrathin planar lenses or optical microscopes with metasurfaces (a kind of artificial material with thicknesses less than a wavelength), open the door to miniaturization and unique methods of "tuning" lenses with the adaptive capacity to correct many kinds of functional vision disorders, simultaneously and automatically.[21]

Also See

Chapter 7, Vision Diet

Chapter 8, Nutrients

Chapter 10-4, Eye Exercises

Chapter 15-4, Computer Eye Syndrome

Chapter 15-13, Keratoconus

Chapter 15-1, Cataracts

---

[1] Mozayan, E., Lee, J.K. (July 2014). Update on astigmatism management. *Curr Op Ophthalmol*, **2** (4):286–90.

[2] Taub, M.B., Harris, P. (2016). When Astigmatism Goes Off-Key, *Rev Opt*, Apr 15.

[3] Wikipedia. Astigmatism. Retrieved May 11 from https://en.wikipedia.org/wiki/Astigmatism.

[4] Vlaicu, V. (2012). Essential features of astigmatism and its correction with excimer laser. *Oftalmologia*, 56(1):27-9.

[5] Harle, D.E., Evans, B.J.W. (2006). The Correlation Between Migraine Headache and Refractive Errors. *Opt Vis Sci*, 83(2): 82–7.

[6] Kivi, R., Boskey, E. (2017). Astigmatism. Retrieved May 16 2018 from https://www.healthline.com/health/astigmatism.

[7] Ibid. Kivi. (2017).

[8] Kocaturk, T., Erkan, E., Egrilmez, S., Cakmak, H., Dundar, S.O., et al. (2015). Surgically Induced Corneal Astigmatism Following Intravitreal Ranibizumab Injection. *Oen Ophthalmol J*, Jul 31:9:121-5.

[99] Alcon. (2017). New data shows astigmatism tends to worsen following cataract surgery with a standard monofocal IOL, while patient awareness about advanced technology treatment options is limited. Retrieved Sep 6 2018 from https://www.alcon.com/news/media-releases/new-data-shows-astigmatism-tends-worsen-following-cataract-surgery-standard.

[10] Holladay, J.T., Lewis, J.W., Allison, M.E., Ruiz, R.S. (1985). Pterygia as cause of post-cataract with-the-rule astigmatism. *J Am Intraocul Implant Soc*, Mar;11(2):176-9.

[11] Ibid. Kivi. (2017).

[12] National Eye Institute. Facts about Astigmatism. Retrieved May 16 2018 from https://nei.nih.gov/health/errors/astigmatism.

[13] Ghoreishi, M., Naderi, B.A., Nadera, B.Z. (2014). Visual outcomes of topography-guided excimer laser surgery for treatment of patients with irregular astigmatism. *Lasers Med Sci*, Jan;29(1):105-11.

[14] Levitz, L., Reich, J., Roberts, K., Hodge, C. (2015). Evaluation of Toric Intraocular Lenses in Patients With Low Degrees of Astigmatism. *Asia Pac J Ophthalmol (Phila)*, Sep-Oct;4(5):245-9.

[15] Landrum, J.T., Bone, R.A., Joa, H., Kilburn, M.D., Moore, L.L., et al. (1997). A one year study of the macular pigment: the effect of 140 days of a lutein supplement. *Exp Eye Res*, Jul;65(1):57-62.

[16] Tong, N., Zhang, W., Zhang, Z., Gong, Y., Wooten, B., et al. (2013). Inverse relationship between macular pigment optical density and axial length in Chinese subjects with myopia. *Graefes Arch Clin Exp Ophthalmol*, Jun;251(6):1495-500.

[17] Piermarocchi, S., Saviano, S., Parisi, V., Tedeschi, M., Panozzo, G., et al. (2012). Carotenoids in Age-related Maculopathy Italian Study (CARMIS): two-year results of a randomized study. *Eur J Ophthalmol*, Mar-Apr;22(2):216-25.

[18] Yazar, S., Hewitt, A.W., Black, L.J., McKnight, C.M., Mountain, J.A., et al. (2014). Myopia is associated with lower vitamin D status in young adults. *Invest Ophthalmol Vis Sci*, Jun 26;55(7):4552-9.

[19] Ibid. Piermarocchi. (2012).

[20] Ibid. Francisco (2015).

[21] She, A., Zhang, S., Shian, S., Clarke, D.R., Capasso, F. (2018). Adaptive metalenses with simultaneous electrical control of focal length, astigmatism, and shift. *Sci Adv*, Feb 23;4(2):eaap9957.

13-2. FARSIGHTEDNESS

Farsightedness is the ability to see clearly at a distance, but near objects are unclear. Early in life, this is called hyperopia. After about age 40, the cause is different, and it is known as presbyopia.

In order to have perfect vision, the eyeball needs to be slightly ovoid (egg-shaped). Newborn children have eyeballs that are nearly spherical; therefore, the ability to focus is limited to about 20 centimeters for the first few months.[1] Their eyes gradually adjust and their hyperopia lessens as they mature. The flexible lens of the eye becomes able to adjust between near and far vision. But after about 40 years old (middle age), the lens becomes less flexible, making it more difficult to see details clearly, up close, without glasses. This is called presbyopia.

In children, more than half of refractive errors (focusing ability) are due to farsightedness.[2] About 8.9% of white children have hyperopia greater than +3D; about 4.4% of African-American children have the same degree of hyperopia.[3] Among adults, 38.2–50.2% have hyperopia of at least +1D, and 6.1–8.8% have hyperopia of +3D. This range is wide due to ethnicity: people of Hispanic origin more often are farsighted.[4]

How the Eye Focuses

The transparent cornea that covers the front of the eye has the most focusing power of the eye. But its curvature, and therefore its focusing capacity, is fixed. It is the flexible lens behind the cornea that fine-tunes total curvature to correctly aim incoming light on the retina. As the retina nerve cells pick up and transmit sensory information to the visual cortex in the brain, fine muscles in the ciliary body cause the lens to flatten or bulge in order to focus on objects near and far.

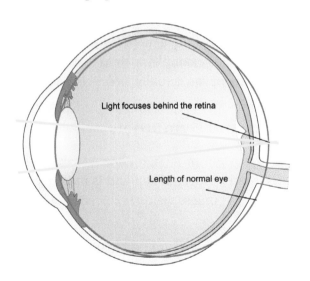

In cases of farsightedness, either because the eyeball is too short (hyperopia) or the lens is too inflexible (presbyopia), the incoming light overshoots the mark and is focused just behind the retina rather than right on it. The result is blurriness.

Hyperopia

Farsightedness is caused by either a smaller than normal length of the eye or a relatively flat curvature of the cornea. It can be overcome somewhat by strengthening the focusing power of the lens of the eye to help see nearby objects more clearly. Ciliary muscles control the flexing of the lens to focus near and far, and eye exercises may help to keep those muscles healthy.

Presbyopia

With aging, the lens itself becomes less flexible. The shape of the eye may still be too short (hyperopia) or too long (myopia), but in addition, the muscles of the ciliary body are less effective, because the lens itself becomes increasingly inflexible.

The human lens grows throughout our life. It is a closed system (although nutrients continue to nourish the living tissue of lens cells) in which continuous restructuring is needed to accommodate additional growth. Increasing density of lens proteins also increases inflexibility. The integrity of the lens depends, at least in part, upon the bioavailability of nutrients and antioxidants that are moved in and out of the lens. The lens has a microcirculation system that operates in place of blood vessels. It has been proposed that this system is a flow of ions that generates a flow of water through the lens. An extracellular flow of water moves nutrients into the lens; an intracellular flow of water moves wastes out of the lens.[5] [6]

As the lens ages, not only does its transparency decrease, but water movement within the lens slows, proteins and aggregates accumulate, glycation (bonding with sugars) increases, lipids accumulate, and glutathione and vitamin C (ascorbic acid) decreases.[7] After about the age of 40, a barrier to transporting glutathione to the interior of the lens develops around the nucleus of the lens, which accounts for lowered glutathione levels. As the nucleus becomes more rigid, presbyopia develops, and in some people, accumulation of aggregates leads to the development of cataracts.[8]

Causes

Causes can include genetics, stress, and age. Emotional considerations at an early age may also factor in. For example, a child who does not want to internalize feelings that are due to their environment can actually affect vision and create farsightedness (not wanting to see things near).

Signs and Symptoms

The symptom of farsightedness is that far vision is good, but near vision is poor. The patient experiences blurry vision and is more easily subject to eyestrain or even headaches when doing close work, unless vision is corrected with eyeglasses.

Conventional Treatment

Glasses or contacts are prescribed to correct the refractive error.

Complementary Approach

Vision is not static and changes over time. Even without any pathology, vision tends to weaken as we age. As eye muscles become weaker, the eye lens becomes less flexible. Compounding these changes, our ability to digest nutrients and deliver them to our eyes gets compromised. Much, however, can be done to maintain healthy vision and reduce the risk of future eye disease through diet, regular exercise (including daily eye exercises), and targeted supplementation. These approaches can also reduce the risk of future eye disease.

Because the literature suggests that risk of cataracts is lessened by diets rich in vitamin C, lutein/zeaxanthin, B vitamins, and omega-3 fatty acids, it may be that such a diet will also help protect the aging lens in other ways.[9]

Nutrients

Very Helpful

Glutathione. 500mg–900mg per day, if taken in capsule or pill form. The sublingual form has 5–10 times greater absorption so the dosage will be smaller. Follow label instructions. Referred to as the anti-aging antioxidant, glutathione is one of the few nutrients that can neutralize all types of free radicals. It plays a central role in protecting the aging lens from cataracts and may be useful in protecting the flexibility of the aging lens.[10] As the lens ages, glutathione levels decrease,[11] reducing its antioxidant protecting capacity.

Lutein. 10mg per day. Lutein is increasingly considered to be important in protecting the lens. In combination with the essential fatty acids, its antioxidant ability may help protect the aging lens from deterioration.[12]

Vitamin C (buffered and ascorbated). 2,000mg per day, split up with meals. As the lens ages, vitamin C decreases,[13] and its antioxidant capacity is lost.

Bilberry. 120–180mg per day. Bilberry is neuroprotective and has been shown to improve microcirculation in the eye. In an animal model, supplementation with bilberry extract helped protect DNA and improve enzyme activity in lens tissue.[14]

Omega-3 fatty acids. 1,000mg–2,000mg per day. Omega-3s may help protect the aging lens.[15]

A wholefood, organic multivitamin.

Helpful

Astaxanthin. 6mg per day. Astaxanthin does help protect the lens crystallins from oxidation and can possibly protect against increasing inflexibility due to its antioxidant effect.[16] [17]

Zeaxanthin. 2mg per day. The risk of cataracts is less when patients have diets rich in nutrients, including zeaxanthin.[18] This antioxidant's ability to protect the lens may have a role in reducing presbyopia risk.

Diet

Eat healthy. Research has verified that a healthy diet that includes daily intake of leafy-green vegetables and whole grains can significantly lower the likelihood of developing eye disease. Follow the Vision diet described in Chapter 7.

Juicing. Choose at least 4–6 items to combine. Favor organic vegetables and fruits.

- Ginger, broccoli, cabbage, carrots, celery, leafy-green vegetables, and berries.
- Do not use too many carrots due to their natural sweetness.

Lifestyle

Eye exercises are good for all eye conditions and overall eye health. We recommend these:

- Palming
- Eye massage of acupressure points around the eyes
- Near and far
- Figure eights
- Hot dog
- Zooming

See Chapter 10 for eye exercises and acupuncture points that may be helpful.

Natural daylight. Some research suggests that natural light exposure may help counter-balance too much indoor/close-up work causing strain on the eyes.

Manage chronic stress. Long-term tension is suspected to be a causative factor in eye conditions.

Exercise. Develop a regular exercise routine, such as a minimum of 20-30 daily walking.

Computer users. See Chapter 15-4 on computer eyestrain.

Magic eye 3D images, which allow the eye to study depth perception, help to increase eye muscle flexibility and relax the eye. See Appendix 8 for more information.

Other Modalities

Chinese Medicine

For General Eye Health

Ming mu di juang wan is a classic formula used in Chinese medicine for eye health, helping to nourish the Kidneys and Liver. It is known to help with blurry vision, tearing against wind, and conjunctive congestion with pain and swelling of eye.

Xiao yao san is a classic Liver tonic used in Chinese medicine. The Liver "opens to the eyes" and is the primary meridian (flow energy) that supports healthy circulation and the free flow of energy in the eyes, as well as throughout the body.

Herbal formula and treatment strategies can vary significantly, based on the Chinese medicine practitioner's evaluation and intake.

On the Horizon

Dynamic lenses. Scientists are searching for feasible dynamic lens replacements with the capacity to respond to existing ciliary body muscles, zonules (ligaments), or the capsule (membrane that encloses the lens), or find a method to reduce the stiffness of the lens.[19]

Pharmacological. In an animal study, researchers found that eyedrops that include pirenoxine, which has been used to treat cataracts, suppressed lens hardening significantly and might slow the progression of presbyopia. However, the changes were less marked with patients aged 60 and over.[20]

A number of other pharmacological avenues are being explored[21] with some degree of success in pilot studies. These involve a variety of methods of improving presbyopia. Some methods include the following:

- Increasing miosis (pupil constriction, like a pin hole camera)[22]
- Stimulating ciliary body action, plus miosis[23]
- Softening the lens, so it retains flexibility[24]

Also See

Chapter 7, Vision Diet

Chapter 8, Nutrients

Chapter 10-4, Eye Exercises

Chapter 12, Drugs

Chapter 15-1, Cataracts

---

[1] University of Calgary. Development of the Visual System. Retrieved May 8 2018 from http://www.ucalgary.ca/pip369/mod9/vision/system.

[2] Rodriguez, N.M., Romero, A.F. (2014). The prevalence of refractive conditions in Puerto Rican adults attending an eye clinic system. *J Optom*, 7:161–7.

[3] Giordano, L., Friedman, D.S., Repka, M.X., Katz, J., Ibironke, J., et al. (2009). Prevalence of refractive error among preschool children in an urban population: the Baltimore Pediatric Eye Disease Study. *Ophthalmology*, 116:739–46.

[4] Pan, C.W., Klein, B.E., Cotch, M.E., Sharger, S., Klein, R., et al. (2013). Racial variations in the prevalence of refractive errors in the United States: the multi-ethnic study of atherosclerosis. *Am J Ophthalmol*, Jun;155(6):1129-1138.

[5] Donaldson, P.J., Musil, L.S., Mathias, R.T. (2010). Point: A Critical Appraisal of the Lens Circulation Model—An Experimental Paradigm for Understanding the Maintenance of Lens Transparency? *Invest Ophthalmol Vis Sci*, My;51(5):2303-2306.

[6] Vaghefi, E., Liu, N., Donaldson, P.J. (2013). A computer model of lens structure and function predicts experimental changes to steady state properties and circulating currents. *Biomed Eng Online*, Aug 30;12:85.

[7] Pescosolido, N., Barbato, A., Giannotti, R., Komaiha, C., Lenarduzzi, F. (2016). Age-related changes in the kinetics of human lenses: prevention of the cataract. *Int J Ophthalmol*, Oct 18;9(10):1506-17.

[8] Michael, R., Bron, A.J. (2011). The aging lens and cataract: a model of normal and pathological aging. *Philos Trans R Soc Lond B Biol Sci*, Apr 27;366(1568):1278-92.

[9] Weikel, K.A., Garber, C., Baburins, A., Taylor, A. (2014). Nutritional modulation of cataract. *Nutr Rev,* Jan;72(1):30-47.

[10] Nye-Wood, M.G., Spraggins, J.M., Caprioli, R.M., Schey, K.L., Donaldson, P.J., et al. (2017). Spatial distributions of glutathione and its endogenous conjugates in normal bovine lens and a model of lens aging. *Exp Eye Res,* Jan;154:70-78.

[11] Ibid. Pescosolido. (2016).

[12] Padmanabha, S., Vallikannan, B. (2018). Fatty acids modulate the efficacy of lutein in cataract prevention: Assessment of oxidative and inflammatory parameters in rats. *Biochem Biophys Res Commun,* Jun 2;500(2):435-442.

[13] Ibid. Pescoslido. (2016).

[14] Aly, E.M., Ali, M.A. (2014). Effects of bilberry on deoxyribonucleic Acid damage and oxidant-antioxidant balance in the lens, induced by ultraviolet radiation. *Malays J Med Sci,* Jan;21(1):11-8.

[15] Ibid. Padmanabha. (2018).

[16] Wu, T.H., Liao, J.H., Hou, W.C., Huang, F.Y., Maher, T.J. et al. (2006). Astaxanthin protects against oxidative stress and calcium-induced porcine lens protein degradation. *J Agric Food Chem,* Mar 22;54(6):2418-23.

[17] Ishikawa, S., Hashizume, K., Nishigori, H., Tezuka, Y., Sanbe, A., et al. (2015). Effect of astaxanthin on cataract formation induced by glucocorticoids in the chick embryo. *Curr Eye Res,* May;40(5):535-40.

[18] Ibid. Weikel. (2014). Nutritional

[19] Charman, W.N. (2014). Developments in the correction of presbyopia II: surgical approaches. *Ophthalmic Physiol Opt,* Jul;34(4):397-426.

[20] Tsuneyoshi, Y., Higuchi, A., Negishi, K., Tsubota, K. (2017). Suppression of presbyopia progression with pirenoxine eye drops: experiments on rats and non-blinded, randomized clinical trial of efficacy. *Sci Rep,* Jul 28;7(1)6819.

[21] Renna, A., Alio, J.L., Vejarano, L.F. (2017). Pharmacological treatments of presbyopia: a review of modern perspectives. *Eye Vis (Lond),* Feb 7;4:3.

[22] Abdelkader, A. (2015). Improved Presbyopic Vision with Miotics. *Eye Contact Lens,* Sept;41(5):323-7.

[23] Renna, A., Vejarano, L.F., De la Cruz, E., Alio, J.L. (2016). Pharmacological treatment of presbyopia by novel binocularly instilled eye drops: a pilot study. *Ophthalmol Ther.* 5(1):63–73.

[24] Crawford, K.S., Garner, W.H., Burns, W. (2014). Dioptin™: A novel pharmaceutical formulation for restoration of accommodation in presbyopes. *Invest Ophthalmol Vis Sci.* 2014;55(13):3765

13-3. NEARSIGHTEDNESS

Nearsightedness (myopia) is the ability to see clearly at a near distance, but far objects are less clear. The conventional belief is that myopia occurs secondary to an excessive curvature of the cornea and/or a longer-than-normal eyeball. The degree of nearsightedness can vary widely, as can the age of onset and the rate of progression. Most myopia develops during the school years[1] and stabilizes in the teenage years.[2]

The widespread use of computers has made the problem worse. In the 1980s, before the present computer-driven world, only 2% of Dutch army recruits from a farming background were myopic, but 32% of those with an advanced education were nearsighted. Presently, in some urban parts of Asia, the percentage is nearing 90%.[3] A third of the world's population is myopic, and half of the world's population will be myopic by 2050, with up to one-fifth of them at a significantly heightened risk of blindness, if current trends continue.[4]

How the Eye Focuses

The cornea actually has the most focusing power of the eye. But its curve, and therefore its focusing ability, is fixed. The flexible lens fine-tunes curvature to aim incoming light on the retina. Fine muscles in the ciliary body cause the lens to flatten or bulge in order to focus on an object.

In cases of nearsightedness (myopia), the eyeball is too long, the incoming light undershoots the mark and the light is focused just before the retina, rather than right on it. The result is vision blurriness.

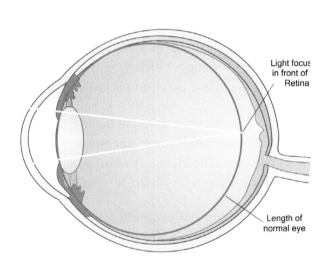

Light focus in front of Retina

Length of normal eye

Types of Myopia

Simple. Most common type is where the eyeball is naturally more oval than round. This is most often related to genetics, but it can be affected by environmental factors as well. This is the easiest form to improve, for example, through eye exercises.

Induced or acquired. This can be caused by certain medications and/or cataracts, which can change the way light is refracted to the retina.

Nocturnal. During the day your distance vision is fine, but at night with low light, seeing distance objects, without glasses, is more difficult.

Degenerative. Called pathological myopia, this is where the length and shape of your eye condition increases over time, ultimately increasing the risk of retinal damage.

Signs and Symptoms

Blurred sight at a distance is the primary symptom of myopia, with the ability to see close-up detail more clearly. Both eyes are usually involved, but one may be worse than the other. Sight tends to be worse at night.

The early signs of myopia tend to occur in the child who has his or her face in a book or electronic device for long periods of time, without ever looking up. That child might experience some blurring of objects in the distance as s/he looks up. School vision screening now catches many of these cases, but not all. Sometimes the discovery may be as simple as a child in the outfield that is unable to catch fly balls but is able to do so after s/he gets prescription glasses.

Myopia is an Epidemic

Optically, nearsightedness is very easy to understand. When refracting perfectly, the cornea and inner lens give you 20/20 vision or better. In the case of being nearsighted, the light is bent to refract in front of the retina, resulting in nearsightedness (distance vision being blurred). This can be corrected through eyeglasses with concave lenses.

This optical explanation of myopia is clear, but how do people develop myopia? It affects more than 80 million people in the U.S. If that's not an epidemic, what is? Are we foolish enough to think that this visual condition is just inherited, or is it also a function of how we use our eyes?

In the U.S., one study found that the incidence of myopia is 1.2% in non-Hispanic school children aged 6–72 months, 3.7% in Hispanics at this age, 3.98% in Asians, and 6.6% in African American school children. The incidence of myopia in school children in East Asia was even higher at 42.7% for 12-year-olds and 59.1% for 17-year-olds.[5]

Our visual system evolved for hunting and gathering and not for long hours of "near work." We are vulnerable to computer eyestrain symptoms and an increase in myopia, due to the weakening, for example, of the ciliary muscles that flex our lenses. Ciliary muscle strain is just one way it is more difficult to relax into a position that enables us to see well at a distance.

Variables affecting myopia in one study included education level, monthly income, housing levels, and jobs related to requiring a lot of "near work." The study also showed the same correspondences in myopic children regarding their parents' higher level of education, higher income, and white collar or professional occupations.[6] Another study that reviewed over 500 research papers concluded that, up to 40% of people with a low level of farsightedness or whose vision does not require eyeglasses (emmetropes, or normal vision people), after entering college and military academies, were likely to become myopic by the age of 25 years. In populations where college graduates are excluded, less than 10% of individuals become myopic as adults.[7]

Causes

The available studies should make it hard for any logical mind to think that nearsightedness can be due to genetics only. After it was recognized that highly educated people are more likely to be myopic, conflicting opinions arose as to whether myopia is genetically caused and/or environmentally caused. Genetics influence how the eye grows, but what causes normal vision (emmetropic) or myopic vision is heavily influenced by other factors.[8]

Hereditary. Certain chromosomes are linked to myopia, nonetheless the genetic effect is larger in people with a higher level of education.[9] Myopic children are likely to have myopic parents.[10] Myopia experienced as a child, in people with myopic parents, and in those who get little outdoor exercise, increases the risk of myopia in adults, especially women.[11]

Education and occupation. Myopia develops during the school years, especially in college students; it is much lower in uneducated or poorly educated people.[12] [13] [14] [15] Occupations that require much close work are more likely to increase the risk of myopia.[16]

Diet. The increase of myopia in undeveloped countries has paralleled the increase of a Western-type diet with a heavy reliance upon sugar and processed ingredients. It has been theorized that this change induces myopia.[17]

Diabetes. Myopia in diabetics appears to be associated with metabolism.[18] A study investigated whether the increasing rate of nearsightedness in diabetics was due to changes in the lens or the length of the eyeball (axial length). The researchers concluded that the changes were due to lens changes, not axial length changes.[19]

Exercise. Physical exercise has a protective effect with respect to nearsightedness.[20] Outdoor physical exercise is especially protective.[21] Researchers have learned that increased stimulation by outdoor light, results in increased dopamine release, which is known to reduce axial elongation.[22]

Premature birth. Children born prematurely are more likely to be nearsighted.[23]

Psychological stress. It is theorized that some children may become nearsighted due to environmental stress factors, such as difficult family situations. Being nearsighted enables them to not "see" or block out, to some extent, what is going on in their family life or environment that is unpleasant.

Oxidative stress. Researchers have found that oxidative stress may alter regulatory mechanisms of eye diseases, which have been linked to myopia, also retinal detachment, glaucoma, cataracts, and macular neovascularization.[24]

High intraocular pressure has been found to be a cause of axial lengthening and consequently, myopia.[25]

Kawasaki disease, which is a condition involving inflammation of arteries, lymph nodes, and mucous membranes, creates a substantially higher risk for developing myopia.[26]

Note. Of trace minerals measured in hair samples in Chinese college students, copper levels increased with the degree of myopia, while zinc, lead, aluminum, iron, and potassium decreased with the myopic degree.[27]

Risks

Patients with myopia, especially if severely nearsighted, are at higher risk for many conditions:

Myopic macular degeneration results in the stretching of the retina and potential vision loss.

Retinal hemorrhage. A study linked the occurrence of lacquer cracks (breaks in the Bruch's membrane) in patients with high levels of myopia and low macular pigment density.[28] These are early warnings of retinal hemorrhage.[29]

Psychological. Being nearsighted often causes a feeling of isolation, especially in adolescents.[30]

Retinal or vitreous detachment, including serous retinal detachment[31]

Macular holes, especially in women[32]

Lattice degeneration

Glaucoma, especially in people who are heavy computer users[33]

Eye floaters

Computer eyestrain

Conventional Treatment

Glasses or contacts are prescribed for correction of the refraction error.

LASIK surgery is another option for some people.

Low-dose atropine (for about two years) is sometimes prescribed for children; its use is controversial since there can sometimes be side effects, and 10% of children do not respond to the treatment.[34] [35]

Other. Pirenzepine drops, cyclopentolate drops, orthokeratology, and special contact lenses are moderately effective.[36]

Complementary Approach

Vision is not static and changes over time. Even without any pathology, vision tends to weaken as we age. As eye muscles become weaker, the eye lens becomes less flexible. Compounding these changes, our ability to break down nutrients and deliver them to our eyes becomes compromised. We can help maintain healthy vision through diet, regular exercise, and targeted supplementation. These approaches can also reduce the risk of future eye disease.

Nutrients

Important

Lutein. 10mg per day. This carotenoid is well researched for retinal support and is essential for supporting macular pigment density.[37] A Chinese study investigating the length from the lens to the retina found that macular pigment density is inversely correlated with axial length.[38] There is a relationship between high blood levels of lutein and lower risk of myopia, but further research is needed.[39] Also, research suggests that oxidative stress is a factor in myopia development.[40]

Zeaxanthin. 2mg per day. As discussed above with lutein, zeaxanthin improves macular pigment density,[41] which in turn is linked to axial length. Likewise, the research implicating oxidative stress[42] makes zeaxanthin's free-radical fighting capacity important.

Bilberry. 120mg–180mg per day. Guinea pigs with a type of myopia called "form deprivation" myopia benefited from a bilberry formulation, with axial length and other markers improving.[43] In addition, fermented bilberry extract improves vision in people who are myopic.[44] Bilberry also has strong antioxidant properties and supports healthy microcirculation.

Helpful

Omega-3 fatty acids. 1,000mg–2,000mg per day. While there has not been any research directly connecting omega-3 with myopia, maintaining overall ocular health is important for nearsighted people because they are more at risk for other conditions. DHA in particular provides protective properties to the retina.[45]

A whole-food, organic multivitamin.

Vitamin D3. 2,000 IU–5,000 IU per day. The research as to whether vitamin D is protective with respect to myopia is contradictory. A study of more than 900 subjects finds that nearsighted people have significantly lower levels of vitamin D3 concentration.[46] However, being outside, which naturally increases vitamin D, is linked to a lower myopia risk. Further research is needed to determine whether vitamin levels are protective, or whether they are simply linked to other consequences of sun exposure on myopia risk.[47]

Astaxanthin. 6mg per day. Researchers conclude that astaxanthin is effective in protecting against damage from light due to its antioxidant effect.[48] Because oxidative stress is a factor in myopia development,[49] astaxanthin's antioxidant capacity is valuable.

Diet

Research has verified that a healthy diet, which includes daily intake of leafy-green vegetables and whole grains, can significantly lower the likelihood of developing eye disease. In particular, diabetics and people consuming Western diets high in sugars are at higher risk of myopia.[50] [51]

Juicing. Choose at least 4-6 items from this suggested list of ingredients.

- Ginger, broccoli, cabbage, carrots, celery, leafy-green vegetables, and berries (preferably all organic)
- You can add your favorite fruits and vegetables as well. Do not use too many carrots or fruit due to their high sugar content.

Lifestyle

Natural daylight. Some research suggests that natural light exposure may counter-balance too much indoor/close-up work that causes strain on the eyes.[52] Even on an overcast day, exposure to natural light for up to 2–3 hours may be helpful. In general, for overall eye and retinal health, you should wear 100% UVA/UVB protecting sunglasses when outdoors.

Exercise. Develop a regular exercise routine. A minimum of 20–30 minutes of vigorous walking, swimming, etc. three or more times a week, for example, is excellent for eye and overall health.

Computer users. Review Chapter 15-4 on computer eyestrain for more information.

Breast-feeding. Several studies have reported that children who are breast-fed have a lower incidence of myopia, though the difference is insignificant.

Vision therapy. Vision therapy can be an effective way to improve vision naturally. Vision therapists are trained in helping people improve vision through individualized eye exercises. Behavioral optometrists are eye doctors trained in vision therapy. To locate a practitioner near you, go to www.oepf.org.

Eye exercises. Eye exercises we recommend include the following (see Chapter 10 for more eye exercises and acupressure eye points to massage):

- Palming
- Eye massage of acupressure points around the eyes
- Near and far
- Figure eights
- Hot dog
- Zooming

Other Modalities

Chinese Medicine

Myopia may be related to patterns such as Kidney yin and/or Liver yang deficiency. Chronic stress, poor diet, and/or lack of exercise are some environmental factors that affect these conditions.

Common Chinese Medical Patterns Related to Myopia

Ba zhen tang. Strengthens qi and nourishes blood

For General Eye Health

Ming mu di juang wan is a classic formula used in Chinese medicine for eye health that helps nourish the Kidneys and Liver. It is also known to help with blurriness of vision, tearing against wind, and conjunctive congestion with pain and swelling of eye.

Xiao yao san is a classic Liver tonic used in Chinese medicine. The Liver "opens to the eyes" and is the primary meridian (flow energy) that supports healthy circulation and the free flow of energy in the eyes, as well as throughout the body.

Herbal formula and treatment strategies can vary significantly, based on the Chinese medicine practitioner's evaluation and intake.

Also See

Chapter 7, Vision Diet

Chapter 10-4, Eye Exercises

Chapter 15-11, Glaucoma

Chapter 15-18, Macular Degeneration

Chapter 15-19, Macular Edema

Chapter 15-25, Retinal Detachment

---

[1] Grosvenor, T. (1987). A review and a suggested classification system for myopia on the basis of age-related prevalence and age of onset. *Am J Optom Physiol Opt*, Jul; 64(7):545-54.

[2] Goss, D.A., Winkler, R.L. (1983). Progression of myopia in youth: age of cessation. *Am J Optom Physiol Opt*, Aug; 60(8):651-8.

[3] O'Brien, G. (2018). Myopia Is on the Rise and Screens May Be to Blame. Retrieved May 10 2018 from http://businesswest.com/blog/myopia-is-on-the-rise-and-screens-may-be-to-blame.

[4] Holden, B.A., Fricke, T.R., Wilson, D.A., Jong, M., Naidoo, K.S., et al, (2016). Global Prevalence of Myopia and High Myopia and Temporal Trends from 2000 through 2050. *Ophthalmology*, May;123(5):1036–1042.

[5] French, A.N., Morgan, I.G., Burlutsky, G., Mitchell, P., Rose, K.A. (2013). Prevalence and 5- to 6-year incidence and progression of myopia and hyperopia in Australian schoolchildren. *Ophthalmology*, Jul;120(7):1482-91.

[6] Xiang, F., He, M., Morgan, I.G. (2012). The impact of parental myopia on myopia in Chinese children: population-based evidence. *Optom Vis Sci*, Oct; 89(10):1487-96.

[7] National Research Council (U.S.) Working Group on Myopia Prevalence and Progression. *Myopia: Prevalence and Progression*. Washington, DC: National Academy Press; 1989.

[8] Goldschmidt, E., Jacobsen, N. (2014). Genetic and environmental effects on myopia development and progression. *Eye (Lond)*, Feb;28(2):126-33.

[9] Ibid. Goldschmidt. (2014).

[10] Morgan, I., Rose, K. (2005). How genetic is school myopia? *Prog Retin Eye Res*, Jan; 24(1):1-38.

[11] Parssinen, O., Kauppinen, M., Viljanen, A. (2014). The progression of myopia from its onset at age 8-12 to adulthood and the influence of heredity and external factors on myopic progression. A 23-year follow-up study. *Acta Ophthalmol*, Dec;92(8):730-9.

[12] Maul, E., Barroso, S., Munoz, S.R., Sperduto, R.D., Ellwein, L.B. (2000). Refractive Error Study in Children: results from La Florida, Chile. *Am J Ophthalmol*, 129:445–454.

[13] Pokharel, G.P., Negrel, A.D., Munoz, S.R., Ellwein, L.B. (2000). Refractive Error Study in Children: results from Mechi Zone, *Nepal. Am J Ophthalmol*, 129:436–444

[14] Zhao, J., Pan, X., Sui, R., Munoz, S.R., Sperduto, R.D., Ellwein, L.B. (2000). Refractive Error Study in Children: results from Shunyi district China. *Am J Ophthalmol*, 129:427–435

[15] He, M., Zeng, J., Liu, Y., Xu, J., Pokharel, G.P., et al. (2004). Refractive error and visual impairment in urban children in southern China. *Invest Ophthalmol Vis Sci*, 45:793–799

[16] Ibid. Goldschmidt. (2014).

[17] Cordain, L., Eaton, S.B., Brand, J., Lindeberg, S., Jensen, C. (2002). An evolutionary analysis of the aetiology and pathogenesis of juvenile-onset myopia. *Acta Ophthalmol Scand. Apr, 80(2):125-35*

[18] Jacobsen, N., Jensen, H., Lund-Andersen, H., Goldschmidt, E. (2008). Is poor glycaemic control in diabetic patients a risk factor of myopia? *Acta Ophthalmol*, Aug;86(5):510-4.

[19] Fledelius, H.C., Miyamoto, K. (1987). Diabetic myopia--is it lens-induced? An oculometric study comprising ultrasound measurements. *Acta Ophthalmol (Copenh), Aug;65(4):469-73.*

[20] Jacobsen, N., Jensen, H., Goldschmidt, E. (2008). Does the level of physical activity in university students influence development and progression of myopia? --a 2-year prospective cohort study. *Invest Ophthalmol Vis Sci*, Apr; 49(4):1322-7.

[21] Rose, K.A., Morgan, I.G., Ip, J., Kifley, A., Huynh, S., et al. (2008). Outdoor activity reduces the prevalence of myopia in children. *Ophthalmology*, Aug; 115(8):1279-85.

[22] French, A.N., Ashby, R.S., Morgan, I.G., Rose, K.A. (2013). Time outdoors and the prevention of myopia. *Exp Eye Res*, Sep; 114():58-68.

[23] Fledeliu, S. H. (1976). Prematurity and the eye. Ophthalmic 10-year follow-up of children of low and normal birth weight. *Acta Ophthalmol Suppl*, 128():3-245.

[24] Francisco, B.M., Salvador, M., Amparo, N. (2015). Oxidative Stress in Myopia. *Oxid Med Cell Longev*, 2015:750637.

[25] Genest, R., Chandrashekar, N., Irving, E. (2012). The effect of intraocular pressure on chick eye geometry and its application to myopia. *Acta Bioeng Biomech*, 2012:14(2):3-8.

[26] Kung, Y.J., Wei, C.C., Chen, L.A., Chen, J.Y., Chang, C.Y., et al. (2017). Kawasaki Disease Increases the Incidence of Myopia, *Biomed Res Int*, 2017:2657913.

[27] Cai, Y. (2011). Determination of select trace elements in hair of college students in Jinzhou, China. *Bio Trace Elem Res*, Dec;144(1-3):469-74.

[28] Benoudis, L. Ingrand, P., Jeau, J., Lichtwitz, O., Boissonnot, M., et al. (2016). Relationships between macular pigment optical density and lacquer cracks in high myopia. *J Fr Ophtalmol*, Sep;39(7):615-21.

[29] Healio. Look for lacquer cracks in high myopes for early warning of retinal hemorrhage. Retrieved May 10 2018 from https://www.healio.com/optometry/retina-vitreous/news/print/primary-care-optometry-news/%7B587d2571-1ee9-42f3-ae39-b6b493b8e2b4%7D/look-for-lacquer-cracks-in-high-myopes-for-early-warning-of-retinal-hemorrhage.

[30] Lazarczyk, J.B., Urban, B., Konarzewska, B., Szulc, A., Bakunowicz-Lazarczyk, A., et al. (2016). The differences in level of trait anxiety among girls and boys aged 13-17 years with myopia and emmetropia. *BMC Ophthalmol*, Nov 14;16(1):201.

[31] Garcia-Ben, A., Garcia-Basterra, I., Gonzalez-Gomez, A., Baquero-Aranda, I., Morillo-Sanchez, M.J., et al. (2018). Comparison of long-term clinical evolution in highly myopic eyes with vertical oval-shaped dome with or without untreated serous retinal detachment. *Br J Ophthalmol*, May 7.

[32] dell'Omo, R., Virgili, G., Bottoni, E., Parolini, B., De Turris, S., et al. (2018). Lamellar macular holes in the eyes with pathological myopia. *Graefes Arch Clin Exp Ophthalmol,* May 3.

[33] Tatemichi, M., Nakano, T., Tanaka, K., Hayashi, T., Nawa, T., et al. (2004). Possible association between heavy computer users and glaucomatous visual field abnormalities: a cross sectional studying Japanese workers. *Epidemiol Community Health,* Dec;58(12):1021-7.

[34] Schittkowski, M.P., Sturm, V. (2018). Atropine for the Prevention of Progression in Myopia - Data, Side Effects, Practical Guidelines. *Klin Monbl Augenheilkd,* Apr;235(4):385-391.

[35] Tran, H.D.M., Tran, Y.HY., Tran, T.D., Jong, M., Coroneo, M., et al. (2018). A Review of Myopia Control with Atropine. *J Ocul Pharmacol Ther,* May 1.

[36] Erdniset, N., Morad, Y. (2017). Treatments for Slowing the Progression of Myopia. *Harefuah,* Nov;156(11):720-724.

[37] Landrum, J.T., Bone, R.A., Joa, H., Kilburn, M.D., Moore, L.L., et al. (1997). A one year study of the macular pigment: the effect of 140 days of a lutein supplement. *Exp Eye Res,* Jul;65(1):57-62.

[38] Tong, N., Zhang, W., Zhang, Z., Gong, Y., Wooten, B., et al. (2013). Inverse relationship between macular pigment optical density and axial length in Chinese subjects with myopia. *Graefes Arch Clin Exp Ophthalmol,* Jun;251(6):1495-500.

[39] Williams, K.M., Bentham, G.C., Young, I.S., McGinty, A., McKay, G.J., et al. (2017). Association Between Myopia, Ultraviolet B Radiation Exposure, Serum Vitamin D Concentrations, and Genetic Polymorphisms in Vitamin D Metabolic Pathways in a Multicountry European Study. *JAMA Ophthalmol,* Jan 1;135(1):47-53.

[40] Ibid. Francisco (2015).

[41] Tanito, M., Obana, A., Gohto, Y., Okazaki, S., Gellermann, W., et al. (2012). Macular pigment density changes in Japanese individuals supplemented with lutein or zeaxanthin: quantification via resonance Raman spectrophotometry and autofluorescence imaging. *Jpn J Ophthalmol,* Sep;56(5):488-96.

[42] Ibid. Francisco (2015).

[43] Deng, H.W., Tian, Y., Zhou, X.J., Zhang, X.M., Meng, J. (2016). Effect of Bilberry Extract on Development of Form-Deprivation Myopia in the Guinea Pig. *J Ocul Pharmacol Ther,* May;32(4):196-202.

[44] Kamiya, K., Kobash, H, Fujiwara, K., Ando, W., Shimizu, K. (2013). Effect of fermented bilberry extracts on visual outcomes in eyes with myopia: a prospective, randomized, placebo-controlled study. *J Ocul Pharmacol Ther,* Apr;29(3):356-9.

[45] Querques, G., Forte, R., Souied, E.H. (2011). Retina and Omega-3. J Nutr Metab, 2011:748361.

[46] Yazar, S., Hewitt, A.W., Black, L.J., McKnight, C.M., Mountain, J.A., et al. (2014). Myopia is associated with lower vitamin D status in young adults. *Invest Ophthalmol Vis Sci,* Jun 26;55(7):4552-9.

[47] Guggenheim, J.A., Williams, C., Northstone, K., Howe, L.D., Tilling, K., et al. (2014). Does vitamin D mediate the protective effects of time outdoors on myopia? Findings from a prospective birth cohort. *Invest Ophthalmol Vis Sci,* Nov 18;55(12):8550-8.

[48] Piermarocchi, S., Saviano, S., Parisi, V., Tedeschi, M., Panozzo, G., et al. (2012). Carotenoids in Age-related Maculopathy Italian Study (CARMIS): two-year results of a randomized study. Eur J Ophthalmol, Mar-Apr;22(2):216-25.

[49] Ibid. Francisco (2015).

[50] Ibid. Cordain. (2002).

[51] Ibid. Jacobsen. (2008).

[52] Ibid. French. (2013).

14-1. BINOCULAR OVERVIEW

Binocular disorders are a group of conditions in which the two eyes have difficulty tracking in sync with each other. We humans have a wide angle of view; we have precise depth perception; and we are able to identify very faint objects. About 20% of the population has some form of binocular imbalance.[1] As many as 56% of those aged 18–38 have some form of binocular limitation,[2] which may be so mild that it is not apparent without testing. The causes range from insufficient development of the vision system in early childhood, to genetically-based nervous-system impairments, to injury, and even to aging.

Vision therapists define various eye movements and orientations systematically as follows:

- **Exophoria** is when the eyes tend to diverge away from the centerline of vision.
- **Esophoria** is when the eyes tend to converge toward the center axis of vision.
- **Convergence** means that the two eyes simultaneously look inward.
- **Accommodation** is the ability of the eye to focus, linked to convergence by a reflex.
- **Fusion** refers to the ability of the visual cortex to convert two images, one input from each eye, into one viewed image.

Binocular Vision Disorders

Amblyopia is the most common type of binocular disorder in which one eye takes in less information than the other.

Strabismus is another binocular disorder in which one eye is misaligned, relative to the other, in a variety of ways. Strabismus can cause amblyopia.[3] [4]

Convergence insufficiency occurs when the eyes have difficulty holding a point of convergence while doing close work. They tend to drift outwards resulting in blurred or double vision.[5]

Accommodative insufficiency simply means that the eye is unable to focus or maintain focus.

Accommodative infacility means that the eye has difficulty changing focus rapidly enough for comfortable functioning.

Fusional vergence dysfunction is the inability to efficiently utilize and/or sustain binocular vision. One diagnostic clue is that the patient will have difficulty using several types of vision therapy prisms. There are positive (convergence) and negative (divergence) types of this disorder.

Complementary Approach

Nutrients and diet can help support overall vision health, but they do not replace the need for vision therapy or recommended procedures.

Diet

Follow the Vision diet described in Chapter 7.

Juicing is a great way to add nutrients to your diet. Choose at least 4–6 items to combine and others that you might enjoy.

- Ginger, broccoli, cabbage, carrots, celery, leafy-green vegetables, and berries (preferably all organic)
- Do not use too many carrots, as they are high in natural sugars.

Lifestyle

Eye exercises. See Chapter 10 for eye exercises and acupuncture points that are good for all eye conditions and overall eye health. We recommend the following:

- Palming
- Hot dog
- Magic eye

Other Modalities

Chinese Medicine

In Traditional Chinese Medicine (TCM), amblyopia, strabismus, and convergence insufficiency may be related to Kidney yin deficiency and/or Kidney essence (jing).

Common Traditional Chinese Medicine Patterns

Kidney yin deficiency or Kidney jing deficiency. TCM treatment is to nourish the Liver and enrich the Kidneys to improve vision.

Ming mu di juang wan is a classic formula used in Chinese medicine for eye health that helps to nourish the Kidneys and Liver. It is known to help with blurriness of vision, tearing against wind, and conjunctive congestion with pain and swelling of eye.

---

[1] Wikipedia. Binocular Vision. Retrieved May 11 2018 from https://en.wikipedia.org/wiki/Binocular_vision.

[2] Montes-Mico, R. (2001). Prevalence of general dysfunctions in binocular vision. *A Opthalmol,* Sep;33(3):205-208.

[3] Stewart, C.E., Fielder, A.R., Stephens, D.A., Moseley, M.J. (2005). Treatment of unilateral amblyopia: factors influencing visual outcome. *Invest Ophthalmol Vis Sci,* Sep; 46(9):3152-60.

[4] Williams, C., Northstone, K., Harrad, R.A., Sparrow, J.M., Harvey, I. (2003). Amblyopia treatment outcomes after preschool screening v school entry screening: observational data from a prospective cohort study. *Br J Ophthalmol,* Aug; 87(8):988-93.

[5] Mayo Clinic. Convergence insufficiency. Retrieved May 11 2018 from https://www.mayoclinic.org/diseases-conditions/convergence-insufficiency/symptoms-causes/syc-20352735.

14-2. AMBLYOPIA

Amblyopia ("lazy eye") is the condition wherein the brain does not fully acknowledge the signals coming in from that eye, so it relies on the other eye, which becomes dominant. When looking at the non-dominant eye, it may look normal to the outside viewer. In some cases, that eye may be misaligned with the dominant eye such as turning inward (endotropia) or outward (esotropia).

Insufficient development of the vision system in early childhood is the cause of amblyopia; it is a significant cause of lifelong vision difficulty.[1] Strabismus is a common cause of amblyopia and can have important effects on social integration.[2][3] Amblyopia is considered to be a cause of blindness that is preventable through early treatment and other treatment options that have been evolving over the years.[4]

Amblyopia Begins in Early Childhood

Amblyopia usually begins in early childhood before the visual system has matured (ages eight to nine). In a study of young Baltimore children (30 months to 71 months) the prevalence of amblyopia was found to be a little less than 2%.[5] Amblyopia also occurs in adults; an Australian study found the condition in about 2.5% of the adult participants.[6] A German study found that 5.6% of adults suffer from the condition.[7]

In the first three years of life, the human eye increases two to three times in size. Eye movement in the newborn develops in steps (saccades) rather than smooth movements. Divergence and convergence movements are not reliable until about three months of age. The curvature of the lens is still nearly spherical, and focusing is limited to about 20 centimeters. At this age, the retina is not fully developed. The rods that perceive shades, peripheral, and night vision are almost as developed as those of adults, but the cones that perceive color and that are responsible for detailed vision are not nearly mature yet. In addition, the visual cortex, which interprets what we are seeing for us, is not mature at birth, though it develops quickly over the first six months of life.[8]

If light is blocked from reaching the retina (form-vision deprivation) as in a congenital cataract, or if there is a neurological dysfunction in the pathways to the retina and to the visual cortex, then the visual system cannot develop properly and amblyopia can result.

Types of Amblyopia

There are three main categories of amblyopia, which are based on the cause of the impairment. These are described as follows:

Strabismic. The brain's visual cortex mis-reads or ignores the sensory signal from the retina. In the case where the amblyopia is due to strabismus, then one will notice one of the child's eyes is misaligned with the other (one eye turns in) or both eyes turn inward (crossed eyes). When the two eyes are not able to align on a target, the child will initially experience double vision. Double vision is intolerable for the brain; one adaptation reduces the turned eye visual acuity so that the brain learns to ignore it.

Refractive is due to unequal focusing (refractive) errors that are significant enough to cause the eyes to not work together. This could include significant differences in near- or far-sightedness or astigmatism.

This inequality, due to discrepancies in image sizes being sent to the brain, makes it difficult for the visual cortex to sort and integrate the two received images. The amblyopic eye is never blind in the sense of being entirely without sight, and the patient typically retains peripheral vision in that eye; but, because the two images the brain "sees" are incompatible, the brain cannot easily blend them into one image (fusion).

When a child's brain cannot blend the images, the brain begins to ignore the blurry image. If this goes on for months or years in a young child, the vision in the eye that sees the blurry image will deteriorate.

Deprivative is due to mechanical obstruction of light, such as a congenital cataract.

Signs and Symptoms

Lazy eye usually does not cause any obvious symptoms. Parents can suspect vision problems in an older baby or toddler if a child squints, cocks her head at an angle to see something, or has obvious crossed eyes. But in the very young children, when one eye focuses more than another, and the brain learns to favor the stronger eye, initially these signs may not be noticeable.

For this reason, vision testing of very young children is recommended, since amblyopia may not be detected without an eye exam.

Amblyopia develops starting at birth and get worse until age 10, but mostly by age 5. Here are signs you might see along the way:[9]

- An eye that wanders toward, or away from, the nose, independently of the other eye, or eyes that don't work in sync with each other
- Poor depth perception, signaled by stumbling or the inability to keep balanced
- Squinting or shutting one eye, especially with double vision experienced
- Tilting of the head

Causes and Risk Factors

- Anisometropia (refractive error) causes 50% of amblyopia instances. Strabismus causes 25% of amblyopia cases. A combination of anisometropia and strabismus causes 16% of amblyopia. [10]
- Genetics may be a risk where lazy eye runs in the family, which may be due to a genetic propensity for cataracts, for significant differences in refraction, or for heredity-related reasons. Researchers are beginning to identify mutations in genes that are needed for

brain stream, ocular motor-neuron development, and connection capacity.[11]

- Premature birth[12] or birth with low body weight is a risk.
- Cataracts upon birth are the most common cause of deprivative amblyopia[13] and are relatively rare.[14]
- Ocular pathologies include the following:
  - o Posterior keratoconus (bulging cornea) is a potential cause.[15]
  - o Uveitis, such as pars plantis (a kind of chronic intermediate uveitis), increases the risk.[16]
  - o Loeys-Dietz syndrome (genetic) puts children at risk for amblyopia.[17]
  - o Duane syndrome is a strabismus syndrome.[18]
  - o Leber's is a genetically based retinal malfunction.[19]
  - o Saethre-Chotzen syndrome is premature fusion of a baby's head bones.[20]
  - o X-linked retinoschisis is a cause of macular degeneration in boys.[21]

Conventional Treatment

Glasses may improve visual acuity to some degree but usually not completely. With amblyopia, the brain is "used to" seeing a blurry image, and it needs to learn how to better see with the lazy eye. Over time the brain may learn to "see" again with the lazy eye.

When a patch is prescribed for the normal eye, it requires the lazy eye to do more work. The extent and duration of the patching depends on the age of the child, the severity of the lazy eye, and the response to treatment. Treatment time can take weeks to months before results are seen. If treatment starts before the age of 7 years old, most children will gain back vision in the lazy eye. Amblyopia becomes much more difficult to treat after about 7–9 years of age.

A 2003 NEI-funded study[22] found that patching the unaffected eye of children with moderate amblyopia for two hours daily works as well as patching for six hours daily. Shorter patching time can lead to better compliance with treatment and an improved quality of life for children with amblyopia. However, a recent study[23] found that with children whose amblyopia persists, despite two hours of daily patching, they might improve if daily patching is extended to 6 hours.

A nationwide clinical trial[24] showed that many children from ages 7 to 17 years benefited from treatment for amblyopia. This is in contrast to what was previously thought possible by professionals, confirming that age alone should not be used as a factor to decide whether or not to treat a child for amblyopia.

In the occasional case where patching cannot be done, a prescribed eyedrop called atropine can be prescribed that temporarily blurs vision in the dominant eye, so that the child will use the eye with amblyopia, especially when focusing on near objects.

Other methods or procedures may be recommended to correct a lazy eye, including eye muscle surgery, vision therapy, or prescription glasses. The surgery, however, only corrects the misalignment of the eye; vision therapy will still be needed afterwards to train the brain to learn to see through that eye again.

Psychological Aspects of Amblyopia

The loss of visual skills related to amblyopia is expanded and reinforced by a person's belief that they are unable to "trust" the information that is coming through the affected eye. When patients are placed in a position where they must use their amblyopic eye, they usually respond by insisting, "I just don't use that eye. It feels old and lazy." When they are shown that the eye has many more abilities than they might perceive, or were led to believe, a "miraculous" increase in vision occurs in that eye.

We see a clear relationship between the eyes and the mind when working with a patient with amblyopia. Getting them to develop trust that their eye is seeing, and breaking down the belief system that it can't see, are powerful tools to improving vision.

Complementary Approach

The complementary approach to all binocular vision problems is to make sure that the basic protocols of good vision are met: good nutrition through diet (also juicing and supplements if needed), drinking pure water, exercise, eye exercises, etc.

- Eye exercises
- Hot dog
- Magic eye

On the Horizon

Dichoptic treatment. By thinking about the development of amblyopia as primarily due to the loss of binocular vision, researchers are testing a way of artificially presenting different images to each eye. The adult patients are able to render the resulting image correctly. The more time spent successfully perceiving the correct image, the more binocular capacity is strengthened and the more the amblyopia resolved.[25]

Binocular zone. In the visual cortex, a region called the binocular zone normally receives input from both eyes, but if one eye is stronger, it takes over the binocular zone, blocking it from the other eye. Researchers have been able to manipulate a specific brain circuit in mice to prevent dominance.[26]

Video game. In a pilot study of children with amblyopia, a custom-made video game allowed children to play either monocularly with the strong eye patched or with both eyes but reduced contrast in the strong eye. Improvements resulted, and most were retained after treatment. [27]

Also See

Chapter 7, Vision Diet

Chapter 10-4, Eye Exercises

[1] Elflein, H.M., Fresenius, S., Lamparter, J., Pitz, S., Pfeiffer, N., et al. (2015). The Prevalence of Amblyopia in Germany. *Dtsch Arztebl Int,* May;112(19):338-344.

[2] Singh, A., Rana, V., Patyal, S., Kumar, S., Mishra, S.K., et al. (2017). To assess knowledge and attitude of parents toward children suffering from strabismus in Indian subcontinent. *Indian J Ophthalmol,* Jul;65(7):604-606.

[3] Jackson, S., Harrad, R.A., Morris, M., Rumsey, N. (2006). The psychosocial benefits of corrective surgery for adults with strabismus. *Br J Ophthalmol,* Jul; 90(7):883-8.

[4] Singh, A., Nagpal, R., Mittal, S.K., Bahuguna, C., Kumar, P. (2017). Pharmacological therapy for amblyopia. *Taiwan J Ophthalmol,* Apr-Jun;7(2):62-69.

[5] Friedman, D.S., Repka, M.X., Katz, J., Giordana, L., Ibrionke, J., et al. (2009). Prevalence of Amblyopia and Strabismus in White and African-American Children Aged 6 through 71 Months: The Baltimore Pediatric Eye Disease Study. *Opthalmology,* Nov;116(11):2128-34.e1-2.

[6] Attebo, K., Mitchell, P., Cumming, R., Smith, W., Jolly, N., et al. (1998). Prevalence and causes of amblyopia in an adult population. *Ophthalmology,* Jan;105(1):154-9.

[7] Ibid. Elflein. (2015).

[8] University of Calgary. Development of the Visual System. Retrieved May 8 2018 from http://www.ucalgary.ca/pip369/mod9/vision/system.

[9] Mayo Clinic. Lazy eye (amblyopia). Retrieved May 8 from https://www.mayoclinic.org/ diseases-conditions/lazy-eye/symptoms-causes/syc-20352391.

[10] Elflein, H.M. (2015). Amblyopia. Epidemiology, causes and risk factors. *Ophthalmologe,* Apr;113(4):283-8.

[11] Engle, E.C. (2006). The genetic basis of complex strabismus. *Pediatr Res,* Mar;59(3):343-8.

[12] Ibid. Elflein. (2016).

[13] Mansouri, B., Stacy, R.C., Kruger, J., Cestari, D.M. (2013). Deprivation amblyopia and congenital hereditary cataract. *Semin Ophthalmol,* Sept-Nov;28(5-6):321-6.

[14] Ibid. Elflein. (2016).

[15] Silas, M.R., Hilkert, S.M., Reidy, J.J., Farooq, A.V. (2017). Posterior keratoconus. *Br J Ophthalmol,* Nov.

[16] Ozdal, P.C., Berker, N., Tugal-Tutkun, I. (2015). Pars Planitis: Epidemiology, Clinical Characteristics, Management and Visual Prognosis. *J Ophthalmic Vis Res,* Oct-Dec;10(4):469-80.

[17] Ibid. Loeys. (2008).

[18] Andrews, C.V., Hunter, D.G., Engle, E.C. (2007). Duane Syndrome. *GeneReviews,* May 25 updated 2015.

[19] Weleber, R.G., Francis, P.J., Trzupek, K.M., Beattie, C. (2004). Leber Congenital Amaurosis. *GeneReviews.* Jul 7 updated 2013.

[20] Gallagher, E.R., Ratisoontorn, C., Cunningham, M.L. (2003). Sethre-Chotzen Syndrome. *GeneReviews,* May 16 updated 2012).

[21] Tantri, A., Vrbec, T.R., Cu-Unjieng, A., Frost, A., Annesley, W.H., et al. (2004). X-linked retinoschisis: a clinical and molecular genetic review. *Surv Ophthalmol,* Mar-Apr;49(2):214-30.

[22] National Eye Institute. (2003). Reduced Daily Eye Patching Effectively Treats Childhood's Most Common Eye Disorder. Retrieved May 1 2018 from https://nei.nih.gov/news/pressreleases/051203.

[23] National Eye Institute. (2013). Extended daily eye patching effective at treating stubborn amblyopia in children. Retrieved May 1 2018 from https://nei.nih.gov/news/briefs/eye_patching.

[24] National Eye Institute. (2005). Older Children Can Benefit From Treatment For Childhood's Most Common Eye Disorder. Retrieved May 1 from https://nei.nih.gov/news/pressreleases/041105.

[25] Hess, R.F. News Medical Life Sciences. (2018). New hope for adults with amblyopia (lazy eye). Retrieved May 8 2018 from https://www.news-medical.net/health/New-hope-for-adults-with-amblyopia.aspx.

[26] National Eye Institute. (2013). NIH-funded study could lead to new treatments for amblyopia. Retrieved May 8 2018 from https://nei.nih.gov/news/pressreleases/082613.

[27] Gambacorta, C., Nahum, M., Vedamurthy, I., Bayliss, J., Jordan, J., et al. (2018). An action video game for the treatment of amblyopia in children: A feasibility study. *Vision Res,* Apr 27.

14-3. CONVERGENCE INSUFFICIENCY

Convergence refers to the ability of the eyes to converge or to direct their independent gaze on a single object. Depending on how close the subject is from the two eyes, each eye must be able to turn inward for both to look directly at the same point. For example, if a finger is held up a few inches in front of the nose, both eyes need to be able to turn sharply inward in order to see the finger.

There are no obvious visual signs that someone has convergence insufficiency; both eyes appear correctly aligned. But because in-school vision exams test only far vision, a child with 20/20 vision insufficiency is not identified. For that reason, teachers have sometimes thought that such instances where a child has trouble reading are the result of dyslexia or learning- or reading disabilities.

Estimates of prevalence vary greatly, from 2.25% to 13%, and there is little information about contributing factors such as age, race, gender, or ethnicity.[1] [2]

What is Convergence Insufficiency?

If the eyes can't maintain this inward gaze toward a finger, then convergence insufficiency (CI) is experienced. When the eyes either cannot focus on a near point, or they have difficulty holding their point of convergence when doing close work, their eyes tend to drift outwards. The result is blurred or double vision for near vision.[3]

At near point viewing, people with convergence insufficiency experience continued or intermittent exophoria, in which the eyes tend to diverge away from the centerline of vision. The point at which the two eyes can focus on a near object is further away than the norm. People with convergence insufficiency may also have difficulty changing or maintaining focus (accommodative insuffiency), or difficulty changing focus rapidly (accommodative infacility). They may also experience fusional-vergence dysfunction, in which they are unable to efficiently utilize the information that their eyes take in.

Symptoms

A number of symptoms are common in both children and adults.[4]

- Asthenopia, vision eyestrain (often accompanies CI in both adults and children)
- Blurred near vision
- Difficulty with reading and close-up work
- Headache while/after reading or doing close work

Causes

The cause is unknown but manifests as a misalignment of the muscles controlling eye movement while focusing on something nearby.[5]

But scientists have identified causes of the resulting eye fatigue:[6]

- The need for continual balance between convergence and accommodation (a reflex of convergence) for near work
- Keeping that balance stable
- Converting the viewed two images into one clear image with increasing difficulty

Conventional Treatment

Most doctors use a number of treatments. Researchers investigated which were the most commonly prescribed. Optometrists and ophthalmologists who responded to a survey, recommended pencil push-up therapy (38–50%), home-based vision therapy (22–21%), and office-based vision therapy (16%); none recommended base-in prism.[7]

A 2008 study funded by the National Eye Institute found that 75% of patients who received therapy in an office setting by a trained therapist, in addition to treatment at home, had the best results. They compared pencil push-up therapy, plus computer vision therapy, and in-office therapy combined with "at home" work. These three therapies, including the placebo therapy, resulted in only 33% to 35% improvement. Interestingly, the placebo therapy was better than pencil push-ups.[8] A 2012 follow-up study confirmed these results.[9]

Surgery is rarely recommended, and then, only for instances where the inability to converge is severe, or where additional refractive problems make vision therapy ineffective.[10]

Vision Therapy

There are several options in vision therapy:[11]

Prism reading glasses. There are various types of prism reading glasses used at home, but they have been found to be no more effective than regular reading glasses.

- Base-in glasses are made with the part of the lens toward the nose thicker, to assist with vision as the eyes converge.[12]
- Base-in glasses plus a progressive-addition lens-design feature, a gradient of increasing lens power, was found to be better than plain base-in glasses.

Home-based exercises. The most common exercise prescribed for at-home use is pencil push-ups.

Home-based therapies. There are therapies that can be performed at home that are more effective than pencil push-ups, including prism glasses, stereoscopes, and computer software programs.

Outpatient vision therapy includes activities prescribed and monitored by a professional vision therapist.[13]

With children, outpatient vision therapy/orthoptics is more effective than exercise (usually pencil push-ups) and/or computer vision therapy at home.[14] With adults, the differences between various therapies are less consistent than with children.[15]

Complementary Approach

Lifestyle factors and diet to support overall vision health are important baseline practices for people with convergence issues. See Chapter 14-1 for an overview of relevant practices. General nutrient support is also helpful.

- Eye exercises
- Hot dog
- Magic eye

On the Horizon

There have been experimental studies evaluating the physiological effects of vision therapy and how brain activity changes. The Oct-Dec, 2016 issue of the *Journal of Optometry* targets new advances in treatments.[16]

Also See

Chapter 10-4, Eye Exercises

Chapter 14-1, Binocular Overview

[1] Scheiman, Mitchell, Gwiazda, J., Li, T. (2014). Non-surgical interventions for convergence insufficiency. *Cochrane Database Syst Rev*, Mar 16;(3):CD006768.

[2] Rouse, M.W., Borsting, E., Hyman, L., Hussein, M., Cotter, S.A., et al. (1999). Frequency of convergence insufficiency among fifth and sixth graders. The Convergence Insufficiency and Reading Study (CIRS) group. *Optom Vis Sci*, Sep;76(9):643-9.

[3] Mayo Clinic. Convergence insufficiency. Retrieved May 11 2018 from https://www.mayoclinic.org/diseases-conditions/convergence-insufficiency/symptoms-causes/syc-20352735.

[4] Westman, M., Liinamaa, M.J. (2012). Relief of asthenopic symptoms with orthoptic exercises in convergence insufficiency is achieved in both adults and children. *J Optom, Apr-Jun;5(2):62-67.*

[5] Mayo Clinic. Convergence Insufficiency. Retrieved May 22 2018 from https://www.mayoclinic.org/diseases-conditions/convergence-insufficiency/symptoms-causes/syc-20352735.

[6] Optometry Students. The Ultimate Guide to Convergence Insufficiency. Retrieved May 22 from http://www.optometrystudents.com/convergence-insufficiency-the-ultimate-guide/.

[7] Ibid. Scheiman. (2014).

[8] National Eye Institute. (2008). More Effective Treatment Identified for Common Childhood Vision Disorder. Retrieved May 22 2018 from https://nei.nih.gov/news/pressreleases/101308.

[9] Ibid. Westman (2012).

[10] Wang, B., Wang, L., Wang, Q., Ren, M. (2014). Comparison of different surgery procedures for convergence insufficiency-type intermittent exotropia in children. *Br J Ophthalmol,* Oct;98(10:1409-13.

[11] Ibid. Scheiman. (2014).

[12] Frames Direct. Understanding Your Glasses Prescription: What the Number Mean. Retrieved May 22 from https://www.framesdirect.com/knowledge-center/understanding-your-prescription.html.

[13] Ciuffreda, K.J. (2002). The scientific basis for and efficacy of optometric vision therapy in nonstrabismic accommodative and vergence disorders. *Optommetry,* Dec;73(12):735-62.

[14] Scheiman, M., Mitchell, G.L., Cotter, S., Cooper, J., Kulp, M., et al. (2005). A randomized clinical trial of treatments for convergence insufficiency in children. *Arch Ophthalmol,* Jan;123(1):14-24.

[15] Ibid. Scheiman. (2014).

[16] Pinero, D.P. (2016). Science-based vision therapy. *J Optom,* Oct-Dec;9(4):203-204.

14-4. STRABISMUS

Strabismus is commonly identified as being crossed-eyed, wall-eyed, or having a wandering eye. One or both of the eyes may turn out (esophoria), in (exophoria), up (hypophoria), or down (hyperphoria), or in rare cases, one eye may rotate (cyclophoria). Damage to the third, fourth, or sixth cranial nerve, due to nerve pressure, head injuries, or poor blood supply can cause strabismus.

Types of Strabismus

Strabismus can be categorized in a number of ways. These include:

Direction of misalignment. This is the most common categorization, involving:

- exophoria (outward divergence),
- esophoria (inward convergence),
- hypophoria (one eye deviates downward),
- hyperphoria (one eye deviates upward), and
- cyclophoria (the vertical axis of one eye rotates right or left compared to the other).

Duration. Strabismus can manifest in a continual or intermittent manner, sometimes it occurs during stressful situations. Doctors recommend that continual/constant strabismus be treated immediately and aggressively.

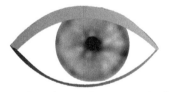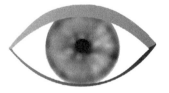

Strabismus due to esophoria

Paralytic or non-paralytic. Damage to one of three of the twelve cranial nerves versus a structural problem is another way of describing the condition.

Comitant versus noncomitant. In patients with comitant strabismus the eye misalignment exists regardless of the direction of their gaze. In noncomitant strabismus, the deviation shifts, depending on the direction of gaze.[1]

Signs and Symptoms

Esotropia

- **Suppression**. The brain blocks all or part of an image.
- **Eyestrain**.
- **Depth perception** problems.
- **Slight head tilt** to right or left, or chin rotated up or downward. Some of these tilts are symptoms of nystagmus, in which the eyes make repeating and uncontrolled movements.[2]

Exotropia

- **Double vision**.
- **Suppression**.
- **Adaptions**. People with intermittent exotropia often develop adaptations that allow them to suppress or ignore the image from the wandering eye and therefore they will not notice the double vision. During the time the eyes are straight, the suppression is absent and both eyes see normally as a team. If the eye-turn is constant, a lazy eye may develop.
- **Light sensitivity.** This is also a common complaint.

Strabismus Causes

Genetic. Researchers have learned that patients' muscles are lacking in certain proteins. Genetic expression of collagens and the enzymes that regulate collagen formation are not sufficiently supported, and genetic expression of collagen-inhibiting enzymes is supported genetically in excess.[3] They have also identified genes with alterations that are implicated.[4]

Nerve disturbances. Strabismus is most often caused by weakness or dysfunction of one or more of the three cranial nerves that regulate eye movement. The cause of infantile strabismus usually comes from the cerebral cortex.[5] Disturbances in the neural-control centers may occur with high fevers and childhood illnesses or for other reasons. This may be why studies show a link between the strabismus onset and delay in a child's learning to sit, walk, talk, and control elimination.

Skill delays. Seemingly, the mind pays more attention to the workings of the visual system between four months and six years (especially until three and a half years). Later, the mind is more involved in other learning skills. Delayed neural growth or nerve protective covering, may put binocular skills out of sync with attention necessary to convert eye coordination skills into conditioned habit patterns. Visual habits are more vulnerable if not firmly fixed. Neurological problems such as cerebral palsy, Down syndrome, hydrocephalus, or brain tumors can cause strabismus.[6]

Trauma. Damage to the visual cortex of the brain, which impacts eye muscle control, can cause strabismus.

Vascular. In adults, strokes or vascular problems can cause strabismus through inadequate blood supply.[7] Microvascular disease is the most common cause of cranial nerve palsy.[8]

Thyroid. In adults, Graves disease and other thyroid disorders can impact eye muscle behavior.[9]

Premature birth. This and low birth weight are linked to the incidence of strabismus.[10]

Myopia. Strabismus has been noted in young adults with myopia, and it may be related to close work for long periods.[11]

Orbital. If there are abnormalities in orbital (eye socket) bones, or masses such as tumors within the orbit, strabismus may indirectly result.[12] In addition, orbital connective tissue links to the muscles that move the eye. Abnormalities in these tissues can cause strabismus in the absence of a neurologic problem.[13]

Eye surgery. Vitreoretinal surgery is a significant cause of strabismus.[14] Refractive surgery is generally effective for exotropia that is related to refractive error. However, patients without apparent strabismus can develop strabismus and/or double vision after surgery.[15] Similarly, surgery to implant an intraocular lens can result in strabismus.[16]

Ocular and related pathologies.

- Duane syndrome is a rare cause of strabismus.[17]
- Sagging eye syndrome, a connective tissue condition, can cause vertical or horizontal strabismus.[18] [19]
- Loeys-Dietz syndrome (genetic) puts children at risk for strabismus.[20]

Conventional Treatment

For esotropia or exotropia, depending on the type and severity, treatment may include surgery, glasses, and/or visual training. Surgery doesn't change the vision, but aligns the eyes by changing the length or position of one or more eye muscles outside the eye. Sometimes botox is used in the stronger muscle and is repeated 3–4 months later. In children, esotropia strabismus is most commonly treated with glasses, but exotropia may require surgical correction.[21] Surgery techniques, such as adjustable sutures,[22] are evolving.

Complementary Approach

Supporting overall vision health through diet, nutrition, exercise, lifestyle, etc. are the basic foundation for the complementary approach to strabismus.

- Eye exercises
- Hot dog
- Magic eye

On the Horizon

Improved methods of imaging and improved understanding of genetics are supporting a number of advances in surgical correction of strabismus. Anterior-chamber optical-coherence tomography and ultrasonic biomicroscopy help detect muscle locations and changes from previous surgery. Also, MRI and diffusion-tensor imaging help evaluate activities in different parts of the brain (brain cluster activation).[23]

Also See

Chapter 7, Vision Diet

Chapter 8, Nutrients

Chapter 10-4, Eye Exercises

Chapter 14-1, Binocular Overview

---

[1] Wikipedia. Strabismus. Retrieved May 11 2018 from https://en.wikipedia.org/wiki/Strabismus.

[2] Teodorescu, L., (2015). Anomalous Head Postures in Strabismus and Nystagmus Diagnosis and Management. *Rom J Ophthalmol,* Jul-Sep;59(3):137-40.

[3] Agarwal, A.B., Feng, C.Y., Altick, A.L., Quilici, D.R., Wen, D., et al. (2016). Altered Protein Composition and Gene Expression in Strabismic Human Extraocular Muscles and Tendons. *Invest Ophthalmol Vis Sci,* Oct 1;57(13):5576-5585.

[4] Kruger, J.M., Mansouri, B., Cestari, D.M. (2013). An update on the genetics of comitant strabismus. *Semin Ophthalmol,* Sep-Nov;28(5-6):438-41.

[5] Tychsen, L. (2012). The cause of infantile strabismus lies upstairs in the cerebral cortex, not downstairs in the brainstem. *Arch Ophthalmol,* Aug;130(8):1060-1.

[6] Ibid. American Association for Pediatric Ophthalmology and Strabismus. Strabismus.

[7] American Association for Pediatric Ophthalmology and Strabismus. Strabismus. Retrieved May 11 2018 from https://www.aapos.org/terms/conditions/100.

[8] Gunton, K.B., Wasserman, B.N., DeBeneditis, C. (2015). Strabismus. *Prim Care,* Sep;42(3):393-407.

[9] Ibid. American Association for Pediatric Ophthalmology and Strabismus. Strabismus.

[10] Gulati, S., Andrews, C.A., Apkarian, A.O., Musch, D.C., Lee, P.P., et al. (2014). Effect of gestational age and birth weight on the risk of strabismus among premature infants. *JAMA Pediatr,* Sep;168(9):850-6.

[11] Zheng, K., Han, T., Han, Y., Qu, X. (2018). Acquired distance esotropia associated with myopia in the young adult. *BMC Ophthalmol,* Feb 20;18(1):51.

[12] Lueder, G.T. (2015). Orbital Causes of Incomitant Strabismus. *Middle East Afr J Ophthalmol,* Jul-Sep;22(3):286-91.

[13] Peragallo, J.H., Pinesles, S.L., Demer, J.L. (2015). Recent advanced clarifying the etiologies of strabismus. *J Neurophthalmol,* Jun;36(2):185-93.

[14] Chaudhry, N.L., Durnian, J.M. (2012). Post-vitreoretinal surgery strabismus-a review. *Strabismus,* Mar;20(1):26-30.

[15] Minnal, V.R., Rosenberg, J.B. (2011). Refractive surgery: a treatment for and a cause of strabismus. *Curr Opin Ophthalmol,* Jul;22(4):222-6.

[16] Park, K.S., Yim, J.H. (2014). Strabismus following implantable anterior intraocular lens surgery. *Int Ophthalmol,* Feb;34(1):117-20.

[17] Kakhandaki, A., Nt, M., Pramila, S. (2014). Duane retraction syndrome: a rare cause of strabismus. *Natl Med J India,* Jan-Feb;27(1):15-6.

[18] Chaudhuri, Z., Demer, J.L. (2013). Sagging eye syndrome: connective tissue involution as a cause of horizontal and vertical strabismus in older patients. *JAMA Ophthalmol,* May;131(5):619-25.

[19] Chaudhuri, Z., Demer, J.L. (2018). Long-term Surgical Outcomes in the Sagging Eye Syndrome. *Strabismus,* Mar;26(1):6-10.

[20] Loeys, B.L., Dietz, H.C. (2008). Loeys-Dietz Syndrome. *GeneReviews.* Feb 28 updated 2018.

[21] Ibid. Gunton. (2015).

[22] Kassem, A., Xue, G., Gandhi, N.B., Tian, J., Guyton, D.L. (2018). Adjustable suture strabismus surgery in infants and children: a 19-year experience. *J AAPOS,* April 21. pii:S1091-8531(17)30431-7.

[23] Sharma, Pradeep, Guar, N., Phujhele, S., Saxena, R. (2017). What's new for us in strabismus? *Indian J Ophthalmol,* May 11;(65):184-90.

15-1. CATARACTS

What are Cataracts?

A cataract can be described simply as an opaque spot on the lens of the eye through which you cannot see. The lens becomes clouded. The degree of opacity depends on how developed the cataract is. At best, you seem to be looking through a cloud or a haze. As this haze can vary in size, density, and location, its effect on vision will vary.

Many people experience a general reduction in vision at first; they need more light to read by, or they have difficulty with street signs when driving. A cataract also can affect depth perception. This is a particular danger to older people at greatest risk for injury from falls and accidents.

Types and Prevalence

Age of Onset

Cataracts are defined less by the age of onset than by the size and location. The age of onset does not determine the cause. Anyone with a genetic marker for cataracts could be more vulnerable to damage due to environmental toxins.[1]

Congenital or **infantile cataract** is visible within the first year of life. Congenital cataracts may be hereditary or secondary to a toxic event while in utero, such as rubella.

Juvenile cataract occurs within the first decade of life. It is also defined as occurring within the first 20 years. Cataracts associated with a systemic or genetic disease such as retinitis pigmentosa, for example, may not present until a person is in their 20s or 30s. Patients with retinitis pigmentosa often develop a type of cataract called a "subcapsular cataract."

Pre-senile cataract occurs before age 45.

Senile or age-related cataract occurs after age 45. Age-related cataracts are generally attributed to multiple environmental insults accumulated over a number of years, including ongoing exposure to sunlight, oxidation in the lens, as well as poor circulation and delivery of essential nutrients to the eyes.

Cataracts in Adults

Cataracts tend to worsen over time and are the major cause of blindness. Almost 40 million people in the U.S. alone, suffer from cataracts. Only 10% of people are affected with cataracts by age 55, but the figure jumps to 50% by age 75, and 70% by age 80+.[2] Cataract removal is the most common surgical procedure covered by Medicare with almost 3,000,000 surgeries performed per year.

Cataracts in Children

Approximately three of every 10,000 children develop cataracts; this is often due to abnormal lens development during the mother's pregnancy. The child may be born with the cataract (congenital) or develop it during childhood. Congenital cataracts can range in degree of severity, resulting in different levels of impact on vision. This type of cataract is responsible for nearly 10% of all vision loss in children worldwide, and it is easily treatable through conventional medicine. However, if the cataract is small and/or off center, it may not have to be removed.

Genetics and Cataracts

Genetics may play a role in cataract development at any stage. According to researchers, there are two mutations in what is termed the heat shock transcription factor gene (HSF4) that have been reported to be associated with hereditary cataracts (HC) in several people. Hereditary cataracts are estimated to account for 8.3–25% of congenital cataracts, and they may be a part of a multisystem genetic disorder.[3][4][5]

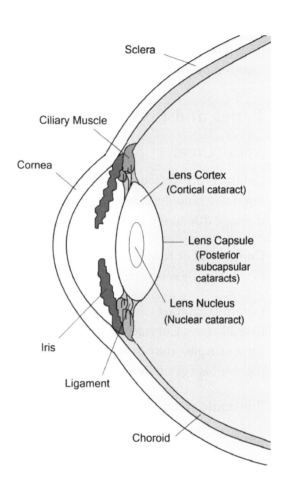

Location of Onset

Nuclear cataracts are those found in the central part of the eye lens. Due to the location of the cataract, these tend to impact vision to a greater degree than those located elsewhere on the eye lens, even in early stages of development.

Cortical cataracts are found on the outside part of the eye lens and are commonly found in people with diabetes. Given the location of this type of cataract, these may have little effect on vision, particularly in the early stage of development, but they can develop quickly in diabetics.

Posterior subcapsular cataracts appear on the back part of the eye lens. Symptoms can include sensitivity to bright light, seeing of halos, and/or difficulty in distance vision.

Secondary cataracts are not technically cataracts; however, they are called this in mainstream medicine. Secondary cataracts occur when old cells of the original lens remain in the eye and collect on the new artificial lens. They may occur in up to 50% of post-cataract surgery patients, and they can result in symptoms similar to the original cataract condition. Doctors use a YAG laser treatment to "burn" off the excess cells from the new lens. This procedure is typically fast, painless, and very effective, and usually done in the eye doctor's office. Immunological and gene therapy approaches to prevent this complication are under development and appear promising.

About the Lens

The healthy eye lens is completely transparent, allowing the maximum amount of light to reach the retina. The lens is comprised of water and a highly concentrated mix of several proteins, including protective proteins that prevent the lens proteins from aggregating and clumping. A cataract results when the proteins start to clump up, clouding the lens, and reducing the amount of light that can pass through. If not treated, the color of the lens starts to change from being clear to yellowish and eventually brownish.

The lens has a microcirculation system which operates in lieu of blood vessels. It has been proposed that this system is a flow of ions that generates a flow of water through the lens. An extracellular flow of water moves nutrients into the lens; an intracellular flow of water removes wastes from the lens.[6]

Signs and Symptoms

Early Stages

Vision blurriness and sensitivity to glare, particularly at night, and/or seeing halos are signs of early stage cataract development. These symptoms can vary depending on the location of the cataract on the eye lens. For example, a cataract located in the center of the eye lens will affect vision more than when located on the outside of the eye lens.

Moderate Stages

At this stage, the eye doctor will usually recommend surgery, particularly if vision cannot be improved better than 20/40 with eyeglasses, due to the cataract. The location of the cataract on the lens also determines whether surgery is recommended at that time. For example, one may have a moderate cataract located on the outside of the lens with little impact on vision, while another's cataract may be small but located directly in the center of the lens causing a more significant effect on vision. Symptoms again, include blurriness of vision, sensitivity to glare (particularly at night), and possibly less color clarity. Double vision, or seeing multiple images, is another common symptom at this stage.

Late Stages

As cataracts get harder and stiffer, they are more difficult to remove. They can also liquefy, and if not removed, can cause substantial inflammation, pain, and possibly infection. At this stage, people often can see shapes, but not detail. While an advanced cataract raises the risk of complications from surgery, unless there is a medical reason to avoid it, surgery should be performed. This is a crucial point in the development of cataracts, and if left unaddressed, further complications could result.

Causes and Risk Factors

Conventional perspective

Here are a few specific known causes of cataracts that most doctors acknowledge:

- Smoking
- Increase in age
- Excessive use of alcohol
- Obesity
- Genetics
- High blood pressure
- Use of pharmaceutical drugs, long term use of steroids
- Diabetes, persistent blood sugar imbalances, even if not diagnosed as diabetes
- Long term exposure to sunlight
- Physical trauma, such as getting hit in the eye with a ball
- Exposure to chemicals

Cell Phone Radiation

Less known to most doctors, but theorized by some researchers is that radiation from cell phones can lead to early cataracts (in addition to causing other ocular problems).[7]

Conventional Treatment

Cataract surgery is performed when the cataract is considered "ripe enough." Typically, eye doctors begin to recommend surgery if one's vision cannot be refracted to 20/40 or better, due to the cataracts. Of all the eye diseases, cataracts are the most amenable to treatment with conventional medical methods. The standard treatment is an outpatient procedure to remove the lens using a technique called phacoemulsification. A surgeon uses an ultrasonic beam to break up the hardened lens, and then vacuums up the pieces from the eye with a suction device. An artificial lens, called an intraocular lens or IOL, is inserted to replace the cataract lens.

Patients who may not be considered good candidates for cataract surgery include those with a history of heart conditions, retinal bleeding, or other health issues considered risky for surgery.

After Surgery

Vision improvement may be noticed immediately after surgery, but there can be initial blurriness due to inflammation, so that improvement is typically noticed within 2–3 days. One may feel itchiness and discomfort for a few days, which should disappear with the antibiotic and anti-inflammatory eye drops prescribed by the eye doctor. An eye patch can help temporarily protect the eye. Complete healing usually occurs within eight weeks after surgery.

Your eye doctor will recommend avoiding physical movements and activities for the first week after surgery. These include bending from the waist, lifting objects weighing more than 10 pounds, straining while on the toilet, or causing any activities that increase pressure in the eyes such as holding one's breath.

Risks After Surgery

Although cataract surgery is typically very successful, it can cause trauma to the eye for a small percentage of people. Such trauma can include choroidal hemorrhage, macula edema, retina tears/detachment, vitreous tears/detachment, flashes, and eye floaters.[8] [9]

Overall, up to 20% of all cataract procedures are for diabetic patients.[10] High levels of sugar in the blood contribute to cataract formation; diabetics are 2–5 times at risk for getting cataracts.[11] [12] [13] Blood sugar interferes with the lens's ability to pump out excess fluid from the eye and maintain its clarity. With too much dietary intake of sugar, this function can become difficult or impossible. Diabetics with severe non-proliferative and proliferative diabetic retinopathy have a higher risk of progressive disease after surgery.[14]

Intraocular Lens Choices

The upside of cataract surgery is potentially huge: a dramatic improvement in vision, and the prevention of further loss of vision. In contrast, the risk of the surgery and complications of surgery are quite low for the healthy population. An intraocular lens is an artificial lens implanted inside the eye to replace the natural lens which has been removed during cataract surgery. The following are various optional IOL choices:

Basic Monofocal Lens. This type of lens is intended to give the recipient 20/20 vision at a specific distance, either close-range or distance. Eye glasses will then be needed for other distances not corrected. Patients decide, with their eye doctor, which will work best for them. If you have a significant astigmatism, you will still need eye glasses for distance viewing.

Multifocal Lenses. Multifocal lenses typically make the patient less dependent on glasses after cataract surgery, as they compensate for near, mid, and far distances. These lenses use a ring design that may cause mild glare for the first month or two after surgery; there may also be less contrast during the day. Common lenses used are RaZoom (best for distance and intermediate vision), Tecnis Multifocal (best for distance and near vision), or ReSTOR lenses (best for distance and near vision).

Crystalens. This is the only intraocular lens approved by the FDA and designed to focus naturally, providing undistorted vision, excellent contrast, and clarification of color and details. These lenses tend to work best for distance and intermediate distances.

The Toric Lens. This lens is often used for cataract patients who also need correction for astigmatism. With Toric lenses, most patients will not need to use eyeglasses for distance vision.

Complementary Approach

Though most conventional physicians attribute cataracts to general aging, we believe that a cataract is often a symptom of an underlying condition due to a metabolic imbalance. It signals that the natural processes of your body are breaking down on some level, and that the normal flow of nutrients into the eyes, and waste products out of the eyes, has been compromised.

While we do recommend cataract surgery for those with moderate to severe vision loss, we prefer to use complementary therapies, including nutritional intervention, where surgery is not considered essential. Through these and other complementary medical treatments, it is possible to slow and even reverse the growth of cataracts.

Even people preparing for cataract surgery should seek to improve their overall health before they go through this invasive procedure, as this will aid in healing times and help protect the retina. Because cataracts typically progress slowly over many years there is often time for preventive measures to work quite successfully.

Nutrients

Essential

Combinations. Studies have also shown that rather than looking at vitamins and nutrients in isolation, combinations tend to decrease cataract risk significantly. For example, a combination of antioxidant group carotenes, vitamins A and C, and an omega-3 group were more effective than those nutrients in isolation.[15] Another study showed a combination of vitamins B1, B2, B3, C, E, and carotene in the diet significantly lessened the risk of all cataract types.[16]

Vitamin C (buffered and ascorbated). 2,000mg per day, split up and taken with meals. The normal healthy lens of the eye contains a higher level of vitamin C than any other organ of the body, except the adrenals. When cataracts are forming there is a decreased level of vitamin C in the aqueous humor as well as in the overall body. Vitamin C has been shown to control sugar imbalances that often play a role in cataract formation.

Source. Good sources are citrus fruits, red peppers, and tomatoes.[17] [18] [19] [20]

Note. When supplementing with vitamin C, for better absorption make sure the formula you take is ascorbated and buffered (to slow the breakdown of vitamin C and extend absorption time in the body) with nutrients such as bioflavonoids, rutin, rosehips, calcium, magnesium, and/or potassium. Plain ascorbic acid flushes out of the body quickly.

Glutathione. 500mg–900mg, if taken in capsule or pill form. The sublingual form has 5–10 times greater absorption so the dosage will be smaller. Follow label instructions. Referred to as the anti-aging antioxidant, glutathione is considered the most important antioxidant made by the body. It is very effective in preventing cataract formation and is crucial in possibly altering free radical damage. Some studies have shown that many lenses with cataracts contain approximately one fifth of the amount of glutathione as compared to normal lenses. Glutathione levels are significantly lower in lenses with cataracts compared to healthy lenses. Glutathione levels are even lower in nuclear cataract lenses compared to cortical cataract lenses.[21] [22]

The rate of childhood cataract, with no known cause, is highest in developing countries where birth weight is low. There is a link between childhood cataract and glutathione depletion in maternal malnutrition.[23]

Source. Food sources that help boost glutathione naturally include milk thistle extract, whey protein, and foods high in sulfur such as arugula, avocado, bok choy, Brazil nuts, broccoli, Brussels sprouts, cabbage, cauliflower, collard greens, dried apricots, eggs, garlic, kale, mustard greens, onions, radishes, roasted peanuts, turnips, and watercress.

The Perfect Pair: Glutathione and Vitamin C

The importance of vitamin C to eye health cannot be understated; concentrations of vitamin C in the lens are 20–30 times higher than those in the plasma.[24] Vitamin C doesn't work alone: it needs glutathione to improve the use of ascorbic acid (the purist form of vitamin C) in the body. Glutathione and vitamin C are thought to work together to promote proper water balance within the lens and prevent the protein clumping that can lead to cataracts.

Very Important

Lutein. 6mg–20mg per day. This powerful antioxidant is found both in the lens of the eye and retina, and it helps protect the eyes from damage due to sunlight exposure by filtering out light.[25] [26] [27] [28] [29]

Zeaxanthin. 2mg–12mg per day. This powerful antioxidant is found in the lens of the eye and the retina, which helps protect the eyes from damage due to sunlight exposure by filtering out light.[30] [31] [32] [33] Zeaxanthin reduces the risk of age-related cataract, especially nuclear cataract.[34] [35]

Alpha-lipoic acid. 120mg–300mg per day. Alpha-lipoic acid has been found to halt complications resulting from blood sugar imbalances and hardening of the lens. Oxidative damage results in cataract formation, and increasing antioxidants, particularly alpha-lipoic acid, can help prevent or stop cataract formation.[36] [37] [38]

Important

An optimal potency **multivitamin** is an important foundation of any cataract prevention program. It should include flavonoids and carotenoids. Scientists found that the risk of cataract formation decreased in the regular users of multivitamin supplements (one-third risk decrease).

Flavonoids. 1,000mg per day. Quercetin and rutin are important antioxidants that are synergistic with vitamin C, meaning they need each other to work efficiently. Of the two, quercetin seems to be one of the most effective flavonoids in the prevention of cataracts.[39] [40]

Carotenoids. These are high in potent antioxidants that support healthy vision and overall health. There are two categories of carotenoids: carotenes and xanthophylls. Read about their role, sources, and research in The Role of Antioxidants, Chapter 5.

Helpful

Green tea extract. 500mg–725mg per day. High in antioxidants, this supplement helps protect the eyes against oxidative damage.[41]

Selenium. 200mcg per day. Patients with senile cataracts were found to have significantly lower blood- and intraocular levels of the mineral selenium than controls.[42]

N-acetyl-carnosine. 500mg per day. Statistical analysis revealed the significant differences over 6 and 24 months in cumulative positive changes of overall characteristics of cataracts in a group taking NAC.[43]

Bilberry, 180mg–240mg per day, *taken along with* **vitamin E**, 400 IU per day. Some studies suggest that bilberry may slow cataract formation. Bilberry combined with vitamin E stopped cataract formation in 48 of 50 patients with senile cortical cataracts.[44] In an animal model supplementation with bilberry extract helped to protect DNA and improve enzyme activity in lens tissue.[45]

Resveratrol. 250mg per day. Resveratrol activates an enzyme called sirtuin type 1 (SIRT1), which protects against oxidative stress in human lens epithelial cells.[46] This enzyme inhibits oxidation in the eye's lens and protects against cataract development.

Melatonin. 1mg–3mg before bedtime. Melatonin can help increase levels of reduced glutathione in the body.[47]

Milk thistle. Suggested dosage 480mg–960mg per day. Milk thistle contains silymarin (its main ingredient), which possesses both anti-inflammatory and antioxidant properties. Because of this, milk thistle may help boost glutathione by preventing glutathione depletion in the liver and helping to cleanse the liver, which is essential for lens health.

Vitamin E. Suggested dosage 400 IU per day. In percentages that were statistically significant, studies have found that high levels of dietary vitamin E, supplemental vitamin E, and high levels of vitamin E in the bloodstream are all tied to a lower risk of cataract. As the levels of vitamin E dropped, the incidence of cataract increased.[48] [49] [50] [51] [52] [53]

Saffron. An interesting and related study found that crocin, a saffron apocarotenoid, was helpful in reducing diabetic cataracts.[54]

Diet

We recommend the Vision diet in Chapter 7.

There is a strong correlation between the risk of cataract onset and the patient's diet. Subjects who ate the most meat had the highest rate of cataracts, and those who ate fish but not meat had a lower rate. Vegetarians had a lower rate and vegans had the lowest rate of cataract incidence.[55] Whenever possible, a nutritional program should be maintained for at least three to four months to help with quicker recovery and retinal support, before considering cataract surgery.

Juicing. Juicing is a great way to deliver nutrients to the body. Our juicing recipe for cataracts is some combination of the following. You can add your favorite fruits and vegetables.

- Fresh apple, endive, carrots, celery, parsley, blueberry, and fresh leafy-green vegetables.
- Not too many carrots because of their high natural sugar content.

This combination helps warm and detoxify the body and provide great nutrients for nourishing the eyes.

Very Important

Reduce or eliminate all types of refined sugars (particularly white sugar, but also fructose, sucrose, fruit juice concentrates, maltose, dextrose, glucose, and refined carbohydrates). This includes "natural" drinks that contain a lot of sugar, including all fruit juices. Those people who are lactose intolerant are at higher risk for cataracts.[56]

Drink eight glasses of water per day (preferably filtered or purified). This is optimally taken as a four-ounce glass of water every half-hour, to equal 16 four-ounce glasses.

Our bloodstream can only effectively handle about four ounces at any one time. When you drink more at a time, this means more work for the kidneys to filter water that hasn't had a chance to travel through the lymph system and to clean body tissues. Adequate water intake helps to maintain the flow of nutrients to the lens and to release wastes and toxins from tissues.

Eat foods high in Vitamin A or beta-carotene, vitamin C, and vitamin E. These substances are called antioxidants, and most of the nutritional components of cataract prevention and reversal are related to boosting antioxidant levels. Antioxidants are one of the most important combatants against free radicals, a major cause of cataract formation (and other eye disease). A good diet supplemented with antioxidant vitamins and minerals can help prevent the damage due to oxidation and free radicals.[57 58 59 60 61 62]

Eat foods high in antioxidants, including leafy-green vegetables, garlic, onions, beans, celery, sea vegetables, apples, carrots, tomatoes, turnips, and oranges.

Important

Eliminate dairy products, at least temporarily. Some foods, particularly dairy products, can exacerbate eye problems by creating mucus and causing sinus congestion, which can impair lymph and blood drainage from the area around the eyes. When lymph and blood can't flow in and out of the eyes, nutrients don't reach the eyes effectively, and toxins and metabolic wastes aren't eliminated as efficiently. Try avoiding dairy for a month to see whether you become less congested and your eye issues clear up.

Note. Many people are lactose intolerant to some degree. Generally, reducing or eliminating dairy from one's diet has innumerable positive benefits on the eyes and the entire body.

Lifestyle

While supplementation is important, nothing replaces a positive, healthy lifestyle that includes regular exercise, daily meditations or walks in nature, and a healthy diet.

The rapid pace of life often interferes with people taking time to care for themselves properly, and on all levels—mental, emotional, spiritual, and physical. However, proper care maximizes the mind/body connection and its inherent healing potential, which is essential for restoring and maintaining health.

Avoid smoking. Researchers have established that smoking cigarettes substantially increases the risk of developing age-related cataracts. Smoking accounts for about 20% of all cataract incidences.[63] [64]

Eye Drop Recommendations

The following eyedrops have either a long history of safe usage for cataract management and/or have research studies showing related benefits to lens health. Take one eyedrop formula to start or any combination of the three. We recommend taking eyedrops for at least 3–6 months to start; this will help you determine their efficacy. Look for a reduction in common symptoms to cataracts, such as related reduction in blurriness and/or less sensitivity to glare, particularly at night.

Cineraria homeopathic eyedrops. 1 drop in each eye, 2–3 times per day, best taken at least 30 minutes apart from other eyedrops. This eyedrop has been listed in the Ophthalmology Physician's Desk Reference herbal section for over 38 years as a treatment for cataracts. They can be taken by themselves or with other eyedrops.[65] [66]

N-acetyl-carnosine eyedrops 1%. 2 drops in each eye, 2 times per day, best to separate each eyedrop by approximately one minute. See Appendix 5 for product recommendations.[67]

Oclumed eyedrops. One drop in each eye, 2 times per day. These eyedrops contain a range of antioxidants including l-carnosine, n-acetyl-l-carnosine, l-glutathione, cysteine ascorbate (providing a source of vitamin C), l-cysteine, taurine, and other nutrients to support the repair of the damaged lens tissues.

Exercise

Long-term regular exercise, as opposed to a burst of exercise training, reduces the risk of cataracts. High levels of inactivity increase cataract risk.[68]

Many therapies promote improved flow of energy and circulation throughout the body. The daily stress that we encounter due to a poor diet, emotional imbalances, lack of regular exercise, and more, can cause areas within the body to tighten up, which restricts circulation. The eyes are the second most biologically active part of the body; only the brain is more active. So, they require a great deal of nutrition and the free flow of blood and energy to remain healthy.

Eye exercises are helpful for maintaining good vision and promoting microcirculation in the eyes. We especially recommend:

- Hopscotch
- Zooming
- Near and far

See Chapter 10-4 for more eye exercises.

Yoga. Inversion poses in yoga have been shown to aid blood flow to the heart and head. It may seem counter-intuitive, but the blood is more freely able to move to the upper extremities, these exercises can be very relaxing to the eyes and face. As such, they are particularly helpful in the prevention of eye conditions. One of the best and safest inversion poses is lying on the floor with your legs up a wall. Beginning, as well as advanced yoga practitioners equally enjoy this posture.

After cataract surgery, avoid inversions. This includes standing forward bends like Uttanasana and Prasarita Padottanasana, and even downward-facing dog. You can still include modified poses like half dog pose at the wall. If you apply the rule of not bending past 90 degrees from vertical, you will minimize the pressure increase to the head and subsequently to the eye. Other rather obvious poses that could have a similar effect are those that require strong, sustained contraction of the abdominal muscles, which would also increase blood pressure in the eyes. Poses like boat pose (navasana), deep held twists (even sitting versions), and arm balances like crow pose also fall into this category.

In a time of healing you want to keep the nervous system quiet, spending more time in the "rest and digest" part of the autonomic nervous system. So, spend the two-week healing period doing gentler practices, including lots of supported restoratives and guided meditations on health and healing.

For more information, go to Chapter 10-7, Yoga and Vision.

Other Modalities

Chinese Medicine

Traditional Chinese Medicine (TCM) views the development of cataracts as often being related to a chronic imbalance in the Kidney meridian, which is related to the emotions of fear and grief. The Liver meridian "opens to the eyes" and is associated with overall eye health, but the Kidney meridian "opens to the eye lens."

Since most of the major meridians (in terms of energy flow) pass through the eyes, the imbalance inherent in eye issues may be related to an imbalance in other meridians that may affect the Kidney and Liver meridians. Where the imbalances lie is best determined through an intake evaluation by an acupuncturist.

Here are the common Chinese medicine patent formulas related to cataracts:

Kidney yin tonic may be taken in a dosage as directed by your practitioner.

Shi hu ye guang wan (dendrobium pill for night vision) nourishes Kidney yin and clears the Liver to improve vision. It is indicated for cataracts as well as red, irritated, or swollen eyes, poor or blurred vision, eyestrain from reading or from computer use, excessive tearing, and pain around the eyes.

Ming mu di huang wan (brighten the eyes) nourishes the Liver, enriches the Kidneys, and improves vision.

Zhu jing wan (preserve vistas pill) tonifies and nourishes the Liver and Kidneys, enriches the yin, and improves vision. Symptoms related to deficiencies in these meridians include weak and aching lower back and knees, excessive thirst, poor memory, cough, asthma, shortness of breath, and wheezing.

Qi ju di huang wan (rehmannia 6 plus chrysanthemum and lycii) nourishes Kidney, Liver blood, and yin. This formula is a classic adaptation of "liu wei di huang wan" (rehmannia 6), with a special emphasis on the eyes. In particular, the formula is helpful for dry eyes, redness, and heat caused by yin (fluid) deficiency.

Celosia 10 was designed for disorders such as cataracts as the lens and cornea tissue that are exposed are easily subject to "wind" disorders.

Essential Oils

Laurel leaf helps with lymph support.

Clary sage helps balance the endocrine system.

Saffron benefits include the following properties: antibacterial, blood purifier, antioxidant, decongestant, and memory enhancer.

Frankincense helps relieve chronic stress and anxiety, reduces pain and inflammation, and boosts immunity.

Carrot seed properties include antiseptic, disinfectant, detoxifier, and antioxidant.

Keep essences away from the mouth, eyes, and mucous membranes; if a few drops get in one of these sensitive areas it may be uncomfortable for 15–30 minutes, but not harmful. You can lessen

discomfort by adding a pure oil like olive or coconut oil to neutralize the irritating effect. For the eye area, dab a few drops around the outside of the eye. Do not put the neutralizing oil in the eye.

Combine ¼ cup of avocado oil with ¼ cup of calendula-infused oil. Slowly add 5 drops each of the essential oils. Then close the bottle and shake well; apply 4 drops of this mixture on your clean face. Massage in gentle circular motions. Leave overnight.

For more information, see Essential Oils in Appendix 9.

Other Therapies

Acupuncture supports the healthy flow of energy and circulation through the eye. There are eight acupressure points around the orbit of the eye, which can be massaged periodically throughout the day to help relax the eyes and stimulate energy and circulation flow. See Chapter 10-4 for recommended eye exercises and acupressure eye points.

On the Horizon

Research on animals using eyedrops containing lanosterol showed reduced severity of cataracts. Future research needs to be done on humans to identify the effectiveness. The application of the molecule lanosterol was shown to dissolve the lens protein buildup that causes cataracts in animal subjects; it may provide a non-surgical treatment for humans in the future.[69]

Using lasers as a pretreatment to cataract surgery is showing potential for improvement in the safety and results of surgery.

Use of stem cells to regrow the eye lens after cataract surgery is another potential treatment of the future. Researchers at the University of California, San Diego School of Medicine, and Shiley Eye Institute, with colleagues in China, have developed a new, regenerative medicine approach to remove congenital cataracts in infants, which permits remaining stem cells to regrow functional lenses.[70]

Also See

Chapter 7, Vision Diet

Chapter 8, Nutrients

Chapter 10-4, Eye Exercises

Appendix 5, Recommended Products

Appendix 7, Additional Therapies

---

[1] Shiels, A., Hejtmancik, J.F. (2007). Genetic Origins of Cataract. *Arch Opthalmol, 125*(2), 165–173.

[2] National Eye Institute. Cataracts. Retrieved Jan 7, 2018 from https://nei.nih.gov/eyedata/cataract.

[3] Francois, J. (1982). Genetics of cataract. *Ophthalmologica.* 18461–71.

[4] Merin, S. (1991). Inherited cataracts. In Merin S. editor. *Inherited Eye Diseases* (pp. 86–120). New York: Marcel Dekker.

[5] Ibid. Shiels. (2007).

[6] Donaldson, P.J., Musil, L.S., Mathias, R.T. (2010). Point: A Critical Appraisal of the Lens Circulation Model—An Experimental Paradigm for Understanding the Maintenance of Lens Transparency? *Invest Ophthalmol Vis Sci,* My;51(5):2303-2306.

[7] Times of India. (2010). Cell phones can damage eyes: Study. Retrieved May 5 2018 from https://timesofindia.indiatimes.com/city/vadodara/Cell-phones-can-damage-eyes-Study/articleshow/6056427.cms.

[8] Patalano, V.J. (2002). The Risks and Benefits of Cataract Surgery. *Dig J Ophthalmol,* Oct 15.

[9] Ibid. National Eye Institute. *Cataracts.*

[10] Hamilton, A.M., Ulbig, M.W., Polkinghorne, P. (1996). Epidemiology of diabetic retinopathy. *Management of Diabetic Retinopathy* (pp. 1–15). London: BMJ Publishing Group.

[11] Kato, S., Shiokawa, A., Fukushima, H., Numaga, J., Kitano, S., et al. (2001). Glycemic control and lens transparency in patients with type 1 diabetes mellitus. *Am J Ophthalmol,* 131:301–304.

[12] Ibid. Hamilton. (1996).

[13] Klein, B.E., Klein, R., Moss, S.E. (1995). Incidence of cataract surgery in the Wisconsin Epidemiologic Study of Diabetic Retinopathy. *Am J Ophthalmol,* (119):295–300.

[14] Somaiyam, M.D., Burns, J.D., Mintz, R., Warren, R.E., Uchida, T., et al. (2002). Factors affecting visual outcomes after small-incision phacoemulsification in diabetic patients. *J Cataract Refract Surg,* 28(8), 1364–1371.

[15] Sedaghat, F., Ghanavati, M., Nezhad, Hajian, P., Hajishirazi, S., Ehteshami, M., et al. (2017). Nutrient patterns and risk of cataract: a case-control study. *Int J Ophthalmol,* Apr 18;10(4):586–592.

[16] Leske, M.C., Chylack, L.T., Wy, S.Y. (1991). The Lens Opacities Case-Control Study. Risk factors for cataract. *Arch Ophthalmol,* Feb;109(2):244–51.

[17] Jacques, P.F., Taylor, A., Hankinson, S.E., Willett, W.C., Mahnken, B., et al. (1997). Long-term vitamin C supplement use and prevalence of early age-related lens opacities. *Am J Clin Nutr,* Oct;66(4):911-6.

[18] Taylor, A., Jacques, P.F., Chylack, L.T., Hankinson, S.E., Khu, P.M., et al. (2002). Long-term intake of vitamins and carotenoids and odds of early age-related cortical and posterior subcapsular lens opacities, *Am J Clin Nutr,* Mar;75(3):540-9.

[19] Ferrigno, L., Aldigeri, R., Rosmini, F., Sperduto, R.D., Maraini, G., et al. (2005). Associations between plasma levels of vitamins and cataract in the Italian-American Clinical Trial of Nutritional Supplements and Age-Related Cataract (CTNS): CTNS Report #2. *Ophthalmic Epidemiol,* Apr;12(2):71-80.

[20] Valero, M.P., Fletcher, A.E., De Stavola, B.L., Vioque, J., Alepuz, V.C. (2002). Vitamin C is associated with reduced risk of cataract in a Mediterranean population. *J Nutr,* Jun;132(6):1299-306.

[21] Brubaker, R.F., Bourne, W.M., Bachman, L.A., McLaren, J.W. (2000). Ascorbic acid content of human corneal epithelium. *Invest Ophthalmol Vis Sci,* Jun;41(7):1681-3.

[22] Mynampati, B.K., Ghosh, S., Muthukumarappa, T, Ram, J. (2017). Evaluation of antioxidants and argpyrimidine in normal and cataractous lenses in north Indian population. *Int J Ophthalmol,* 10(7): 1094–1100.

[23] Kumar, D., Lim, J.C., Donaldson, P.J. (2013). A link between maternal malnutrition and depletion of glutathione in the developing lens: a possible explanation for idiopathic childhood cataract? *Clin Exp Optom,* Nov;96(6):523-8.

[24] Ravindran, R.D., Vashist, P., Gupta S.K., Young, I.S., Maraini, G., et al. (2011). Inverse Association of Vitamin C with Cataract in Older People in India. *Ophthalmology,* Oct;118(10):1958-1965.

[25] Olmedill, B., Granado, F., Blanco, I., Vaquero, M. (2003). Lutein, but not alpha tocopherol, supplementation improves visual function in patients with age-related cataracts: A 2 year double-blind, placebo controlled study. *Nutrition,* Jan;19(1):21-4.

[26] Yeum, K.J., Taylor, A., Tang, G., Russell, R.M. (1995). Measurement of Carotenoids, Retinoids, and Tocopherols in Human Lenses. *Invest Ophthalmol Vis Sci,* Dec;36(13):2756-61.

[27] Chasan-Taber, L., Willett, W.C., Seddon, J.M., Stampfer, M.J., Rosner, B., et al. (1999). A prospective study of carotenoid and vitamin A intakes and risk of cataract extraction in US women. *Am J Clin Nutr,* Oct;70(4):509-16.

[28] Brown, L., Rimm, E.B., Seddon, J.M., Giovannucci, E.L., Chasen-Taber, L., et al. (1999). A prospective study of carotenoid intake and risk of cataract extraction in US men. *Am J Clin Nutr,* Oct;70(4):517-24.

[29] Liu, X.H., Yu, R.B., Liu, R., Hao, Z.X., Han, C.C., et al. (2014). Association between lutein and zeaxanthin status and the risk of cataract: a meta-analysis. *Nutrients,* Jan 22;6(1):452-65.

[30] Ibid. Chasan-Taber. (1999).

[31] Ibid. Brown. (1999).

[32] Li, Y., Liu, Y.Z., Shi, J.M., Jia, S.B. (2013). Alpha lipoic acid protects lens from H(2)O(2)-induced cataract by inhibiting apoptosis of lens epithelial cells and inducing activation of anti-oxidative enzymes. *Asian Pac J Trop Med*, Jul;6(7):548-51.

[33] Ibid. Liu. (2014).

[34] Ma, L., Hao, Z.X., Liu, R.R., Yu, R.B., Shi, Q., et al. (2014). A dose-response meta-analysis of dietary lutein and zeaxanthin intake in relation to risk of age-related cataract. *Graefes Arch Clin Exp Ophthalmol*, Jan;252(1):63-70.

[35] Liu, X.H., Yu, R.B., Liu, R., Hao, Z.X., Han, C.C., et al. (2014). Association between lutein and zeaxanthin status and the risk of cataract: a meta-analysis. *Nutrients*, Jan 22;6(1):452-65.

[36] Packer, L., Witt, E.H., Tritschler, H.J. (1995). alpha-Lipoic acid as a biological antioxidant.

Free Radic Biol Med, Aug;19(2):227-50

[37] . Chen, Y., Yi, L., Yan, G., Fang, Y., Jang, Y., et al. (2010). alpha-Lipoic acid alters post-translational modifications and protects the chaperone activity of lens alpha-crystallin in naphthalene-induced cataract. *Curr Eye Res*, Jul;35(7):620-30.

[38] Kan, E., Kilickan, E., Ayar, A., Colak, R. (2015). Effects of two antioxidants; α-lipoic acid and fisetin against diabetic cataract in mice. *Int Ophthalmol*, Feb;35(1):115-20.

[39] Cornish, K.M., Williamson, G., Sanderson, J. (2002). Quercetin metabolism in the lens: role in inhibition of hydrogen peroxide induced cataract. *Free Radic Biol Med*, Jul 1;33(1):63-70.

[40] Du, L., Hao, M., Li, C., Wu, W., Wang, W., et al. (2017). Quercetin inhibited epithelial mesenchymal transition in diabetic rats, high-glucose-cultured lens, and SRA01/04 cells through transforming growth factor-β2/phosphoinositide 3-kinase/Akt pathway. *Mol Cell Endocrinol*, Sep 5;452:44-56.

[41] Sheng, Y., He, F., Lin, J.F., Shen, W., Qiu, Y.W. (2015). Tea and Risk of Age-Related Cataracts: A Cross-Sectional Study in Zhejiang Province, China. *J Epidemiol*, 26(11): 587–592.

[42] Karakucuk S, Ertugrul, M.G., Faruk, E.O., Saraymen, R., Karakucuk, I., et al. (1995). Selenium concentrations in serum, lens and aqueous humour of patients with senile cataract. *Acta Ophthalmol Scand*, Aug;73(4):329-32.

[43] Babizhayev, M.A., Deyev, A.I. Yermakova, V.N., Semiletov, Y.A., Daydova, N.G., et al. (2001). N-Acetylcarnosine, a natural histidine-containing dipeptide, as a potent ophthalmic drug in treatment of human cataracts. *Peptide*, Jun;22(6):979-94

[44] Bravetti, G. (1989). Preventive medical treatment of senile cataract with vitamin E and anthocyanosides: clinical evaluation. *Ann Ottalmol Clin Ocul*,115:109

[45] Aly, E.M., Ali, M.A. (2014). Effects of bilberry on deoxyribonucleic Acid damage and oxidant-antioxidant balance in the lens, induced by ultraviolet radiation. *Malays J Med Sci*, Jan;21(1):11-8.

[46] Zheng, T., Lu, Y. (2016). SIRT1 Protects Human Lens Epithelial Cells Against Oxidative Stress by Inhibiting p53-Dependent Apoptosis. *Curr Eye Res*, Aug;41(8):1068-1075.

[47] Abe, M., Reiter, R.J., Orhii, P.B., Hara, M., Poegeler, B. (1994). Inhibitory effect of melatonin on cataract formation in newborn rats: evidence for an antioxidative role for melatonin. *J Pineal Res*, Sep;17(2):94-100.

[48] Vitale, S., West, S., Hllfrisch, J., Alston, C., Wang, F., et al. (1993). Plasma antioxidants and risk of cortical and nuclear cataract. *Epidemiology*, May;4(3):195-203.

[49] Bantseev, V., Bhardwaj, R., Rathbun, W., Nagasawa, H., Trevithick, J.R. (1997). Antioxidants and cataract: (cataract induction in space environment and application to terrestrial aging cataract). *Biochem Mol Biol Int*, Sep;42(6):1189-97.

[50] Zhang, Y., Jiang, W., Xie, W., Wu, W., Zhang, D. (2015). Vitamin E and risk of age-related cataract: a meta-analysis. *Public Health Nutr*, Oct;18(15):2804-14.

[51] Ibid. Zhang. (2015).

[52] Ibid. Bantseev. (1997).

[53] Ibid. Babizhayev. (2001).

[54] Bahmani, F., Bathaie, S.Z., Aldavood, S.J., Ghahghaei, A. (2016). Inhibitory Effect of Crocin(s) on Lens α-Crystallin Glycation and Aggregation, Results in the Decrease of the Risk of Diabetic Cataract. *Molecules*, Jan 26;21(2):143.

[55] Appleby, P.N., Allen, N.E., Key, T.J. (2011). Diet, vegetarianism, and cataract risk. *Am J Clin Nutr*, May;93(5):1128-35.

[56] Birlouez-Aragon, I., Ravelontseheno, L., Villate-Cathelineau, B., Cathelineau, G. Abitbol, G. (1993). Disturbed galactose metabolism in elderly and diabetic humans is associated with cataract formation. *J Nutr*, Aug;123(8):1370-6.

[57] Leske, M.C.; Chylack, L.T., He, Q, Wu, S.Y., Schoenfeld, E, et al. (1998). Antioxidant vitamins: the longitudinal cataract study, *Ophthalmology*, May;105(5):831-6.

[58] Taylor, A. (1993). Cataract: relationship between nutrition and oxidation. *J Am Coll Nutr*, Apr, 12(2):138-46.

[59] Cumming, R.G., Mitchell, P., Smith, W. (2000). Diet and cataract: the Blue Mountains Eye Study. *Ophthalmology*, Mar;107(3):450-6

[60] Leske, M.C., Chylack, L.T., Wu, S.Y. (1991). The Lens Opacities Case-Control Study. Risk factors for cataract. *Arch Ophthalmol*, Feb;109(2):244-51.

[61] Hankinson, S.E., Stampfer, M.J., Sedden, J.M., Colditz, G.A., Rosner, B., et al. (1992). Nutrient intake and cataract extraction in women: a prospective study. *BMJ*, Aug 8;305(6849):335-9.

[62] Wang, A., Han, J., Jiang, Y., Zhang, D. (2014). Association of vitamin A and β-carotene with risk for age-related cataract: a meta-analysis. *Nutrition*, Oct;30(10):1113-21.

[63] Christen, W.G., Glynn, R.J., Ajani, U.A., Schaumberg, D.A., Buring, J.E., et al. (2000). Smoking cessation and risk of age-related cataract in men. *JAMA*, 2000 Aug 9;284(6):713-6

[64] Kar, T., Ayata, A., Aksoy, Y., Kaya, A., Unal, M. (2014). The effect of chronic smoking on lens density in young adults. *Eur J Ophthalmology*, Sep-Oct;24(5):682-7.

[65] Anitha, T.S., Annadurai, T., Thomas, P.A., Geraldine, P. (2011). Prevention of selenite-induced cataractogenesis by an ethanolic extract of Cineraria maritima: an experimental evaluation of the traditional eye medication. *Biol Trace Elem Res*, Oct;143(1):425-36.

[66] Anitha, T.S., Muralidharan, A.R., Annadurai, T., Jesudasan, C.A., Thomas, P.A., et al. (2013). Putative free radical-scavenging activity of an extract of Cineraria maritima in preventing selenite-induced cataractogenesis in Wistar rat pups. *Mol Vis*, Dec 16;19:2551-60.

[67] Ibid. Babizhayev. (2001).

[68] Zheng, S.J., Orsini, N., Ejdervik, L.B., Wolk, A. (2015). Long-term physical activity and risk of age-related cataract: a population-based prospective study of male and female cohorts. *Ophthalmology*, Feb;122(2):274-80.

[69] Zhao L, Chen XJ, Zhu J, Xi, Y.B., Yang, X. et al. (2015). Lanosterol reverses protein aggregation in cataracts. *Nature*, Jul 30;523(7562):607-11.

[70] Lin, H., Ouyang, H., Zhu, J., Huang, S., Liu, Z, et al. (2016). Lens regeneration using endogenous stem cells with gain of visual function. *Nature*, Mar 17;531(7594):323-8.

15-2. COLOR BLINDNESS

Color blindness or color deficiency means that a person has trouble seeing red, green, or blue, or a mix of these colors. Approximately 8% of men and only one-half of 1% of women in the U.S. have a problem with color perception.[1] Most colorblind people have lost only part of their color vision and are therefore termed as color deficient.

Very rarely a person sees no color at all. This most severe form of color blindness is known as achromatopsia. Unlike genetically based color blindness, this condition results after damage to the cerebral cortex such as trauma, tumor growth, or internal cortex bleeding.

What is Color Blindness?

The eye contains photoreceptor cells in the form of both rods and cones; however, the three types of cones are the cells responsible for giving us color vision, and these are mostly found in the macula (central portion of the retina). Color blindness is an indication that a person's photoreceptor cones are either absent or not functioning fully.

Long wavelength-sensitive L-cones, peaking about 560nm, detect red light. Medium wavelength-sensitive M-cones, peaking about 530nm, detect green light. Short wavelength-sensitive S-cones, peaking about 420nm, detect blue light.[2]

Typically, only one or two types of cones are absent or not functioning optimally. For example, if the dysfunction occurs in the L-cones that perceive the color green, a person is deficient picking up green. However, red and blue[3] colors, and combinations of red and blue are seen.

The cone cells contain different kinds of photopsins or pigments, which filter light and detect different colors. They respond to color variations in different ways. Being color blind changes how they respond or whether they respond at all.[4]

Types of Color Blindness

The cones of the eye constitute several different types, each responsible for receiving input from different wavelengths of light. Deutan defects make the person less sensitive to green light, protan defects make the person less sensitive to red light, and tritan defects make the person less sensitive to green-blue and yellow-violet light.

Additionally, researchers have discovered that the thickness of the macular pigment affects the quality of color discrimination.

Deuteranopia: Green Insensitive (red-green)

Deutan defects are the most common kind of color blindness. People with deutan color blindness are less sensitive to green light. It affects more men than women and usually in a mild form. There are some related colors that are difficult to distinguish, such as greenish blue-green and purple.

Deuteranopia. This is also known as green-blind color blindness. While people with normal vision can distinguish seven different colors of light, people with deuteranopia can only see two or three. The cones that receive input from green medium wavelength light are entirely missing.[5]

Deuteranomoly. This is also known as green-weak color blindness. People with deuteranomoly have green mid-wavelength cones present, but they are more sensitive to red than green light.

Deutan Defect Causes

Genetics. Red-green color blindness is genetic and is a sex-linked trait associated with the X chromosome. Because women have two X chromosomes and men have only one, women are less likely to have deutan defects.[6]

Normal Color Vision Perception

700 650 600 550 500 450 400

Deuteranopia

700 650 600 550 500 450 400

Protanopia

700 650 600 550 500 450 400

Tritanopia

700 650 600 550 500 450 400

Protanopia: Red-Insensitive (red-green)

This form of red-green color blindness varies from deutan defects because the cones (L-cones) are insensitive to long wave red light. People with protan defects have difficulty seeing the difference between blue and green and between red and green.

Drivers with protan color blindness are particularly vulnerable to driving problems since they are unable to correctly see red lights. Some researchers consider protan defects to be the equivalent of having a blood alcohol level of .05–.06%.[7]

Protanopia. The long wavelength cones are missing entirely. This form is sometimes called red-dichromacy.

Protanomaly. In this case the L-cones are present, but are somewhat insensitive to red light.

Protan Defect Causes

Genetics. Like deutan defects, this form of color blindness is congenital, coming from malformations of L-cone encoding on the X chromosome. Because men have only one X chromosome, the condition is more common in men than in women.

Tritan: Blue Insensitive (blue-yellow)

This type of color blindness exists from birth or can be acquired during one's lifetime, in which case it may be reversible. Tritan defects affect about 1 in 10,000 people, men and women equally.

Tritanopia. People affected by tritan color blindness have trouble distinguishing blue from green and yellow from violet. S-cones that receive short wave light are missing entirely.

Tritanomaly. In this partial form of blue-yellow color blindness, the S-cones are present but are mutated in some way.

Tritan Defect Causes

- The lens of the eye becomes less transparent with age; very mild tritanopia may develop.[8]
- Alcoholics have a higher rate of tritanopia. Excessive alcohol consumption is associated with a higher rate of blue-yellow color errors as compared to red-green.[9]
- Inhalation of organic solvents, even at very low concentrations, primarily impairs blue-yellow color vision.[10]
- Physical trauma to the cerebral cortex can cause blue-yellow color blindness.[11]
- Genetic causes are due to mutations on the OPN1SW gene chromosome 7 encoding.[12]

Monochromacy

The most severe form of color blindness is monochromacy, in which no colors can be distinguished. It is also called achromotopsia. It is quite rare, affecting 1 in 40,000 people.

Monochromacy Causes

Genetic. Cone cells are unable to detect light input due to mutations in several different genes (CNGA3, CNGB3, CNAT2, and PDE6C).

Tumor growth. Tumors can cause damage to the thalamus or the cerebral cortex, both of which receive information from the eye's nervous system.

Trauma to, or **hemorrhage** within, the cerebral cortex. This damages the same information-receiving process.

Conventional Treatment

There are a number of lenses in the market today that have shown to be helpful for correcting color blindness. Each of these lenses has shown that they are effective for the following:

- Improving general color perception
- Making colors brighter and clearer
- Allowing shades of color, previously unseen, to be observed
- Improving the ability to name colors correctly

The quality of life for a person struggling with color deficiency or color blindness can be greatly enhanced. For example, a person has improved safety through more accurate identification of hazard warning lights and brake lights on the roads. They can also experience greater ease in daily living; for example, distinguishing traffic lights by color rather than their position on the post. Ask your ophthalmologist for more information on the following:

A single pink contact lens for one eye only. This seems to facilitate the discernment of colors for some people.

Dr. Thomas Azman Color Correction System[TM13] claims to be the world's only color blindness treatment with a 100% success rate. It works by using customized filters to change the wavelength of each color that goes into the eyes. The filters are designed uniquely for each individual and can be worn as colorblind glasses or colorblind contact lenses.

ChromaGen[14] is a unique system of colored lenses of a specific density and hue that are worn as either contact lenses or spectacles. ChromaGen haploscopic filters also work by changing the wavelength of each color going into one or both eyes, which enhances color perception and color discrimination. In trials, over 97% of color blind people reported a significant enhancement to their color vision.

ColorView[15] is made for people with red-green color-vision deficiency, a deficiency which is most associated with genetics. ColorView adjusts the amount of each of the three prime colors (red, green, and blue) entering the eye, since these are the only colors of light that the eye can perceive.

Complementary Approach

Complementary therapies cannot replace missing cone cells or damaged cells due to heredity, but they can stimulate and support the cells that may be either dormant or active, possibly enabling the person to see colors more clearly.

Nutrients

There is a link between acquired (not congenital) color blindness and other conditions such as macular degeneration and diabetic retinopathy. Because these conditions damage the retina, any nutrients that help support retinal health will help support the photoreceptor cells.

Essential

Lutein. 6mg–20mg per day. Red-green (but not yellow-blue) vision for people is somewhat strengthened by supplementation with lutein. This is because the carotenoid improves thickness of the macular pigment, and macular pigment thickness is associated with better red-green vision.[16] Furthermore, lutein helps to protect the retina generally, which helps to protect the photoreceptor cells.

Zeaxanthin. 2mg–12mg per day. Red-green (but not yellow-blue) vision for people is somewhat strengthened by supplementation with zeaxanthin. Zeaxanthin supports macular pigment thickness that is linked to better red-green vision sensitivity.[17] Additionally, zeaxanthin supports retinal health and the photoreceptor cells that are part of the retina.

Astaxanthin. 6mg–12mg per day. Astaxanthin protects pigment cells from oxidative stress.[18]

Bilberry. 180mg–240mg per day. Along with supporting night vision, bilberry is neuroprotective and has been shown to improve microcirculation.[19] [20] [21]

Vitamin A (palmitate). 5,000 IU–15,000 IU per day. Helps support the photoreceptor cells.[22]

> **Note**. Vitamin A is contra-indicated for those suffering from Stargardt disease (see Stargardt's chapter for more information).

Taurine. 750mg–1,000mg per day. Deficiency of taurine, an amino acid, has been shown to lead to retinal degeneration, and supplementing with it has been used with some success toward preventing, treating, and stabilizing retinal changes.[23] [24] [25]

Very Important

CoQ10 (100mg–200mg per day), *along with* **N-acetyl-carnitine** (500mg–1,000mg per day), *and* **omega-3 fatty acids** (2,000mg–3,000mg per day). Study findings strongly suggest that an appropriate combination of acetyl-L-carnitine, omega-3 fatty acids, and coenzyme Q10 (which affect mitochondrial lipid metabolism) may improve and subsequently stabilize visual functions, and it may also support a healthy fundus, which includes the retina and photoreceptor cells.[26]

Helpful

Green tea. 500mg–750mg per day. Green teas and its extracts are potentially neuroprotective in the photoreceptor outer segment and retinal pigment epithelium (RPE).[27]

Ginkgo biloba. 120mg per day. Ginkgo extracts support vision quality.[28]

Diet

The Vision diet described in Chapter 7 is a carotenoid-rich, nutrient-rich, balanced pH diet that supports both vision health and general heath.

Juicing. Choose at least 4-6 items to combine, as well as adding your favorite fruits and vegetables. Do not use too many carrots and beets due to their natural sweetness.

- Ginger, parsley, beets, cabbage, carrots, endive, green-leafy vegetables, chlorophyll, wheatgrasses, and berries, (preferably all organic)
- Don't use cold fruit or ice since this arrests the digestive fires.
- In the winter, you may have warm soups or stews instead.

Lifestyle

Recommended eye exercises. See Chapter 10-4 for eye exercises and acupuncture points that are good for all eye conditions and overall eye health. These exercises may be helpful:

- Palming
- Eye massage of acupressure points.

Other Modalities

Chinese Medicine

In Chinese medicine, the Liver "opens to the eyes," and is the primary meridian for supporting overall flow of energy and circulation through the eyes. The Kidney meridian nourishes the blood to the eyes. The Spleen meridian nourishes the blood and helps keep fluids from leaking from blood vessels. Other meridians may be out of balance as well, which can affect eye health, so an evaluation by an acupuncturist can best determine where the out-of-balances are located and offer the optimal treatment strategy.

As long as there are cones active in the eyes that can pick up the range of colors needed to see the red, blue, and green wavelengths, these can be supported and nourished through acupuncture and specific herbs. Acupuncture treatments are typically done by inserting needles below the knees and elbows, then in specific points along the orbit of the eye.

Herbal Formulas

Xiao yao san (rambling powder) is a classic Liver tonic used in Chinese medicine. The Liver "opens to the eyes" and is the primary meridian (flow energy) that supports healthy circulation and the free flow of energy in the eyes (as well as throughout the body).

Ming mu di huang wan (brighten the eyes) contains a blend of herbs, specifically designed to improve eyesight by nourishing two main organs that are energetically responsible for vision: the Liver and Kidney. This results in improved blood availability to the eyes and better circulation.

On the Horizon

Successful gene therapy has been done on adult male monkeys that are all born with a gene that makes red photopigment, or the gene that makes green photopigment, but never both. In this NEI-supported study, researchers injected the red photopigment gene into the retinas of male monkeys that were born without it. The gene was targeted to green cones and allowed those cells to respond to red light. The monkeys were able to see with full three-color (trichromatic) vision. This shows that even though the monkeys' red cones had been absent from birth, the brain circuitry for detecting red was still in place. The hope is that this approach will work with humans as well.[29]

Also See

Chapter 7, Vision Diet

Chapter 8, Nutrients

Chapter 10-4, Eye Exercises

Chapter 15-5, Cone-Rod Dystrophy

Appendix 5, Recommended Products

1 Colblinder. Colorblind Population. Retrieved Oct 21 2017 from http://www.color-blindness.com/2006/04/28/colorblind-population.

2 Wikipedia. Cone cell. Retrieved Nov 22 2017 from https://en.wikipedia.org/wiki/Cone_cell

3 Rodriguez-Carmona, M., Kvansakul, J., Harlow, J.A., Kopcke, W., Schalch, W., et al. (2006). The effects of supplementation with lutein and/or zeaxanthin on human macular pigment density and colour vision. *Ophthalmic Physiol Opt*, Mar;26(2):137-47.

4 Ibid. Wikipedia. Cone Cell.

5 Colblinder. Deuteranopia - Red Green Color Blindness. Retrieved Nov 21 2017 from http://www.color-blindness.com/deuteranopia-red-green-color-blindness/

6 Ibid. Colblinder. Deuteranopia

7 Colblinder. Protanopia - Red-Green Color Blindness. Retrieved Nov 21 2017 from http://www.color-blindness.com/protanopia-red-green-color-blindness/

8 Colblinder. Tritanopia - Blue-Yellow Color Blindness. Retrieved Nov 21 2017 from http://www.color-blindness.com/tritanopia-blue-yellow-color-blindness/.

9 Ibid. Colblinder. Tritanopia

10 Ibid. Colblinder. Tritanopia.

11 Ibid. Colblinder. Tritanopia.

12 Deuteranopia. Hereditary Ocular Disease. Retrieved Nov 21 2017 from http://disorders.eyes.arizona.edu/category/alternate-names/deuteranopia

13 Colormax. About the Doctor. Retrieved Nov 21 2017 from https://colormax.org/about-the-doctor/

14 WebMD. Chromagen Capsule. Retrieved Nov 21 2017 from https://www.webmd.com/drugs/2/drug-1172/chromagen-oral/details.

15 CertainTeed. Color View. Retrieved 10/20/2017 from https://www.certainteed.com/gsearch/color%2Bview.

16 Ibid. Rodriguez-Carmona.

17 Ibid. Rodriguez-Carmona.

18 Li, Z, Dong, X., Liu, H., Chen, X., Shi, H., et al. (2013). Astaxanthin protects ARPE-19 cells from oxidative stress via upregulation of Nrf2-regulated phase II enzymes through activation of PI3K/Akt.*Mol Vis*, Jul 25;19:1656-66.

19 Matsunaga, N., Imai, S., Inokuchi, Y., Shimazawa, M., Yokata, S., et al. (2009). Bilberry and its main constituents have neuroprotective effects against retinal neuronal damage in vitro and in vivo. *Mol Nutr Food Res*, Jul;53(7):869-77.

20 Zhu, Y., Xia, M., Yang, Y., Liu, F., Li, Z., et al. (2011). Purified anthocyanin supplementation improves endothelial function via NO-cGMP activation in hypercholesterolemic individuals. *ClinChem*, Nov;57(11):1524-33.

21 Yao, Y., Vieria, A., (2013). Protective activities of Vaccinium antioxidants with potential relevance to mitochondrial dysfunction and neurotoxicity. *NeuroToxicology*, 28:93–100

22 Berson, E.L., Rosner, B., Sandberg, M.A., Hayes, K.C., Nicholson, B.W. (1993). *A randomized trial of vitamin A and vitamin E supplementation for retinitis pigmentosa*. Arch Ophthalmol Jun;111(6):761-72.

23 Birdsall, T.C. (1998). Therapeutic applications of taurine. *Altern Med Rev*, Apr;3(2):128-36.

24 Shpak, N.I., Naritsyna, N.I., Konovalova, N.V. (1989). Taufon and emoksipin in the combined treatment of sclerotic macular dystrophies. *Oftalmol Zh*, (8):463-5

25 Lombardini, J.B. (1991). Taurine: retinal function. *Brain Res Brain Res Rev*, May-Aug;16(2):151-69

26 Feher, J., Kovacs, B., Kovacs, I., Schveoller, M., Papale, A., et al. (2005). Improvement of visual functions and fundus alterations in early age-related macular degeneration treated with a combination of acetyl-L-carnitine, n-3 fatty acids, and coenzyme Q10. *Ophthalmologica*, May-Jun;219(3):154-66

27 Jarrett, S.G., Boulton, M.E. (2012). Consequences of oxidative stress in age-related macular degeneration *Aspects Med*, 2012 Aug;33(4):399–417

28 Lebuisson, D.A., Leroy, L., Rigal, G. (1986). Treatment of senile macular degeneration with Ginkgo biloba extract. A preliminary double-blind drug vs. placebo study. *Presse Med*, Sep 25;15(31):1556-8

[29] National Eye Institute. Facts About Color Blindness. Retrieved 10/20/2017 from https://nei.nih.gov/health/color_blindness/facts_about.

15-3. CENTRAL SEROUS CHOROIDOPATHY

Central serous choroidopathy (CSCR), also referred to as central serous retinopathy (CSR), is characterized by fluid leaking from tissues behind the retina, primarily into the central macula area, resulting in the macula detaching from the tissue that supports it. The separation results in a fairly sudden distortion or blurriness, usually in one eye. It is thought to be associated with stress, type A personality, steroid use, and hypertension; in other words, it appears more frequently in those who tend towards hyperactivity.

One local population study from 2001 to 2006 showed that for men, the mean annual incidence was 0.27%. The highest rate was for 35–39 year old men, followed by the 40–44 year old men.[1] CSCR generally affects middle-aged men between the ages of 20 and 50 years,[2][3][4] at rates nearly 2 times[5] to almost 6 times that of women, depending on the study methodology.

Pathology

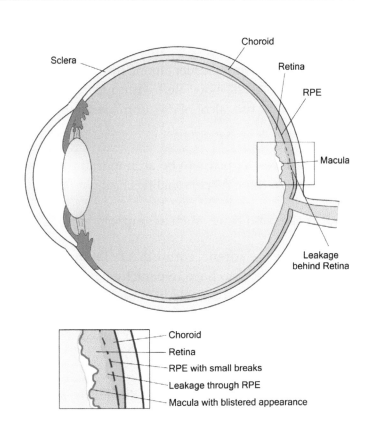

Leakage due to CSCR comes mostly from the fine capillaries in the choroid layer, through, and because of, small breaks in the retinal pigment layer. Advances in technology have allowed researchers to identify poor multifocal choroidal hyperpermeability and hypofluorescent areas suggestive of focal choroidal vascular compromise. Some investigators believe that initial choroidal vascular compromise subsequently leads to secondary dysfunction of the overlying retinal pigment epithelium (RPE).

Researchers have linked macular thickness with CSCR, finding that these patients have low macular pigment optical density.[6][7][8]

Classic CSCR is caused by isolated leaks in the RPE that are visible via a technology known as florescein angiography. But ophthalmologists now understand that the condition can also take other forms.

Diffuse RPE dysfunction, known as diffuse retinal pigment epitheliopathy, occurs when the leakage and changes to the RPE are widespread.[9]

Chronic CSCR is the term given to CSCR that endures for six months or more, compared to the normal duration of about 3 months.[10]

Decompensated RPE is described as retinal detachment, combined with RPE atrophy and pigment mottling that continue to degenerate with time. [11]

Signs and Symptoms

- A fairly sudden onset of blurry vision in one eye
- Dimmer colors
- Images appearing in miniature in the affected eye
- A blind spot in the center of vision, or distortion of straight lines in Amsler Grid.

Causes and Risk Factors

The cause is unproven, but below are some likely contributors. Chief among these are high levels of stress, particularly in type "A" personalities (also often associated with hypertension), and ongoing use of steroids. One study also noted antibiotic use, alcohol use, untreated hypertension, and allergic respiratory disease as risk factors.[12]

Stress and trauma. Both physical and emotional stress appears to be an important risk factor. Most patients are young men (20-45) with aggressive "type A" personalities.[13] [14]

Use of stimulants. These include cigarettes, caffeine, and drugs such as amphetamines.

High cortisol levels. Cortisol, a hormone secreted by the adrenal cortex that helps the body cope with stress, is linked to CSCR. Patients older than 50 tend to have hyperactivity in the adrenals (bilateral disease), high blood pressure, and a history of corticosteroid use.[15] A higher risk is associated with those exposed to corticosteroids taken for conditions such as asthma, autoimmune disorders, skin problems, and allergies. A higher risk is also linked to receiving epidural steroids for degenerative disc disease. [16]

Epinephrine used for various conditions such as asthma or obstructive sleep apnea.[17]

Ischemia, an inadequate blood supply to an organ or part of the body, especially the heart muscles, or **inflammation** may contribute.[18]

Other drugs may include decongestants, erectile dysfunction drugs, and some anti-cancer agents.

Smokers are more vulnerable to CSCR and need a longer period for healing.[19]

Helicobacter pylori. There is evidence that this bacterium, which naturally occurs in the body, is associated with CSCR.[20] Gastritis, which is an inflammation of the stomach lining, sometimes caused by Helicobacter pylori, may play a role in the development of CSCR.

Type II kidney-disease patients are at higher risk. Glomeruli are clusters of capillaries in the kidneys that help to filter waste from your blood. When these structures become inflamed because of the accumulation of "dense deposits," a condition known as glomerulonephritis (GN) develops. These patients can similarly develop a variety of retina problems, including CSCR, due to the same type of accumulated deposits that damage the kidney membranes.[21] [22]

Pregnancy. In women, pregnancy is a known risk factor.

Anti-anxiety drugs. One study provides nationwide, population-based data on the incidence of idiopathic CSCR in adult Asians, and suggests that exposure to anti-anxiety drugs is an independent risk factor for idiopathic CSCR among males.

Testosterone treatment. Chronic CSCR has developed from long-term testosterone treatment.[23]

Conventional Treatment

CSCR is usually a self-limiting disease with spontaneous resolution within 3–4 months and with overall good visual outcome.[24] [25] [26] Patients who are using steroid drugs (for example, to treat autoimmune diseases) should discontinue using them, if medically feasible. However, any change in steroid drug use MUST be under the supervision of a physician.

Because of limited or poor study design, which interventions are most effective is debatable, but photodynamic therapy or micropulse laser treatment appears to be the most promising.[27]

Photodynamic therapy. A photosensitizing drug is injected into the bloodstream and fills the abnormal, bleeding-blood vessels in the choroid. Then, a low-level laser light is applied to activate the drug, converting it into a substance that destroys the abnormal blood vessels without damaging surrounding tissue. In one large series of case studies, no patient developed severe visual loss or complications derived from PDT within an average follow-up of 12 months. However, nine cases developed reactive RPE hypertrophy after PDT.[28] Possible side effects include temporary visual abnormalities, pain, swelling, bleeding, photosensitivity reactions (such as sunburn), inflammation at the site of the injection, joint pain, or muscle weakness.

Laser treatment. Treatment with laser photocoagulation or hot laser that uses heat to seal or destroy abnormal, leaking blood vessels in the retina, may help patients with more severe leakage and visual loss, or longer persistence of the disease. The procedure is typically performed in the office, and a small number of patients will experience complications. The laser may permanently impair some central vision, due to the burning of parts of the retina, or reduced night vision, and a decreased ability to focus. The risks versus benefits are assessed on an individual basis, considering overall health, lifestyle, medications taken, etc. and must be discussed with your ophthalmologist. The risks need to be weighed against the dangers of allowing bleeding to continue or of trying other procedures.

Low-level heat laser therapy (transpupillary thermotherapy, or TTT). This treatment delivers less power for longer periods of time and is typically thought to be a lower risk alternative to hot laser. It introduces specific wavelengths of light through the pupil to the retinal pigmented epithelium and choroid tissues. It is thought to help accelerate the healing process while limiting the risk of damage to the retinal pigment epithelium. TTT may be helpful in CSR that lasts over three months, as it may help the RPE reabsorb subretinal fluid. Anti-vascular growth-factor injections have mixed results, but in theory, may help, such as through the upregulation of tight junctions between endothelial cells and the reduction of abnormal vascular channels. [29] [30] [31] [32]

Methotrexate was shown to have potential as a treatment strategy.[33] Finasteride is a safe and effective treatment for CSCR, and it may be a possible new option for the initial management of patients with CSCR.[34]

Complementary Approach

The goal of the complementary approach is to nourish the retina, strengthen circulation and blood vessels, reduce inflammation naturally, and support overall eye health through targeted eye supplements, diet, and lifestyle modifications—all with the goal of preventing or reducing the risk of recurring CSCR. A range of nutrients has been well researched for helping improve circulation to the retina, improving retinal thickness, reducing inflammation, strengthening related blood vessels, and eliminating waste. Researchers have demonstrated that the following nutrients support retinal health and help improve retinal thickness.

Nutrients

Essential

Lutein. 10mg–20mg per day. In a study of patients with CSCR, short-term lutein supplementation did not increase the macular pigment thickness; however in CSCR patients who had low blood levels of lutein, such supplementation prevented an additional loss of macular pigment thickness.[35] In other studies of patients with chronic CSCR, lutein supplementation, used because of its antioxidant capacity, significantly reduced accumulation behind the retina.[36] Another study reported that 6mg of lutein may not be sufficient to improve retinal thickness. Even so, that level of supplementation did improve contrast and retinal sensitivity.[37]

Zeaxanthin. 2mg–12mg per day. Along with lutein, zeaxanthin is a potent antioxidant found in the retina that helps maintain the health of the retina (and reduce the risk of AMD.)[38]

Astaxanthin. 6mg–12mg per day. Researchers conclude that astaxanthin is effective in protecting against damage from light, due to its antioxidant effect.[39] [40]

Omega-3 fatty acids. 2,000mg–3,000mg per day. Researchers have found that omega-3 fatty acids have the capacity to actually regulate formation of blood vessels,[41] and along with lutein and zeaxanthin, they help preserve vision.

Vitamin D3. 2,000 IU–5,000 IU per day. This study found people with low levels of Vitamin D were at a higher risk for retinopathy. Additional studies investigating the link between vitamin D and indices of microvascular disease have shown that vitamin D deficiency is associated with poor coronary microcirculation.[42]

Resveratrol. 150mg–175mg per day (trans-resveratrol is a well absorbed form). This is a powerful antioxidant with anti-inflammatory properties and can inhibit formation of extra blood vessels.[43]

Grapeseed extract. 300mg per day, *and/or* **pycnogenol**[44] (pine bark extract, 50mg, 3 times per day). These have similar benefits, in that they help strengthen blood vessels while reducing inflammation. They can be taken along with resveratrol and help protect vision for those with a history of, or at high risk for, retinal bleeding. Grapeseed extract protects the central nervous system from reactive oxygen species.[45]

Vitamin C (buffered and ascorbated). 2,000mg–3,000mg per day. As an antioxidant, vitamin C scavenges free radicals in the body and protects tissues from oxidative stress.[46] [47]

Meriva, a curcumin-phosphatidylcholine complex. 500mg, 1-2 times per day. This is an effective and safe anti-inflammatory compound.[48]

Very Important

Bilberry 120mg–180mg per day. Along with supporting night vision, bilberry is neuroprotective and has been shown to improve microcirculation.[49] [50] [51] [52]

Ginkgo biloba. 120mg per day. Ginkgo extracts support vision quality.[53]

Taurine. 500mg–1,000mg per day. Taurine deficiency is linked to retinal degeneration; it has been used with some success to prevent, treat, and stabilize retinal changes.[54] [55] [56]

Multivitamin. Take a high-quality, whole-food, organic multivitamin.

Helpful

Green tea. 500mg–750mg per day. Green teas and their extracts are potentially neuroprotective in the photoreceptor outer segment and retinal pigment epithelium.[57]

A cortisol balancing formula. A study shows that idiopathic central serous chorioretinopathy is associated with morning elevated serum cortisol levels.[58] Adaptogen herbs may help; these include ginseng, ashwaganda, holy basil, cordyceps mushrooms, astragalus, licorice root, and rhodiola. Two products that also may help include AdrenaVen from Premiere Research and Cortisol Manager from Pure Encapsulations.

Diet

For general vision support we recommend the Vision diet described in Chapter 7.

Juicing. This juicing recipe is designed to help strengthen the retina and related blood vessels. Consume at least 6 oz. of juice per day of vegetables and fruits (preferably organic), and not too much fruit. Our recipe for this condition is some combination of the following. You can add your favorite fruits and vegetables.

- Ginger, garlic, leeks, parsley, beets, cabbage, carrots, celery, spinach, kale, collard greens, apples, grapes, raspberries, lemon, chlorophyll, and wheatgrasses

The juicing recipes are geared toward supporting healthy blood and blood flow, as well as providing a wide range of antioxidants that help keep your eyes and blood vessels healthy.

Lifestyle

Eye exercises are helpful for reducing strain and fatigue and improving circulation around the eyes. See Chapter 10-4 for eye exercises and acupuncture points that are good for eye conditions and overall eye health. We recommend you include these exercises:

- Palming and eye massage
- Near and far
- Hot dog

Exercise regularly. Daily aerobic exercise (speed walking, light jogging, hiking, using the elliptical machine at the gym, weightlifting with light weights and increasing repetitions, swimming, etc.) increases circulation, which helps deliver important nutrients to the eyes.

It is important not to over-exercise since excessive exercise releases cortisol that can reduce immunity and the body's ability to heal.

Other Modalities

Chinese Medicine

In Chinese medicine, the Liver "opens to the eyes" and is the primary meridian for supporting overall flow of energy and circulation through the eyes. The Kidney meridian nourishes the blood to the eyes. The Spleen meridian nourishes the blood while also helping to keep fluids from leaking from blood vessels.

Herbal Medicine:

Ming mu di huang wan (brighten the eyes) treats what is known as Kidney and Liver yin deficiency. Typical symptoms of yin deficiency include dryness, dizziness, night sweats, insomnia, and constipation, with the addition of dry eyes, blurry vision, sensitivity to light, photophobia (extreme light sensitivity), excessive tearing (specifically with exposure to wind), eye pain and/or swelling, and dizziness.

Zhu jing wan (preserve vistas pill) tonifies and nourishes the Liver and Kidneys, enriches the yin energy that includes supporting essential fluids in the body, and improves vision.

Gui pi tang (restore the Spleen decoction) increases qi, tonifies blood, strengthens the Spleen, nourishes the heart, and helps the Spleen control the blood. In traditional Chinese medicine, the heart controls the blood and stores shen (the spirit). The Spleen absorbs the nutrients from food and transports them to the blood. Poor transport of blood and the inability to completely absorb nutrients can affect eye health and contribute to a wide range of eye conditions, including ERM (epiretinal membrane) and macular degeneration.

Other herbal formulas to consider depending upon the underlying imbalance:

Hua jian er chen wan (decoction of two herbs: citrus and pinellia) treats phlegm-stasis congestion by strengthening and harmonizing the Spleen and stomach, drying dampness and transforming phlegm.

Si wu zi wan (four substance decoction) treats Liver and Kidney yin deficiency. It regulates the Liver, nourishes the blood, and improves blood circulation.

Sheng pu huang tang (pollen typhae) addresses yin deficiency fire. It helps to stop bleeding, invigorates the blood, and dispels blood stasis.

Xiao yao san (free and easy wanderer) calms the Liver and disperses Liver qi. It strengthens the Spleen to nourish the blood and harmonizes the Liver and Spleen.

San ren tang (three seed decoction) clears damp-heat and disperses and regulates qi.[59]

Other Therapies

Acupuncture, craniosacral, and gentle chiropractic treatments may offer some help. Also consider ayurvedic medicine, homeopathic remedies, and reiki. (See Appendix 7 for details of these therapies.)

Essential Oils

Carrot seed essential oil improves the eyes by protecting the retina, detoxifying blood vessels, toning the liver, relieving stress and anxiety, and providing nourishing vitamins and minerals.

Frankincense has been around since antiquity; it can be helpful in showing us our visual blind spots. Frankincense tells us to "open up that third eye."

Keep essences away from the mouth, eyes, and mucous membranes; if a few drops get in one of these sensitive areas it may be uncomfortable for 15–30 minutes, but not harmful. You can lessen

discomfort by adding a pure oil like olive or coconut oil to neutralize the irritating effect. For the eye area, dab a few drops around the outside of the eye. Do not put the neutralizing oil in the eye.

Combine ¼ cup of avocado oil with ¼ cup of calendula-infused oil. Slowly add 5 drops each of the essential oils. Then close the bottle and shake well; apply 4 drops of this mixture on your clean face. Massage in gentle circular motions. Leave overnight.

For more information, see Essential Oils in Appendix 9.

Also See

Chapter 7, Vision Diet

Chapter 8, Nutrients

Chapter 10-4, Eye Exercises

Chapter 15-18, Macular Degeneration

Appendix 5, Recommended Products

Appendix 6, Amsler Test

[1] Tsai, D.C., Chen, S.J., Huang, C.C., Chou, P., Chung, C.M., et al. (2013). Epidemiology of Idiopathic Central Serous Chorioretinopathy in Taiwan, 2001–2006: A Population-based Study. *PLoS One*, Jun 10.1371/journal.pone.0066858

[2] Gass, J.D. (1977). Photocoagulation treatment of idiopathic central serous choroidopathy. *Trans Sect Ophthalmol Am Acad Ophthalmol Otolaryngol*, 83(3 Pt 1):456–467.

[3] Yannuzzi L.A. (1986). Type A behavior and central serous chorioretinopathy. *Trans Am Ophthalmol Soc.* 84:799–845.

[4] Gilbert C.M., Owens S.L., Smith P.D., Fine S.L. (1984). Long-term follow-up of central serous chorioretinopathy. *Br J Ophthalmol*, 68(11):815–820.

[5] Ibid. Tsai. (2013).

[6] Dinc, U.A., Yenerel, M., Tatlipinar, S., Gorgun, E., Alimgil, L. (2010). Correlation of retinal sensitivity and retinal thickness in central serous chorioretinopathy. *Ophthalmologica*, 224(1):2-9

[7] Sasamoto, Y., Gomi, F., Sawa, M., Tsujikawa, M., Hamasaki, T. (2010). Macular pigment optical density in central serous chorioretinopathy. *Invest Ophthalmol Vis Sci*, Oct;51(10):5219-25.

[8] Putnam, C.M., Kinerk, W.T., Bassi, C.J. (2013). Central serous chorioretinopathy produces macular pigment profile changes. *Optom Vis Sci*, Jul;90(7):e206-12.

[9] Cohen, D., Gaudric, A., Coscas, G., Quentel, G., Binaghi, M. (1983). Diffuse retinal epitheliopathy and central serous chorioretinopathy. *J Fr Ophtalmol*, 6(4):339-49.

[10] Lin, H.Y., Peng, K.L. (2015). Bilateral Chronic Central Serous Chorioretinopathy (CSCR) Induced by Long-Term Testosterone Treatment. *J Clin Exp Ophthalmol*, 6:509.

[11] Jalkh, A.E., Jabbour, N., Avila, M.P., Trempe, C.L., Schepens, C.L. (1984). Retinal pigment epithelium decompensation. I. Clinical features and natural course. *Opthalmology*, Dec;91(12):1544-8.

[12] Haimovici, R., Koh, S., Gagnon, D.R., Lehrfeld, T., Willik, S. (2004). Risk factors for central serous chorioretinopathy: a case-control study. Ophthalmology, Feb;111(2):244-9.

[13] Ibid. Yannuzzi. (1986).

[14] Yannuzzi, L.A. (1987). Type-A behavior and central serous chorioretinopathy. *Retina*, 7(2):111–131.

[15] Spaide, R.F., Campeas, L., Haas, A., Yannuzzi, L.A., Fisher, Y.L., et al. (1996). Central serous chorioretinopathy in younger and older adults. *Ophthalmology*, Dec;103(12):2070-9.

[16] Polak, B.C., Baarsma, G.S., Snyers, B. (1995). Diffuse retinal pigment epitheliopathy complicating systemic corticosteroid treatment. *Br J Ophthalmol*, 79(10):922–925

[17] Carvalho-Recchia, C.A., Yannuzzi, L.A., Negrao, S., Spaide, R.F., Freund, K.B., et al. (2002). Corticosteroids and central serous chorioretinopathy. *Ophthalmology*, 109:1834-1837.

[18] Yannuzzi, L.A. (2010). Central serous chorioretinopathy: a personal perspective. *Am J Ophthalmol*, 149:361–363

[19] Türkcü, F.M., Yüksel, H., Sahin, A. (2014). Effects of smoking on visual acuity of central serous chorioretinopathy patients. *Cutan Ocul Toxicol*, 33(2):115–119

[20] Giusti, C. (2004). Association of Helicobacter pylori with central serous chorioretinopathy: hypotheses regarding pathogenesis. *Med Hypotheses*, 63(3):524-7.

[21] Colville, D., Guymer, R., Sinclair, R.A., Savige, J. (2003). Visual impairment caused by retinal abnormalities in mesangiocapillary (membranoproliferative) glomerulonephritis type II ("dense deposit disease"). *Am J Kidney Dis*, Aug;42(2):E2-5.

[22] Ibid. Colville. (2003).

[23] Ibid. Tsai. (2013).

[24] Klein, M.L., Van Buskirk, E.M., Friedman, E., Gragoudas, E., Chandra, S. (1974). Experience with nontreatment of central serous choroidopathy. *Arch Ophthalmol*, 91(4):247–250.

[25] Mudvari, S.S., Goff, M.J., Fu, A.D. (2007). The natural history of pigment epithelial detachment associated with central serous chorioretinopathy. *Retina*, 27(9):1168–1173

[26] Aggio, F.B., Roisman, L., Melo, G.B., Lavinsky, D., Cardillo, J.A., et al. (2010). Clinical factors related to visual outcome in central serous chorioretinopathy. *Retina*, 30(7):1128–1134.

[27] Salehi, M., Wenick, A.S., Law, H.A., Evans, J.R., Gehlbach, P. (2015). Interventions for central serous chorioretinopathy: a network meta-analysis. *Cochrane Database Syst Rev*, Dec 22;(12):CD011841.

[28] Ruiz-Moreno, J.M., Lugo, F.L., Armadá, F. (2010). Photodynamic therapy for chronic central serous chorioretinopathy. *Acta Ophthalmol*, 88(3):371–376

[29] Witkin, A.J., Brown, G.C. (2011). *Update on nonsurgical therapy for diabetic macular edema. Curr Opin Ophthalmol*, 22:185-9.

[30] Chiang. A, Regillo, CD. (2011). Preferred therapies for neovascular age-related macular degeneration. *Curr Opin Ophthalmol*, 22:199-204.

[31] London, N.J., Brown, G. (2011). Update and review of retinal vein occlusion. *Curr Opin Ophthalmol* 22:159-65.

[32] Mathur, V., Parihar, J.K.S., Maggon, R., Mishra, S.K. (2009). Role of Transpupillary Thermotherapy in Central Serous Chorio-Retinopathy. *Med J Armed Forces India*, Oct; 65(4): 323–327.

[33] Kurup, S.K., Oliver, A., Emanuelli, A., Hau, V., Callanan, D. (2012). Low-dose methotrexate for the treatment of chronic central serous chorioretinopathy: a retrospective analysis. *Retina*, 32(10):2096–2101.

[34] Moisseiev, E., Holmes, A.J., Moshiri, A., Morse, L.S. (2016). Finasteride is effective for the treatment of central serous chorioretinopathy. *Eye (Lond)*, Jun; 30(6): 850–856.

[35] Sawa, M., Gomi, F., Hara, C., Nishida, K. (2014). Effects of a lutein supplement on the plasma lutein concentration and macular pigment in patients with central serous chorioretinopathy. *Invest Ophthalmol Vis Sci*, Jul 29;55(8):5238-44

[36] Shinojima, A., Sawa, M., Sekiryu, T., Oshima, Y., Mori, R., et al. (2017). A Multicenter Randomized Controlled Study of Antioxidant Supplementation with Lutein for Chronic Central Serous Chorioretinopathy. *Ophthalmologica*, 237(3):159-166

[37] Sasamoto, Y., Gomi, F., Sawa, M., Tsujikawa, M., Nishida, K. (2011). Effect of 1-year lutein supplementation on macular pigment optical density and visual function. Graefes Arch Clin Exp *Ophthalmol*, Dec;249(12):1847-54.

[38] National Eye Institute. (2013). NIH Study provides clarity on supplements for protection against blinding eye disease. Retrieved Dec 10 2017 from https://nei.nih.gov/news/pressreleases/050513.

[39] Otsuka, t., Shimazawa, M., Nakanishi, T., Ohno, Y. Inoue, Y. et al. (2013). Protective effects of a dietary carotenoid, astaxanthin, against light-induced retinal damage. *J Pharmacol Sci*, 123(3):209-18.

[40] Ibid. Otsuka. (2013).

[41] Yanai, R., Mulki, L., Hasegawa, E., Takeuchi, K., Sweigard, H., et al. (2014). Cytochrome P450-generated metabolites derived from omega-3 fatty acids attenuate neovascularization. *Proc Natl Acad Sci USA*, Jul 1;111(26):9603-8.

[42] Capitanio S, Sambuceti G, Giusti M, et al. (2013). 1,25-Dihydroxy vitamin D and coronary microvascular function. *Eur J Nucl Med Mol Imaging*, 40:280–9.

[43] Wang, Z., Wang S., Yang, S., Yin, T., Zhang, Y., et al. (2017). Tissue Distribution of trans-Resveratrol and Its Metabolites after Oral Administration in Human Eyes, *J Ophthalmol*, Mar:4052094.

[44] Steigerwalt, R., Belcaro, G., Cesarone, M.R., Di Renzo, A., Grossi, M.G., et al. (2009). Pycnogenol improves microcirculation, retinal edema, and visual acuity in early diabetic retinopathy. *J Ocul Pharmacol Ther*, Dec;25(6):537-40.

[45] Balu, M., Sangeetha, P., Murali, G., Pnneerselvam, C. (2005). Age-related oxidative protein damages in central nervous system of rats: modulatory role of grape seed extract. *Int J Dev Neurosci*, Oct;23(6):501-7.

[46] Du, J., Cullen, J.J., Buettner, G.R., (2012). Ascorbic acid: chemistry, biology and the treatment of cancer. *Biochem Biophys Acta*, Dec;1826(2):443-57.

[47] Cangemi, R., Angelico, F., Loffredo, L., Del Ben, M., Pignatelli, P., et al. (2007). Oxidative stress-mediated arterial dysfunction in patients with metabolic syndrome: Effect of ascorbic acid. *Free Radic Biol Med*, Sep 1;43(5):853-9.

[48] Belcaro, G., Cesarone, M.R., Dugall, M., Pellegrini, L., Ledda, A., et al. (2010). Efficacy and safety of Meriva®, a curcumin-phosphatidylcholine complex, during extended administration in osteoarthritis patients. *Altern Med Rev*, Dec;15(4):337-44.

[49] Matsunaga, N., Imai, S., Inokuchi, Y., Shimazawa, M., Yokota, S., et al. (2009). Bilberry and its main constituents have neuroprotective effects against retinal neuronal damage in vitro and in vivo. *Mol Nutr Food Res*, Jul;53(7):869-77.

[50] Zhu, Y., Xia, M., Yang, Y., Liu, F., Li, Z., et al. (2011). Purified anthocyanin supplementation improves endothelial function via NO-cGMP activation in hypercholesterolemic individuals. *Clin Chem*, Nov;57(11):1524-33.

[51] Cohen-Boulakia, F., Valensi, P.E., Boulahdour, H., Lestrade, R., Dufour-Lamartinie, J.F., et al. (2000). In vivo sequential study of skeletal muscle capillary permeability in diabetic rats: effect of anthocyanosides. *Metabolism*, Jul;49(7):880-5.

[52] Yao, Y., Vieria, A. (2007). Protective activities of Vaccinium antioxidants with potential relevance to mitochondrial dysfunction and neurotoxicity. *NeuroToxicology*, 28 93–100.

[53] Lebuisson, D.A., Leroy, R., Rigal, G. (1896). Treatment of senile macular degeneration with Ginkgo biloba extract. A preliminary double-blind drug vs. placebo study. *Presse Med*, Sep 25;15(31):1556-8.

[54] Birdsall, T.C., (1998). Therapeutic applications of taurine. *Altern Med Rev*, Apr;3(2):128-36.

[55] Shpak, N.I., Naritsyna, N.I., Konovalova, N.V. (1989). Taufon and emoksipin in the combined treatment of sclerotic macular dystrophies. *Oftalmol Zh*, (8):463-5.

[56] Lombardini, J.B. (1991). Taurine: retinal function. *Brain Res Brain Res Rev*, May-Aug;16(2):151-69.

[57] Jarrett, S.G., Boulton, M.E. (2012). Consequences of oxidative stress in age-related macular degeneration. *Mol Aspects Med*, 2012 Aug;33(4):399–417.

[58] Zakir, S.M., Shukla, M., Simi, Z.U., Ahmad, J., Sajid, M. (2009). Serum cortisol and testosterone levels in idiopathic central serous chorioretinopathy. *Indian J Ophthalmol*, Nov-Dec; 57(6): 419–422.

[59] Qing-hua, P., Frank, C. O. (2014). TCM *Case Studies: Eye, Ear, Nose and Throat Disorders*. People's Medical Publishing House, Beijing, China.

15-4. COMPUTER VISION SYNDROME

Computer vision syndrome (CVS) is more commonly known as computer eyestrain; the medical term is asthenopia. This condition is the #1 vision complaint in the U.S. It consists of a combination of vision problems, typically noticed during and after long hours on the computer.

According to The Vision Council, 60% of Americans report eyestrain in the form of eye fatigue, dry eyes, headache, blurry vision, or shoulder and neck pain.[1] We spend an average of more than 8 hours a day using these digital devices.[2] Over 70% percent of American adults are now using a smartphone on a daily basis, compared with 50% three years ago. Smartphone and tablet use per day has nearly doubled in the last three years.[3] Americans aged 18 and older spend more than 11 hours a day engaged in a combination of digital-based activities: watching TV, watching videos, or using smartphones and other electronic devices.[4]

One thing is certain, digital devices are here to stay. They permeate so many aspects of American life today; yet, so few users are aware of the dangers they pose to eye health.

How the Eye Stays Rested

Eye Movement: The Saccade

Our eyes move constantly. They engage in incredibly rapid movements (hundreds of thousands a day) and jump around to take in parts of the seemingly endless number of scenes before us. The information taken in through this continual scanning movement is known as saccade or micro-saccade, and is transmitted to the brain so that we are able to perceive what is before us, without looking at every detail. The continual saccade is both involuntary and efficient, as the eyes travel from one bit of information to the next, forming a rapid understanding of the whole.

The function of the saccade is to continually refresh the information sent to the brain. Each saccade causes the image you see to shift to a different part of the retina, which allows the image to adapt to a new neuron in your eye and brain, and in turn, for the brain to interpret the scene afresh. So, these micro-saccades keep every changing thing visible for you.

However, when we blink, the saccade is interrupted. And when we are focusing intently, we do not want to interrupt that focus. Therefore, we tend to unknowingly stop blinking. And this is part of the problem causing computer eye vision.

Blink Rate and Eye Moisture

The tear film and the blinking process also make vision possible. Tear film is the moisture-laden surface of the eye, consisting of three layers (mucous layer, aqueous layer, and lipid layer). These interrelated layers work together to remove debris from the surface of the eye, to lubricate it, and protect it. Blinking, normally about 10–12 times a minute, helps to maintain the tear film.

Blinking momentarily disrupts the saccade. However, when we are intensely focused on one subject, whether on a computer screen in front of us or on a deer in the distance, blinking slows to an average of 3–4 times a minute. This allows us to maintain focus on the subject, since the information-gathering saccade is not interrupted.

A slower rate of blinking and/or incomplete blinking means that the tear film is not distributed across the surface of the eye, and we experience irritation and fatigue. The tear film begins to become unstable and thin *after only 10 seconds* without complete blinking. Since the tear film is so quickly dissipated, we recommend that you consciously engage your eyes in blinking when working at a computer.

Muscles of the Eye

In order to perform close work, several sets of muscles in the eye are active.

Extraocular muscles cause the eyes to converge to a specific location.

Ciliary muscles flex fibrous strands known as the "zonules of Zinn" that fine-tune the shape of the lens. When you look at your computer screen for a long time, the ciliary muscles remain contracted and eventually lose their ability to remain contracted. As the ciliary muscles loosen, their natural tension on the zonules of Zinn decrease, focus becomes blurry, pain sets in, and headaches and other symptoms result.

Pupillary muscles, cause the diameter of the pupil to constrict so that light rays hit only the center of the retina.

Furthermore, if you wear glasses or contacts, then your focus is locked into a specific range. Your eye muscles, not needing to shift for clearer focus, lose their muscle tone, their flexibility, and their ability to focus accurately.

Pathology of Computer Eyestrain

There are two main issues that cause computer eye fatigue and contribute to potentially serious vision problems, eye movement and distance, and blue light.

Eye Movement and Distance

Our daily activities form a tremendous shift from how our parents and grandparents lived. Since humans evolved as hunters and gatherers, our vision was designed for distance. Yes, there was some close-up work; but most of the time our ancestors needed to gaze afar to decide where they could most easily access food and water and to keep themselves safe from potential predators.

Our eye muscles are most relaxed when we are using our distance vision. In the absence of mostly close-up work, our grandparents' eyes flexed continually during the day, from near to far, from far to near. Vision problems arose when long hours of close work in poor light brought eyestrain.

Furthermore, we are also designed to move. Sitting all day in one position is unnatural and has consequences for both vision and general health. Studies show that digital device users blink about half as frequently, and the surface of their eyes gets drier.

Blue Light

While patients may be familiar with vision damage from UVA and UVB light from the sun, few are aware of the damage to the retina from blue light, or HEV light, which is emitted by digital screens, electronic devices, fluorescent energy-saving light bulbs, and LED lighting. The sun also emits blue light, so we are at risk for exposure while outdoors as well.

Because blue light is a short wavelength, it has more energy and "flickers" more easily than longer, weaker wavelengths. While not superficially noticeable, blue light creates glare, reduces visual contrast, affects vision acuity, and causes general eyestrain, headaches, and fatigue. The damaging effects of blue light are more serious in low light conditions when the pupil is enlarged and takes in more light. Consequently, the retina receives a larger dose of blue light.

Note. In natural light, blue light is combined with other spectrums of light that helps us maintain our circadian-rhythm. Artificial light at night can confuse out brains into thinking it is still daytime, affecting our ability to sleep well. The lack of blue light at night stimulates the pineal gland that produces adequate amounts of melatonin, which helps us sleep.

Consequences

Computer eyestrain is a contributing cause to a host of eye conditions including glaucoma, dry eye, advanced macular degeneration, damage to rods and cones, damage to the retinal pigmented layer of macula, and eye cancer.

In one study with university students regarding computer use and eye problems, many exhibited eye issues including the following: headache (53.3%), burning sensation in the eyes (54.8%) and tired eyes (48%).[5] While studies on the effects of computer eyestrain are not yet prevalent, taking a look at data related to repetitive strain injuries (RSIs) can help put this problem into perspective.

Glaucoma

Researchers found, in a 2004 study of more than 9,000 computer-based employees in Japan, that many of them were experiencing peripheral vision problems, and a third of those patients had visual field abnormalities (VFA), such as glaucoma. The incidence of glaucoma was higher when the workers also were nearsighted.[6] A 2017 study followed more than 2,000 workers (from the 2004 study group) who originally had no VFA for an additional seven years. There was a significant increased risk of VFA among this group.[7]

Dry Eye Syndrome

The innermost layer of the surface of the eye is an aqueous mucous layer that forms the bulk of the tears, and contains electrolytes, a variety of proteins, and water. This layer is vital to a stable ocular surface, since it allows the tear film to actually adhere to the eye.[8] Workers spending the most time on the computer have the lowest concentrations of an essential component of the mucous layer of the tear film, mucin 5AC, which contributes to their dry eye syndrome.[9] [10]

Photoreceptor Damage

The shortest wavelengths of light (UV and blue light), directly cause damage to the macula, retina, and photoreceptors. The retina contains cells that are impacted by blue light in both the photoreceptors and the retinal pigment epithelium layer (RPE). Photoreceptors contain photo-pigmented cells that change and trigger other functions when they are struck by a photon of light. In the RPE, pigmented cells absorb light and perform a number of functions. Both types of cells are vulnerable to blue light damage.[11]

Blue Light Damages Rods and Cones

Recent research using mice helps explain just how and why the eye is damaged by blue light. Mice that were exposed to high levels of blue light displayed the following characteristics:

- Massive irreversible cell death that was identified as shrinkage of protein, DNA, and RNA from both the inner and outer layers of photoreceptor rods and cones[12]
- Leaking and rupture of fine capillaries in retina cone photoreceptors
- Edema or swelling of the retina
- Development of cystoid spaces (cysts) further indicating edema
- Changes in expression of certain proteins
- Inner blood-retinal barrier damaged

In humans, this translates to widespread leaking and rupture of tiny blood vessels in the photoreceptor level of the macula, in turn, damaging the remainder of the macula. This may be expressed in a number of vision conditions, such as macular degeneration, choroid neovascularization, macular edema, retinitis pigmentosa, macular pucker, Stargardt's, cone-rod dystrophy, and diabetic retinopathy.

Rod Cell Protein

There's a light-sensitive protein called rhodopsin that is found in photoreceptor rod cells that supports vision in dim light. Rhodopsin levels are low in bright light and high in dim light. This protein triggers retinal damage by blue light during dim lighting conditions.[13] Furthermore, rods are more sensitive to blue light than cones, exacerbating the problem.[14] This is the reason that it is important to not use computers or smartphones emitting blue light during dim light conditions.

Retinal Pigment Epithelium (RPE)

Retinal pigment epithelium is a single-cell layer within the retina that provides nourishment to the photoreceptor cells and protects the division between the retina and the rest of the eye. It contains pigmented granules that absorb scattered light; it secretes a number of signaling photochemicals; it forms an immune-safe barrier between the photoreceptors and blood vessels; and it is an essential part of the vision process. Blue light harms the RPE, but just how is somewhat obscure. It is clear that such damage does occur, and that filtering, as with amber glasses, prevents such damage.[15]

Eye Cancer

Blue light is associated with significantly increased rates of cell division (mitosis), implicating it in uveal cancers. In some animal models, blue light was found to markedly increase the rate of cancer cell proliferation. In other animal studies where no uvea melanomas previously existed, exposure to blue light contributes to development of such cancers. Blue light stimulates the development of DNA lesions, especially in the presence of free radicals.[16]

Biochemical Change

A study published in 2018 found that blue light changes and damages a signaling biochemical, phosphatidylinositol 4,5 bisphosphate (PIP2), causing cell death; alpha-tocopherol reduces the change.[17]

Insomnia

The pineal gland secretes the hormone melatonin; this is the body's biochemical signal of biological darkness, in other words, the signal that you are ready for sleep. Blue light suppresses production of melatonin[18] to a surprisingly profound degree.[19] If you are exposed to blue light right before bedtime (e.g. checking your email one more time), it throws off the internal rhythm that allows you to get adequate sleep. Nearly 75% of children now use some sort of electronic device in their bedroom. The use of these devices markedly impacts sleep quality, which in turn, contributes to social adjustment problems, behavioral problems in school and at home, and surprisingly, weight gain.

While most research on the effects of smartphones on sleep and circadian rhythms have involved children and teens, adults are also adversely impacted. One Flemish study included more than 800 adults, 50% of whom owned smartphones, and 60% of whom used their smartphone during the night. Nighttime phone use and texting at night markedly increased how long it took to fall asleep and markedly decreased the quality, duration, and efficiency of sleep.

- In younger adults, nighttime electronic-device use was tied to more fatigue and later rising time.
- In older adults, it was associated with shorter sleep duration and earlier rise time.[20]

Similarly, it has been found that sleeping in a room that is not dark, also disrupts sleep, or makes it less effective in reducing fatigue and alleviating the accumulated stress of the day. Most studies found that exposure to light in the room, during sleep, reduces melatonin production by 50%.

Damage to Macula

Ongoing exposure to blue light increases the risk of neovascular (wet) macular degeneration, particularly associated with low levels of antioxidants, and especially low levels of vitamin C, zeaxanthin, and vitamin E.[21] Another study suggested that extended exposure to sunlight outdoors may be associated with age-related maculopathy.[22]

Blue Light Worsens Other Problems

Blue light in low-light conditions

The damaging effects of blue light are more serious in low-light conditions. The reason is simple. In low light conditions the pupil enlarges to take in more light, and consequently the retina receives a larger dose of blue light. This is one reason to not use computers, smartphones, and handheld devices (and TVs!) without other sources of light in the room.

Children under age 9 are particularly vulnerable to damage to the retina's RPE and photoreceptor cells from blue light emitted by computers, smartphones, and other handheld devices. This creates a dilemma for parents who find that providing children with handheld devices makes for peace in the family during long road trips, at the restaurant, and other places where children get impatient with adult activities.

Until about age 9, young children's eyes have not fully developed the protective pigment to help filter harmful blue light. Babies have little, if any melanin pigment in their eyes. The only pigment in our eyes is brown melanin. Whether we have blue, green, hazel, or brown eyes, depends simply on how much melanin is present—not whether there is blue pigment instead of brown pigment. Melatonin is important for filtering out blue light, and when there is little or no melatonin, then blue light is more dangerous. Additionally, in young children, blue light appears to retard the development of retinal nerve cells.

For this reason, it is very important that you restrict the use of handheld devices in young children. It is even more important that you restrict the use of such devices in dim light such as in the car at nighttime and the bedroom before lights are out. Similarly, it is very important that you make sure your children consume plenty of fresh fruits and vegetables, with plenty of important carotenoids that help protect the eyes from blue light damage.

Blue Light Damage in People with Blue Eyes

For the very same reason that young children are more susceptible to damage from blue light, adults with paler eyes are more vulnerable. People with blue eyes are the most vulnerable; people with green eyes are slightly less so; those with hazel colored irises are less at risk; and people with brown eyes are the least at risk. This is why blue eyes are considered a risk factor for conditions such as cataracts and macular degeneration.

Blue Light Flicker Phenomenon

One symptom of computer vision syndrome is caused in part by the blue light component of the visible light spectrum. Due to blue light's short-wavelength nature, it "flickers" more easily than longer, weaker wavelengths.[23] Such flickering, not superficially noticeable, creates glare, reduces visual contrast, affects vision acuity, and causes general eyestrain, headaches, and fatigue. This is yet another reason to take care with the number of hours you sit in front of your computer. If you have to spend long hours in front of the computer, make sure to take regular breaks to stretch and do some eye exercises. See Chapter 10-4 for more information.

Signs and Symptoms

Ways to reduce these symptoms and help preserve healthy vision are discussed in the Complementary Care section below. Symptoms can include:

- Eyestrain and fatigue
- Blurred or fuzzy vision
- Dizziness, upset stomach
- Difficulty focusing (concentrating) on work
- Headaches, including migraine headaches
- Dry, red, or irritated eyes
- Increased myopia (nearsightedness)
- Slow ability to refocus
- Excessive tiredness of the eyes, overall body fatigue
- Neck strain, shoulder, and upper and lower back pain
- Occasional double vision, eye-coordination problems

Causes and Risk Factors

We can experience computer eyestrain when we sit too close to the computer, spend too many hours at the computer, blink less, have poor posture, have poor lighting, or work in conditions with excessive glare.

The nature of these symptoms, whether acute or chronic, and their level of intensity, depends on a number of factors that include:

- How much time one spends overall on a digital device per day
- Length of sessions between breaks
- Whether the device and related lighting is set up properly (ergonomics)
- Whether prescription eyeglasses are needed to prevent eyestrain (not needed if one sees 20/20 without glasses at the distance needed from the computer)
- Number and frequency of breaks a person takes from the computer to relax his/her eyes, and potentially to do eye exercises
- Type of computer screen in use:
    - Most people use LCD screens today, a significant improvement over screens of the past.
    - In general, looking at monitors for long periods of time is not good for overall eye health.
    - The contrast and brightness settings matter more than the nature of the lighting efficiency.

- o In selecting the monitor, first choose an LCD panel (if you need it—IPS panel vs. TN panels vs. VA panels), then choose a backlight (color range, power use).
- o All monitors use LCD technology to create the image but may use either LEDs or CCFLs to backlight the LCD. An LED backlight recovers full brightness immediately upon being turned on or waking from sleep mode, and it uses less power than a CCFL backlight.
- o LEDs have ecological benefits and picture quality advantages, but emit blue light that damages the retina, circadian physiology and cognitive performance.[24]
- Text size
  - o The size should be three times the smallest size you can read from a normal viewing position, 20–30 inches from your monitor.
- Backgrounds and colors
  - o When it comes to color combinations, your eyes prefer black text on a white background or other dark-on-light combination. Avoid low contrast text/background color schemes.
- Eye problems
  - o If you have uncorrected eye problems such as astigmatism, farsightedness, or eye-related aging issues such as presbyopia, see your eye doctor to get the proper eyeglass prescription for computer use.

Less serious symptoms may temporarily clear up after a couple of weeks away from using the computer and other digital devices. For some, the symptoms can become chronic and intense enough that they can no longer use the computer for work.

When our eyes get tired, two things happen: the muscles of the eye become tired, and the surface of the eyes becomes too dry.

Computer Eyestrain in Children

Your child likely spends a lot more time on the computer than you realize. Depending on their age, they may use computers as much as you do, when considering time at school and at home. This can have a detrimental impact, so here are some points to be aware of:

- Your child can experience computer eyestrain and musculoskeletal disorders as a result of their computer use, especially with laptops and mobile devices.
- Extensive use can lead to eye tiredness, blurred vision, and headaches, which can increase irritability, as with adults.
- Some of the ways children use computers can make them even more susceptible.

Why? The American Optometric Association reports that:

- Children have the ability to keep playing or working on the computer with great concentration and without realizing that they are getting tired. True, adults are perfectly capable of the same actions, but they tend to have more self-awareness, and can recognize when they are getting tired.

- After we focus on one target and viewing distance, "accommodation problems" may result. The muscles of the eye become trained to a particular "setting" and have difficulty adjusting to other settings. A child may be unable to easily or smoothly focus on something else, like reading a book or doing homework, even long after they've left the computer.
- Blinking, which is necessary to keep the surface of the eyes moist and comfortable, is often compromised or inhibited when a person is staring at a computer screen. Gaming, in particular, promotes staring behavior; the smallest distraction may cause one to lose.
- Since the field of view is more upward when a child is engaged with a computer monitor or television than when working at a table or reading, the upper eyelids are more retracted than normal. Therefore, eyes experience more than the normal dryness and irritation.

Children are adaptable by nature, and tend not to think in terms of health. A child viewing a computer screen with a lot of glare may not even notice or think about creating a change to their environment; we have to teach them to do this.

There are other factors that contribute to eye fatigue and dryness; screen glare is one. Nearsightedness (myopia), farsightedness (hyperopia), and astigmatism are others. Because they have no comparison, children often think that their blurred vision is normal. So, unless a child's vision challenges are accompanied by headaches or other physical symptoms which they are able to communicate to an adult, eye issues may go unnoticed.

To exacerbate the situation, most computer workstations that a child uses are arranged for adult use. A child using a computer on a typical desk, looks up farther than an adult, which, over time, creates eye and neck strain. The best viewing angle is slightly downward—about 15 degrees. In addition, children may have difficulty reaching the keyboard or placing their feet on the floor, causing arm, neck, and back discomfort. Again, children are less aware of these physiological concerns, since their bodies are suppler and more flexible. They also tend to heal more rapidly than adults do, and they may not experience lingering symptoms due to physical discomfort.

Finally, children as well as adults often use computers with less than optimum lighting. The lighting level for proper computer use is about half as bright as that normally found in a classroom. Increased light levels can contribute to excessive glare and problems associated with the eye's adjustments to different levels of light.

Conventional Treatment

The conventional treatment is to set up your workstation properly to reduce eyestrain, and get evaluated by your eye doctor annually to make sure your prescription (if needed) is accurate. You will want to ensure proper lighting, viewing angles, the use of anti-glare screens, seating that supports correct posture, taking regular rest breaks, and remembering to blink frequently.

A program of vision therapy may be needed to treat eyestrain symptoms. Vision therapy, also called visual training, is a structured program of visual activities prescribed to improve visual abilities. To find a local vision therapist near you, you can go to www.oepf.org

Eyeglass lenses are available to help filter out blue light (including computer eyeglasses). These can be part of prescription glasses, or used by those who have 20/20 vision. This is particularly important for children and young adults, as they are more prone to eye lens and retinal damage over time from excessive exposure to blue light; their melanin production is not yet at 100%.

Software does exist that enables you to adjust the intensity of brightness and level of blue light emitted from the computer. Some computers may already have this built in.

Complementary Approach

Along with the ergonomic recommendations above, there are excellent supplements one can take to help protect the retina and lens from blue light, sun damage, and overall, help protect vision.

Nutrients

Lutein. 6mg–20mg per day. Combined with **zeaxanthin** and **black currant seed oil**, lutein helps protect the retina and eye lens from damage by filtering out light, and it has been shown to help reduce eyestrain.[25]

Zeaxanthin. 2mg–12mg per day. Carotenoid nutrients such as lutein and specific forms of zeaxanthin make up your macular pigment. This part of your retina protects underlying photoreceptor cells from the harmful effects of excess blue and ultraviolet light.[26][27][28]

Black currant seed oil. 200mg–500mg per day. Black currant seed oil has been shown to help symptoms associated with dry eyes.[29]

Astaxanthin. 6mg–12mg per day.[30] Test groups taking 6mg of astaxanthin improved significantly better at week 2 and 4 of the test period. Other research confirmed the previous findings that astaxanthin supplementation at 6mg for 4 weeks improves symptoms associated with tiredness, soreness, dryness, and blurry vision.[31][32][33]

Omega-3 fatty acids. 1,000mg–2,000mg per day.[34] Orally administered O3FAs alleviate dry eye symptoms, decrease tear evaporation rate, and improve Nelson grade in patients suffering from computer-vision-syndrome related dry eye.[35] Another study with older women showed reduced risk of dry eye syndrome with a high dietary intake of omega-3 fatty acids.[36]

Eye fatigue homeopathic pellets taken orally. Recommended dosage is 1–3 pellets dissolved in mouth 2–3 times per day (see Appendix 5).

Dry-eye eyedrops (no preservatives). Take as needed to keep eyes lubricated (see Appendix 5).

Diet

Follow the Vision diet in Chapter 7. This diet promotes proper circulation to and from the eyes, which helps keep the eyes well lubricated, and it provides essential nutrients such as lutein and zeaxanthin that are used both in the retina and the eye lens to help filter out UVA/UVB light.

Juicing. We recommend a combination of 4–6 of the nutrients below, along with your favorite fruits and vegetables (organic is preferable).

- Ginger, leeks, garlic, parsley, cabbage, beets, carrots, green-leafy vegetables, apples, celery, grapes, lemon, berries, wheatgrasses, (not too much fruit due to their high natural sugar content)

Lifestyle

Over time, too much computer use has negative effects that add up. Beyond the threat of direct damage to the retina from HEV blue light, other effects include the development of farsightedness (presbyopia), nearsightedness (myopia), astigmatism, poor eye coordination, and ability-to-focus disorders such as adjusting near to far vision quickly. In addition, sitting in the same position for hours causes potentially chronic neck, back, and shoulder stiffness, and tension headaches, which in turn, can cause TMJ (temporomandibular joint) pain.

Rest. Like other muscles in the body, our eye muscles need frequent rest in order to perform at their highest levels. One of the key aspects for preventing eyestrain is effective rest; see 10-4 for exercises and suggestions that alleviate eye stress.

Amber-colored lenses. These are the best color lenses for computer eyewear and sunglasses, because this particular color neutralizes blue light. Over time, UVA light affects the macula and contributes to the onset of macular degeneration and cataracts. The cornea and the lens absorb most UVB rays, so these rays may cause even more damage to your eyes than UVA rays.

Environmental light. Don't use computers, smartphones, and other handheld devices as well as televisions, without other sources of light in the room because dilated pupils allow more blue light from electronic devices to reach the retina.

20/20/20 rule. For adults, use the 20/20/20 rule: look away from your computer at least every 20 minutes and gaze at a distant object at least 20 feet away for at least 20 seconds. Then take a short 2-minute break every 30 minutes to stretch and do eye exercises.

Breathing. Poor posture and breathing habits reduce available oxygen that in turn adds stress to the physiology.

- Nose breathing allows for 20% more oxygenation than mouth breathing as breathing through the nose accesses the lower lobes of the lungs as well as releases nitric oxide.
- Correctly aligned posture that expands the lung can also increase oxygenation by at least 20%. Reduced breathing occurs due to a hunched over posture which compresses the lungs. This results in shallow breathing, which causes an imbalance in the oxygen and carbon dioxide ratio and a reduction in the ability of oxygen to enter into the body's cells (additionally activating the sympathetic nervous system and causing stress). This hunched posture can eventually become habitual, so even when standing, the person maintains a slouched posture. Additionally, a hunched posture collapses the lungs, which reduces the capacity of oxygen.

A humidifier in the winter helps keep your eyes more comfortable.

Remember to blink, full-blinks so that the eyelids touch briefly.

Check your medications for any side effects that may cause dry eyes.

Gently massage your eyelids several times a day to stimulate the tear glands.

Try reading from hardcopy books rather than from the computer or electronic readers.

Drink plenty of water throughout the day (non-caffeinated teas are fine as well).

Help Your Computer-Using Child

According to the American Optometric Association (AOA), infants should have their first comprehensive eye exam at 6 months of age. A follow-up exam should occur at age 3, and just before they enter the first grade, at about age 5 or 6. For school-aged children, the AOA recommends an eye exam every two years if no vision correction is required. Children who need eyeglasses or contact lenses should be examined annually, or as recommended by their optometrist or ophthalmologist; this will detect any hidden conditions that may contribute to eyestrain.

Time limits. Enforce strict time limits for computer use.

Computer arrangement. Check the height and arrangement of the computer. The child's size should determine how the monitor and keyboard are positioned. Use an adjustable chair that can be raised for comfort, and make sure the monitor is not too high for their field of view. Also, ensure that your child's arms are somewhat level to the desk as they reach for the mouse and keyboard. If your child's feet do not reach the floor, add a footstool under the desk that allows their legs and feet to relax, or get a chair that has comfortable rungs so they can rest their feet.

Glare. Check the desk and room lighting for glare on the computer screen from their viewing angle. Windows or other light sources should not be directly visible when sitting in front of the monitor. Glare is a common cause of eyestrain and headaches that can cause discomfort and loss of productivity, so glare filters for monitors can help reduce eyestrain.

Adjust lighting. Reduce the amount of lighting in the room to match that of the computer screen. Install a smaller light, or use a dimmer bulb, or dimmer switch to create adjustable lighting.

Also See

Chapter 15-7, Dry Eyes

Chapter 15-11, Glaucoma

Appendix 5, Recommended Products

---

[1] The Vision Council. (2017). Digital Eye Strain. Retrieved Dec 5 2017 from www.thevisioncouncil.org/content/digital-eye-strain.

[2] Nielson. (2017). The Neilson Total Audience Report, Q2, 2017. Retrieved Dec 5 2017 from www.nielson.com.

[3] Ibid. Nielson. (2017).

[4] Nielson. (2014). Content is King but Viewing Habits Vary by Demographic. Retrieved Oct 10 2017. http://www.nielsen.com/us/en/insights/news/2014/content-is-king-but-viewing-habits-vary-by-demographic.html.

[5] Shantakumari, N., Eldeeb, R., Sreedharan, J., Gopal, K. (2014). Computer Use and Vision-Related Problems Among University Students In Ajman, United Arab Emirate. *Med Health Sci Res,* 4 Mar-Apr; 4(2): 258–263.

[6] Tatemichi M, Nakano T, Tanaka K, Hayashi, T., Nawa, T. et al. (2004). Possible association between heavy computer users and glaucomatous visual field abnormalities: a cross sectional study in Japanese workers. *J Epidemiol Community Health,* Dec;58(12):1021-7.

[7] Nakano, T., Hayaski, T., Nakagawa, T., Honda, T., Owada, S., et al. (2017). Increased Incidence of Visual Field Abnormalities as Determined by Frequency Doubling Technology Perimetry in High Computer Users Among Japanese Workers: A Retrospective Cohort Study. *J Epidemiol,* Nov 25.

[8] JAMA Ophthalmol. 2014;132(8):985-992. doi:10.1001/jamaophthalmol.2014.1008

[9] Uchino, Y., Uchino, M., Yokoi, N. (2014). Alteration of Tear Mucin 5AC in Office Workers Using Visual Display Terminals: The Osaka Study. *JAMA Ophthalmol,* 132(8):985-992.

[10] Gipson, I.K., Hori, Y., Argueso, P. (2004). Character of ocular surface mucins and their alteration in dry eye disease. *Ocul Surf,* 2(2):131-148.

[11] Hunter, J.J., Morgan, J.I., Merigan, W.H., Sliney, D.H., Sparrow, J.R., et al. (2012). The susceptibility of the retina to photochemical damage from visible light. *Prog Ret Eye Res,* Jan;31(1):28-42.

[12] Geiger, P., Barben, M., Grimm, C., Samardzija, M. (2015). Blue light-induced retinal lesions, intraretinal vascular leakage and edema formation in the all-cone mouse retina. *Cell Death Dis,* Nov 19;6:e1985.

[13] Grimm, C., Wenzel, A., Williams, T., Rol, P., Hafezi, F., et al. (2001). Rhodopsin-mediated blue-light damage to the rat retina: effect of photoreversal of bleaching. *Invest Ophthalmol Vis Sci,* Feb;42(2):497-505.

[14] Anstis, S., Macleod, D. (2015). Why hearts flutter: Distorted dim motions. *J Vis,* 15(3): 23.

[15] Narimatsu, TI, Negishi, K., Miyake, S., Hirasawa, M., Osada, H., et al. (2015). Blue light-induced inflammatory marker expression in the retinal pigment epithelium-choroid of mice and the protective effect of a yellow intraocular lens material in vivo. *Exp Eye Res,* Mar;132:48-51.

[16] Logan, P., Bernabeu, M., Ferreira, A., Burner, M.N. (2015). Evidence for the Role of Blue Light in the Development of Uveal Melanoma. *J Ophthalmol,* 2015:386986.

[17] Ratnayake, K., Payton, J.L., Lakmal, O.H., Karunarathne, A. (2018). Blue light excited retinal intercepts cellular signaling. *Sci Rep,* Jul 5;8:10207

[18] Gooley, J.J., Chamberlain, K., Smith, K.A., Khalsa, S.B., Rajaratnam, S.M., et al. (2011). Exposure to Room Light before Bedtime Suppresses Melatonin Onset and Shortens Melatonin Duration in Humans. *J Clin Endocrinol Metab,* Mar;96(3):E463-72.

[19] Vartanian, G.V., Li, B.Y., Chervenak, A.P., Walch, O.J., Pack, W., et al. (2015). Melatonin Suppression by Light in Humans Is More Sensitive Than Previously Reported. *J Biol Rhythms,* Aug;30(4):351-4

[20] Exelmans, L., Van den Bulck, J. (2016). Bedtime mobile phone use and sleep in adults. *Soc Sci Med,* Jan;148:93-101.

[21] Fletcher, A.E., Bentham, G.C., Agnew, M., Young, I.S., Augood, C., et al. (2008). Sunlight exposure, antioxidants, and age-related macular degeneration. *Arch Ophthalmol,* Oct;126(10):1396-403.

[22] Cruickshanks, K.J., Klein, R., Klein, B.E. (1993). Sunlight and age-related macular degeneration. The Beaver Dam Eye Study. *Arch Ophthalmol,* 111(4):514-518.

[23] Blue Light Exposed. Where is the Increased Exposure to Blue Light Coming From? Retrieved Sep 20 2017 from http://www.bluelightexposed.com/where-is-the-increased-exposure-to-blue-light-coming-from.

[24] Cajochen, C., Frey, S., Anders, D., Spati, J., Bues, M., et al. (2011). Evening exposure to a light-emitting diodes (LED)-backed computer screen affects circadian physiology and cognitive performance. *J Appl Physiol,* May;110(5):1432-8.

[25] Yagi, A., Fujimoto, K., Michihiro, B., Goh, D., Tsi, H. (2009). The effect of lutein supplementation on visual fatigue: A psychophysiological analysis. *Appl Ergon,* Nov;40(6):1047-54.

[26] Piermarocchi, S., Saviano, S., Parisi, V., Tedeschi, M., Panozzo, G., Scarpa, G. et al. (2012). Carotenoids and antioxidants in age-related maculopathy. *Eur J Ophthalmol,* Mar-Apr;22(2):216-25

[27] Krinksy, N.I., Landrum, J.T., Bone, R.A. (2003). Biologic mechanisms of the protective role of lutein and zeaxanthin in the eye. *Annu Rev Nutr,* 23:171-201.

[28] Semba, R.D., Dagnelie, G. (2003). Are lutein and zeaxanthin conditionally essential nutrients for eye health? *Med Hypotheses,* Oct;61(4):465-72.

[29] Ibid. Yagi. (2009).

[30] Nagaki, Y, Hayasaka, S, Yamada, T, Hayasaka, Y, Sanada, M, et al. (2002). Effects of astaxanthin on accommodation, critical flicker fusions, and pattern evoked potential in visual display terminal workers. *J Trad Med,* 19(5):170-173.

[31] Astaxanthin for Eye Health. Retrieved Oct 10 2017 from http://ccres-aquaponics.blogspot.com/ 2014/04/the-effects-of-astaxanthin-eye-health.html.

[32] Nakamura, A., Isobe, R., Otaka, Y., Abematsu, Y., Nakata, D., et al. (2004). Changes in Visual Function Following Peroral Astaxanthin. *Japan J Clin Opthal,* 58(6):1051-1054.

[33] Takahashi, N., Kajita, M. (2005). Effects of astaxanthin on accommodative recovery. *J Clin Therap Med,* 21(4):431-436.

[34] Gatell-Tortajada, J. (2016). Oral supplementation with a nutraceutical formulation containing omega-3 fatty acids, vitamins, minerals, and antioxidants in a large series of patients with dry eye symptoms: results of a prospective study. *Clin Interv Aging,* May 19;11:571-8.

[35] Bhargava, R., Kumar, P., Phogat, H., Kaur, A., Kumar, M. (2015). Oral omega-3 fatty acids treatment in computer vision syndrome related dry eye, *Con Lens Ant Eye,* Jun;38(3):206-10.

[36] Ribelles, A., Galbis-Estrada, C., Parras, M.A., Vivar-Llopis, B. Marco-Ramirez, C., et al. (2015). Ocular Surface and Tear Film Changes in Older Women Working with Computers, *Biomed Res Int,* 2015:467039.

15-5. CONE-ROD DYSTROPHY

Cones and rods are the photoreceptor cells that enable us to see. The cones and rods change light into electric nerve impulses that travel to our brain via our optic nerve. Cone-rod (or rod-cone) dystrophy is the condition in which these critical cells degenerate. Most sources estimate the incidence as approximately 1 in 40,000 in the general population.[1]

What is Cone-Rod Dystrophy?

The term cone-rod dystrophy (CRD) describes a group of rare photoreceptor disorders affecting first, the cones, and then the rods of the retina.

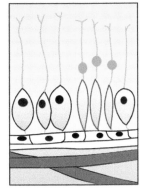
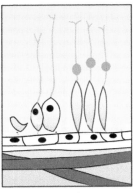
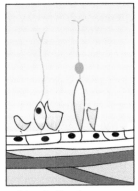

Healthy Rods   Fewer, Shorter   Next, Rods are
and Cones   Abnormal Cones   Damaged

Cone-rod dystrophy is a disorder caused by the malfunction or degeneration of rod and cone cells. Cone receptors, which are important for color vision and detail, are lost first, followed by rods. The severity of symptoms associated with cone-rod dystrophy vary significantly. Many cases are genetically based, while others are idiopathic (doctors don't know why they develop). Cone-rod dystrophy may first appear in childhood with the failing of some photoreceptor cells, though symptoms may not appear until adulthood.

Although complete blindness from cone-rod dystrophy is rare, vision can worsen to 20/200, or less, for those with the progressive form of cone-rod dystrophy.

Cones and Rods

The back of the eyeball is covered with the thin layer called the retina, which is responsible for collecting information from light and conveying it to the optic nerve. At the front of the retina is a thin layer of neurons connected to photoreceptor cells: cones and rods. Cone and rod photoreceptor cells have distinctive functions; they help us detect different things.

Cones are clustered near the macula at the center of the retina. They are good at "seeing" the following:

- Objects that are not moving
- Objects in daylight
- Colors and subtleties of color
- Objects in fine detail, including reading and recognizing faces

Rods are found all over the retina except in the macula. They are good at "seeing" the following:

- Objects that move, but only in black and white
- In the dark and in very dim light
- Objects to either or both of our sides (peripheral vision)

Types of Cone-Rod Dystrophy

There are two broad groups of CRD[2]:

Stationary CRD begins to develop during infancy or childhood and symptoms remain stationary for most of life.

Progressive CRD usually develops a little later, in late childhood or early adulthood. The symptoms progressively worsen to legal blindness, but usually not complete blindness unless the rods also deteriorate.

Signs and Symptoms

Symptoms of cone-rod dystrophy are similar to those of a number of other conditions and include the following:

- Gradual loss of night vision
- Gradual loss of peripheral vision
- Sensitivity to bright light
- Best vision at dusk
- Errors in color vision in both red-green and blue-yellow ranges

Young children may develop the following:

- A condition called **nystagmus** wherein the eyes make repetitive, uncontrolled movements, which can result in reduced vision and depth perception
- **Roving eye movements**, where the eyes appear to slowly wander without fixing or remaining still on objects
- **Eye poking**, where the child touches their eyes with their fingers

For an accurate diagnosis, an exam is necessary. Cone-rod dystrophy displays a distinct electroretinogram (ERG) pattern that an eye doctor can identify.

Related Conditions

- Retinitis pigmentosa. With this condition, photoreceptors and RPE deteriorate. Early cone-rod dystrophy typically shows up as loss of the cones, as distinct from retinitis pigmentosa, which starts with the loss of the rods, affecting peripheral and night vision. The effect of CRD is generally more severe and rapid than that of RP, leading to earlier legal blindness and disability. At end stage, however, CRD does not differ from RP.
- Leber's congenital amaurosis in which many different genes are to be involved.
- Stargardt disease. A rare juvenile form of macular degeneration.
- Syndromic cone dystrophy. An umbrella term that includes a range of eye diseases, such as Refsum disease, Bardet-Biedl syndrome, NARP syndrome, Batten disease, and spinocerebellar ataxia type 7.[3]

Causes and Risk Factors

Most causes are genetically based and result from "misprints" in a child's genes. These misprints are typically carried forward from the parents' genes; although sometimes by chance, a misprint occurs in a child's genes when the parents' genes are normal.

There are over 30 types of cone-rod dystrophy caused by mutations in several different genes that can be inherited. Mutations occur in genes that are responsible for making proteins, which are critical in the development, functioning, and health of the photoreceptors.[4] There are several classifications of genetically-based CRD.[5]

Dominant. Autosomal dominant means that a mutated gene from only one parent is necessary to cause cone-rod dystrophy. For example, the father may have a mutated gene but the mother does not. Each parent gives two genes to children; the mother gives two normal genes; the father gives one normal and one mutated gene and that gene is dominant.

Recessive. Autosomal recessive means that gene mutations must come from both parents. Each parent has one mutated gene and one normal gene. Children may get two mutated (they are affected); one normal and one mutated (they are carriers); or two normal genes and they do not have the mutation.

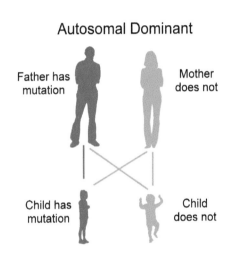

Autosomal Dominant

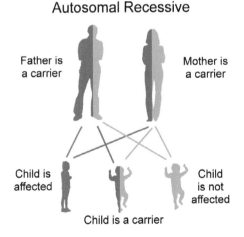

Autosomal Recessive

X-linked recessive. Mutations of the X chromosomes can occur in either the mother or the father, and both can pass the mutation to their children. If the mother carries the recessive gene she does not exhibit the mutation. But half of her sons can inherit the mutated x chromosome, and half of her daughters will inherit and be a carrier, but not have the disease. If the father has the mutation, his son is not affected, but his daughter can be a carrier. Men can pass the mutation to their daughters, but not their sons. Usually only men have this form of CRD.

X-Linked Recessive

This is just one example of x-linked; there are both recessive and dominant mutations, and either men or women can be affected.

Father has mutation

Mother does not

Son is not affected

Daughter is a carrier

Autosomal Dominant

- Gene CRX,[6] known as the cone-rod homeobox gene, is also implicated in Leber's and retinitis pigmentosa. The CRX gene influences cells in the pineal gland.[7]
- Gene GUCY2D is triggered by abnormal sensitivity to calcium regulation.[8] There has been some investigation into links between this mutation and oxidative stress.[9] [10]
- Gene GCAP1 mutations also cause severe, abnormal-calcium sensitivity and regulation.
- Gene HRG4 is a protein in photoreceptor nerve synapses.[11]
- Loci CRD, the term "loci" refers to the position of genes on chromosomes, and CORD7.

Autosomal Recessive

- Gene ABCA4 causes Stargardt Disease and also 30–60% of autosomal recessive CRDs.[12] [13] Some research suggests that in the absence of healthy ABCA4, tissue is vulnerable to acute oxidative stress.[14] Another researcher mentions the increased oxidative environment in ABCA4 mutations.[15]
- Loci CORD9 and CORD8.

X-Linked (CORDX1, 2 and 3)

- RPGR mutations cause CORDX1 which is about two-thirds of X-linked retinitis pigmentosa and is also an undetermined percentage of X-linked cone-rod dystrophy.
- An unknown gene (at location xq27) causes CORDX2.
- CACNA1F causes CORDX3. Mutations in this gene also cause night blindness.
- When no cause of CRD can be identified, the case is labeled as idiopathic (cause not known). Also, environmental factors may contribute to causes.

Conventional Treatment

There is no effective conventional treatment for stopping sight loss due to cone-rod dystrophy, nor is there any conventional way to slow down the progression of vision loss for those with the progressive form of cone-rod dystrophy. Eye doctors may recommend using red-tinted lenses or dark sunglasses in bright environments, magnifying devices to assist in reading, and other similar activities. They may also recommend targeted vitamins.

Complementary Approach

The body is always trying to maintain optimal health even in the face of genetic disorders. There is a wide range of research available that identifies the nutrients used in the retina that are needed to support photoreceptors and vision health. Targeted supplements that have been shown to help protect the photoreceptor cells from damage may be helpful.

It has been recognized by scientists that oxidative stress is a key factor in many eye diseases and in gene mutation. Links have been made between oxidative stress and gene mutations. While there is no direct evidence in the case of genes and loci linked to CRD, oxidative stress may well be a factor, and it therefore seems reasonable to support the body's antioxidant functions.[16] [17]

Nutrients

Although research for nutrients that specifically help with cone-rod dystrophy is limited, there are many studies showing the benefit for related retinal diseases, including retinitis pigmentosa and macular degeneration. Some of the following nutrients are antioxidants or support antioxidant functioning. In addition, researchers have suggested that it can be useful for patients with retinal degeneration, including retinitis pigmentosa, to supplement with nutrients such as vitamin A, lutein, omega-3 fatty acids, zeaxanthin, and astaxanthin. While these nutrients are not a cure, they may slow progression[18] [19] [20] and vision loss.[21] [22] [23]

Essential

Lutein. 10mg-20mg per day. This is an essential antioxidant for maintaining the health of the retina and protecting the retina and lens from sunlight damage.[24] [25] [26]

Vitamin A palmitate. 5,000 IU–15,000 IU per day is essential for the proper functioning of the photoreceptor cells in processing light and rebuilding.[27] [28]

> **Note**. Vitamin A is contra-indicated for those suffering from Stargardt disease (see Stargardt's chapter for more information). Pregnant women should not take vitamin A.

Zeaxanthin. 2mg–12mg per day. Carotenoid nutrients such as lutein and specific forms of zeaxanthin make up your macular pigment. This part of your retina protects underlying photoreceptor cells from the harmful effects of excess blue and ultraviolet light.[29] [30]

Omega-3 fatty acids. 3,000 IU–4,500 IU per day. DHA from omega-3 fatty acids accounts for approximately 50–60% of the total fatty acid content within outer segments of photoreceptor rods. OFAs tend to be very deficient in today's diet[31] [32] but are needed for maintaining retinal health.[33]

Taurine. 750mg–1,000mg per day. When taurine levels are deficient, a variety of vision problems can occur, such as retinal ganglion cell degeneration.[34]

Bilberry. 180mg–240mg per day. Bilberry extracts have antioxidative properties that are not only neuroprotective, but also help suppress photooxidative processes. They improve capillary integrity. Bilberry's anthocyanosides may be especially beneficial for night vision.[35] [36] [37] [38]

Vitamin C (buffered and ascorbated). 1000mg–2,000mg per day. Nerve cells in the eye require vitamin C in order to function properly[39] and have been found to be bathed in vitamin C.[40] As an antioxidant, vitamin C scavenges free radicals and protects tissues from oxidative stress.[41]

Grapeseed extract. 300mg per day. Grapeseed extract, a bioflavonoid, is a potent antioxidant and protects the central nervous system from reactive oxygen species.[42]

Ginkgo biloba. 120mg per day. Ginkgo biloba improves microcapillary circulation in the eye and slows deterioration of the macula through its antioxidant effects.[43][44] It improves overall circulation,[45] stabilizes capillaries, and makes capillaries less fragile.[46][47]

Saffron. 20mg per day. Saffron helps protect photoreceptor cells from damage and supports healthy circulation in the retina.[48][49]

Very Important

Mesozeaxanthin. 10mg per day. A combination of lutein, zeaxanthin, and mesozeaxanthin may be needed for healthy retinal vision for people with abnormal retinal pigmentation.[50]

Multivitamin (whole-food and organic). Take daily and include the range of B vitamins, which have neuroprotective properties that support vision health. By taking a good multivitamin, you are supporting overall body health. As the health of the eyes is directly connected to overall body health, keeping the body nourished is essential for maintaining healthy vision.

Vitamin D3. 2,000 IU–5,000 IU per day. Studies investigating the link between vitamin D and indices of microvascular disease have shown that vitamin D deficiency is associated with poor coronary microcirculation.[51]

Astaxanthin. 6mg–12mg per day. This nutrient is a red-orange carotenoid from microalgae, fish, and crustaceans. Astaxanthin is also unique among the antioxidants in that it spans both layers of the cell membrane, allowing it to trap free radicals, outside and inside the cell. Astaxanthin's powerful antioxidant benefits help prevent retinal damage[52] and protect against sun damage.[53][54]

Trans-resveratrol. 150mg–250mg per day. Studies indicate that resveratrol may be the most effective compound for maintaining optimal health and promoting longevity. This study shows that resveratrol may be effective in the microcirculation of the eye.[55]

Helpful

Zinc. 30mg–60mg per day, with copper in an approximate 15:1 ratio. Zinc supports cardiovascular and neurological health and helps maintain vision in the elderly.[56]

Diet

Juicing. Choose at least 4-6 items to combine.

- Broccoli, yellow and orange bell pepper, apples, blueberries, raspberries, green-leafy vegetables, carrots (preferably all organic)

- Add your favorite fruits and vegetables, but not too many sweet fruits and vegetables.

See the information on Vision diet in Chapter 7.

Lifestyle

Eye exercises. We recommend these eye exercises:

- Eye massage of acupressure points
- Near and far
- Palming

See the information in Chapter 10 on Eye Exercises.

Other Modalities

Chinese Medicine

The following are common Chinese medicine patterns related to cone-rod dystrophy and retinitis pigmentosa:

You gui wan. Restore the right decoction helps warm the body by warming and tonifying the Kidney yang-heat meridians, which raises warmth and energy to the eyes.

Gui pi tang. Restore the Spleen decoction increases qi, tonifies blood, strengthens the Spleen, nourishes the Heart, and helps the Spleen control the blood.

Bu zhong yi qi tang. Central qi tea is a popular formula used for coordinating Spleen and Stomach, which supports healthy digestion and the distribution of nutrients through the body.

Zhu jing wan. Preserve vistas pill tonifies and nourishes the Liver and Kidneys, enriches the yin, and improves vision.

Ming mu di huang wan (brighten the eyes) nourishes the Liver, enriches the Kidneys, and improves vision.

Xiao yao san (free and easy wanderer) calms the Liver and disperses Liver qi. It strengthens the Spleen to nourish the blood and harmonizes the Liver and Spleen.

Herbal formula and treatment strategies can vary significantly based on the Chinese medicine practitioner's evaluation and intake.

On the Horizon

There are future treatments on the horizon for gaining lost vision such as stem cells to regenerate lost rods and cones,[57] implants of electronic chips to imitate the function of rods and cones,[58] retinal transplants, and genetic defect repair through gene therapy.[59]

Also See

Chapter 7, Vision Diet

Chapter 8, Nutrients

Chapter 10-4, Eye Exercises

Chapter 15-15, Leber's Disease

Chapter 15-18, Macular Degeneration

Chapter 15-27, Retinitis Pigmentosa

Chapter 15-29, Stargardt Disease

1 Hamel, C. P. (2007). Cone rod dystrophies. *Orphanet J Rare Dis,* 2007; 2:7.

[2] Heckenlively, J. Cone Dystrophy. Retrieved Mar 28 2018 from https://rarediseases.org/rare-diseases/cone-dystrophy/

[3] Ibid. Heckenlively. RareDiseases.org.

[4] Ibid. Heckenlively. RareDiseases.org.

[5] Ibid. Heckenlively. RareDiseases.org.

[6] Griffith, J.F., DeBenedictis, M.J., Traboulsi, E.I. (2018). A novel dominant CRX mutation causes adult-onset macular dystrophy. *Ophthalmic Genet,* Jan-Feb:39(1):120-124.

[7] Rovsing, L., Clokie, S., Bustos, D.M., Rohde, K., Coon, S.L. (2011). CRX broadly modulates the pineal transcriptome. *J Neurochem,* Oct;119(2):262-74.

[8] Sato, S., Peshenko, I.V., Olshevkaya, E.V., Kefalov, V.J., Dizhoor, A.M. (2018). GUCY2D Cone-Rod Dystrophy-6 Is a "Phototransduction Disease" Triggered by Abnormal Calcium Feedback on Retinal Membrane Guanylyl Cyclase 1. *J Neurosci,* Mar 21;38(12):2990-3000.

[9] Lustremant, C., Habeler, W., Plancheron, A., Goureau, O, Grenot, L., et al. (2013). Human induced pluripotent stem cells as a tool to model a form of Leber congenital amaurosis. *Cell Reprogram,* June; 15(3):233-46.

[10] Boye, S.L., Peterson, J.J., Choudhury, S., Min, S.H., Ruan, Q., et al. (2015). Gene Therapy Fully Restores Vision to the All-Cone Nrl−/−Gucy2e−/− Mouse Model of Leber Congenital Amaurosis-1. *Hum Gene Ther,* Sept 1; 26(9):575-592.

[11] Kobysaki, A., Higashide, T., Hamasaki, D., Kubota, S., HRG4 (UNC119) Mutation Found in Cone–Rod Dystrophy Causes Retinal Degeneration in a Transgenic Model. *Invest Ophthalmol Vis Sci,* Oct;41(11): 3268-77.

[12] Maugeri, A., Klevering, B.J., Rohschneider, K., Blankenagel, A., Brunner, H.G., et al. (2000). Mutations in the ABCA4 (ABCR) Gene Are the Major Cause of Autosomal Recessive Cone-Rod Dystrophy. Am J Hum Genet, Oct; 67(4): 960-966.

[13] Ducroq, D., Rozet, J.M., Gerber, S., Perrault, I., Barbet, F., et al. (2002). The ABCA4 Gene in Autosomal Recessive Cone-Rod Dystrophies. *Am J Hum Genet,* Dec; 71(6); 1480-1482.

[14] Parmar, T., Parmar, V.M., Arai, E., Sahu, B., Perusek, L., et al. (2016). Acute Stress Responses Are Early Molecular Events of Retinal Degeneration in Abca4-/-Rdh8-/- Mice After Light Exposure. *Invest Ophthalmol Vis Sci,* June 1;57(7):3257-67.

[15] Radu, R.A., Hu, J., Yuan, Q., Welch, D.L., Makshanoff, J., et al. (2011). Complement System Dysregulation and Inflammation in the Retinal Pigment Epithelium of a Mouse Model for Stargardt Macular Degeneration. *J Biol Chem,* May 27; 286(21):8593-18601.

[16] Ibid. Ducroq. (2002).

[17] Ibid. Parmar. (2016).

[18] Berson, E. L., Rosner, B., Sandberg, M. A., Hayes, K. C., Nicholson, B. W., et al. (1993). A randomized trial of vitamin A and vitamin E supplementation for retinitis pigmentosa. *Arch Ophthalmol,* Jun;111(6):761-72.

[19] Berson, E.L., Rosner, B., Sandberg, M.A., Weigel-DiFranco, C., Moser, A., et al. (2004). Further evaluation of docosahexaenoic acid in patients with retinitis pigmentosa receiving vitamin A treatment: subgroup analyses. *Arch Ophthalmol,* Sep; 122(9): 1306-14.

[20] Hoffman, D.R., Locke, K.G., Wheaton, D.H., Fish, G.E., Spencer, R., et al. (2004). A randomized, placebo-controlled clinical trial of docosahexaenoic acid supplementation for X-linked retinitis pigmentosa. *Am J Ophthalmol,* Apr;137(4):704-18.

[21] Aleman, T.S., Duncan, J.L., Bieber, M.L., de Castro, E., Marks, D.A., et al. (2001). Macular pigment and lutein supplementation in retinitis pigmentosa and Usher syndrome. *Invest Ophthalmol Vis Sci,* Jul;42(8):1873-81.

[22] Bahrami, H., Melia, M., Dagnelie, G. (2006). Lutein supplementation in retinitis pigmentosa: PC-based vision assessment in a randomized double-masked placebo-controlled clinical trial [NCT00029289]. *BMC Ophthalmol,* Jun 7;6:23.

[23] Berson, E.L., Rosner, B., Sandberg, M.A., Weigel-DiFranco, C., Brockhurst, R.J., et al. (2010). Clinical trial of lutein in patients with retinitis pigmentosa receiving vitamin A. *Arch Ophthalmol,* Apr;128(4):403-11.

24 Bernstein, P. S., Zhao, D., Wintch, S. W., Ermakov, I. V., McClane, R. W. (2002). Resonance Raman Measurement of Macular Carotenoids in Normal Subjects and in Age-related Macular Degeneration Patients. *Ophthalmology,* Oct; 109(10): 1780–1787.

25 Ibid. Berson. (2010).

26 Ibid. Bahrami. (2006).

27 Saari, J. C. (2012). Vitamin A metabolism in rod and cone visual cycles. *Annu Rev Nutr,* Aug 21;32:125-45.

28 Ibid. Berson. (1993).

29 Piermarocchi, S., Saviano, S., Parisi, V., Tedeschi, M., Panozzo, G., Scarpa, G., Boschi, G. (2012). Carotenoids in Age-related Maculopathy Italian Study (CARMIS): two-year results of a randomized study. *Eur J Ophthalmol,* Mar-Apr;22(2):216-25.

30 Krinsky, N., Landrum, J. T., Bone, R.A. (2003). Biologic mechanisms of the protective role of lutein and zeaxanthin in the eye. *Annu Rev Nutr,* 23:171-201.

31 Bush RA, Malnoe A, Reme CE, Williams TP. (1994). Dietary deficiency of N-3 fatty acids alters rhodopsin content and function in the rat retina. *Invest Ophthalmol Vis Sci,* 35(1):91–100.

32 Stillwell, W., Wassall, S.R. (2003). Docosahexaenoic acid: membrane properties of a unique fatty acid. *Chem Phys Lipids,* 126(1):1–27

33 Elner, V. M. (2002). Retinal pigment epithelial acid lipase activity and lipoprotein receptors: effects of dietary omega-3 fatty acids. *Trans Am Ophthalmol Soc,* 100:301–338.

34 Froger, N., Cadetti, L., Lorach, H., Martins, J., Bemelmans, A.P. (2012). Taurine provides neuroprotection against retinal ganglion cell degeneration. *PLoS One,*7(10):e42017.

35 Muth, E. R., Laurent, J. M., Jasper, P. (2000). The effect of bilberry nutritional supplementation on night visual acuity and contrast sensitivity. *Altern Med Rev,* Apr;5(2):164-73.

36 Matsunaga, N., Imai, S., Inokuchi, Y., Shimazawa, M., Yokota, S., et al. Bilberry and its main constituents have neuroprotective effects against retinal neuronal damage in vitro and in vivo. *Mol Nutr Food Res,* Jul;53(7):869-77.

[37] Yao, Y., Vieira, A. (2007). Protective activities of Vaccinium antioxidants with potential relevance to mitochondrial dysfunction and neurotoxicity. *Neurotoxicology,* Jan;28(1):93-100.

38 Fiorini, G., Biancacci, A., Graziano, F. M. (1965). Perimetric and adaptometric modifications after ingestion of myrtillin associated with betacarotene. *Ann Ottalmol Clin Ocul,* 1965;91:371-86.

39 Calero, C. I., Vickers, E., Moraga Cid, G., Aguayo, L. G., von Gersdorff, H., et al. (2011). Allosteric Modulation of Retinal GABA Receptors by Ascorbic Acid. *J Neurosci,* Jun 29;31(26):9672-82.

40 OHSU News. OHSU scientists discover new role for vitamin C in the eye - and the brain. Retrieved Dec 04 2017 from https://news.ohsu.edu/2011/07/14/ohsu-scientists-discover-new-role-for-vitamin-c-in-the-eye-and-the-brain

41 Du, J., Cullen, J.J., Buettner, G.R. (2012). Ascorbic acid: chemistry, biology and the treatment of cancer. *Biochem Biophys Acta,* Dec;1826(2):443-57.

42 Balu, M., Sangeetha, P., Murali, G., Panneerselvam, C. (2005). Age-related oxidative protein damages in central nervous system of rats: modulatory role of grape seed extract. *Int J Dev Neurosci,* Oct;23(6):501-7.

43 Droy-Lefaix, M.T., Cluzel, J., Menerath, J.M., Bonhomme, B., Doly, M. (1995). Antioxidant effect of a Ginkgo biloba extract (EGb 761) on the retina. *Antint J Tissue React,* 17(3):93-100.

44 Thiagarajan, G., Chandani, S., Harinarayana Rao, S., Samuni, A.M., Chandrasekaran, K., (2002). Molecular and cellular assessment of ginkgo biloba extract as a possible ophthalmic drug. *Exp Eye Res,* Oct;75(4):421-30.

45 Wu, Y.Z., Li, S.Q., Zu, X.G., Du, J., Wang, F.F. (2008). Ginkgo biloba extract improves coronary blood flow in healthy elderly adults: role of endothelium-dependent vasodilation. *Phytomedicine,* Mar;15(3):164-9.

46 Welt, K., Weiss, J., Martin, R., Hermsdorf, T., Drews, S., et al. (2007). Ginkgo biloba extract protects rat kidney from diabetic and hypoxic damage. *Phytomedicine*, Feb;14(2-3):196-203.

47 Qiu, Y., Rui, Y.C., Li, T.J., Zhang, L., Yao, P.Y. (2004). Inhibitory effect of extracts of Ginkgo biloba leaves on VEGF-induced hyperpermeability of bovine coronary endothelial cells in vitro. *Acta Pharmacol Sin,* 2004 Oct;25(10):1306-11.

48 Marangoni, D., Falsini, B., Piccardi, M., Ambrosio, L., Minnella, A.M., Savastano, M.C., (2013). Functional effect of Saffron supplementation and risk genotypes in early age-related macular degeneration: a preliminary report. *J Transl Med,* Sep 25;11:228.

49 Falsini, B., Piccardi, M., Minnella, A., Savastano, C., Capoluongo, E., et al. (2010). Influence of saffron supplementation on retinal flicker sensitivity in early age-related macular degeneration. *Invest Ophthalmol Vis Sci,* Dec;51(12):6118-24.

50 Bone, R.A., Landrum, J.T., Cao, Y., Howard, A.N., Alvarez-Calderon, F. (2007). Macular pigment response to a supplement containing meso-zeaxanthin, lutein and zeaxanthin. *Nutr Metab (Lond),* 4:12.

51 Capitanio S, Sambuceti G, Giusti M, et al. (2001). 1,25-Dihydroxy vitamin D and coronary microvascular function. Retrieved Dec 04 2017 from https://moh-it.pure.elsevier.com/en/publications/125-dihydroxy-vitamin-d-and-coronary-microvascular-function

52 Nakajima, Y., Inokuchi, Y., Shimazawa, M., Otsubo, K., Ishibashi, T. (2008). Astaxanthin, a dietary carotenoid, protects retinal cells against oxidative stress in-vitro and in mice in-vivo. *J Pharm Pharmacol,* Oct;60(10):1365-74.

53 Ibid. Piermarocchi. (2012).

54 Otsuka T., Shimazawa, M., Nakanishi, T., Ohno, Y., Inoue, Y., et all. (2013). Protective effects of a dietary carotenoid, astaxanthin, against light-induced retinal damage. *J Pharmacol Sci,* 123(3):209-18

55 Bola, C., Bartlett, H., Eperjesi, F., (2014). Resveratrol and the eye: activity and molecular mechanisms. *Graefes Arch Clin Exp Ophthalmol,* May;252(5):699-713.

56 Rasmussen, H.M., Johnson, E.J. (2013). Nutrients for the aging eye. *Clin Interv Aging,* 2013;8:741-8.

57 Blenkinsop, T.A., Corneo, B., Temple, S., Stern, J.H. (2012). Ophthalmologic stem cell transplantation therapies. *Regen Med,* Nov;7(6 Suppl):32-9.

58 MacLaren, R.E., (2017). Electronic retinal implant surgery. *Eye (Lond),* Feb;31(2):191-5.

59 Petit, L., Khanna, H., Punzo, C. (2016). Advances in Gene Therapy for Disease of the Eye. *Hum Gene Ther,* Aug 1;27(8):563-79.

15-6. DIABETIC RETINOPATHY

Diabetic retinopathy (DR) is a potentially blinding complication of diabetes that damages the eye's retina; it is a leading cause of vision loss in the world. Of an estimated 285 million people with diabetes mellitus worldwide, approximately one-third have symptoms, and of these, a further one-third have vision-threatening DR, including diabetic macular edema. It has been considered to be a disease caused primarily by the deterioration of tiny capillaries in the retina. However, in recent years it has also being recognized as a neurodegenerative condition.[1]

Because diabetic retinopathy often goes unnoticed until vision loss occurs, those with diabetes should get a comprehensive dilated eye exam at least once a year. With timely treatment, many of those with advanced diabetic retinopathy can be saved from going blind.

How Diabetes Affects Vision

In patients with diabetes, the global prevalence of non-proliferative diabetic retinopathy is about 35.4% and proliferative diabetic retinopathy is about 7.5%.[2] Type 1 diabetes prevalence has been increasing at a rate of about 3% per annum in the U.S., especially in young children from 5 to 9.

Types of Diabetes

An estimated 23.1 million people, or 7.2% of the U.S. population, have diagnosed diabetes.[3] This total includes 132,000 children and adolescents younger than age 18 and 193,000 children and adolescents younger than 20. Diabetes is ranked as the 7th leading cause of death in America.

Type 1 diabetes (formerly called juvenile-onset or insulin-dependent diabetes) is a condition where the body's immune system destroys the cells that release insulin, eventually eliminating insulin production from the body. It is a very serious, potentially life-threatening condition. Without insulin the body's cells cannot absorb glucose to produce the energy that we need to live. Type 1 diabetes generally begins in childhood; however, it does affect adults, and at increasing rates today. For some time, only a small portion of diabetes sufferers were diagnosed with type 1 diabetes (5–10%). But for over a decade, reports have been showing that type 1 diagnoses are rising by 3% annually in the U.S., and particularly in children between the ages of 5 and 9.[4]

Type 2 diabetes (formerly called adult-onset diabetes or non-insulin-dependent diabetes) is the more prevalent type of diabetes, comprising 90-95% of the cases. It typically develops over many years, and it is characterized by the body's inability to use insulin in the correct way; this is called insulin resistance. As type 2 diabetes worsens, the pancreas may make less and less insulin (insulin deficiency). Type 2 diabetes is typically diagnosed during adulthood; however, the incidence of type 2 diabetes in children is rising dramatically.

Note. There is another type of diabetes called "gestational diabetes" which occurs only during a woman's pregnancy. Researchers don't know why some women develop gestational diabetes, but it may have to do with the placenta producing insulin-blocking hormones, impairing the action of insulin in the mother's cells, resulting in raising her blood sugar. Gestational diabetes mellitus (GDM), although a temporary condition during pregnancy, increases the life-long risk of developing type 2 diabetes in both mother and baby. The risk does not go away. Every year, approximately 7% of all pregnant women are affected by GDM, and of those, 5–10% of these women go on to have type 2 diabetes. In fact, women who have had GDM have a 20–50% chance of becoming diabetic sometime in their life.[5]

The Four Stages of Diabetic Retinopathy

Diabetic retinopathy develops as a complication of uncontrolled or poorly controlled diabetes. While there is only one type of diabetic retinopathy, there are four stages associated with this disorder.[6] An eye does not necessarily pass through all of these stages in the following order:

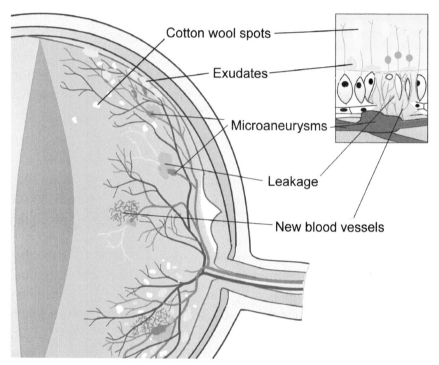

Mild non-proliferative form. Tiny capillaries in the retina swell and leak. These are called "microaneurysms."

Moderate non-proliferative form. Some of these capillaries are completely blocked, depriving the retina of nourishment.

Severe non-proliferative form. Many capillaries are blocked and more of the retina does not receive needed nutrients. This triggers neovascularization, a condition where the body grows new blood vessels in abnormal areas in order to supply the eyes with blood and nutrients. These new blood vessels are weak, and tend to leak blood and fluids that can cause severe vision loss if not treated.

In addition, "cotton wool" spots may appear on the retina, evidence of nerve fiber damage. These are a hallmark of pre- or non-proliferative diabetic retinopathy. These look like fluffy white spots that develop as a result of diabetic retinopathy or hypertension.[7] In addition to cotton wool spots are hard exudates which are similar to the drusen seen in macular degeneration.

Proliferative form (advanced stage of diabetic retinopathy). New, fragile capillaries grow within and along the surface of the retina and into the vitreous of the eye. The additional growth, in and of itself, may not cause vision loss, although portions of the retina can become distorted, thereby altering vision. Because the new capillaries have thin walls, they are fragile, and they are at great risk of leaking which can result in vision loss if not treated.

Ketosis may also develop if insulin production is insufficient. Ketosis occurs when the body starts burning fat instead of carbohydrates for energy. It arises from profound reduction in beta-cell mass (the cells that produce insulin) and results in ketone formation. Ketosis can become dangerous when ketones accumulate to too-high levels, leading to dehydration and changes to the chemical balance of your blood.

Signs and Symptoms

Blurred vision. High glucose levels can cause blurry vision as long as glucose levels remain high.

Diabetes symptoms. Diabetic retinopathy is difficult to detect. It is also important to watch for other symptoms typically related to diabetes, which include:

- Dark floaters looking like strings or spots floating around in your visual field
- Dark or empty areas in your vision
- Impaired color vision
- Fluctuating vision and vision loss

Reactive hypoglycemia (insulin resistance). Many people may not recognize reactive hypoglycemia (low blood sugar) as a symptom. It is a symptom of pre-diabetes. Reactive hypoglycemia occurs in people who regularly consume sugars and refined carbohydrates (including refined foods, sweetened beverages, bread, pasta, rice, and white potatoes).

Symptoms of reactive hypoglycemia include low blood sugar symptoms such as fatigue, weakness, sleepiness, blurry vision, dizziness, feeling cold and/or sweating, shakiness, palpitations, anxiety, nausea, hunger, and brain fog or difficulty in concentrating.

One of the jobs of insulin is to get glucose into the cells for energy production. When fast carbohydrates are ingested, the result is a quick release of a lot of insulin from the pancreas. Insulin is very efficient at doing its job of either getting the glucose into the cells, or storing the excess as fat. When a lot of insulin is produced in response to a high sugar/refined carbohydrate meal, the result is a drop in blood sugar, and then the need arises for quick energy in the form of more sugar/refined carbohydrates. This cycle of high and low blood sugar and insulin levels eventually causes the cells to become resistant or insensitive to insulin; this is diabetes.

Reactive hypoglycemia can be diagnosed based on symptoms and high blood insulin levels. High insulin results in increased belly fat, inflammation, muscle loss, fatigue, and is linked to high blood pressure, heart disease, stroke, elevated cholesterol and triglycerides, low HDL, low libido, infertility, depression, dementia, and cancer.

Causes and Risk Factors

Key Factors

High blood sugar. Chronically high levels of blood sugar associated with diabetes are the primary cause of diabetic retinopathy.

Poor diet. A diet high in refined carbohydrates and sugar and low in whole foods and antioxidants is a big contributor to the development of type 2 diabetes.

Inadequate exercise. Lack of regular exercise is also a key factor. So, it is possible to avoid type 2 diabetes by staying physically active and maintaining a healthy, largely plant-based diet, high in complex carbohydrates, such as whole fruits, vegetables, grains, and healthy fats (see Chapter 7, Vision diet). However, even if you do not make all of the necessary lifestyle changes, controlling diabetes by staying consistent with prescribed medications can prevent or delay vision loss.

Additional Factors

Factors related to the development of diabetes include:

- Obesity and overweight conditions (inherent conditions of chronic inflammation)
- Family history
- Race/people of color (affected by diabetes more than their Caucasian counterparts)
- Polycystic ovary syndrome (common condition affecting women, characterized by irregular menstrual periods, excess hair growth, and obesity)[8]
- High blood pressure (sustained levels of blood pressure, over 140/90 millimeters of mercury, mm Hg, linked to an increased risk of type 2 diabetes.[9]
- Abnormal cholesterol and triglyceride levels[10]

Diabetic Retinopathy Factors

For patients with diabetes, there are other factors that increase the risk of diabetic retinopathy.

- Depression[11]
- Low magnesium levels in the blood[12]
- Low vitamin C levels[13]
- Low folic acid levels[14]
- Kidney disease[15]
- Vitamin D deficiency[16]
- Inflammation (insulin treatment does not alleviate inflammation nor improve the

integrity of the capillaries and nerve function in the retina)[17]

- High homocysteine levels[18]

Conventional Treatment

Laser Surgery

Argon-laser photocoagulation is a type of laser surgery used to treat macular edema and proliferative retinopathy (advanced diabetic retinopathy). Generally, laser surgery is used to stabilize vision, not necessarily to improve it.[19] Laser surgery includes focal and scatter laser treatment. Focal laser treatment seals leaking vessels.[20] Scatter laser treatment (used for proliferative retinopathy) shrinks the abnormal blood vessels. Both of these treatments can often result in loss of peripheral vision.

Anti-VEGF (vascular endothelial growth factor) Injections

These include drugs such as Lucentis, Avestin, Regeneron, and/or Eylea. They are administered via injection for retinal bleeding or edema, and help to shrink new blood vessels. Treatment using these injections can last up to five years, with a gradual decrease of injections over time. Recovery time depends on the extent of the diabetic retinopathy. Depending on the extent of the blood leakage, it may take weeks or up to months for the blurriness to improve; full vision does not always return. As a side note, dilated eye exams may be needed less often as the disease stabilizes. However, it is important to note, that if the underlying mechanism is not addressed, these treatments are a temporary solution. The signals (VEGF) in the body to create new blood vessels are still present, so eventually more new blood vessels will develop.

Vitrectomy

Vitrectomy is the surgical removal of the vitreous gel in the center of the eye. In some people with proliferative diabetic retinopathy, bleeding into the vitreous (vitreous hemorrhage) makes laser photocoagulation treatment impossible because the blood obscures the surgeon's view of the retina. Vitrectomy, which is performed under local or general anesthesia, typically on an outpatient basis, removes the cloudy vitreous and replaces it with a salt solution, or air (which is a mixture of gases—mainly nitrogen and oxygen), but also small amounts of carbon dioxide and substantially lower amounts of many other inert gases such as argon, neon, and helium. Eye drops are used for a few weeks after the surgery. This solution has a low surface tension and therefore does not have a negative effect on the retina.

The surgery typically includes steroid drops to minimize inflammation, antibiotic drops to prevent infection, and dilating drops to provide comfort and minimize scarring of the pupil. The gases from air are reabsorbed by the body in a week to two months and are replaced by natural vitreous fluid that the eye is constantly producing. Silicone oil is also sometimes used and may result in a quicker visual recovery after surgery, no restriction on air travel, no special head positioning after surgery, and longer duration of effect. But it needs to be removed later in a procedure similar to vitreous humor removal.

Side Effects of Vitrectomy

- Short-term sensitivity to glare and/or double vision.
- 5-10% risk of needing further retinal surgery
- 30-43% likelihood of developing a cataract[21]
- Elevated pressure inside the eye especially in people who have glaucoma
- Further bleeding into the vitreous gel
- Retinal detachment
- Fluid buildup in the clear covering of the eye (corneal edema)
- Infection inside the eye (endophthalmitis)[22]

Intravitreal Corticosteroids

Corticosteroids have been successfully used in the eyes of patients with persistent diabetic macular edema (DME), similar to diabetic retinopathy.[23] The epidemiology of DME is not well studied and the diagnosis is challenging since proper diagnosis and classification is not possible with non-stereoscopic retinal photos.

Complementary Approach

Eye health is directly related to healthy circulation, which enables the body to deliver essential nutrients to the eyes. Targeted supplements can reduce the risk of damage resulting from excessive free radical activity that is due to inflammation both in the eyes and body, as well as helping manage and reduce chronic inflammation, supporting circulation, blood sugar balancing, insulin sensitivity, strong capillaries, and overall eye health.

Nutrients

Generally, the carotenoids help prevent vascular complications of diabetes such as diabetic retinopathy. Because inflammation, oxidative damage, and the production of sugars bonded to fats, proteins, and nucleic acids are all reduced through the carotenoids; they are potentially very useful in treating and preventing diabetic retinopathy.[24] [25]

Essential

See Appendix 5 for products that contain a number of the recommended nutrients below.

Alpha-lipoic acid. 300mg–600mg per day. This antioxidant compound improves insulin sensitivity in individuals with type 2 diabetes, and it may prevent diabetic retinopathy by reducing damage to fine capillaries due to mitochondrial overproduction.[26] Alpha-lipoic acid has potent antioxidant actions.[27] [28]

Astaxanthin. 6mg–12mg per day. Astaxanthin supplementation reduces cataract formation and diabetic retinopathy (both preventable forms of blindness in people with diabetes) and has protective actions of microalgae against endogenous and exogenous advanced glycation end products (AGEs) in human retinal pigment epithelial cells.[29] [30]

Bilberry. 180mg–240mg per day. Bilberry and extracts may lessen neovascularization in the retina, which complicates retinopathy.[31] Bilberry is also used to improve night vision and to decrease vascular permeability and capillary fragility; most interest has been focused on its anthocyanin-related antioxidant effects.[32] [33] [34] [35]

CoQ10. 100mg–200mg per day. CoQ10 has strong antioxidant properties[36] and protects proteins and mitochondrial DNA from oxidative damage. CoQ10 levels in your body deplete over time.[37]

DHA/EPA. 1,400mg EPA and 1,000mg DHA daily. DHA, a component of omega-3s, reduces inflammation and so may reduce stress caused by inflammation in the retina seen in diabetic retinopathy. DHA is also a precursor for a biochemical compound known as neuroprotectin D1, which also helps protect against damage from inflammation and reduces cell death within the retina.[38] [39] [40] [41] Alternatively, take high-quality liquid fish oil 2000mg-3000mg per day with a meal.

Ginkgo biloba. 120mg per day. Ginkgo biloba helps protect retinal cells from oxidative damage due to toxic chemicals. It contains antioxidant flavonoids such as quercetin and kaempferol.[42] [43]

Glutathione (reduced form). 500mg–900mg per day. Take preferably in an intraoral or sublingual form (the dosage would be lower as the absorption rate is 5–10 times higher than in capsules), as glutathione (GSH) does not get absorbed well through the digestive system. Glutathione is one of the super antioxidants that neutralizes the full range of free radicals. Patients with uncontrolled type 2 diabetes are unable to adequately synthesize glutathione because of a lack of natural precursors in the body. Supplementing with amino acids, which are GSH precursors, supports GSH synthesis and reduces oxidative damage and inflammation.[44] [45]

Grapeseed extract. 200mg per day. Grapeseed extract helps platelets form properly in the circulatory system, protecting the retina from capillary leakage, and protecting against cell death.[46] It also helps to protect the central nervous system from free radicals.[47]

Lutein/zeaxanthin/lycopene. By addressing inflammation, oxidative damage, and glycation end products (sugars bonded to other molecules), these carotenoids are generally helpful.[48] This combination of carotenoids are found naturally in the eye and is essential for normal vision, protecting the eye from UV radiation and oxidative stress. People with diabetic retinopathy have lower levels of lycopene, lutein, and other carotenoids compared to diabetics without retinopathy.

- **Lutein.** 6mg–20mg per day[49]
- **Zeaxanthin.** 2mg–12mg per day[50]
- **Lycopene.** 3mg per day[51]

Taurine. 750mg–1,000mg per day. Taurine has been reported to protect visual function during diabetes and to help prevent damage due to oxidative stress[52] and inflammation.[53]

Trans-resveratrol. 175mg per day. Trans-resveratrol helps protect nerve cells from damage, promotes healthy insulin sensitivity, encourages enhanced mitochondrial function, promotes a healthy inflammatory response, and protects against the effects of a high-fat diet.[54] [55] [56] [57]

Vitamin A palmitate. 5,000 IU per day. This acts like an antioxidant and is important for vision and protection from oxidative stress,[58] especially for non-proliferative diabetic retinopathy.[59]

> **Note**. Vitamin A is contra-indicated for those suffering from Stargardt disease (see Stargardt's chapter for more information). Pregnant women should not take vitamin A.

Vitamin B12. 1,000mcg per day. B12 works synergistically with B6 and folate to regenerate the amino acid methionine, which helps to maintain already healthy homocysteine levels within normal range. This is important for diabetics.[60] [61] We suggest the methylcobalamin form.

Vitamin D3. 2,000 IU–5,000 IU per day. Low levels of vitamin D is a risk factor in diabetes. Vitamin D deficiency is associated with retinopathy in both children and adolescents with type 1 diabetes.[62] [63] [64] The D3 form is the most readily absorbed.

Very Important

Curcumin. 500mg daily. Taken as a highly absorbable phospholipid blend, [65] curcumin is the active chemical component of the Indian herb turmeric, commonly used in Indian food preparations. Curcumin prevents some of the complications of diabetes, including retinopathy, through reducing inflammation and inhibiting growth of new blood vessels.[66] It helps protect retinal pigment cells against oxidative stress.[67]

Green tea extract. 725mg per day. Green tea extract supports the integrity of retinal cells.[68] It may also be able to help diabetics improve their blood sugar control while protecting against glycation end products, the compounds formed when sugars bond with fats, proteins, or nucleic acids.[69]

Magnesium. 300mg–500mg per day. Low levels of magnesium present an increased risk of diabetes complications.[70] Magnesium reduces the risk of developing diabetes and diabetic retinopathy. It assists in the metabolism of carbohydrates and modulates insulin release that in turn, supports normal blood sugar levels. Studies show that for every 100mg increase in daily magnesium intake, there is a 15% decrease in the risk of developing type 2 diabetes.[71]

French maritime pine bark. 50mg, 3 times per day. Pycnogenol, taken at an early stage of retinopathy, may enhance retinal blood circulation and reduce swelling.[72]

Helpful

Astragalus. 250mg–500mg of standardized extract, 2–4 times per day. Astragalus may improve vision and prevent diabetic retinopathy, in part, by inhibiting the formation of AGEs (advanced glycosylated end products).[73] [74]

Chromium. 200mcg per day. Chromium reduces and maintains glucose levels in the blood.[75] It is one of several nutrients which may improve micro-vascular damage.[76]

Gymnema sylvestre. 400mg per day. This herb has the potential to repair and regenerate pancreas beta cells.[77]

N-acetyl-carnosine. (NAC) 500mg per day. NAC is an amino acid that helps slow down protein molecules bonding to sugar molecules, resulting in AGEs. It is believed that NAC acts as an antioxidant in the body against glycation.[78]

Vanadyl sulfate. 75mg–150mg per day, with or without food. Research indicates vanadyl sulfate may improve tissue sensitivity and promote already healthy glucose metabolism for those within normal range.[79] [80]

Benfotiamine. 300mg per day, along with 300mg per day of alpha-lipoic acid. Vitamin B1 (thiamin) and its natural derivative benfotiamine is one of the most important natural anti-AGE compounds; reduces AGE-triggered damage in the retina and throughout the body.[81] Benfotiamine has actually been found to be better than thiamine at penetrating cell membranes and protecting AGE-vulnerable tissues from harmful glucose-protein and glucose-lipid reactions, helping to protect nerve, retinal, kidney, and other cells. [82]

> **Note.** Supplementing with 300mg of benfotiamine *along with* 600mg of alpha-lipoic acid, taken twice daily for 28 days, also reduces AGE accumulation in type 1 diabetics.[83]

Diet

Avoid foods containing AGEs. AGEs are biochemical compounds that form naturally within the body through enzyme reactions involving sugars, proteins, fats, or nucleic acids. If too-high levels of AGEs form, they cause oxidative damage and inflammation. AGEs are found in some foods and are formed by cooking these foods. High heat methods of cooking meat and cheese such as grilling, searing, roasting, and frying hasten formation of additional AGEs. High fat, aged cheeses contain more AGEs than low fat cheeses (low fat mozzarella, cheddar, and cottage cheese). Other foods high in AGEs include butter and processed foods such as cream cheese and mayonnaise. Oils and nuts contain lower quantities.[84]

Anti-inflammatory diet. Tight control of both blood glucose levels and hypertension is essential to slow or stop progression of DR. There are a number of treatments available to help control it. See the Vision diet, an anti-inflammatory diet, described in Chapter 7.

Juicing. Below are some suggestions for your juicing recipe. Select some combination of the following, as well as adding your favorite fruits and vegetables.

- Ginger, asparagus, garlic, leeks, Jerusalem artichokes, spinach, parsley, beets, pumpkin, celery, carrots, cabbage, berries, wheatgrass, (not too much fruit)

Lifestyle

Stop smoking. If you smoke, it is also essential that you quit, as smoking results in restricted blood flow to the eyes, as well as being a source of AGEs.[85]

Exercise. Get regular exercise such as a 20–30 minute brisk walk daily. Research indicates that 90 minutes of yoga twice a week reduces inflammation, depression, and fatigue.[86] But activities such as heavy weight lifting, excessive sports, and contact sports can promote retinal bleeding.

Manage stress. Manage chronic stress through relaxation, meditation, exercise, or yoga.

Eye exercises. We recommend palming and eye massage eye exercises for diabetic retinopathy. See Chapter 10-4 for more information.

Other Modalities

Chinese Medicine

According to Traditional Chinese Medicine (TCM), diabetes mellitus is a disorder characterized by yin deficiency (essential fluids) with dryness, heat, and dampness that is reflected in increased blood glucose. Diabetes mellitus is most closely related to wasting (*xiao ke*) syndrome, which is generally categorized as:

- **Upper (Lung heat)**, characterized by excessive thirst
- **Middle (Stomach dryness)**, characterized by excessive hunger
- **Lower (Kidney yin and jing deficiency)**, characterized by excessive urination

This is a simplistic explanation as there are many syndromes that can result in diabetic retinopathy, so only a certified TCM or acupuncture practitioner can ascertain the root cause and treat it. At some point, most people with diabetes show symptoms of all three types.

With that said, diabetes mellitus is a complicated condition, particularly related to the change in the American diet over the last 50 years that is significantly different than a person's diet before then. For obese people for example, the pattern may be more Liver and Stomach heat stagnation syndrome. Type 2 diabetes can occur because of any number of imbalances, which are also connected to lifestyle choices.

In Traditional Chinese Medicine, the Spleen and Stomach meridians can be damaged by consuming too much greasy food and alcohol or an excessive amount of sweets. Even over-consuming hot drinks, such as coffee or tea, can create an imbalance. A constitutional yin deficiency (characterized by fatigue, weakness, lethargy, and pale complexion) could cause a depletion of Spleen energy, marked by difficulty in transporting and digesting food. The result is a buildup of interior heat associated with sluggish digestive capabilities that can lead to diabetes.

Deficiency in Kidney energy caused by an overactive sex life, or some congenital Kidney meridian issue, can be a cause. In these cases, the Kidney qi can trigger the Bladder to malfunction, resulting in polyuria (excessive urination), which is linked to diabetes.

Chronic emotional imbalances such as ongoing anxiety, anger, stress, depression, etc. injures the Liver (meridian), causing the Liver qi to stagnate. If this happens for long periods of time, excessive heat can build up, consuming body fluids rapidly, which can eventually lead to diabetes.

In treating diabetes, the acupuncturist will take these types into consideration in determining the best treatment strategy at any given time. A typical acupuncture treatment for diabetes involves

8–16 points and allowing the needles to remain in place for approximately 20–30 minutes, usually weekly. It is recommended to start with 10–14 treatments, then continue with herbs, while ongoing weekly treatments may be recommended.

In Chinese medicine, common patterns of imbalance related to diabetic retinopathy are: disharmony between the Gallbladder and Stomach with phlegm-heat, Kidney yang weakness, spleen and stomach weakness with damp accumulation, central (Spleen) qi weakness, and heart blood deficiency.

Common Patent Formulas

Er chen tang helps dry dampness, promoting the healthy function of the Stomach, resulting in improved digestion, and less gurgling and nausea.

Wen dan tang nourishes Kidney and Liver yin, and "brightens the eyes." This is specifically formulated for disharmony between Gallbladder and Stomach and the resulting phlegm heat, enabling the free flow of qi (energy). When qi in these meridians are blocked, phlegm can develop, which inhibits proper digestion and elimination, often resulting in frequent nausea and vomiting.

You gui wan (restore the right decoction) helps warm the body (warms and tonifies the Kidney yang heat), raising warmth and energy to the eyes. Common deficiency symptoms include fatigue, cold limbs, incontinence, and infertility.

Celosia 10 was designed on the basis of formulas described in Chinese research reports for the treatment of retinal disorders.

These are just examples of formulas that might be helpful in the treatment of diabetic retinopathy. It is best for herbal formulas to be prescribed by TCM practitioners, as the formulas and treatment strategies can vary significantly, based on a person's specific symptoms and the practitioner's evaluation.

Oxygen Therapy

A small pilot study of patients with diabetic retinopathy, who had all had conventional laser treatment, showed that supplemental oxygen improved symptoms related to post-operative issues, including edema. In particular, excess thickness of the fovea, the part of the eye responsible for the sharpest vision, was reduced by 42%, and macular volume dropped by 54%; three of the eyes tested had better visual acuity, and most of the eyes gradually worsened when the oxygen was withdrawn. Four of the eyes maintained stability, suggesting that supplemental oxygen has a stabilizing effect on the possible side effects of laser surgery for retinopathy. In fact, the researchers believed that when the retina received a decrease in oxygen, the body releases vascular endothelial growth factor (VEGF) and other substances that cause retinal blood vessels to become leaky and ultimately stimulate the growth of new blood vessels.[87]

Micro Acupuncture

This treatment, which is a form of acupuncture, uses a particular system of points and a specific number of needlets (smaller needles than typically used in acupuncture) in the hands and feet, for the purpose of reversing the effects of diabetic retinopathy, specifically retinal bleeding and inflammation. Each treatment lasts around 20 minutes, and it is common to expect a number of treatments each day over the course of a week. See Chapter 9-4 for more information.

Eyedrop Recommendations

There is a close link between diabetes and cataracts. An estimated 20% of cataract procedures are for diabetic patients.[88] Eyedrops containing 1% N-acetyl-carnosine solutions help prevent glycation (the binding of sugar and protein molecules together) in the lens of the eye. For diabetic patients, these daily eyedrops can help prevent the onset of cataracts or help manage them.

On the Horizon

Gene therapy. Researchers have been able to completely reverse fat content, inflammation, and liver fibrosis in rodents through gene therapy. These changes increased insulin sensitivity.[89]

Vitrectomy. Researchers have been investigating new possible solutions to substitute for the vitreous humor in a vitrectomy. One is a cross-linked hyaluronic acid solution that has the advantages of having good transparency and viscosity. It also has hydrophilic (mixes with water) properties and a tamponade (closure of blockage) effect. This solution lasts for more than 4 weeks and has limited tissue inflammatory and toxic reactions. Using hydrogels such as polyvinyl alcohol is also being investigated. Implantation of a new type of polyvinyl has been experimented with in rabbit models and vitreous regeneration techniques.

Optigenics. European researchers have found that optogenics (a gene therapy designed to reactivate dormant cones by making them light-sensitive) may be helpful in treating retinal degenerative conditions like diabetic retinopathy. With the treatment, proteins are introduced into the eye, causing the sustained production of halorhodopsin, a light-sensitive protein. It has been shown to restore light sensitivity as well as vision for people who have very little.[90]

Caesalpinia pulcherrima. Lab animals treated with an extract of this tropical plant displayed better antioxidant levels and lowered blood sugar alcohol levels. It is a flowering plant in the pea family often known as Red or Mexican Bird of Paradise. More research is needed to determine its viability in humans.[91]

Envisia™ Therapeutics. Envisia, an ophthalmology therapeutics research company, is researching more efficient delivery systems of next generation ophthalmology drugs using micro- and nanoparticles to address ocular conditions such as macula edema due to diabetes, glaucoma, and macular degeneration.[92]

Also See

Chapter 7, Vision Diet

---

[1] Ren, X., Lu, H., Wang, N., Zhang, C., Ji, Y., et al. (2017). Thioredoxin is implicated in the anti apoptotic effects of grapeseed proanthocyanidin extract during hyperglycemia. *Mol Med Rep*, Nov;16(5):7731-7737.

[2] Lee, R., Wong, T.Y., Sabanayagam, C. (2015). Epidemiology of diabetic retinopathy, diabetic macular edema and related vision loss. *Eye Vis*, 2:17.

3 Ibid. Lee. (2015).

[4] Egro, F.M. (2013). Why is type 1 diabetes increasing? *J Mol Endocrinol*, August 1, 51 R1-R13.

5 NIH. (2006). History of Gestational Diabetes Raises Lifelong Diabetes Risk in Mother and Child. Retrieved Nov 2 2017 from https://www.nih.gov/news-events/news-releases/history-gestational-diabetes-raises-lifelong-diabetes-risk-mother-child.

6 Weir, G.C., Bonner-Weir, S. (2004). Five stages of evolving beta-cell dysfunction during progression to diabetes. *Diabetes*, Dec;53 Suppl 3:S16-21.

[7] Wikipedia. Cotton wool spots. Retrieved Jul 28 2018 from https://en.wikipedia.org/wiki/Cotton_wool_spots.

8 Celik, C., Tasdemir, N., Abali, R., Bastu, E., Yilmaz, M. (2014). Progression to impaired glucose tolerance or type 2 diabetes mellitus in polycystic ovary syndrome: a controlled follow-up study. *Fertil Steril*, Apr;101(4):1123-8

[9] Campbell, N.R.C., Gilbert, R.E., Leiter, L.A., Larochelle, P., Tobe, S., et al. (2011). Hypertension in people with type 2 diabetes

Hypertension in people with type 2 diabetes. *Can Fam Physician,* Sep; 57(9): 997–1002.

[10] Bitzur, R., Cohen, H., Kamari, Y., Shaish, A., Horats, D. (2009). Triglycerides and HDL Cholesterol. Stars or second leads in diabetes? *Diabetes Care*, Nov; 32(Suppl 2): S373–S377.

11 Sieu, N., Katon, W., Lin, E.H., Russo, J., Ludman, E., et al. (2011). Depression and incident diabetic retinopathy: a prospective cohort study. *Gen Hosp Psychiatry*, Sep-Oct;33(5):429-35

[12] McNair, P., Christiansen, C., Madsbad, S., Lauritzen, E. Faber, O., et al. (1978). Hypomagnesemia, a risk factor in diabetic retinopathy. *Diabetes*, Nov; 27(11):1075-7.

[13] Afkhami-Ardekani, M., Shojaoddiny-Ardekani, A. (2007). Effect of vitamin C on blood glucose, serum lipids & serum insulin in type 2 diabetes patients. *Indian J Med Res,* Nov;126(5):471-4.

[14] Malaguarnera, G., Gagliano, C., Salomone, S., Giordano, M., Bucolo, C., et al. (2015). Folate status in type 2 diabetic patients with and without retinopathy, *Clin Ophthalmol*, Aug 7;9:1437-42

[15] Hammes, H.P., Welp, R., Kempe, H.P., Wagner, C., Siegel, E., et al. (2015). Risk Factors for Retinopathy and DME in Type 2 Diabetes-Results from the German/Austrian DPV Database. *PLoS One*, Jul 15;10(7):e0132492

[16] Alcubierre, N., Valls, J., Rubinat, E., Gao, G., Esquerda, A., et al. (2015). Vitamin D Deficiency Is Associated with the Presence and Severity of Diabetic Retinopathy in Type 2 Diabetes Mellitus. *J Diabetes Res*, 2015:374178.

17 Bixler, G.V., VanGuilder, H.D., Brucklacher, R.M., Kimball, S.R., Bronson, S.K., et al. (2011). Chronic insulin treatment of diabetes does not fully normalize alterations in the retinal transcriptome. *MBC Medical Genomics*, 4:40.

[18] Goldstein, M., Leibovitch, I., Yeffimov, I., Gavendo, S., Sela, B.A., et al. (2004). Hyperhomocysteinemia in patients with diabetes mellitus with and without retinopathy. *Eye,* 18:460–465.

[19] Takamura, Y., Arimura, S., Miyake, S., Matsumura, T., Gozawa, M., et al. (2017). Panretinal Photocoagulation Using Short-Pulse Laser Induces Less Inflammation and Macular Thickening in Patients with Diabetic Retinopathy. *J Ophthalmol*, 2017:8530261

[20] Crosson, J.N., Mason, L., Mason, J.O., (2017). The Role of Focal laser in the Anti-Vascular Endothelial Growth Factor Era. Ophthalmol Eye Dis, Nov 21;9:1179172117738240

[21] WebMD. Vitrectomy. Retrieved Dec 12 2017 from http://www.webmd.com/eye-health/vitrectomy.

[22] Ibid. WebMD. Vitrectomy.

[23] Sarao, V., Veritti, D., Boscia, F., Lanzetta, P. (2014). Intravitreal Steroids for the Treatment of Retinal Diseases. *Sci World J*, 2014:989501.

[24] Murillo, A.G., Fernandez, M.L. (2016). Potential of Dietary Non-Provitamin A Carotenoids in the Prevention and Treatment of Diabetic Microvascular Complications. *Adv Nutr*, Jan 15;7(1):14-24.

[25] Moshetova, L.K., Vorob'eva, I.V., Alekseev, I.B., Mikhaleva, L.G. (2015). Results of the use of antioxidant and angioprotective agents in type 2 diabetes patients with diabetic retinopathy and age-related macular degeneration. *Vestn Oftalmol*, May-Jun;131(3):34-44.

[26] Lin, J., Bierhaus, A., Bugert, P., Dietrich, N., Feng, Y., et al. (2006). Effect of R-(+)-alpha-lipoic acid on experimental diabetic retinopathy. *Diabetologia*, May;49(5):1089-96.

[27] Hultberg, M. Hultberg, B. (2006). The effect of different antioxidants on glutathione turnover in human cell lines and their interaction with hydrogen peroxide. *Chem Biol Interact*, Nov 7;163(3).

[28] Nebbioso, M., Pranno, F., Pescosolido, N. (2013). Lipoic acid in animal models and clinical use in diabetic retinopathy. *Expert Opin Pharmacother,* Sep;14(13):1829-38.

[29] Nakano, M., Orimo, N., Katagirim N., Tsubata, M., Takahashi, J., et al. Inhibitory effect of astaxanthin combined with Flavangenol on oxidative stress biomarkers in streptozotocin-induced diabetic rats. *Int J Vitam Nutr Res*, 2008 Jul-Sep;78(4-5):175-82.

[30] Ibid. Murillo. (2016).

[31] Ghadiri, S. E., Arbabi-Aval, M., Rezaei, K.M., Ahmadieh, H. (2015). Anti-inflammatory properties of resveratrol in the retinas of type 2 diabetic rats. *Clin Exp Pharmacol Physiol,* Jan;42(1):63-8.

[32] Kim, J., Kim, C.S., Lee, Y.M., Sohn, E., Jo, K., et al. (2015). Vaccinium myrtillus extract prevents or delays the onset of diabetes--induced blood-retinal barrier breakdown. *Int J Food Sci Nutr,* Mar;66(2):236-42.

[33] Camire M.E. (2000). Herbs Botanicals and Teas. *Bilberries and blueberries as functional foods and nutraceuticals*, pp. 289–319. Lancaster, PA: Technomic Publishing Company.

[34] Upton, R, editor. (2001). American Herbal Pharmacopoeia and Therapeutic Compendium. *Bilberry Fruit Vaccinium myrtillus L. Standards of Analysis, Quality Control, and Therapeutics*. Santa Cruz, CA.

[35] Mazza, G., Kay, C.D., Correll, T., Holub, B.J. (2002). Absorption of anthocyanins from blueberries and serum antioxidant status in human subjects. *J Agric Food Chem*, 50:7731–7.

36 Domanico, D., Fragiotta, S., Cutini, A., Carnevale, C., Zompatori, L., et al. Circulating levels of reactive oxygen species in patients with nonproliferative diabetic retinopathy and the influence of antioxidant supplementation: 6-month follow-up. *Indian J Ophthalmol*, Jan;63(1):9-14.

[37] Littarru, G.P., Tiano, L. (2007). Bioenergetic and antioxidant properties of coenzyme Q10: recent developments. *Mol Biotechnol*, Sep;37(1):31-7.

[38]. Bazan, N.G. (2006). Survival signaling in retinal pigment epithelial cells in response to oxidative stress: significance in retinal degenerations. *Adv Exp Med Biol*, 572:531-40.

[39] Bazan, N.G., Molina, M.F., Gordon, W.C. (2011). Docosahexaenoic acid signalolipidomics in nutrition: significance in aging, neuroinflammation, macular degeneration, Alzheimer's, and other neurodegenerative diseases. *Annu Rev Nutr*, Aug 21;31:321-51.

40 Mukherjee, P.K., Marcheselli, V.L., Serhan, C.N., Bazan, N.G. (2004). Neuroprotectin D1: a docosahexaenoic acid-derived docosatriene protects human retinal pigment epithelial cells from oxidative stress. *Proc Natl Acad Sci USA*, Jun 1;101(22):8491-6

[41] Chen, W., Esselman, W.J., Jump, D.B., Busik, J.V. (2005). Anti-inflammatory effect of docosahexaenoic acid on cytokine-induced adhesion molecule expression in human retinal vascular endothelial cells. *Invest Ophthalmol Vis Sci,* Nov;46(11):4342-7.

[42] Feng, X., Zhang, L., Zhu, H. (2009). Comparative anticancer and antioxidant activities of different ingredients of Ginkgo biloba extract (EGb 761). *Planta Med,* Jun;75(8):792-6.

[43] Droy-Lefaix, M.T., Cluzel, J., Menerath, J.M., Bonhomme, B., Doly, M. (1995). Antioxidant effect of a Ginkgo biloba extract (EGb 761) on the retina. *Int J Tissue React*, 17(3):93-100.

[44] Gurler, B., Vural, H., Yilmaz, N., Oguz, H., Satici, A., et al. (2000). The role of oxidative stress in diabetic retinopathy. *Eye (Lond),* Oct;14 Pt 5:730-5.

[45] Sekhar, R.V., McKay, S.V., Patel, S.G., Guthikonda, A.P. Reddy, V.T., et al. (2011). Glutathione Synthesis Is Diminished in Patients With Uncontrolled Diabetes and Restored by Dietary Supplementation With Cysteine and Glycine. *Diabetes Care,* Jan; 34(1):162–167.

46 Ren, X., Lu, H., Wang, N., Zhang, C., Ji, Y., et al. (2017). Thioredoxin is implicated in the anti-apoptotic effects of grapeseed proanthocyanidin extract during hyperglycemia. *Mol Med Rep*, Nov;16(5):7731-7737.

47 Vitseva, O., Varghese, S., Chakrabarti, S., Folts, J.D., Fredman, J.E. (2005). Grape seed and skin extracts inhibit platelet function and release of reactive oxygen intermediates. *J Cardiovasc Pharmacol,* Oct;46(4):445-51.

48 Ibid. Murillo. (2016).

49 Koushan, K., Rusovici, R., Li, W., Ferguson, L.R., Chalam, K.V. (2013). The Role of Lutein in Eye-Related Disease. *Nutrients*, May; 5(5): 1823–1839.

50 Neelam, K., Goenadi, C.J., Lun, K., Yip, C.C., Au Eong, K.G. (2017). Putative protective role of lutein and zeaxanthin in diabetic retinopathy. *Br J Ophthalmol,* May;101(5):551-558.

51 Li, Z.Z., Lu, X.Z., Ma, C.C., Chen, L. (2010). Serum lycopene levels in patients with diabetic retinopathy. *Eur J Ophthalmol,* Jul-Aug;20(4):719-23.

52 Yu, X., Xu, Z., Mi, M., Xu, H., Zhu, J., et al. (2008). Dietary taurine supplementation ameliorates diabetic retinopathy via anti-excitotoxicity of glutamate in streptozotocin-induced Sprague-Dawley rats. *Neurochem Res,* Mar;33(3):500-7.

53 Sarkar, P., Basak, P., Ghosh, S., Kundu, M., Sil, P.C. (2017). Prophylactic role of taurine and its derivatives against diabetes mellitus and its related complications. *Food Chem Toxicol,* Dec;110:109-121.

54 Abu-Amero, K.K., Kondkar, A.A., Chalam, K.V. (2016). Resveratrol and Ophthalmic Diseases. *Nutrients,* Apr; 8(4): 200.

55 Timmers, S., Konings, E., Bilet, L., Houtkooper, R.H., van de Weijer, T., et al. (2011). Calorie restriction-like effects of 30 days of resveratrol supplementation on energy metabolism and metabolic profile in obese humans. *Cell Metab,* Nov 2;14(5):612-22.

56 Crandall, J.P., Oram, V., Trandadirescu, G., Reid, M. Kishore, P., et al. (2012). Pilot study of resveratrol in older adults with impaired glucose tolerance. *J Gerontol A Biol Sci Med Sci,* Dec;67(12):1307-12.

57 Anderson, G., Burkon, A., Sulzmaier, F.J., Walker, J.M., Leckband, G. (2011). High dose of dietary resveratrol enhances insulin sensitivity in healthy rats but does not lead to metabolite concentrations effective for SIRT1 expression. *Mol Nutr Food Res,* Aug;55(8):1197-206.

58 Valdes-Ramos, Guadarrama-Lopez, A.L., Martinez-Carrillo, B.E. and Benitez-Archiniega, A.D. (2015). Vitamins and Type 2 Diabetes Mellitus. *Endocr Metab Immune Disord Drug Targets*, 15(1):54–63.

59 Smolek, M.K., Notaroberto, N.F., Jaramillo, A.G., Pradillo, L.R. (2013). Intervention with vitamins in patients with nonproliferative diabetic retinopathy: a pilot study. *Clin Ophthalmol*, 7: 1451–1458.

60 Fotiouu, P., Raptis, A., Apergis, G., Dimitriadis, G., Vergados, I., et al. (2014). Vitamin status as a determinant of serum homocysteine concentration in type 2 diabetic retinopathy. *J Diabetes Res*, 2014:807209.

61 Satyanarayana, A., Balakrishna, N., Pitla, S., Reddy, P.Y., Mudili, S., et al. (2011). Status of B-vitamins and homocysteine in diabetic retinopathy: association with vitamin-B12 deficiency and hyperhomocysteinemia. *PLoS One,* 6(11):e26747

62 Ibid. Alcubierre. (2015).

63 Targher, G., Bertolini, L., Padovani, R., Zenari, L., Scala, L., et al. (2006). Serum 25-hydroxyvitamin D3 concentrations and carotid artery intima-media thickness among type 2 diabetic patients. *Clin Endocrinol (Oxf),* 65:593–597.

64 Aksoy, H., Akçay, F., Kurtul, N., Baykal, O., Avci, B. (2000). Serum 1,25 dihydroxy vitamin D (1,25(OH)2D3), 25 hydroxy vitamin D (25(OH)D) and parathormone levels in diabetic retinopathy. *Clin Biochem*, 33:47–51.

65 Jeenger, M.K., Shrivastava, S., Yerra, V.G., Naidu, V.G., Ramakrishna, S., et al. (2015). Curcumin: a pleiotropic phytonutrient in diabetic complications. *Nutrition,* Feb;31(2):276-82.

66 Aldebasi, Y.H., Aly, S.M., Rahmani, A.H. (2013). Therapeutic implications of curcumin in the prevention of diabetic retinopathy via modulation of anti-oxidant activity and genetic pathways. *Int J Physiol Pathophysiol Pharmacol*, Dec 15;5(4):194-202.

67 Kowluru, R.A., Kanwar, M. (2007). Effects of curcumin on retinal oxidative stress and inflammation in diabetes. *Nutr Metab (Lond),* Apr 16;4:8.

68 Ma, Q., Chen, D., Sun, H.P., Yan, N., Xu, Y., et al. (2015). Regular Chinese Green Tea Consumption is Protective for Diabetic Retinopathy: A Clinic-Based Case-Control Study. *J Diabetes Res*, 2015:231570.

69 Silva, K.C., Rosales, M.A., Hamassaki, D.E., Saito, K.C., Faria, A.M., et al. (2013). Green tea is neuroprotective in diabetic retinopathy. *Invest Ophthalmol Vis Sci,* Feb 15;54(2):1325-36.

70 Lu, J., Gu, Y., Guo, M., Chen, P., Wang, H., et al. (2016). Serum Magnesium Concentration Is Inversely Associated with Albuminuria and Retinopathy among Patients with Diabetes. *J Diabetes Res*, 2016:1260141

71 NIH. Magnesium: Fact Sheet for Health Professionals. Retrieved Dec 14 2017 from https://ods.od.nih.gov/factsheets/Magnesium-HealthProfessional/.

72 Steigerwalt, R., Belcaro, G., Cesarone, M.R., Di Renzo, A., Grossi, M.G., et al. (2009). Pycnogenol improves microcirculation, retinal edema, and visual acuity in early diabetic retinopathy. *J Ocul Pharmacol Ther*, Dec;25(6):537-40.

73 Behl, T., Kotwani, A. (2017). Chinese herbal drugs for the treatment of diabetic retinopathy. *J Pharm Pharmacol*, Mar;69(3):223-235.

[74] Cheng, L., Zhang, G., Zhou, Y., Lu, X., Zhang, F., et al. (2013). Systematic Review and Meta-Analysis of 16 Randomized Clinical Trials of Radix Astragali and Its Prescriptions for Diabetic Retinopathy. *Evid Based Complement Alternat Med*, 2013:762783.

75 McCarty, M.F. (1997). Exploiting complementary therapeutic strategies for the treatment of type II diabetes and prevention of its complications. *Med Hypothesis*, Aug;49(2):143-52

[76] Rajendran, K., Manikandan, S., Nair, L.D., Karuthodiyil, R., Vijayarajan, N., et al. (2015). Serum Chromium Levels in Type 2 Diabetic Patients and Its Association with Glycaemic Control. *J Clin Diagn Res*, Nov;9(11):OC05-8

77 Kimura, I. (2006). Medical benefits of using natural compounds and their derivatives having multiple pharmacological actions. *Yakugaku Zasshi*, Mar;126(3):133-43.

78 Pfister, F., Riedl, E., Wang, Q., von Hagen, F., Deinzer, M. et al. (2011). Oral carnosine supplementation prevents vascular damage in experimental diabetic retinopathy. *Cell Physiol Biochem*, 28(1):125-36.

79 Srivastava, A.K., Medhi, M.Z., (2005). Insulino-mimetic and anti-diabetic effects of vanadium compounds. *Diabet Med*, Jan;22(1):2-13.

80 Tas, S., Sarandol, E., Ayvalik, S.Z., Serdar, Z., Dirican, (2007). Vanadyl sulfate, taurine, and combined vanadyl sulfate and taurine treatments in diabetic rats: effects on the oxidative and antioxidative systems. *M. Arch Med Res*, 2007 Apr;38(3):276-83

81 Thorne Research. (2006). Benfotiamine. Monograph. Altern Med Rev. Sep;11(3):238-42.

82 Ibid. Thorne Research. (2006).

83 Ibid. Thorne Research. (2006).

84 Sharma, Y., Saxena, S., Mishra, A., Saxena, A., Natu, S. (2012). Advanced glycation end products and diabetic retinopathy. *J Ocul Biol Dis Infor*, Dec 5(3-4).

85 Uribarri, J., Woodruff, S., Goodman, S., Cai, W., Chen, X., et al. (2010). Advanced Glycation End Products in Foods and a Practical Guide to Their Reduction in the Diet. *J Am Diet Assoc*, Jun; 110(6):911–16.e12.

86 Kiecolt-Glaser, J.K., Bennett, J.M., Andridge, R., Peng, J., Shapiro, C.L. (2014). Yoga's impact on inflammation, mood, and fatigue in breast cancer survivors: a randomized controlled trial. *J Clin Oncol*, Apr 1;32(10):1040-9.

87 Nguyen, Q.D., Shah, S.M., Van Anden, E., Sung, J.U., Vitale, S., et al. (2004). Supplemental Oxygen Improves Diabetic Macular Edema: A Pilot Study. *Invest Ophthalmol Vis Sci*, Feb;45(2):617-24.

88 Javadi, M.A., Zarei-Ghanavati, S. (2008). Cataracts in Diabetic Patients: A Review Article. *J Ophthalmic Vis Res*, Jan; 3(1): 52–65.

[89] Jimenez, V., Jambrina, C., Casana, E., Sacristan, V., Munoz, S., et al. (2018). FGF21 gene therapy as treatment for obesity and insulin resistance. *EMBO Mol Med*, Aug;10(8):e8971.

90 Busskamp, V., Duebel, J., Balya, D., Fradot, M., Viney, T.J., et al. (2010). Genetic reactivation of cone photoreceptors restores visual responses in retinitis pigmentosa. *Science*, Jul 23;329(5990):413-7

91 Kumar, M.P., Sankeshi, V., Naik, R.R., Thirupathi, P. Das, B., et al. (2015). The inhibitory effect of Isoflavones isolated from Caesalpinia pulcherrima on aldose reductase in STZ induced diabetic rats. *Chem Biol Interact*, Jul 25;237:18-24.

92 Envisia. Retrieved Dec 7 2017 from http://www.envisiatherapeutics.com/.

15-7. DRY EYES

The most frequent complaint to eye doctors is dry eyes, known as aqueous insufficiency, meibomian gland dysfunction, or dry eye syndrome. Twenty-five percent of patients who visit ophthalmic clinics report symptoms of dry eye, making it a growing public health problem and one of the most common conditions seen by eye care practitioners.[1] In the U.S., moderate and/or severe dry eye affects more than 3.2 million of the female population and 1.6 million of male, at or over the age of 50.[2]

Anatomy of Dry Eye

Three Layers

The moisture-laden surface of the eye contains three interrelated layers known as the **tear film**. Stable continuity of that surface and the production of tears rely on the function of these three layers, which need to be produced in proper balanced amounts by the body to avoid dry eye syndrome:

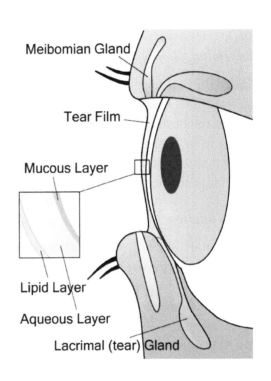

1. The innermost layer of the surface of the eye is a **mucous layer** that forms the bulk of the tears and contains electrolytes, a variety of proteins, and water. It also has some anti-microbial properties.
2. On top, on the outside of the mucous layer, is a mildly alkaline **aqueous layer** (watery) comprising up to 90% of the thickness of the tear film.
3. Outside the watery layer is an oily **lipid layer** that slows evaporation of the tear film. This thin layer is made up of meibum, produced by the meibomian gland.

Mucous Membrane

The mucous layer is the innermost layer of the tear film, closest to the surface of the cornea. "Goblet cells," floating in the conjunctiva, are gland-like cells that produce mucin. Mucin interacts with the watery layer of the tear film to form the thin mucous layer of the tear film that coats the cornea and allows for even distribution of the tear film. Goblet cells can be stimulated to greater production of mucin when the eye is irritated by environmental pollutants. Irritants such as some solvents can destroy goblet cells.

Eye surgery, which holds the eyelids open, can damage the conjunctiva and destroy goblet cells. This may be why many patients experience severe dry eyes after eye surgery.

The Tear Glands

The aqueous (watery) layer makes up to 90% of the thickness of the tear film. It is created by lacrimal glands, one for each eye, which lie along the orbit (bone) of the eyes above the lateral (outside) part of the eye. The slightly alkaline (pH-7.4) liquid produced by the lacrimal glands flows through canals into the lacrimal sac that is located on the inside of each eye beside the bridge of the nose. The action of blinking pumps tears onto and across the surface of the eye. In addition, tears flow from this sac into the nose. This is the reason you get a runny nose when there is too much fluid to stay on the surface of the eyes.

Nerves connect to the lacrimal glands, providing sensory stimulation (as when you cut an onion) to stimulate tears. Blood vessels also connect to the lacrimal glands, distributing nutrients and oxygen to the gland. These glands are also tied to the lymph system and as such, help drain toxins and impurities from the surface of the eye.

Meibomian Glands

A very thin oily (lipid) layer covers the outside of the tear film and helps slow evaporation of moisture. The meibomian glands, located on the upper and lower eyelids between the eye lashes, secretes meibum. Meibum is also produced by the Zeis and Moll glands. Meibum is fluid at body temperature. It slows tear film evaporation and lowers tear-film surface tension so that the tear film remains contoured to the surface of the eye and tears don't spill down to the cheeks. When the eyelids are closed, it is meibum that makes the eye within airtight.

Blink Function

The normal blinking process acts as a pump on the lacrimal sac to move more fluid to the eye and distribute it across the surface of the eye. Blinking brings material from the watery and oily layers and helps to remove debris. It is an essential part of eye comfort because the tear film naturally begins to degrade after about 10 seconds and needs renewal. Therefore, we normally blink automatically about 10-12 blinks a minute. When focused intently on something, our blink rate slows, as when working on the computer, which can result in dry eye syndrome.

After about 10 unblinking seconds, tear film becomes unstable, leading to tired, dry eyes. This is also partially true when the blink is incomplete and does not fully cover the cornea. The cornea tells the brain to send messages to the body to produce more or less tears and when to blink.

Symptoms

Symptoms of dry eye syndrome may include:

- Dryness and irritation
- Grittiness and a feeling that something is in your eye
- Burning and itching
- The seeming contradiction of excessive watering or tearing

Risk Factors and Causes

Meibomian dysfunction. Most dry eye symptoms have to do with meibomian gland dysfunction (MGD).[3] This occurs when natural oil produced by the lacrimal gland is either (a) blocked by the ducts along the upper and lower lids (25–30 in each lid), or (b) blocked along the openings at the lid margin. These oils produce the top layer of the tear film called the oil layer. When not secreted properly, tears evaporate more quickly causing dry eyes.

Tear film changes. Any condition that reduces the production, alters the composition, or impedes the distribution of the tear film may result in dry eyes. A problem with the eyelid can prevent the tears from distributing over the eyes properly.

Computer use. Mucin 5AC is a key component of the mucous layer and is essential in protecting the ocular surface by removing debris.[4] Workers spending the most time on the computer have the lowest concentrations of mucin 5AC, which contributes to their dry eye syndrome.[5]

Other health conditions. Like most eye conditions, dry eye syndrome often is related to health conditions in the rest of the body. It is commonly associated with dryness of other mucous membranes and brittle nails.

Dry eye syndrome also can be a sign of digestive imbalances or of more serious autoimmune diseases such as rheumatoid arthritis, Sjogren's syndrome, or lupus erythematosus. Such diseases trigger an immune response generating lymphocytes (white blood cells) that slowly destroy the cells that are responsible for tear production and secretion. As a result, tear volume decreases, cells in the conjunctiva decrease, and corneal cells can be lost. This can create dry spots.

In post-menopausal women, dry eyes also can be a sign of Sjogren's syndrome, commonly misdiagnosed. In Sjogren's syndrome, dry eyes are accompanied by dryness in other parts of the body: dry mouth, dry joints (arthritis), sore throat, dry skin, dry cracked lips, dry scalp (dandruff), and brittle nails. This is an autoimmune process in which antibodies attack fluid secreting cells and produce this pattern of symptoms. Fatigue and dental cavities often are present.

Inflammation. Dry eye syndrome is considered to be an inflammatory condition. In Sjogren's syndrome, for instance, the entire lacrimal gland that is responsible for 90% of tear production, may be destroyed by inflammatory lymphocytes. Drops to decrease inflammation are often used along with specific supplements.

Hormonal levels. Dry eyes are a health problem mainly for women and seems to be related to fluctuations in hormone levels, particularly estrogen and androgens. Pregnant women, women who use birth control pills, and peri-menopausal, menopausal, and post-menopausal women frequently report dry eyes.

Aging. Dry eyes also can be an isolated problem. As we age, our eyes produce about 40% less lubrication; seniors naturally have drier eyes. Free radicals are partly to blame; they take their toll over time, damaging body tissues and increasing the prevalence of dry eye symptoms.

Contact lenses. Long-term contact lens use, especially soft lens, also can contribute to dry eyes,[6] because over time, contact lenses can reduce corneal sensitivity. The sensitivity of the cornea and the entire ocular surface determines how many tears the lacrimal gland will secrete. The less sensitive the cornea, the fewer tears, or more in some cases.

Environmental issues. Tobacco smoke, environmental allergens, air conditioning, and wind might also cause dry eyes. A 5-year study showed that cigarette smokers were more likely to have dry eyes by a factor of 1.44 compared to sex and age-matched nonsmokers.[7]

Medications. Many medications trigger dry eyes, most commonly antihistamines, codeine, decongestants, diuretics, morphine, oral contraceptives, and even eyedrops such as Visine and Murine used for "getting the red out."

Migraines. Researchers have long suspected that there may be a connection between dry eyes and migraine headaches. One study investigates that tie by investigating the relationship between tear capacity and migraine symptoms in patients.[8]

Conventional Approach

First, a careful review is done on the patient history, and then diagnostic testing measures how salty the tear content is (**osmolarity**). Schirmer testing measures tear volume. InflammaDry is a rapid in-office test that detects MMP-9, an inflammatory marker that is consistently elevated in the tears of patients with dry eye disease. Standard medical treatment for dry eyes includes the following options: artificial tear preparations in the form of eyedrops or a procedure called punctal occlusion after which you retain more tears in your eyes by reducing tear drainage.

Treatment often includes Blephex, an instrument used to scrub the bacterial biofilm across the eyelid where approximately 50 gland openings are, probing glands as necessary, and MiBoflo treatment. MiBoflo is a 108 degree, heated, double pad with ultrasound gel to heat the lids and melt lipids, so that they flow thru the openings. With this system, eyedrops can be customized for each patient.

Sometimes the eye doctor will prescribe an eyedrop such as Restasis or Xiidra for helping, over time, to produce more tears. These eyedrops can be helpful, but do have potential side effects, so these should be discussed with your eye doctor. For the more severe dry eye problems, many doctors use an amniotic membrane on the eye for healing purposes, such as Prokera.

Artificial tears

Although many people find temporary relief by using artificial tear preparations, these merely palliate the symptoms. Worse, the preservatives in many of these products can aggravate the condition and can even kill corneal cells. Eyedrops called vasoconstrictors that promise to "get the red out" reduce circulation in the eye, decrease production of the tear film, and eventually make your eyes even drier. Once the effects of the vasoconstrictors wear off, the blood vessels that were constricted re-dilate, causing a "rebound red eye" that can trap you in a cycle of constantly having to use the drops.

Punctal Occlusion

Many people tire of using eyedrops and turn to punctal occlusion that might provide longer-term relief. Punctal occlusion is a procedure based on the theory that if the tear outflow is limited by occluding (blocking) the area from which the tears flow, the amount of tearing will increase. This, in turn, increases the overall length of time that tears are in contact with the cornea and may be more comfortable to dry-eye sufferers.

Punctal occlusion closes the drain that draws away excess fluids from the eyes. Here is how it works: there are tear drainage canals on the margins of the upper and lower eyelids near the nose. Tiny pumps inside the drainage opening suck away fluid from the surface of the eyes. In punctal occlusion, the doctor closes the drain with silicone plugs, which keep most of the fluids from being pumped away. In one mega study analysis, the conclusion was that plug placement resulted in ≥50% improvement of symptoms, improvement in ocular-surface health, reduction in artificial tear use, and improved contact lens comfort in patients with dry eye. Serious complications from plugs were infrequent.[9]

Home Treatment

Also utilized is a home treatment including heat goggles and occasionally moisture goggles. Information can be collected using digital photography and video, to show the patient the difference prior to, and after, treatment.

Cyclosporine and Lifitegrast are prescription medications approved by the U.S. Food and Drug Administration for treating dry eyes. Corticosteroid eyedrops also may be prescribed short-term to reduce eye inflammation.[10] New formulations of eye lubricant drops contain substances such as hyaluronic acid (absorbs up to 10 times its weight in water), vitamin A, E, and omega-3 oils.

Complementary Approach

Only use eyedrops without preservatives. These have been shown to enhance corneal healing and improve dry eye problems. Several recommended brands are Thera Tears, Oasis Plus, Natural Ophthalmics' Tear Stimulation Forte eyedrops, and/or Similisan #1, 2, or 3. Thera Tears has been shown to aid in the healing of dry eyes after eight weeks of treatment. In several studies, users have reported 90% improvement. Similisan and Natural Ophthalmics have homeopathic formulations that help stimulate the eyes to produce tears naturally. We recommend eyedrops that not only help relieve dry eyes but have the potential to contribute to eye healing (see Appendix 5 for product suggestions).

As dry eye syndrome is often related to other issues, using only eyedrops can help relieve symptoms, but it can also be very important to take supplements. Supplements can help internally moisten the body related to dry eyes, as well as reduce inflammation that may be related to dry eye symptoms. Some supplements help with natural tear production as well.

Nutrients

Essential

Omega-3 fatty acids. 3,000 IU–4,500 IU per day. In an evaluation of diet and dry-eye incidence in nearly 40,000 people, researchers noted that high intakes of omega-3s taken in foods (like fish) contribute as much as 66% reduction in dry eye syndrome. These women ate 5–6 servings of tuna weekly.[11] Other subjects receiving omega-3 supplementation showed significantly reduced osmolarity. Additionally, **tear break up time** (TBUT) was reduced, which is a measure of how fast the tear film protecting the surface of the cornea begins to break up. Lowered levels of inflammation were observed. Of particular interest was that many of the signs and symptoms of chronic dry eye improved relatively quickly, as early as 6 weeks.[12]

Note 1. We do not recommend 5-6 servings of tuna weekly as these fish may contain high levels of mercury and there are other ways such as taking supplements from low level fish including sardines and mackerel.

Note 2. Because of mixed results in research, more analysis needs to be done. Eating whole fish, as well as paying attention to the omega-3 and omega-6 ratio may be important. One double-blind study involving about 350 people found that taking only omega-3 fatty acids did not, by itself, improve dry eye.[13]

Homeopathic eyedrops for dry eyes

Preservative free eyedrops help keep the eyes lubricated.

Castor oil eyedrops (used before bedtime) help to keep the eyes lubricated and have natural anti-inflammatory and healing properties. They are particularly good for dry eyes symptoms that are more severe during the night and early morning.

Dry eye formulas containing mucopolysaccharides (mucin complex) are sugar complexes that help with natural tear production. Mucin is the primary component of the mucous or innermost layer of the tear film. See Appendix 5 for more information.

Important

Evening primrose or black current oil. 500mg per day. Black currant oil increases prostaglandin PGE1. PGE1 is a fatty compound with hormone-like effects that stimulates aqueous tear secretion and reduces the production of another prostaglandin, PGE2, which causes inflammation that contributes to dry eyes.[14]

Vitamin D (vitamin D3 recommended). 2,000 IU–5,000 IU per day. Not only is dry eye syndrome associated with low levels of vitamin D, but the evaporative type of dry eye syndrome is linked to changes in cornea structure (which may be linked to vitamin D deficiency).[15] [16] [17]

Helpful

Vitamin A (palmitate). 2,000 IU–5,000 IU per day. Vitamin A is an essential nutrient for the health of the epithelial cells of the eye's cornea and conjunctiva, and it is required for the manufacture of mucin, the primary component of the mucous (innermost) layer of the tear film.[18]

> **Note**. Vitamin A is contra-indicated for those suffering from Stargardt disease (see Stargardt's chapter for more information). Pregnant women should not supplement with vitamin A.

Green tea extract. Patients with malfunctioning meibomian glands improved significantly compared to a control group when supplementing with this extract.[19]

Kidney yin tonic. The Kidney meridian helps with water metabolism throughout the body, supports overall energy, and helps with overall dryness (dry eyes, dry skin, dry scalp, etc.) See VisionTone formula in Appendix 5. This tonic is particularly recommended for women entering or going through menopause.

Liver tonic. In Chinese medicine the Liver "opens to the eyes" and supports overall eye health. It also helps with natural tear production (see ReVision formula in Appendix 5).

Diet

Follow the Vision diet described in Chapter 7.

Limit or avoid sugar and artificial sweeteners. It is thought that excess sugar in one's diet results in too much glucose making its way to the eyes, making it difficult for the eyes to utilize all the glucose. This may result in more dry eye symptoms and can cause diabetes. 54.3% of diabetics suffer from dry eye syndrome.[20] Know what you are putting into your body.

Avoid toxic fats in commercial red meats, dairy products, fried foods, and hydrogenated oils (such as margarine and shortening). These fats interfere with the proper metabolism of essential fatty acids in the body and, indirectly, cause dry eye syndrome.

Gut issues may contribute to dry eye. Try taking a high-quality probiotic to replenish the healthy flora in your gut, particularly if you have been on long-term antibiotics. Once your symptoms are under control, try switching from probiotics in pill form to real food ferments such as sauerkraut, pickles, miso, kefir, kombucha, kimchi, etc. Not only do they provide a greater variety of beneficial bacteria than can be found in a pill, but they contain many vitamins and minerals.

If inflammation is a contributing factor in your dry eye, then it is imperative to look at the possibility that your gut (leaky gut) may be the source of the inflammation, as well as imbalances in gut flora. Chronic inflammatory conditions have been tied to dry eye syndrome.[21]

Juicing is an excellent way to deliver nutrients to your body. Our juicing recipe includes:

- Parsley, beets, carrots, cucumber, tomatoes, persimmons, lemon, green-leafy vegetables,

(preferably all organic)

Choose at least 4-6 items to combine. Do not use too many carrots. Add your favorite fruits and vegetables.

Lifestyle

Exercise such as a brisk daily walk is important for all eye conditions and overall health.

A Japanese study concluded that an increase in the level of physical activity can be an effective intervention for the prevention of and/or treatment of dry eye disease, as well as helping alleviate other disorders including pain in the neck, shoulders, and/or low back, and chronic depression.[22]

Daily eye exercises include:

- Palming
- Eye massage of acupressure points
- Near and far
- Hot dog

See Chapter 10-4 for more ideas.

Other Modalities

Chinese Medicine

Although there are a number of conditions and circumstances that can result in dry eyes, acupuncture and Chinese herbal formulas often help manage the dry eye problem and reduce symptoms. The Liver "opens to the eyes" and is the primary meridian for supporting overall flow of energy and circulation through the eyes. It also helps with natural tear production.

The Kidney meridian nourishes the blood to the eyes and helps with internal water metabolism often related to dry eye syndrome. Other meridians may be out of balance as well that can affect eye health, so an evaluation by an acupuncturist can best determine where the out-of-balances are, and offer the optimal treatment strategy. Acupuncture treatments are typically done by inserting needles below the knees and elbows, then in specific points along the orbit of the eye and under the eye (not in the eye). An evaluation by an acupuncturist is the best way to determine where the imbalances are.

Chinese Medicine Patent Formulas

Preserve vistas pill (zhu jing wan). Tonifies and nourishes the Liver and Kidneys, enriches the yin and improves vision.

Ming mu di huang wan (rehmannia pills to brighten the eyes). This is related to the patterns of Liver blood deficiency, Kidney yin deficiency, and/or Liver yin deficiency

Xiao yao san (rambling powder). Classic Liver tonic supports the flow of the Liver meridian energy.

Herbal Tea

Chrysanthemum and goji berry tea. Chrysanthemum flowers have heat-clearing properties that are important in helping cool off red, dry eyes. Goji berries are beneficial for the kidneys, the lungs, the liver, and build yin fluids such as tears. Brew the chrysanthemum flowers like you would any loose tea and then put a small handful of goji berries into the made tea. After drinking the tea, you can eat the berries

Essential Oils

Carrot seed essential oil has antiseptic, disinfectant, detoxifier, and antioxidant properties.

Frankincense helps relieve chronic stress and anxiety, reduces pain and inflammation, and boosts immunity.

Clary sage helps balance the endocrine system.

Keep essences away from the mouth, eyes, and mucous membranes; if a few drops get in one of these sensitive areas it may be uncomfortable for 15–30 minutes, but not harmful. You can lessen discomfort by adding a pure oil like olive or coconut oil to neutralize the irritating effect. For the eye area, dab a few drops around the outside of the eye. Do not put the neutralizing oil in the eye.

Combine ¼ cup of avocado oil with ¼ cup of calendula-infused oil. Slowly add 5 drops each of the essential oils. Then close the bottle and shake well; apply 4 drops of this mixture on your clean face. Massage in gentle circular motions. Leave overnight.

For more information, see Essential Oils under Appendix 9.

On the Horizon

The MiBoFlo Thermoflo is a therapeutic device providing an alternative therapy for dry eyes. It uses a proprietary thermoelectric heat pump to help maximize liquefaction of meibum, thus improving the preservation and function of the evaporative component of the tear film. This therapy is aimed at improving function of the meibomian component of the tear film.

A small pilot study found that a standardized maqui berry extract increased tear production and relieved dry eye.[23]

Also See

Chapter 7, Vision Diet

Chapter 8, Nutrients

Chapter 10-4, Eye Exercises

Appendix 5, Recommended Products

[1] O'Brien, P.D., Collum, L.M. (2004). Dry eye: diagnosis and current treatment strategies. *Curr Allergy Asthma Rep*, 4:314–319.

[2] Schaumberg, D.A., Sullivan, D.A., Buring, J.E., Dana, M.R. (2003). Prevalence of dry eye syndrome among US women. *Am J Ophthalmol*, Aug; 136(2):318-26.

[3] Nowinska, A., Wylegala, E., Tarnawska, D., Janiszewska, D., Dobrowolskia, D. (2012). Meibomian gland dysfunction—review. *Klin Oczna*, 114(2):147-52.

[4] Gipson, I.K., Hori, Y., Argueso, P. (2004). Character of ocular surface mucins and their alteration in dry eye disease. *Ocul Surf*, 2(2):131-148.

[5] Uchino, Y., Uchino, M., Yokoi, N. (2014). Alteration of Tear Mucin 5AC in Office Workers Using Visual Display Terminals: The Osaka Study. *JAMA Ophthalmol,* 132(8):985-992.

[5] Kastelan, S., Lukenda, A., Salpek-Rabatic, J., Pavan, J., Gotovac, M. (2013). Dry eye symptoms and signs in long-term contact lens wearers. *Coll Antropol*, Apr;37 Suppl 1:199-203

[7] Moss, S.E., Klein, R., Klein, B.E. (2000). Prevalence of and risk factors for dry eye syndrome. *Arch Ophthalmol*, Sep; 118(9):1264-8.

[8] Koktekir, B.E., Celik, G., Karalezli, A., Kal, A. (2012). Dry eyes and migraines: Is there really a correlation? *Cornea*, Dec;31(12):1414-6.

[9] Marcet, M.M., Shtein, R.M., Bradley, E.A., Deng, S.X., Meyer, D.R., et al. (2015). Safety and efficacy of lacrimal drainage system plugs for dry eye syndrome. *Ophthalmology*, Aug;122(8):1681-7.

[10] National Eye Institute, Facts about dry eye. Retrieved Dec 17 2017 from https://nei.nih.gov/health/dryeye/dryeye.

[11] Epitropoulous, A.T., Donnenfeld, E.D., Shah, Z.A., Holland, E.J., Gross, M., et al. (2016). Effect of Oral Re-esterified Omega-3 Nutritional Supplementation on Dry Eyes. *Cornea*, Sep;35(9):1185-91.

[12] Miljanovic, B., Trivedi, K.A., Dana, M.R., Gilbard, J.P., Buring, J.E., et al. (2005). Relation between dietary n-3 and n-6 fatty acids and clinically diagnosed dry eye syndrome in women. *Am J Clin Nutr*, Oct;82(4):887-93.

[13] Dry Eye Assessment and Management Study Research Group. (2018). n−3 Fatty Acid Supplementation for the Treatment of Dry Eye Disease. *N Engl J Med*, Apr 13.

[14] Baudouin, C. (1986). Dry eye: An unexpected inflammatory disease. Arch Soc *Esp Oftalmol*, 76: 205-206.

[15] Shetty, R. Sethu, S., Deshmukh, R., Despande, K., Ghosh, A., et al. (2016). Corneal dendritic cell density is associated with sub-basal nerve plexus features, ocular surface disease index, and serum vitamin D in evaporative dry eye disease. *BioMed Res Int*, 2016:4369750.

[16] Denurcum, G., Karaman, E.S., Ozsutcu, M., Eliacik, M., Olmuscelik, O., et al. (2016). Dry eye assessment in patients with vitamin D deficiency. *Eye Contact Lens*, Sep 22.

[17] Nejabat, M., Reza, S.A., Zadmehr, M., Yasemi, M., Sobhani, Z. (2017). Efficacy of green tea extract for treatment of dry eye and meibomian gland dysfunction; A double-blind randomized controlled clinical trial study. *J Clin Diagn Res*, Feb;11(2):NC05-NC08.

[18] Tei, M., Spurr-Michaud, S.J., Tisdale, A.S., Gipson, I.K. (2000). Vitamin A deficiency alters the expression of mucin genes by the rat ocular surface epithelium. *Invest Ophthalmol Vis Sci*, Jan;41(1):82-8.

[19] Ibid. Nejabat. (2017).

[20] Masoud, R.M., Rashidi, M., Afkhami-Ardekani, M., Shoja, M.R. (2008). Prevalence of dry eye syndrome and diabetic retinopathy in type 2 diabetic patients. *BMC Ophthalmol*, Jun 2;8:10.

[21] Ibid. Baudouin. (1986).

[22] Kawashima, M., Uchino, M., Yokoi, N., Uchino, Y., Dogru, M., et al. (2014). The Association between dry eye disease and physical activity as well as sedentary behavior: Results from the Osaka study. *J Ophthalmol*, 2014:943786.

[23] Hitoe, S., Tanaka, J., Shimoda, H. (2014). MaquiBright™ standardized maqui berry extract significantly increases tear fluid production and ameliorates dry eye-related symptoms in a clinical pilot trial. *Panminerva Med*, Sep;56(3 Supple 1):1-6.

15-8. EPIRETINAL MEMBRANE

Epiretinal membrane (ERM) is more commonly known as "macular pucker." It is identified as well with the following terms of very similar conditions: epimacular membrane, surface-wrinkling retinopathy, cellophane maculopathy, and pre-retinal macular fibrosis.

ERM gets its common name from scar tissue that has formed on the macula, creating a very thin, nearly transparent layer of fibrous tissue that spreads across the retinal surface. When this thin fibrous layer contracts, the retinal surface is wrinkled or puckered. Other names come from its similarity in appearance to a layer of cellophane, where folding and puckering has not yet developed.[1]

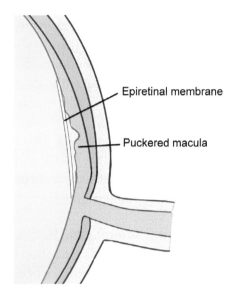
Epiretinal membrane

Puckered macula

This condition is seen most in elderly persons over 75 and is often associated with other eye problems such as vitreous or retinal detachment, diabetic retinopathy, trauma to the eye, and other conditions. Based on one study, the prevalence of ERM was 1.9% in persons younger than 60 years of age, 7.2% in persons 60 to 69 years of age, 11.6% in persons 70 to 79 years of age, and 9.3% in persons 80 years of age and older, with slightly higher rates in women. Strong associations were shown for this with diabetes, as well as with past cataract surgery and retinal disease.[2]

In a study done with Chinese adults in 2015, the prevalence rate of ERM in mainland Chinese individuals of 50 years of age or older was estimated to be 7.3%. The prevalence of ERM in elderly urban Chinese was similar to that in Caucasians. Risk factors for idiopathic ERM were older age, female gender, myopia, and hyperlipidaemia (medical term for abnormally high levels of fats/lipids in the blood).[3]

For most people, visual acuity remains stable and does not get progressively worse. Usually macular pucker affects one eye, although it may affect the other eye later.

Pathology

Epiretinal membranes do not contain blood vessels. They are comprised of fibrocellular cells: glial cells (cells that surround neurons), retinal pigment epithelial cells (lining tissue cells), macrophages (large white blood cells), fibrocytes (cells that produce connective tissue), and collagen (structural protein in connective tissue).[4] This composite is attached to the retina and contracts, distorting the retina. The degree of visual distortion can vary, depending on the amount of, and the location of, the pucker.

Macular pucker is typically a slow-progressing problem that affects the central vision by causing blurring and distortion. As it progresses, pulling of the membrane on the macula (central part of the retina) may cause swelling. An epiretinal membrane will not cause total blindness and will typically and only affect the central vision in the affected eye. Peripheral or 'side' vision remains unaffected. The vast majority of those with ERM are asymptomatic. For most people, vision remains stable and does not get progressively worse. Usually macular pucker affects one eye, although it may affect the other eye later.

Types of Epiretinal Membrane

IEMM. Idiopathic epiretinal macular membrane (IEMM) is one of the most common forms of epiretinal membrane. Membranes that are comprised of glial cells (cells that surround nerve cells, insulating them) apparently develop spontaneously or from idiopathic (unknown) causes.[5] Posterior vitreous detachment results in 75–93% of these cases.

Retinal detachment-related. This is the other common type of epiretinal membrane in relation to breaks or tears in the retina, detached retina, or surgical reattachment of the retina to the pigmented layer that uses laser photocoagulation and cryopexy.[6] These membranes are mostly comprised of retinal pigment epithelial cells.

Vitreous traction-related. If there is no posterior vitreous detachment, then patients may experience vitreomacular traction syndrome (VMT).[7] The vitreous contains millions of fine fibers that are attached to the surface of the retina. As we age (over 50 years old commonly), the vitreous that keeps the shape of the back of our eyes begins to shrink, causing a pulling on the retina.

Interior limiting membrane. Sometimes the interior of the retinal surface is affected, in which case the membrane forms prior to a vitreous detachment.[8]

Signs and Symptoms

An epiretinal membrane can be minor and may have no noticeable effect on vision at all. In other cases, the epiretinal membrane may worsen over time, causing blurring and distortion to the central part of your vision. In some cases, macular edema occurs (in which fluid is retained in a cyst under the macula) or retinal detachment.

If a macular hole occurs as a result of the ERM, the size of the hole determines how much it will reduce vision. Larger holes cause greater vision loss. Vision often is reduced to 20/200 or less if the hole is not repaired. In worst-case scenarios, one will not lose all vision. Peripheral or side vision is still retained.

Causes and Risk Factors

Age. Epiretinal membranes occur more frequently in older patients with a 20% rate in people over age 75.

Vitreous detachment. Sixty-five percent of people over the age of 65 will experience a posterior vitreous detachment (PVD).[9] The vitreous keeps the shape of the back of the eye and is attached to the retina. As one ages (particularly 50 years of age and older), the vitreous starts to shrink, which causes pulling on the retina that often results in a PVD and sometimes a macula pucker.

Conventional Treatment

IEMM. A procedure called internal limiting membrane peeling is commonly used in the idiopathic form of ERM. It is considered safe and effective.[10]

Vitreous traction related. Though often not requiring any medical intervention, sometimes vision deteriorates due to the pulling on the retina, to the point where it affects daily routine activities. In these cases, a surgical procedure called a vitrectomy may be recommended. The retinal surgeon removes the vitreous gel to prevent it from further pulling on the retina and replaces it with a salt solution (because the vitreous is mostly water, you will notice no change between the salt solution and the normal vitreous). The surgeon also removes the scar tissue causing the wrinkling. Usually half of the vision lost can be restored and the vision distortion improved.

Cataracts often develop as a result of the surgery within a few years afterward. Less common complications are **retinal detachment** either during or after surgery, and/or **infection** after surgery.

Recurring pucker. The macular pucker may grow back, but this is rare.

Complementary Approach

We believe that vision conditions like epiretinal membrane are a reflection of the health of the entire physiology and vision system. Lifestyle choices, including a high-quality diet and taking targeted supplements can make a big difference in preventing and managing this condition. Proper nutrition is essential for eye health, as it promotes proper circulation, bringing nutrients to, and removing toxins from, the eyes. Also, getting daily exercise, avoiding smoking, and avoiding other toxins such as food additives are crucial.

Nutrients

These nutrients have been found to support the health of the retina.

Essential

Lutein. 6mg–20mg per day. This carotenoid is well researched for retinal support and essential for supporting the retinal pigment.[11] Taking lutein along with zeaxanthin and astaxanthin improves visual acuity (vision sharpness).[12]

Zeaxanthin. 2mg–12mg per day. Along with lutein, zeaxanthin is a potent antioxidant found in the retina to help maintain the health of the retina.[13]

Omega-3 fatty acids. 2,000mg–3,000mg per day. Studies found that omega-3 fatty acids, along with lutein and zeaxanthin help preserve vision. Researchers have found that omega-3 fatty acids have the capacity to actually regulate formation of blood vessels, and along with lutein and zeaxanthin in helping preserve vision and supporting people to maintain independent living.[14]

Vitamin D3. 2,000 IU–5,000 IU per day. Lower levels of vitamin D are associated with retinal microvascular damage, suggesting that the link with cardiovascular risk may partly run through changes in the microvasculature.[15]

Astaxanthin. 6mg–12mg per day. Researchers concluded that astaxanthin was effective in protecting against damage from light due to its antioxidant effect.[16] [17]

Trans-resveratrol. 150mg–175mg per day. **Grapeseed extract** (300mg per day) and **pycnogenol** (100mg–200mg per day) can also be used; they have similar benefits of helping to strengthen blood vessels and reduce inflammation. All these antioxidants have been found to support blood vessels and healthy circulation, modulate the inflammatory response, and neutralize free radicals. One study noted that resveratrol has antioxidant and anti-inflammatory abilities.[18] Take one of the above, or all three.

Vitamin C (buffered and ascorbated). 2,000mg–3,000mg per day. Vitamin C is a powerful antioxidant that is essential for overall eye health. Vitamin C supports blood and lymph circulation, waste elimination, and connective tissue integrity. As an antioxidant, vitamin C scavenges free radicals in the body and protects tissues from oxidative stress.[19] [20]

Very Important

Bilberry. 120mg–180mg per day. Bilberry is neuroprotective and has been shown to improve microcirculation.[21] [22] [23] [24] It is widely used to decrease vascular permeability and capillary fragility; moreover, the berry has various other reputed health benefits, although most interest has been focused on anthocyanin-related antioxidant effects.[25]

Ginkgo biloba. 120mg per day, *and/or* **vinpocetine** at 10mg–30mg per day. Ginkgo contains many different flavonoids, including polyphenolic flavonoids, which have been proven to exert antioxidative properties by delivering electrons to free radicals.[26] It improves overall circulation.[27]

Taurine. 500mg–1,000mg per day. Taurine deficiency leads to retinal degeneration, and supplementing with taurine helps to prevent and stabilize retinal changes.[28] [29] [30] [31]

A good, whole-food, organic **multivitamin.**

Helpful

Green tea. 500mg–750mg per day. Green tea has excellent capacity for scavenging reactive oxygen species such as superoxide and the hydroxyl and peroxyl radical.[32] [33] [34] [35]

Hyaluronic acid. 100mg per day. Hyaluronic acid is found in high concentrations in the vitreous and may be related to helping maintain the integrity of the vitreous and related connective tissue to the retina.[36] Hyaluronic acid (hyaluronan) is a large molecule found in the vitreous gel that is believed to contribute to the vitreous' gel-like quality, and which also may support related connective tissue.[37] It is a component of the tissue healing process. As we age, the amount of hyaluronan in the body decreases. Common foods that contain hyaluronic acid include bone broth, organ meat, soy foods, red wine, and root vegetables.

Diet

Make sure you have a healthy diet with lots of fresh vegetables and fruits (preferably organic).

Juicing. Daily juicing of organic vegetables and fruits is ideal. Include any combination of the following. Add your favorite fruits and vegetables.

- Ginger, leeks, garlic, parsley, cabbage, beets, carrots, green, leafy vegetables including spinach, kale, and swiss chard, apples, celery, grapes, lemon, raspberries, or wheatgrasses
- Don't include too much fruit, beets, or carrots because of their high natural sugar content.
- Try to use room temperature vegetables and fruit and do not add ice or very cold liquids since cold foods and liquids will eventually extinguish the stomach's digestive fire.
- Do not juice too often during the cooler months of the year, and instead, switch to vegetable soups or stews.

Lifestyle

Exercise. Get some exercise daily; a brisk walk is a great idea, though we recommend being careful with bouncing exercises, head down yoga postures, or lifting heavy weights without your doctor's permission. Light exercise may include daily aerobic exercise such as speed walks, light jogging, hiking, elliptical machine use at the gym, light weights with more reps, swimming, etc.

Eye exercises can include:

- Palming
- Near and far
- Hot dog

See Chapter 10-4 for more information on eye exercises.

Other Modalities

Chinese Medicine

In Chinese medicine, the Liver "opens to the eyes" so it is the primary meridian for supporting overall flow of energy and circulation through the eyes. The Kidney meridian nourishes the blood to the eyes. The Spleen meridian also nourishes the blood while also helping to keep fluids from leaking from blood vessels. Other meridians may be out of balance as well, which can affect eye health, so an evaluation by an acupuncturist can best determine where the out-of-balances are and offer the optimal treatment strategy.

Ming mu di huang wan (brighten the eyes), taken by mouth in pill form, treats what is known as Kidney and Liver yin deficiency. It helps treat symptoms typical of yin deficiency (dryness, dizziness, night sweats, insomnia, constipation, etc.) with the addition of dry eyes, blurry vision, sensitivity to light, as well as photophobia, excessive tearing (specifically with exposure to wind), eye pain, and/or swelling, and dizziness.

Zhu jing wan (preserve vistas pill) tonifies and nourishes the Liver and Kidneys, enriches the yin energy which includes supporting essential fluids in the body, and improves vision.

Gui pi tang (restore the Spleen decoction) increases qi, tonifies blood, strengthens the Spleen, nourishes the Heart, and helps the Spleen control the blood. In Traditional Chinese Medicine (TCM), the Heart controls the blood and stores Shen (the spirit). The Spleen absorbs the nutrients from food and transports them to the blood. Poor transport of blood and inability to completely absorb nutrients can affect eye health and contribute to a wide range of eye conditions, including ERM and macular degeneration.

Also See

Chapter 7, Vision Diet

Chapter 8, Nutrients

Chapter 10, Self Help Tips and Eye Exercises

Chapter 15-19, Macular Edema

Chapter 15-20, Macular Hole

Chapter 15-25, Retinal Detachment

Chapter 15-32, Vitreous Detachment

Appendix 5, Recommended Products

[1] Delcourt, C., Korobelnik, J.F., Barberger-Gateau, P., Delyfer, M.N., Marie-Benedicte, R., et al. (2010). Nutrition and Age-Related Eye Diseases: The ALIENOR (Antioxydants, Lipides Essentiels, Nutrition et Maladies OculaiRes) Study. *J Nutr Health Aging*, 14(10): 854–861.

[2] Mitchell, P., Smith, W., Chey, T., Wang, J.J., Chang, A. (1997). Prevalence and associations of epiretinal membranes. The Blue Mountains Eye Study, Australia. *Ophthalmology*, Jun;104(6):1033-40

[3] Ye, H., Zhang, Q., Liu, X., Cai, X., Yu, W., et al. (2015). Prevalence and associations of epiretinal membrane in an elderly urban Chinese population in China: the Jiangning Eye Study. *Br J Ophthalmol*, Dec;99(12):1594-7.

[4] Oh, K.T. (2016). Epiretinal Membrane: Pathophysiology. *Medscape*. Retrieved Jan 24 2018.

[5] Ibid. Oh. (2016).

[6] Ibid. Oh. (2016).

[7] Chang, L.K., Fine, H.F., Spaide, R.F., Koisumi, H., Grossniklaus, H.E. (2008). Ultrastructural correlation of spectral-domain optical coherence tomographic findings in vitreomacular traction syndrome. *Am J Ophthalmol*, Jul;146(1):121-7.

8 Bovey, E.H., Uffer, S. (2008). Tearing and folding of the retinal internal limiting membrane associated with macular epiretinal membrane. *Retina*, Mar;28(3):433-40.

9 Scott, I.U., Smiddy, W.E., Merikansky, A., Feuer, W. (1997). Vitreoretinal surgery outcomes: impact on bilateral visual function. *Ophthalmology*, 104:1041-8

[10] Ondrejkova, M., Gajdosova, M., Kyselova, P. (2015). Surgical Treatment for Idiopathic Epiretinal Membrane. *Cesk Slov Oftalmol*, Aug;71(4):204-8.

[11] Landrum, J.T., Bone, R.A., Kilburn, M.D., Moore, L.L., et al. (1997). A one year study of the macular pigment: the lutein supplement. *Exp Eye Res*, Jul;65(1):57-62

[12] Piermarocchi, S., Saviano, S., Parisi V, Tedeschi, M., Panozzo, G., et al. (2012.) Carotenoids in age-related maculopathy Italian study, *Eur J Ophthalmol*, Mar-Apr:22(2):216-25.

[13] National Eye Institute. (2013) NIH study provides clarity on supplements for protection against blinding eye disease. Retrieved Feb 18 2018 from https://nei.nih.gov/news/pressreleases/ 050513

[14] Goodnight, S.H. (1989). The vascular effects of omega-3 fatty acids. *J Invest Dermatol*, Aug;93(2 Suppl):102S-106S

[15] Mutlu, U., Ikram, M.A., Hofman, A., de Jong, P.T., Uiterlinden, A.G., et al. (2016). Vitamin D and retinal microvascular damage: The Rotterdam Study. *Medicine (Baltimore)*, Dec; 95(49): e5477.

[16] Otsuka, T., Shimazawa, M., Nakanishi, T., Ohno, Y., Inoue, Y., et al. (2013). Protective effects of a dietary carotenoid, astaxanthin, against light-induced retinal damage, *J Pharmacol Sci*, 123(3):209-18.

[17] Piermarocchi, S., Saviano, S., Parisi, V., Tedeschi, M., Panozzo, G., et al. (2012). Carotenoids in Age-related Maculopathy Italian Study (CARMIS): two-year results of a randomized study. *Eur J Ophthalmol*, Mar-Apr;22(2):216-25.

[18] Wang, Z. Wang S., Yang, S., Yin, T., Zhang, Y., et al. (2017). Tissue Distribution of trans-Resveratrol and Its Metabolites after Oral Administration in Human Eyes, *J Ophthalmol*, 4052094.

[19] Du, J., Cullen, J.J., Buettner, G.R. (2012). Ascorbic acid: chemistry, biology and the treatment of cancer. *Biochem Biophys Acta*, Dec;1826(2):443-57.

[20] Cangemi, R., Angelico, F., Loffredo, L., Del Ben, M., Pignatelli, P., et al. (2007). Oxidative stress-mediated arterial dysfunction in patients with metabolic syndrome: Effect of ascorbic acid. *Free Radic Biol Med*, Sep 1;43(5):853-9

[21] Matsunaga, N., Imai, S., Inokuchi, Y., Shimazawa, M., Yokota, S., et al. (2009). Bilberry and its main constituents have neuroprotective effects against retinal neuronal damage in vitro and in vivo. *Mol Nutr Food Res*, Jul;53(7):869-77.

22 Zhu, Y., Xia, M., Yang, Y., Liu F., Li, Z. et al. (2011). Purified anthocyanin supplementation improves endothelial function via NO-cGMP activation in hypercholesterolemic individuals. *Clin Chem*, Nov;57(11):1524-33.

23 Cohen-Boulakia, F., Valensi, P.E., Boulahdour, H., Lestrade, R., Dufour-Lamartinie, J.R., et al. (2000). In vivo sequential study of skeletal muscle capillary permeability in diabetic rats: effect of anthocyanosides. *Metabolism*. Jul;49(7):880-5.

24 Yao, Y., Vieira, A., (2007). Protective activities of Vaccinium antioxidants with potential relevance to mitochondrial dysfunction and neurotoxicity. *NeuroToxicology*, 28 (2007) 93–100

25 Pool-Zobel, B.L, Bub, A., Schrader, N., Rechkemmer, G. (1999). Anthocyanins are potent antioxidants in model systems but do not reduce endogenous oxidative DNA damage in colon cells. *Eur J Nutr*, 227-34;38

26 Ou, H.C., Lee, W.J., Lee, I.T., Chiu, T.H., Tsai, K.L., et al. (2009). Ginkgo biloba extract attenuates oxLDL-induced oxidative functional damages in endothelial cells. *J Appl Physiol*, 106:1674–85.

27 Chung, H.S., Harris, A., Kristinsson, J.K., Ciulla, T.A., Kagemann, C., et al. (1999). Ginkgo biloba extract increases ocular blood flow velocity. *J Ocul Pharmacol Ther*, 15:233–40.

28 Birdsall, T.C. (1998). Therapeutic applications of taurine. *Altern Med Rev*, Apr;3(2):128-36.

29 Shpak, N.I., Naritsyna, N.I., Konovalova, N.V. (1989). Taufon and emoksipin in the combined treatment of sclerotic macular dystrophy. *Oftalmol Zh*, (8):463-5

30 Lombardini, J.B. (1991). Taurine: retinal function. *Brain Res Rev*, May-Aug;16(2):151-69

31 Imaki, H., Maretz, R., Wisniewski, H., Neuringer, M., Sturman, J. (1987). Retinal degeneration in 3-month rhesus monkey infants fed a taurine-free human infant formula. *J Neurosci Res*, 18(4):602-14

32 Chen, L., Yang, X., Jiao, H., Zhao, B. (2003). Tea catechins protect against lead-induced ROS formation, mitochondrial dysfunction, and calcium dysregulation in PC12 cells. *Chem Res Toxicol*, Sep;16(9):1155-61.

33 Kondo, K., Kurihara, M., Miyata, N., Suzuki, T., Toyoda, M. (1999) Mechanistic studies of catechins as antioxidants against radical oxidation. *Arch Biochem Biophys*, Feb 1;362(1):79-86.

34 Sinha, D., Roy, S., Roy, M. (2010). Antioxidant potential of tea reduces arsenite induced oxidative stress in Swiss albino mice. *Food Chem Toxicol*, Apr;48(4):1032-9.

35 Sun, Y., Hung, W.C., Chen, F.Y., Lee, C.C., Huang, H.W. (2009). Interaction of tea catechin (-)-epigallocatechin gallate with lipid biolayers. *Biophys J*, Feb;96(3):1026-35

36 Jumper, J.M., Chang, D.F., Hoyt, C.S., Hall, J.L., Stern, R., Schwartz, D.M. (1997). Aqueous hyaluronic acid concentration: comparison in pediatric and adult patients. *Curr Eye Res*, Oct;16(10):1069-71.

37 Ibid. Jumper. (1997).

15-9. FLOATERS

Floaters are a good name for the small dark shapes that float before our eyes. They are common as we age. These spots may look like squiggles, strands, or any of a hundred other shapes. Though they can be annoying (sometimes excruciatingly so), floaters are physiologically harmless to the eyes. But if you suddenly become aware of floaters, particularly accompanied by bright flashes of light, it may signal a tear or detachment, or a more serious condition such as a retinal tear or detachment, so you should contact your eye doctor ASAP.

What are Floaters?

As we age two things begin to happen:

The **vitreous gel** that keeps the shape of the back of our eyes starts to liquefy and/or clump and shrink, which creates a pulling on the retina.

The protein-based **connective tissue** attaching the vitreous lining weakens, and tiny pieces of connective tissue may float free in the vitreous.

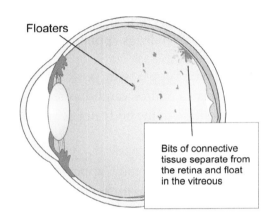

Floaters

Bits of connective tissue separate from the retina and float in the vitreous

Signs and Symptoms

- Visual spots appear in the form of specks, strings, clusters, and any combination of these.
- The spots move as you move your eyes.
- The spots tend to drift out of your line of vision when you are not moving your eyes.

Caution. Sudden appearance of floaters might be an indication of retinal tear or detachment or vitreous detachment. Contact your eye doctor right away, particularly if combined with flashes and/or loss in vision.

Causes and Risk Factors

Age. Most vitreous eye floaters are age-related and are due gradual shrinking and/or clumping of vitreous gel. This results in the release of connective tissue proteins into the vitreous gel. More than 50% of people over 70 see these proteins. Shrinking of the vitreous due to liquification of the gel that occurs with aging is called vitreous syneresis.[1]

Nearsightedness. Those who are nearsighted are more likely to develop eye floaters, particularly if at 6 diopters or over, due to chronic pulling on the retina combined with weakening of the connective tissue to the retina.[2] The greater the level of nearsightedness, the higher the risk of vitreous tears and detachments (often resulting in eye floaters), and a higher risk of retinal tears and detachments.

Cataract surgery. After cataract surgery, patients often report floaters, which are considered complications. One study assessing types of cataract surgery determined that patients receiving a "hinged capsulotomy" reported fewer floaters.[3]

Diabetes. Floaters are common in people with diabetes because this condition causes a number of weakened capillaries in the retina that can leak blood. The blood clots and can leak into the vitreous, appearing as floaters.[4]

Drugs. Some prescription and other drugs can cause floaters.

Eye trauma. Trauma to the eye or head may also cause spots and floaters. Floaters can over time break down or float out of view, though for some, they remain for many years.

Food allergies. People with food allergies are at higher risk of developing floaters. One paper describes topical drugs applied to the eyes that cause allergic reactions and floaters.[5]

Candidiasis. People with yeast infections are at higher risk of developing floaters.[6] Regarding food allergies and/or candidiasis, these issues can result in poor absorption of nutrients from food, resulting in the body not being able to deliver the essential nutrients to the eyes to maintain eye health and integrity.

Pre-birth. Floaters may appear in babies during pregnancy as a result of hyaloid artery degradation. Prior to birth, the eyes of the unborn child contain an artery that regresses during the last three months of pregnancy. Sometimes cell material is left behind and is experienced as floaters. Pregnant mothers can take prenatal supplements to help support the development of the baby, along with essential fatty acids for brain development.[7]

Stress. We believe that chronic stress may contribute to the generation of floaters, as well as any other health condition one may be prone to. Studies show that physical or emotional stress can contribute to the onset of posterior vitreous detachment.[8] Developing a daily routine of meditation, or relaxation is essential for overall well-being.

Inflammation in the uvea or vitreous body can result in increased eye floaters.[9] [10]

Vitreous anomalies. Retinal tears, detachments, leaky blood vessels, and other vitreous anomalies can be experienced as floaters. Pulling on the retina that may result in vitreous tears and detachments may also result in bright flashing lights. In one study, 11% of the population ages 64-69, experience a vitreous detachment.[11] The risk increases with age.

Related Conditions

Scheerer's phenomenon. This experience features small bright dots, lasting for less than a second, which are often seen when looking at the sky. The bright dots are actually white blood cells in the retina's capillaries that cannot absorb the blue light and therefore are seen as white specks.

Vitreous tear/detachment. Part or all of the vitreous pulls away from the retina, often resulting in sudden increases in eye floaters.

Premacular bursa floaters. Children and teens can experience a floater-like phenomenon which occurs within the premacular bursa, an area of liquified vitreous located in front of the macula. Although these "floaters" appear like a translucent web or spot in the eye, these are not real floaters since they are not within the vitreous. They are microscopic in size and appear large only because they are very close to the retina.

Conventional Treatment

There are no conventional treatments; patients are usually told they must learn to live with them. In more serious eye floater conditions, a vitrectomy surgery may be recommended, although there is the risk of a number of side effects. A few eye doctors in the U.S. have provided laser treatments, but this procedure has not yet become a conventional floater treatment.

Complementary Approach

Maintaining a healthy diet can help prevent the onset of floaters, particularly with foods that contain vitamin C, silica, glucosamine sulfate, MSM, omega-3 fatty acids, and other nutrients listed below to help maintain the integrity of the retina, vitreous, and connective tissue.

Diet, exercise, and targeted supplementation can go a long way in strengthening the retina and supporting the vitreous. Research has determined that the body supplies certain nutrients in the eye such as hyaluronic acid that helps support the vitreous and connective tissue.[12]

Nutrients

Essential

Vitamin C (buffered and ascorbated). 2,000mg–3,000mg per day. Vitamin C is a powerful antioxidant that is essential for overall eye health. Since floaters are often the result of vitreous tears, detachments, and/or clumping of the vitreous due to aging, vitamin C plays an essential role in its health. Vitamin C supports blood and lymph circulation, waste elimination, and connective tissue integrity. Vitamin C is found in high concentrations in the eyes and helps neutralize the effect of oxygenation in the ocular fluids.[13] [14] [15]

Hyaluronic acid. 100mg–200mg per day. Hyaluronic acid (hyaluronan) is a large molecule found in the vitreous gel[16] that is believed to contribute to the vitreous' gel-like quality and possibly support connective tissue at the retina.[17] As we age, the amount of hyaluronan in the body decreases.

Liver tonic. We recommend the classic Chinese liver formula *xiao yao san*, which contains rehmannia, milk thistle and dandelion. Additionally, see Appendix 5 for the recommended ReVision formula. In Chinese medicine, the Liver "opens to the eyes" and stimulates energy and blood circulation throughout the eyes and body.

Floater homeopathic pellets. 1-3 pellets 3 times per day (dissolve in mouth), preferably away from meals. Herbs prepared in a homeopathic preparation can be found in the homeopathy Physicians Desk Reference, and may include Physostigma HPUS 12x, Phosphorus HPUS 12x, Silica HPUS 10x, Kali Phos. HPUS 10x, Kali Sulph. HPUS 10x, and Nat. Mur. HPUS 10x.

Very Important

Nutrients recommended below do not directly relate to eye floaters, but may protect against future eye floaters by supporting a healthy retina.

Lutein. 6mg–20mg per day. Lutein is an essential nutrient for strengthening the retina.[18]

Zeaxanthin. 2mg–12mg per day. Zeaxanthin is an essential nutrient for strengthening the retina.[19]

Omega-3 fatty acid. 2,000mg–3,000mg per day with a meal. Omega-3s generally support retinal health, reducing the incidence and progression of retinal diseases.[20]

Helpful

Multivitamin. Whole-food, organic multivitamin for eye and overall body health.

Lifestyle

Eye exercises. See Chapter 10-4 for eye exercises and acupressure points that are good for all eye conditions and overall eye health. For floaters, we recommend that you regularly do:

- Palming
- Effortless focus
- Near and far
- Hot dog

Sunglasses. Invest in a good pair of ultra-violet protecting lenses (100% UVA/UVB filtering); amber or brown colored (polarized lenses are preferred). Exposure to ultraviolet light, the blue light from sunlight, and blue light from computers/phones causes oxidative stress in the eye. Wearing sunglasses is an especially important part of eye care for older people because vitreous detachments are associated with weakening connective tissue between the retina and vitreous, more common with age in seniors.

Diet

We recommend the Vision diet described in detail in Chapter 7.

Juicing. Choose 4-6 of these, plus any of your favorite fruits and vegetables.

- Garlic, parsley, beets, carrots, celery, parsnip, apple, raspberries (preferably all organic); not too many carrots due to their sweetness
- Try to use room temperature vegetables and fruit.
- Do not add ice or very cold liquids since cold foods and liquids will eventually extinguish the stomach's digestive fire.

- Do not juice as often during the cooler months of the year, and instead, switch to vegetable soups or stews.

Other Modalities

Chinese Medicine

Eye floaters can be related to a number of different imbalances in the body, including:

- Poor circulation and storage of blood (often related to Liver imbalances)
- Poor absorption and distribution of essential nutrients (often related to Spleen deficiency)
- Poor production of blood (commonly related to Kidney and Spleen deficiencies)
- Congestion in the Kidney, Liver, and Colon

Common patent formulas

Zhu jing wan (preserve vistas pill) tonifies and nourishes the Liver and Kidneys, enriches the yin, and improves vision.

Ming mu di huang wan (rehmannia pills to "brighten the eyes") addresses problems related to the following patterns: Liver blood deficiency, Kidney yin deficiency, and Liver yin deficiency.

Gui pi tang (restore the Spleen decoction) increases qi, tonifies blood, strengthens the Spleen, nourishes the Heart, and helps the Spleen control the blood.

Xiao yao san (rambling powder) is a classic Liver tonic used in Chinese medicine. The Liver "opens to the eyes" and is the primary meridian (flow energy) that supports healthy circulation, the free flow of energy in the eyes, and free flow of energy throughout the body.

Based on the Chinese medicine practitioner's evaluation and intake, herbal formula and treatment strategies can vary significantly.

Also See

Chapter 7, Vision Diet

Chapter 8, Nutrients

Chapter 10-4, Eye Exercises

Chapter 15-1, Cataracts

Chapter 15-6, Diabetic Retinopathy

Appendix 5, Recommended Products

---

[1] Gauger, E., Chin, E.K., Sohn, E.H. (2014). Vitreous Syneresis: An Impending Posterior Vitreous Detachment (PVD). Retrieved Jan 29 2018 from https://webeye.ophth.uiowa.edu/ eyeforum/cases/196-PVD.htm.

[2] Milston, R., Madigan, M.C., Sebag, J. (2016). Vitreous floaters: Etiology, diagnostics, and management. *Surv Ophthalmol*, Mar-Apr;61(2):211-27.

[3] Alipour, F., Jabbarvand, M., Hashemian, H., Hosseini, S., Khodaparast, M. (2015). Hinged Capsulotomy – Does it Decrease Floaters After Yttrium Aluminum Garnet Laser Capsulotomy? *Middle East Afr J Ophthalmol.* Jul-Sep; 22(3): 352–355.

[4] Haddrill, M., Diabetic Retinopathy. Retrieved Jan 29 2018 from http://www.allaboutvision.com/conditions/diabetic.htm.

[5] Lyle, W.M., Hopkins, G.A. (1977). The unwanted ocular effects from topical ophthalmic drugs. Their occurrence, avoidance and reversal. *J Am Optom Assoc.* Dec;48(12):1519-23.

[6] Sallam. A., Lynn, W., McCluskey, P., Lightman, S. (2006). Endogenous Candida endophthalmitis. *Expert Rev Anti Infect Ther*, Aug; 4(4):675-85.

[7] Oken, E., Bellinger, D.C. (2008). Fish consumption, methylmercury and child neurodevelopment. *Curr Opin Pediatr*, Apr; 20(2):178-83.

[8] Flammer, J., Konieczka, K., Bruno, R.M., Virdis, A., Flammer, A.J., et al. (2013). The eye and the heart. *Eur Heart J*, May 1; 34(17): 1270-1278.

[9] National Eye Institute. Facts About Uveitis. Retrieved Mar 29 2018 from https://nei.nih.gov/health/uveitis/uveitis.

[10] Ibid. National Eye Institute. Facts About Uveitis.

[11] Weber-Krause, B., Eckardt, C. (1997). Incidence of posterior vitreous detachment in the elderly. *Ophthalmologe*, Sept;94(9):619-23.

[12] Stolyszewski, I., Niemcunowicz-Janica, A., Pepinski, W., Spolnicka, M. Zbiec, R., et al. (2007). Vitreous humour as a potential DNA source for postmortem human identification, Fola *Histochem Cytobiol*, 45(2):135-6.

[13] Pirie, A. (1965). A light-catalysed reaction in the aqueous humor of the eye. *Nature*, 205:500–501.

[14] Takano, S., Ishiwata, S., Nakazawa, M., Mizugaki, M., Tamai, M. (1997). Determination of ascorbic acid in human vitreous humor by high-performance liquid chromatography with UV detection. *Curr Eye Res*, 16(6):589–594.

[15] Eaton, J.W. (1991). Is the lens canned? *Free Radic Biol Med*, 11(2):207–213.

[16] Brewton, R.G., Mayne, R. (1992). Mammalian vitreous humor contains networks of hyaluronan molecules: electron microscopic analysis using the hyaluronan-binding region (G1) of aggrecan and link protein. *Exp Cell Res*, Feb;198(2):237-49.

[17] Jumper, J.M., Chang, D.F., Hoyt, C.S., Hall, J.L., Stern, R., et al. (1997). Aqueous hyaluronic acid concentration: comparison in pediatric and adult patients. *Curr Eye Res*, Oct;16(10):1069-71.

[18] Piermarocchi, S., Saviano, S., Parisi, V., Tedeschi, M., Panozzo, G., et al. (2012). Carotenoids in Age-related Maculopathy Italian Study (CARMIS): two-year results of a randomized study. *Eur J Ophthalmol*, Mar-Apr;22(2):216-25.

[19] Richer, S.P., Stiles, W., Graham-Hoffman, K., Levin, M., Ruskin, D., et al. (2011). Randomized, double-blind, placebo-controlled study of zeaxanthin and visual function in patients with atrophic age-related macular degeneration: the Zeaxanthin and Visual Function Study (ZVF) FDA IND #78, 973. *Optometry*, Nov;82(11):667-680.e6.

[20] Querques, G., Forte, R., Souied, E.H. (2011). Retina and Omega-3. *J Nutr Metab*, Oct 31:748361.

15-10. FUCHS' DYSTROPHY

The most common cause of cornea swelling (edema) is due to Fuchs' dystrophy, occurring most frequently in people ages 30 to 40. This disease rarely affects vision until people reach ages 50-60.

The condition is 2-4 times more common and more severe in women. Prevalence in the U.S. is approximately 897 per million.[1] The exact prevalence is not known but has been found to be uncommon in Saudi Arabia, the Singaporean Chinese, and Japan. Approximately 40,000 corneal transplants are performed in the U.S. every year.

Fuchs' dystrophy is a slowly progressing disease that usually affects both eyes. The inner cell layer of the cornea deteriorates, inner layers thicken, and blisters form in other layers. When these tiny blisters or cysts burst, they are extremely painful.

The Cornea

The cornea consists of a number of layers that have been identified by scientists. Changes in these layers are indicative of Fuchs'. There is some evidence showing that the likelihood of the onset of Fuchs' can be significantly reduced through lifestyle choices and nutrients. Researchers have determined that free radicals in the cornea may contribute to Fuchs'.[2]

Corneal layers

The following layers of tissue have been identified, each with unique functions.

The epithelium is filled with thousands of tiny nerve endings that make the cornea extremely sensitive to pain. Its function is to block foreign material, while providing a nutrient-absorbing, oxygen-absorbing surface, and signaling the brain to activate tear production.

The Bowman's layer contains collagen fibers that maintain the cornea's shape.

The stroma consists of regularly arranged collagen fibers along with sparsely distributed interconnected keratocytes, which are the cells for general repair and maintenance.

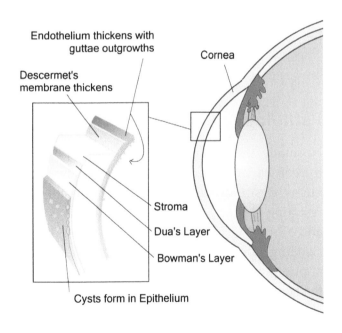

Endothelium thickens with guttae outgrowths

Descermet's membrane thickens

Cornea

Stroma

Dua's Layer

Bowman's Layer

Cysts form in Epithelium

Descemet's membrane is a base layer for the growth of endothelium cells.

The endothelium is a single layer of cells that pumps excess water out of the stroma.

The thin Dua's layer, recently discovered, is the sixth layer in the cornea. It is located at the back of the cornea between the stroma and Descemet's membrane. This layer is thought to play a vital role in the structure of the tissue that controls the flow of fluid from the eye. New research indicates that this makes an important contribution to the sieve-like meshwork—the trabecular meshwork (TM)—in the periphery of the cornea. A poor functioning trabecular meshwork can lead to glaucoma.[3]

Corneal Function

The cornea is clear and seems to lack substance, but these layers and groups of cells and proteins are highly organized. Unlike other parts of the body, the cornea does not contain any blood vessels to nourish or protect the tissue against infection. The cornea instead, receives its nourishment from the tears and aqueous humor, a fluid in the anterior portion (front) of the eye that fills the chamber behind the cornea. The cornea must remain transparent to refract light properly and enable clear vision. The presence of even the tiniest blood vessels can interfere with this process. To see well, all layers of the cornea must be free of any cloudy or opaque areas.

The cornea plays several essential roles, both for protecting the eye and for beginning the focusing process.

- It helps to shield the rest of the eye from germs, dust, and other harmful matter. The cornea shares this protective task with the eyelids, the eye socket, tears, and the white part of the eye (sclera).
- The cornea acts as the eye's outermost lens. It functions like a window and is part of the system that controls and focuses light entering the eye, directing light to accurately land on the retina. The cornea contributes 65–75% of the eye's total focusing power.
- It alerts the brain to signal the tear-related glands as to when more tears need to be produced or not.

Pathology of Fuchs' Dystrophy

Normally, the cells lining the inside of the cornea help maintain a healthy balance of fluids within the cornea, preventing the cornea from swelling, and helping to keep the cornea clear. But with Fuchs' dystrophy, the endothelial cells slowly die off and probably do not function correctly, resulting in fluid buildup within the cornea (swelling or edema). This causes corneal thickening and blurred vision. The changes to the endothelium and Descemet's membrane lead to corneal swelling, known as edema. This is a condition where the cells of the cornea become less efficient at pumping water out of the stroma, and fluid is retained. With accumulated water, the layers of the cornea swell, distorting vision.

The endothelium, the inner cell layer of the cornea that normally pumps water out of the stroma, deteriorates and thickens as outgrowths called guttae form. Descemet's membrane also thickens and cysts develop in the epithelium. When these cysts (or tiny blisters on the inner side of the corneal surface) burst, they are extremely painful.

Corneal swelling damages vision in two ways: it changes the cornea's normal curvature affecting how light gets focused onto the back of the eye, and it causes sight impairment in the form of a haze. Because there is excess fluid buildup in the cornea tissue, it's like trying to look through a wet and foggy window.

Types of Fuchs'

Early-onset. A gene in chromosome 1 has been discovered that is responsible for early-onset Fuchs' (COL8A).[4] The guttae that form in early-onset Fuchs' are coarser and more distinct than those of late-onset Fuchs'. The cysts or excrescences that form in early-onset Fuchs' have sharp margins and areas where there are many cysts. These areas are distinctly different from the areas with no cysts.[5]

Late-onset. Mutations in chromosomes 13 and 18 are linked to late-onset Fuchs'.[6][7] The guttae in late-onset Fuchs' are finer and patchier than those of early-onset, and they are associated with individual endothelial cells. The cysts are uniformly elevated and spread out over the cornea.[8]

Signs and Symptoms

The first symptom is blurry vision, which clears up during the day in the early stages of the disease. This occurs because the cornea is normally thicker in the morning. It retains fluids during sleep that evaporate in the tear film while we are awake. As the disease worsens, this swelling will remain constant and reduce vision throughout the day.

Causes and Risk Factors

Genetics. Fuchs' dystrophy can be inherited. The genetic basis of the disease is complex. Family members can be affected to varying degrees, although sometimes other members are not affected.

Free radicals. Free radicals damage the eyes. They are formed when the ultraviolet and blue light of sunlight passes through the crystalline lens. Free radicals are also natural byproducts of metabolism. These highly reactive chemicals cause oxidation and can destabilize healthy cells in the back of the cornea and the retina as well. Moreover, free radical damage is accelerated by smoking, chronic fatigue, poor diet, chronic stress, and excessive exposure to sunlight and blue light from electronic devices.

Compromised immune system. Conditions that cause chronic inflammation such as autoimmune diseases and diabetes particularly, result in increased production of free radicals.

Conventional Treatment

Patients who have Fuchs' endothelial dystrophy but still have clear corneas, do not typically need treatment. When the cornea starts to change, medical treatment is needed. However, there is no conventional treatment that can actually halt or reverse the course of this disease, just ways to help manage it. If the condition worsens, then the eye doctor may recommend surgery.

In the early stages of Fuchs', doctors will try to reduce corneal swelling with soft contact lenses or ointments targeted to reducing the swelling. They may also instruct a person to use a hair dryer directed across the face at arm's length for 5–10 minutes upon wakening (to dry out the surface of the cornea and tear film). As a dehydrating agent, sodium chloride 5% solution eye drops are used 4–6 times daily, especially in the morning and less frequently in the evening. Sodium chloride ointment is used at bedtime.[9]

Glycerine is used diagnostically, and for some patients it can be therapeutic as well. Glycerine causes rapid dehydration of the cornea and clears vision.[10] Another intervention is to lower the intraocular pressure which helps reduce pressure on the cornea.[11]

If painful sores develop on the cornea, soft contact lenses, or surgery to create flaps over the sores, may help reduce pain.

Corneal Transplants

According to the Mayo Clinic,' only a small percentage of those with Fuchs' require corneal transplants. According to the Eye Bank Association of American, that's about 40,000 per year.

As visual distortion becomes more severe, a corneal transplant may be recommended as the only alternative for returning impaired vision. The two options currently available are Penetrating Keratoplasty (PK) and Descemet's Stripping with Endothelial Keratoplasty (DSEK). With PK, the patient's cornea is carefully removed, and then a healthy donor cornea is sewn into place, if possible.[12] With DSEK, instead of replacing the entire cornea, only the back half (the endothelium and Descemet's membrane) of the cornea is replaced.[13]

Surgery risk factors include bleeding, cataract onset, leakage of fluids from the incision, and damage or, rarely, infection to other parts of the eye. In addition, new vision problems may result as the surgery can cause astigmatism, nearsightedness, and farsightedness, requiring thick lenses on eyeglasses or contact lenses.[14]

The short-term success rate of corneal transplantation is quite good for people with Fuchs' dystrophy. But some studies do suggest that the long-term survival of the donor cornea can be a problem. In addition, the age of the donor appears to have a slight effect, with corneas from donors aged 66–75 years having a 75% loss.[15] One study found that corneal survival rates were about 66% after five years with the following problems: keratoconus (98%), viral keratitis (86%), recurrence of Fuchs' (85%), pseudophakic bullous keratopathy (84%), regrafts required (55%), and other conditions (57%).[16]

If the transplant gets rejected, topical corticosteroids (for example, dexamethasone 0.1% or prednisolone acetate 1%) are prescribed 4–6 times a day until the signs of rejection resolve, followed by a slow tapering of the topical medication. In more severe cases, the eye doctor may inject a higher concentration of the corticosteroids. If the transplant cannot be preserved, then once again there will be severe vision loss as the rejected cornea clouds and vision deteriorates.

Complementary Approach

Because free radicals in the cornea are considered one of the major contributors of Fuchs' dystrophy,[17] a way to help the body neutralize free radicals is by making sure there are adequate antioxidants in the body to support healthy vision. Antioxidants can be acquired through both diet and targeted supplementation. This is a general approach for helping to prevent and manage most eye and body diseases.

Nutrients

Important

Glutathione (GSH). 500mg–900mg (tablet or capsule form). It is preferable to take intraorally or sublingually (follow lower dosage on label), as glutathione is not absorbed well through the digestive system. Glutathione is one of the super antioxidants that neutralize the full range of free radicals.[18] With age, GSH levels decline in human eyes.[19] Normally present in high levels in the ocular lens, cornea, aqueous humor, and retina, it performs multiple roles, including maintaining normal tissue hydration and lens transparency, and protecting against oxidative damage.

Glutathione eyedrops. These drops should contain reduced glutathione. Take 1 drop in each eye 2 times per day, or as directed by your healthcare professional. Glutathione is one of the super antioxidants that can neutralize the full spectrum of free radicals and is known to be essential for maintaining eye lens health.

Helpful

Omega-3 fatty acids. 2,000 IU–3,000 IU per day with a meal. Research shows that this essential nutrient for retinal health has anti-inflammatory properties.[20] [21]

Green tea. 500mg–750mg per day. Green tea has a potent antioxidant property for eye and general health.[22] [23] [24]

MSM capsules. 2,000mg per day split up with meals or with water. MSM helps nourish and strengthen body tissues and has natural anti-inflammatory properties.[25]

Castor oil eyedrops. 1 drop in each eye before bedtime. One study found that these eyedrops help maintain eye lubrication by improving tear stability, preventing tear evaporation, and supporting meibomian gland function.[26] It may have natural anti-inflammatory and healing properties as well.

Caution. Ensure the castor oil is formulated and approved for use in the eye.

Lubricating eyedrops (preservative free) containing glycerin. As mentioned above, glycerin-containing eyedrops are used therapeutically as it causes rapid dehydration of the cornea and clears the vision.

Multivitamin. A high-quality, whole food, organic multivitamin is recommended.

Bilberry. 180mg–240mg per day. Bilberry is neuroprotective and has been shown to improve microcirculation.[27] [28] [29]

Eyedrops. Homeopathic eye drops containing cineraria maritima help with circulation and reduce opacities in the lens.

Diet

Pay attention to the dietary recommendations in Chapter 7, particularly related to maintaining an alkaline (anti-inflammatory) diet with lots of healthy fruits and vegetables.

Juicing. We recommend some combination of the following (select at least 4-6), plus your favorite fruits and vegetables:

- Ginger, leeks, garlic, beets, parsley, carrots, cabbage, celery, apples, spinach, raspberries, grapes, lemon, wheatgrasses, chlorophyll, (not too much fruit)
- Try to use room temperature vegetables and fruit.
- Do not add ice or very cold liquids since cold foods and liquids will eventually extinguish the stomach's digestive fire.
- Do not juice as often during the cooler months of the year, and instead, switch to vegetable soups or stews.

Lifestyle

Eye exercises. Gently massage upper and lower lids a few of times a day. This helps stimulate the free flow of energy and blood throughout the eyes and helps the body nourish and maintain the health of the eye tissues. See Chapter 10-4 for eye exercises and acupressure points.

Lymphatic massage. Another good practice is to gently massage food grade castor oil along the bones of the eyebrows, and down along the side of the face in front of the ears. Then continue behind the earlobe and down the side of the neck to the collarbone. Do this at least once a day for several repetitions. Self-lymphatic massage will assist the movement of the sluggish lymphatic drainage system around the eyes, helping to remove waste products and toxins.

Wear UV sunglasses. If you are in sunlight for more than 20 minutes, wear these to protect your eyes from UV radiation.

Avoid allergens. These include air contaminants and known food allergies.

Do not smoke.

Other Modalities

Chinese Medicine

In Chinese medicine, the Liver "opens to the eyes" and "rules over the cornea," so a good Liver supporting formula can be helpful for corneal issues.

Xiao yao san (rambling powder) is a formulation that supports the Liver meridian. Also, see the ReVision formula in Appendix 5, which is based on this formula plus added antioxidants for eye health.

On the Horizon

Gene Therapy

Several genes have been associated with early-onset or late-onset Fuchs'.[30] One gene (transcription factor 4) increased the risk of developing Fuchs' by five times.[31] Gene therapy may one day offer treatment for Fuchs' dystropy.

In a mouse model of early-onset Fuchs', N-acetyl-cysteine (NAC) increased survival of corneal endothelial cells.[32]

Also See

Chapter 7, Diet

Chapter 8, Nutrients

Chapter 10, Self Help and More

Appendix 5, Recommended Products

[1] Musch, D.C., Niziol, L.M., Stein, J.D., Kamyar, R.M., Sugar, A. (2011). Prevalence of Corneal Dystrophies in the United States: Estimates from Claims Data. *Invest Ophthalmol Vis Sci*, Aug; 52(9): 6959–6963.

2 Jurkunas, U.V., Bitar, M.S., Funaki, T., Azizi, B. (2010). Evidence of oxidative stress in the pathogenesis of Fuch's endothelial corneal dystrophy. *Am J Pathol*, Nov;177(5):2278-89.

3 Dua, H.S., Faraj, L.A., Branch, M.J., Yeung, A.M., Elalfy, M.S., et al. (2014). The collagen matrix of the human trabecular meshwork is an extension of the novel pre-Descemet's layer (Dua's layer). *Brit J Ophthalmol*, May;98(5):691-7.

4 Gottsch, J.D., Sundin, O.H., Liu, S.H., Jun, A.S., Broman, K.W., et al. (2005). Inheritance of a novel COL8A2 mutation defines a distinct early-onset subtype of Fuch's corneal dystrophy. *Invest Ophthalmol Vis Sci*, Jun;46(6):1934-9.

5 Wilmer Eye Institute. Types of Fuchs. Retrieved Jan 24 2018 from https://www.hopkinsmedicine.org/wilmer/conditions/Fuchs/about/typesfuchs.html.

6 Sundin, O.H., Jun, A.S., Broman, K.W., Liu, S.H., Sheehan, S.E. (2006). Linkage of late-onset Fuchs corneal dystrophy to a novel locus at 13pTel-13q12.13. *Invest Ophthalmol Vis Sci*, Jan;47(1):140-5.

7 Li, Y.J., Minear, M.A., Rimmler, J., Zhao, B., Balajonda, E., et al. (2011). Replication of TCF4 through association and linkage studies in late-onset Fuchs endothelial corneal dystrophy. *PLoS One*, Apr 20;6(4):e18044.

8 Ibid Wilmer Eye Institute.

9 Singh, D. (2016). Fuchs Endothelial Dystrophy Treatment & Management. Retrieved Jan 24 2018 from https://emedicine.medscape.com/article/1193591-treatment.

10 Ibid. Singh (2016).

11 Ibid. Singh (2016).

12 University of Iowa Healthcare, Ophthalmology and Visual Sciences. Penetrating keratoplasty. Retrieved Jan 24 2018 from https://webeye.ophth.uiowa.edu/eyeforum/ tutorials/Cornea-Transplant-Intro/2-PK.htm.

13 University of Iowa Healthcare, Ophthalmology and Visual Sciences. Descemet Membrane Endothelial Keratoplasty (DMEK). Retrieved Jan 24, 2018 from https://webeye.ophth.uiowa.edu/ eyeforum/tutorials Cornea-Transplant-Intro/5-DMEK.htm.

14 Mayo Clinic. Cornea Transplant. Retrieved Jan 24 2018 from https://www.mayoclinic.org/ tests-procedures/cornea-transplant/about/pac-20385285

15 Cornea Donor Study Investigator Group, Lass, J.H., Gal, R.L., Dontchev, M., Beck, R.W., et al. (2008). Donor age and corneal endothelial cell loss 5 years after successful corneal transplantation. Specular microscopy ancillary study results. *Ophthalmology*, Apr;115(4):627-632.

16 Beckingsale, P., Mavrikakis, I., Al-Yousuf, N., Mavrikakis, E., Daya, S.M. (2006). Penetrating keratoplasty: outcomes from a corneal unit compared to national data. *Br J Ophthalmol*, Jun;90(6):728-31.

17 Jurkunas, U.V., Bitar, M.S., Funaki, T., Azizi, B. (2010). Evidence of oxidative stress in the pathogenesis of Fuch's endothelial corneal dystrophy. *Am J Pathol*, Nov;177(5):2278-89.

18 Dringen, R. (2000). Glutathione metabolism and oxidative stress in neurodegeneration. *Eur J Biochem,* Aug; 267(16):4903.

19 Harding JJ. (1970). Free and protein-bound glutathione in normal and cataractous human lenses. *Biochem J,* May; 117(5):957-60.

20 Udell, I.J., Abelson, M.B. (1983). Chemical mediators of inflammation. *Int Ophthalmol Clin*, 23:1:15-26.

21 Abelson, M.B., Butrus, S.I., Kliman, G.H., Larson, D.L., Corey, E.J., et al. (1987). Topical arachidonic acid: A model for screening anti-inflammatory agents. *J Ocul Pharmacol*, 3:63-75.

22 Chen, L., Yang, X., Jiao, H., Zhao, B. (2003). Tea catechins protect against lead-induced ROS formation, mitochondrial dysfunction, and calcium dysregulation in PC12 cells. *Chem Res Toxicol*, Sep;16(9):1155-61.

23 Skrzydlewska, E., Ostrowska, J., Stankiewicz, A., Farbiszewski, R. (2002). Green tea as a potent antioxidant in alcohol intoxication. *Addict Biol*, Jul;7(3):307-14.

24 Kondo, K., Kurihara, M., Miyata, N., Suzuki, T., Toyoda, M. (1999). Mechanistic studies of catechins as antioxidants against radical oxidation. *Arch Biochem Biophys*, Feb 1;362(1):79-86.

25 Butawan, M., Benjamin, R.L., Bloomer, R.J. (2017). Methylsulfonylmethane: Applications and Safety of a Novel Dietary Supplement. *Nutrients*, Mar 16;9(3).

26 Goto, E., Shimazaki, J., Monden, Y., Takano, Y., Yagi, Y., et al. (2002). Low-concentration homogenized castor oil eye drops for noninflamed obstructive meibomian gland dysfunction. *Ophthalmology*, Nov;109(11):2030-5.

27 Matsunaga, N., Imai, S., Inokuchi, Y., Shimazawa, M., Yokota, S., et al. (2009). Bilberry and its main constituents have neuroprotective effects against retinal neuronal damage in vitro and in vivo. *Mol Nutr Food Res*, Jul;53(7):869-77.

28 Cohen-Boulakia, F., Valensi, P.E., Boulahdour, H., Lestrade, R. Dufour-Lamarinie, J.F., et al. (2000). In vivo sequential study of skeletal muscle capillary permeability in diabetic rats: effect of anthocyanosides. *Metabolism*, Jul;49(7):880-5.

29 Yao, Y., Vierra, A. (2007). Protective activities of Vaccinium antioxidants with potential relevance to mitochondrial dysfunction and neurotoxicity. *NeuroToxicology*, Jan;28(1):93-100.

30 Baratz, K.H., Tosakulwong, N., Ryu, E., Brown, W.L., Branham, K. (2010). E2-2 Protein and Fuchs's Corneal Dystrophy. *N Engl J Med,* Sep 9;363(11):1016-24.

31 Ibid. Baratz. (2010).

32 Kim, E.C., Meng, H., Jun, A.S. (2014). N-Acetylcysteine increases corneal endothelial cell survival in a mouse model of Fuchsendothelial corneal dystrophy. *Exp Eye Res,* Oct;127:20-5.

15-11. GLAUCOMA

Glaucoma is a symptom-free condition that is thought to be caused by damage to the optic nerve, which robs the patient of peripheral vision and can cause blindness. It is often referred to as the "silent thief." In 2010, 2.7 million people in the United States had glaucoma. The number is expected to increase to over four million by 2030. African Americans had the highest prevalence rate (3.4%), followed by other races (2.1%), whites (1.7%), and Hispanics (1.5%).[1]

What is Glaucoma?

Glaucoma can be difficult to detect without a regular eye exam until a significant amount of vision is lost. The reason it is so dangerous is that most people with glaucoma have no symptoms. Many feel no pain, and most have 20/20 visual acuity, although possibly only straight-ahead vision. But left untreated, glaucoma can slowly steal your peripheral vision until you think you are peering through a tunnel (at best) or until you go blind (at worst). Most frightening, 70% of the vision lost to glaucoma occurs before diagnosis. Glaucoma may be due to the result of the loss of retinal ganglion cells and axons (nerve cells that pass along information) in the optic nerve and retina.[2] Thinning of the optic nerve may occur as well.

Neurodegeneration

Researchers now view glaucoma as a disease of the brain (a neurodegenerative disease) rather than simply an eye disease. Recent research has shown that the complex connection between the eye and the brain is an important key to the disease. The retina and optic nerve are both made up of brain tissue and are part of the brain. Glaucoma shares a number of features with degenerative brain diseases such as Alzheimer's, Parkinson's, and Lou Gehrig's disease. In these diseases, age and family history are major risk factors, and specific areas of the brain are damaged over time.

In glaucoma, changes occur in the back of the eyes. The optic nerve continues to be a focus for researching the underlying causes of glaucoma. Whether due to mechanical trauma, decreased blood flow, or other causes, optic nerve axon injury causes changes in retinal ganglion cells, eventually resulting in cell death. Researchers have observed that specific areas of injured optic nerve axons and retinal ganglion cell loss match the peripheral vision damage from glaucoma.[3]

Neuroinflammation

Glaucoma, especially if acute, may be largely an inflammatory condition. Researchers believe that high intraocular pressure triggers an inflammatory response.[4] In experiments, inflammation occurs in the central nervous system and at early stages of glaucoma. Inhibiting the process through which inflammation develops appears to protect the neurons from damage.[5] Researchers have been investigating the precise role of neuroinflammation in causing glaucoma. Cells known as microglia behave like sensors to damage the nervous system and play a role in the inflammatory response. The process contributes to beta-amyloid accumulations, implicated in Alzheimer's disease. Similarly, the eye, actually part of the brain, also accumulates beta-amyloid in the retina and optic nerve. Microglia activity and the inflammatory response are linked to protein clumping and nerve cell degeneration.[6]

Oxidative Stress

Increased oxidative stress is a risk factor. Antioxidant drugs and nutrients that reduce enzymes involved in oxidation are reported to be helpful in animals with glaucoma. Although targeting IOP has been a prime therapy, researchers are increasingly looking to provide antioxidants for targeting oxidative stress.[7] Damage to DNA in the tissue layers that regulate aqueous humor outflow is linked to oxidative damage, as well as damage to neurons and the optic nerve.[8][9]

Anatomy of Glaucoma

Aqueous humor is produced by the ciliary body, a ring of tissue right behind the iris. It flows into the small space between the iris and the lens, then through the pupil into the front of the eye and between the iris and the cornea. Next the liquid passes through little sieve-like openings between the iris and the cornea, the **trabecular meshwork**, into a circular canal called the **Schlemm's canal**. From there, it continues into the blood system.[10]

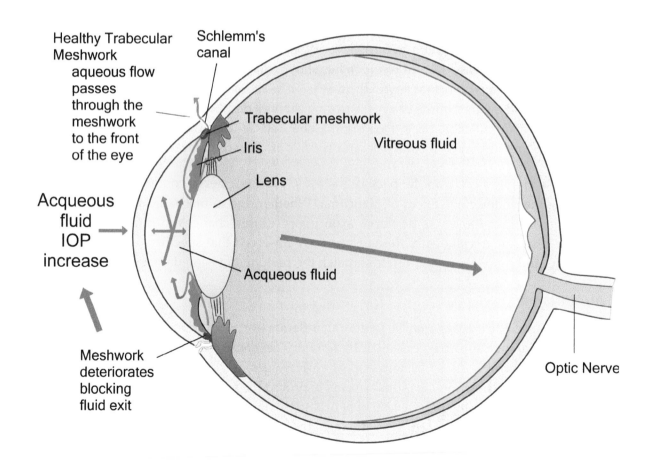

Pathology

Technically, glaucoma is diagnosed based on a number of factors, including changes in the optic nerve, increased intraocular pressure (IOP), and/or changes in peripheral vision. In the healthy eye, aqueous humor is produced and drained from the eye into the bloodstream at a constant rate so that you always have a fresh supply in the right amount. Aqueous humor drains through the trabecular meshwork.

Sometimes, too much aqueous humor is produced, and the eye can't get rid of it fast enough to maintain what is called "normal intraocular pressure." Sometimes the drainage mechanism is faulty, the fluid can't escape fast enough to keep pressure at normal levels. Blockage in the trabecular meshwork or in the canal itself may occur. Either way, the abnormal high-pressure that results is called intraocular hypertension. The increased pressure can damage the optic nerve, first affecting side or peripheral vision, leaving central or straight-ahead vision perfectly normal. If left untreated, the high-pressure can eventually affect central vision, leading to blindness.

What is considered to be normal intraocular pressure (IOP) for a patient may vary. People may have signs of damage yet have normal or even low IOP. Corneal thickness and corneal hysteresis also play a role in determining the proper IOP for a patient. For example, a patient with a thicker cornea is more resistant to glaucoma, and higher than normal eye pressure may be normal for them, but a thinner cornea in the mid-to-upper normal IOP range may be considered dangerous and too high for that patient.

Corneal hysteresis also plays a role, which is how well the cornea absorbs and dissipates energy. These measures are considered in the diagnosis and management of glaucoma.

Types of Glaucoma

Glaucoma Suspect

A patient deemed a glaucoma suspect typically has higher than normal eye pressure (IOP) but has not developed other symptoms as compared to prior visits. Other considerations would be changes to the optic nerve that the eye doctor would see, such as cupping, or thinning of the optic nerve, or changes in the visual field test for peripheral vision. Glaucoma suspects may include people with a family history of glaucoma, diabetes, hypertension, heart disease, heavy computer use, and people with extreme nearsightedness or farsightedness. They also include people who suffer from obesity, hyperthyroidism, and African Americans. Glaucoma suspects should have glaucoma testing regularly.

Open-Angle or Chronic Glaucoma

Open-angle glaucoma (OAG) is the most common form of glaucoma. It develops when the trabecular meshwork, acting as a filter for the aqueous fluid in the eye, becomes clogged or obstructed and does not filter the fluid efficiently. This, in turn, leads to high ocular pressure.

Typically, eye pressure is over 20–21mm Hg in chronic (open-angle) glaucoma. Even though elevated eye pressure is one of the diagnostic tests used for glaucoma, approximately 30–40% of patients with glaucoma develop optic nerve changes and progressive vision loss, yet they maintain normal or low eye pressure.

Narrow-Angle Glaucoma

Narrow-angle or closed-angle glaucoma occurs when the angle of the drainage area (trabecular meshwork) is too small to allow the drainage of the aqueous fluid to drain as quickly as it is produced. This can be a more acute version of glaucoma, as it can result in an eye stroke, so it needs to be watched carefully by your eye doctor. Topiramate (Topamax) is used to treat epilepsy and migraine headaches, and it is used off-label for weight loss. It can cause narrow-angle glaucoma.[11]

This condition may be considered an ocular emergency if the eye pressure gets too high. If the eye pressure gets excessively high, you might experience sudden red eye(s), eye pain, headache, visual halos, and sometimes also vomiting and nausea. If you have these symptoms, treat it as an emergency, and call your eye doctor.

Low-Tension Glaucoma

Low-tension or normal-tension glaucoma is generally an indicator of poor circulation. Not enough oxygen-carrying blood and essential nutrients reach the optic nerve, and it becomes damaged. Normal tension glaucoma is generally defined as the appearance of glaucoma with an IOP in the normal range of 8-21mm Hg.

Thin corneas can mask accurate reading of eye pressure. In some cases, the changes in the optic nerve may be the result of thin corneas. Thin corneas (less than 555 micrometers) may cause artifically low eye pressure readings which would equate to high eye pressure for someone with normal corneal thickness.[12] Optic nerve damage results from thin corneas. Many conditions, including brain tumors, heart problems, or toxic substances can cause optic nerve damage to appear to be glaucoma.

Secondary Glaucoma

Secondary Glaucoma arises as a side result to other health conditions such as injury to the eye, inflammation of the eyes, or various drug side effects including steroids.

Pseudoexfoliation Glaucoma

Pseudoexfoliation syndrome (PEX) is a systemic disease that is diagnosed by the presence of white flake-like deposits on the lens, iris, ciliary body, corneal epithelium, and trabecular meshwork. These deposits originate from the lens, trabecular meshwork, iris, ciliary processes, conjunctiva, and periocular tissue. They are an insoluble material that floats in the aqueous humor and eventually is deposited in, and clogs, the trabecular meshwork. The resulting outflow decrease and IOP increase potentially leads to PEX with optic nerve damage.[13] PEX can be due to a genetic condition or due to eye exposure to too much of the sun's ultraviolet (UV) light. People who live in some northern parts of the world, such as Scandinavia, are more at risk for this type of glaucoma. This could be due to genetic heritage and/or higher altitude with thinner air and more UV radiation exposure.

Increased plasma homocysteine has also been reported in pseudo-exfoliation.[14] [15] [16]

Congenital Glaucoma

Congenital glaucoma is that which begins within the first months after birth.

Causes and Risk Factors

Genetics. There is a strong genetic correlation related to the onset of glaucoma.[17] [18] [19]

High blood pressure. Although high blood pressure is not a direct cause of glaucoma, many studies have found it to be related.[20] [21] In a 2011 study, researchers examined medical records of over two million people older than 40 who were enrolled in a U.S. managed care network. Those with hypertension had a 17% increased risk.[22]

Hypertension may be implicated because high blood pressure can result from poor circulation. Poor circulation can also lead to a compromised delivery of nutrients to the eyes, possibly resulting in poor eye drainage, leading to an increase in ocular pressure. Poor circulation also can reduce the supply of critical nutrients to the optic nerve. Perhaps this is why glaucoma can result in vision loss at any level of eye pressure if the optic nerve is weak, due to poor circulation and lack of oxygen and essential nutrients.

Mitochondrial dysfunction. Researchers propose that a mitochondrial complex I defect is linked to the deterioration of trabecular meshwork cells, and that antioxidants and MPT (mitochondrial permeability transition inhibitors) can reduce such degeneration.[23]

Damage to blood vessels. Increased eye pressure (IOP) can be caused by endothelial dysfunction and vascular structural changes. This can substantially alter blood flow within the tissues and elevate IOP, leading eventually to open-angle glaucoma.[24] Vascular changes, such as low blood pressure, and vascular obstruction (poor circulation), have been linked to glaucoma.[25] [26]

Homocysteine. High levels of homocysteine have also been identified as a risk factor for open-angle glaucoma.[27] Other studies link high levels of homocysteine to the onset of pseudoexfoliation glaucoma.[28] [29]

Diabetes. Research has also shown that glaucoma is closely related to diabetes, indicating a link to circulation and possibly inflammation. Examination of medical records of over 2 million people older than 40 found a 35% increased risk for open-angle glaucoma in people with diabetes.[30]

Thyroid disease. According to a study of 12,376 participants from the CDC's 2002 National Health Interview Survey, an association has also been drawn between thyroid disease and glaucoma. Researchers found that the prevalence of glaucoma was almost double in people with thyroid problems versus those without thyroid problems.[31]

Helicobacter pylori. Medical researchers believe that H. pylori, which is the cause of many cases of stomach ulcers, may be implicated in a number of non-digestive conditions. These conditions include cardiovascular disorders, cerebrovascular disorders (blood circulation in the brain), and vascular dysfunctions. This organism may be involved in the pathology of the eye, specifically glaucoma. Meta-analysis suggested a statistically significant association between H. pylori infection and open-angle glaucoma,[32] uveitis, and central serous maculopathy.

Drugs and medications. Non-steroidal anti-inflammatory drugs (NSAIDs) may interfere with effectiveness of IOP-lowering medications such as latanoprost.[33] Ongoing use of corticosteroids such as prednisone, used for reducing inflammation, could increase IOP.[34] Topiramate (Topamax) can increase IOP and cause acute glaucoma, as well as medications prescribed for depression, Parkinson's disease, and allergies. These medications can cause the pupil to dilate, resulting in a smaller angle for drainage of the aqueous fluid.[35]

Allergies. One study showed allergic rhinitis is associated with open-angle glaucoma.[36]

Impaired signaling. Increasingly, researchers are discovering that impaired signaling between different receptors is linked to poor functioning of structures controlling IOP levels. For example, the proper signaling of a protein growth factor, angiopoietin, and a corresponding receptor, Angpt Tie2, is critical for Schlemm's canal integrity.[37] See further discussion in the "On the Horizon" section at the end of this chapter.

Obesity. Health problems such as obesity can also increase risk of glaucoma.[38] [39] [40]

Diagnosing Glaucoma

How does a person know if they have glaucoma?

The tests for glaucoma are simple and painless. The doctor will first check your eye pressure with an instrument called a tonometer. There are two types. The first is called an applanation tonometer, which measures the pressure with a touch of a tiny probe to the cornea. The second type is called a non-contact tonometer, which blows a little puff of air at your eyes.

IOP tends to increase slightly after the eyelids have been closed. For this reason, one test used in evaluating therapies for glaucoma is the closed-eyelid test,[41] which is a predictive test for glaucoma.

The doctor will also look into your eyes with an instrument called a biomicroscope to evaluate the health of both the anterior chamber of the eye and the posterior chamber, or back of the eye. If the anterior chamber is shallow, or if there is a presence of debris, drainage may not be as efficient as with a deep or clear chamber.

In addition, the doctor will examine the optic nerve, which is about the size and shape of the head of a pencil, for a condition called cupping. Cupping may indicate that the optic nerve has been pushed out of shape by too much pressure from the aqueous humor, or that nerve cells have been lost, leaving empty space behind. Also, your doctor will look at the abundance, or lack, of nerve fibers coming from healthy retinal cells. Loss of nerve fibers is analogous to thinning of hair. Over time, a certain amount of thinning is to be expected, but in the retina, a large amount of nerve fiber loss indicates problems.

Finally, the doctor will check your peripheral vision with a machine called a visual field analyzer. This machine detects blind spots in your side vision, an indicator of glaucoma damage. Additionally, other tests such as optical coherence tomography (OCT) or Heidelberg retinal tomography (HRT) may be ordered, if your doctor feels it is necessary.

Only a complete exam of the eye pressure, the drainage angle of the anterior chamber, optic nerve, nerve fiber layer, and the peripheral vision can help determine your risk of developing or having glaucoma.

Conventional Treatment

People with glaucoma are typically put on medications that lower intraocular pressure (IOP) in the eyes. Sometimes surgery is appropriate to address structural issues.

Medications to lower intraocular pressure

There are basically two categories of glaucoma eyedrops prescribed by eye doctors: 1). Beta-blockers that lower eye pressure by reducing the amount of aqueous fluid in the eye, and 2). alpha-agonists and prostaglandin analogs that improve the outflow of the aqueous fluid; these modern eyedrops tend to have fewer side effects than the beta-blockers.

Important. Patients must be told to evaluate how they feel after beginning any medication or herbal formulas and report any changes or side effects. These changes will give the medical practitioner information on how to adjust the medication or the formulas, if necessary.

Types of Preservatives

The most common eye drop preservative is Benzalkonium chloride that is known to cause inflammation and cell damage." More recently, other preservatives including stabilized oxychloro complex (Purite) found in Alphagan-P (Allergan) and ionic-buffered preservatives (sofZia) found in Travatan Z (Alcon) have been used. Clinical studies demonstrate improved patient comfort when using the same active ingredient but switching from benzalkonium chloride (BAK) to Purite as the preservative. While significantly less toxic than BAK, sofZia still causes some negative effects, and interestingly, clinical trials have not demonstrated much difference in patient *comfort* when compared to BAK."[42]

Preservative-free Options

Preservative-free eyedrops are recommended for glaucoma because patients notice less discomfort compared to eyedrops with preservatives, and because they lower the risk of ocular surface disease.[43] Several drugs, timolol, adorzolamide/timolol fixed combination, and a prostaglandin analog, tafluprost, are available preservative-free. Ocular surface disease can include dry eye syndrome with redness, irritation, burning, sensitivity to light, and even blurred vision. As many as 60% of glaucoma patients suffer from ocular surface disease.

Beta-Blockers

Beta-blockers inhibit aqueous humor formation. They include Timoptic, Timoptic XE (timolol maleate), and Betimol (timolol hemihydrate). They cause about a 25% drop in IOP. Ten to 20% of patients do not respond to beta-blockers.

They can have side effects since their activity extends beyond the eye. Through the nervous system they can interfere with breathing, heart rate, worsening asthma, emphysema, and lung disease. Beta-blockers can lower blood pressure, slow the heart rate, and induce heart rhythm abnormalities, causing problems for vulnerable elderly patients. Betimol is less likely to negatively affect heart rhythm. Timolol can upset the cholesterol HDL/LDL (cholesterol) ratio. Beta-blockers also can lead to emotional depression.

Fortunately, the side effects disappear when the beta-blocker is discontinued. Treating with CoQ10 appears to mitigate at least some of the negative effects of timolol.[44]

Betaxol (Betoptic). Betaxol may be the safest beta-blocker; it does not decrease IOP as effectively as other beta-blockers but may do a better job at protecting the visual field.

Carteolol (Ocupress). Unlike other beta-blockers, this drug does not cross the blood-brain barrier very well, which helps protect against common side effects like depression or changes in cholesterol ratios.

Pilocarpine. This is a drug that operates through the parasympathetic nervous system (the nerves that connect the brain and spinal cord with internal organs), hormonal system, and circulatory system. This drug pulls the iris out of the chamber angle (see narrow-angle glaucoma above), and so it increases trabecular meshwork outflow. It also opens the chamber angle and constricts the pupil and the ciliary body, limiting aqueous humor production. Possible side effects include slower heart beat, decreased stamina, and increased fatigue.

Alpha-Agonists

The alpha-agonists reduce production of aqueous humor through changes to the ciliary epithelium. A recent study in twenty healthy eyes showed that the alpha-agonist Apraclonidine (1%) can actually increase the blood flow to the retina.

However, alpha-agonists can cause serious allergic reactions in 10–30% of patients. Brimonidine (Alphagan) produces fewer allergic reactions and is becoming a first line drug; its effectiveness is approximately the same as timolol, 0.5% twice a day, reducing IOP by 20–25%, but it is safer. Its main side effects are dry mouth and fatigue.

Alpha-agonists eyedrops include apraclonidine (Iopidine), brimonidine (Alphagan), dipivefrin (Propine), and epinephrine (Epifrin).

Possible side effects of alpha-agonists include:

- Red eyes
- Allergic conjunctivitis
- Headache
- Dry mouth
- Tachycardia
- Tremors
- Hypertension
- Allergic reactions

Caution. Monamine oxidase inhibitors (used to treat depression) should not be used in conjunction with alpha-agonist drugs.

Prostaglandin Analogs

These drugs generally take about two weeks to achieve maximum or near maximum therapeutic effect.

Note. IOP generally is reduced physiologically during the sleep cycle. Therefore, the first dose of the medication is taken after awakening, and if a second drop is used, it is taken in mid-to-late afternoon. This hopefully lowers IOP when it is at its highest, during waking hours. Some doctors prefer to use beta-blockers in the morning and prostaglandins at bedtime. In terms of timing:

- For a drop that is taken once a day, there are some medications that are better taken in the morning and others that are better taken in the evening. For example, one class of medications, the prostaglandin analogues (including latanoprost, bimatoprost, and travoprost) should be instilled at bedtime once a day.
- For drops that are required twice a day, the ideal dosing regimen is every 12 hours.
- For drops that are dosed three times a day, the ideal dosing regimen is every 8 hours.
- The most important thing is to make sure you take the drops the correct number of times each day

Latanoprost (Xalatan). Prostaglandin analogs are drugs with hormone-like effects. They enhance drainage of aqueous humor via the uveoscleral pathway. That route passes from the anterior chamber into the anterior chamber angle without requiring the trabecular meshwork channels. This route is not a distinct path with channels but instead is transported as seepage passing through, around, and between various tissues. It is also known as the unconventional outflow pathway.[45] Normally as much as 10% of aqueous humor passes through this route. Xalatan is believed to loosen the intracellular spaces on the face of the ciliary body to enhance uveoscleral aqueous outflow.

Studies have shown that Xalantan 0.005% at one drop per day, reduces the IOP more than timolol 0.5% twice a day, with better safety. About 90% of patients respond to this drug.

Xalatan can be used with all other glaucoma drugs. The combined use of two or more prostaglandins, or prostaglandin analogs, including Xalatan is not recommended. It has been shown that administration of these prostaglandin drug products more than once per day, may decrease the IOP lowering effect or cause paradoxical elevations in IOP.[46]

Travatan (Travoprost ophthalmic solution 0.004%). Travatan Z is a new prostaglandin analog to reduce IOP. However, it is contraindicated in pregnant women or in women who are attempting to become pregnant.

Travatan causes hyperemia (red eyes) in 35–50% of users.

Zioptan (Tafluprost) reduces IOP by increasing the quantity of fluid that drains from the eye. It is used to treat open-angle glaucoma or other causes of elevated IOP. It may cause a gradual change in the color of eyes, eyelids, or eyelashes, which may be permanent after drug use ceases.

Possible side effects of prostaglandin analogs include:

- One-third of patients with mixed color or hazel irises experience a darkening or browning of the iris. These changes are cosmetic and have no known pathological implications. The pigment changes represent an enhanced production of melanin pigment.
- Iritis occurs in two percent of patients.
- Cystoid macular edema occurs in about 3-4% of users.
- Skin rashes
- Bronchitis
- Hair loss
- Memory loss and impotence
- Depression
- Increased cholesterol and other blood lipids
- Eyelash growth and periorbital fat-cell shrinkage in the eye.[47] Note: the effect of eye shrinkage can occur even with cosmetic use of bimatoprost 0.03%/Latiss.

Surgical Options for Glaucoma

In addition to traditional glaucoma surgery, there are a number of surgical options for specific areas of concern: argon laser trabeculoplasty (ALT), selective laser trabeculoplasty (SLT), laser peripheral iridotomy (LIP), or cycloablation. Traditional surgery includes trabeculectomy, drainage implant surgery, and nonpenetrating surgery.

Trabeculectomy. This standard surgical procedure opens a small hole in the sclera, leaving it covered by a flap to permit drainage of excessive aqueous fluid. This reduces pressure on the optic nerve.[48]

Laser therapy. Laser trabeculoplasty is performed in the eye surgeon's office for open-angle glaucoma. A laser beam opens clogged channels in the trabecular meshwork to enhance drainage. After several weeks, the full effect of the procedure becomes apparent.[49]

Filtering surgery. Part of the trabecular meshwork is removed surgically.[50]

Drainage tubes. The eye surgeon inserts a small tube in your eye to support better drainage.[51]

Electrocautery. This procedure is minimally invasive. It removes tissue from the trabecular meshwork using a small electrocautery device called a trabectome.[52]

Caution. *Note that acute angle-closure glaucoma must be monitored closely by your eye doctor as it can result in an eye stroke.* If you're diagnosed with this condition, you'll need urgent treatment to reduce the pressure in your eye. This generally will require both medication and laser or other surgical procedures. You may have a procedure called a laser peripheral iridotomy in which the doctor creates a small hole in your iris using a laser to allow drainage.

Complementary Approach

Through nutrition, diet, and lifestyle modification we can help nourish and support the health of the optic nerve for those with glaucoma or at risk of developing glaucoma.

Nutrients

Oxidative stress and free radicals may play an important role in the onset of glaucoma by causing damage to the trabecular meshwork responsible for effective outflow of the aqueous fluid, and the retinal ganglion cells.[53] [54] [55] [56] [57] The optic nerve requires healthy circulation to the eyes and essential nutrients to maintain cell integrity and good vision. Research has shown that circulation to the optic nerve is poorer for those with glaucoma, particularly for normal or low-tension glaucoma.[58] Glaucoma is not just a matter of normal IOP but also of keeping the optic nerve properly nourished. There are numerous nutrients that have been well researched as supporting circulation to the optic nerve and being neuroprotective as well (see causes above). Antioxidants play many roles to help reduce oxidative stress and damage due to free radicals,[59] protect the trabecular meshwork,[60] and support healthy circulation to the optic nerve.

Nutrients Related to Type of Glaucoma

Open-angle glaucoma. If you are already on eye medications for lowering eye pressure, but would like to lower it further and lower it naturally, recommended nutrients include the following (any changes in medication should receive your eye doctor's approval and management):

- **For circulation:** Ginkgo biloba *and/or* vinpocetine. Also, a good Liver tonic such as Revision, which is based on the classic Chinese medical model, helps support healthy circulation and movement of energy in the eyes.
- **For optic nerve health:** Coleus forskohlii, taurine, bilberry, grapeseed extract, magnesium, folate, vitamin B6, vitamin B12, N-acetyl-cysteine, alpha-lipoic acid, CoQ10, omega-3 fatty acids, and vitamin C.
- **For helping reduce eye pressure:** Coleus forskohlli, vitamin C, and alpha-lipoic acid.

A number of these nutrients can be found in the optic nerve formulas (see Appendix 5).

Narrow or closed-angle glaucoma. If surgery is not needed and your eye doctor is monitoring your condition, then the following nutrients can be helpful in supporting optic nerve health:

- **For circulation**: Ginkgo biloba and vinpocetine. Also, a good Liver tonic such as Revision, based on the classic Chinese medical model (this formula was based on "rambling powder" of *xiao yao san*), helps support healthy circulation and movement of energy.
- **For optic nerve support**: Taurine, bilberry, grapeseed extract, magnesium, vitamin B12, N-acetyl-cysteine, alpha-lipoic acid, CoQ10, pyrroloquinoline quinone (PQQ), omega-3 fatty acids, and vitamin C.
  - A number of these nutrients can be found in eye formulas such as Viteyes Optic Nerve Support formula, Pure Focus, and a high-quality fish oil such as Carlsons fish oil or Nordic Natural.
- **Eyedrops:** Cineraria homeopathic eyedrops and Pleo Muc homeopathic eyedrops can help support circulation in the outer layer of the eyes.

Low or normal-tension glaucoma (the appearance of glaucoma is present with normal IOP). Changes resulting in thinning of the cornea, damage due to poor circulation, and/or lack or availability of essential nutrients may be improved using the same nutrients as in chronic glaucoma, but without the nutrients that can help lower eye pressure.

- **For circulation**: Ginkgo biloba *and/or* vinpocetine.
- **Optic nerve support**: Combination of ginkgo biloba *and* bilberry,[61] as well as taurine, grapeseed extract, folate, vitamin B6, vitamin B12 (methylcobalamin), N-acetyl-cysteine, CoQ10, and pyrroloquinoline quinone (PQQ).[62]

Pseudoexfoliative glaucoma (PEX) is distinguished by clumps of amyloid protein that accumulate in the eye and ultimately end up blocking the outflow of aqueous humor by clogging the trabecular network. Recommended nutrients are those that are both natural anti-inflammatories and supporters of optic nerve health.

- **Natural anti-inflammatories:** These include omega-3 fatty acids, astaxanthin, vitamin D3, MSM, and herbs such as turmeric (curcumin), holy basil, resveratrol, ginger, digestive enzymes, and rutin.
- **For optic nerve support:** Taurine, bilberry, grapeseed extract, magnesium, vitamin B9, vitamin B12, N-acetyl-cysteine, alpha-lipoic acid, CoQ10, pyrroloquinoline quinone (PQQ), omega-3 fatty acids, Vitamin C.
  - Many of these can be found in quality eye formulas (see Appendix 5 for more information on specific products).
- **Eyedrops:** Pleo Muc homeopathic eyedrops, MSM drops (used as eyedrops), castor oil eyedrops, and cineraria maritima homeopathic eyedrops.

Review of Individual Nutrients

Essential

Antioxidants. Oxidative free radicals and reactive oxygen species (ROS) appear to damage the trabecular network, a key cause of glaucoma. It is well established that antioxidants are effective in reducing the presence of these antagonists. Treatment with the antioxidants vitamin E or N-acetyl-cysteine induced decreased ROS production in glaucoma trabecular meshwork (GTM) cells.[63] We recommend 200 IU vitamin E or 600mg n-acetyle-cysteine three times daily.

Alpha-lipoic acid. 150mg–300mg per day. Alpha-lipoic acid is the only antioxidant that is both fat and water soluble. Studies have shown that it benefits people with glaucoma by enhancing color vision, general vision sensitivity, and helps protect nerve cells from damage.[64] Alpha-lipoic acid is an ideal substance in the treatment of oxidative brain and neural disorders involving free radical processes. It is a powerful antioxidant and supports other antioxidants such as vitamin C and vitamin E. It helps to raise glutathione levels within cells.[65] It has also been found to reduce neuronal damage due to over-stimulation by cyanide, glutamate, and iron ions, and protects nerve tissue.[66]

Aminoguanidine. 75mg, 3 times per day. This is an anti-glycating agent that inhibits the 'cross-linking' or glycosylation of proteins. Glycosylation may cause, or at least contribute to, many of the problems of old age, such as cataracts, glaucoma, and macular degeneration. In an animal study, aminoguanidine was shown to help protect the optic nerve from damage.[67]

Bilberry (vaccinium myrtillus). 180mg–240mg per day. The anthocyanin antioxidants contained in bilberry have long been confirmed to benefit vision. The combination of bilberry and ginkgo biloba was found to be very helpful in a study involving over 300 patients with normal tension glaucoma. Another study of treatment finds that a combination of bilberry and French maritime pine bark (pycnogenol) could lower IOP up to 24%.[68]

Ginkgo biloba. 120 mg per day. Found to improve the visual field in some patients with normal-tension glaucoma,[69] ginkgo biloba supports vascular cell integrity, providing better delivery of antioxidants and nutrients to the optic nerve and related cell tissue.[70] Ginkgo stabilizes cell tissue on the mitochondrial level (where our cells' energy is manufactured). The mitochondria play a major role in several diseases, particularly neurodegenerative diseases, including glaucoma.[71] Several studies have shown mitochondrial irregularities in glaucoma patients.[72] Finally, ginkgo supports microcirculation.[73]

Taurine. 500mg–1,000mg per day. Taurine is an amino acid that protects the eyes against neurotoxin damage. Nerve-damaging toxins include excessive levels of glutamate, which may be responsible for ganglion cell death and optic nerve damage seen in open-angle glaucoma.[74] It is recommended for glaucoma and retinal disease for its valuable antioxidant properties.[75]

Curcumin. 500mg per day. Curcumin's antioxidative capacity provides good protection for the nervous system, due to its anti-inflammatory, antioxidant, and anti-protein-clumping capacity.[76]

Vitamin B1 (thiamine). 50mg–100mg per day. Glaucoma patients tend to have low levels of vitamin B1.[77]

Vitamin B6. 100mg daily. A combination of B6, B9 and B12 helps to lower homocysteine levels that are linked to higher risk of developing glaucoma.[78] This is taken in divided dosages with food, often part of a vitamin B complex formulation.

Vitamin B9 (folate form). 800mcg or more per day. Supplementing with folate may be helpful to those with the pseudoexfoliation (PEX) form of glaucoma.[79]

> **Caution**. See Chapter 8, regarding supplementing with folic acid or folate.

Vitamin B12 (methylcobalamin): 1,000mcg per day. Supplementing with vitamin B12 (up to 1,000mcg–1,500mcg per day) may help protect vision in glaucoma patients.[80] [81]

Vitamin C (buffered and ascorbated). 2,000mg per day, divided amongst several meals. Whole fruit, natural vitamin C with bioflavonoids is preferred as opposed to vitamin C synthesized from corn. The eyes of open-angle glaucoma patients were found to have significantly lower vitamin C levels.[82] Several studies have determined that low vitamin C levels in blood and in the vitreous humor inside the eye can contribute to meshwork outflow blockage due to aging, and it can contribute to development of glaucoma.[83] Supplementation with large doses (10,000mg daily) can significantly lower IOP by 10 points.[84]

- For some people, a lower dose is recommended if the larger dose causes loose stools.

In many parts of the world, vitamin C is routine for glaucoma patients because it has the capacity to both decrease aqueous fluid production and improve drainage. In addition, vitamin C supports collagen metabolism, which may be linked to glaucoma.

Vitamin E. 200 IU three times per day (d-alpha-tocopherol and preferably with tocotrienols and not synthetic dl-alpha-tocopherol). Vitamin E is also found in the vitreous humor and provides antioxidant capacity to the eyes. It is most effective when combined with **vitamin C,** which helps regenerate vitamin E.[85] One study showed that patients who supplement with 300 IU–600 IU of vitamin E per day, improved blood flow and reduced vision loss. Non-treated subjects showed a significant reduction in their visual field at 6 and 12 months.[86] Another study compared non-treated subjects with those receiving vitamin E. The non-treated showed a statistically significant reduction in visual field (change in mean deviation) at 6 and 12 months.[87] [88]

Vitamin E combined with **CoQ10** is also more effective than vitamin E alone; CoQ10 increases mitochondrial alpha-tocopherol concentration which improves mitochondrial-mediated neuroprotection and inhibits astrocyte activation (a biomarker for neurodegenerative disease).[89]

CoQ10. 100mg-200mg per day. CoQ10 provided neuroprotection against mitochondrial DNA alternations in an animal model of pre-glaucoma. CoQ10 protected against retinal ganglion cell death, prevented upregulation of certain protein biomarkers, improved other biomarkers, and protected mitochondria and mitochondrial transcription factor A.[90]

DHA, B complex, and vitamin E. DHA 200mg–400mg per day, B complex and vitamin E 400 IU. Another study showed that the fatty acid DHA (abundant in fish oil), along with B complex and vitamin E, were helpful in preventing or delaying vision loss associated with glaucoma.[91]

Essential fatty acids. 3,000 IU per day. Essential fatty acids can help reduce the chronic inflammatory processes associated with glaucoma. Fish and fish oils are rich in omega-3 fatty acids (as well as DHA and EPA). The best sources of omega-3 fatty acids are cold-water fish such as salmon, mackerel, sardines, anchovies, and codfish. Black currant seed oil and flaxseed oil are also good sources of essential fatty acids. One study showed patients with primary open-angle glaucoma had reduced levels of plasma DHA and EPA compared with healthy siblings. These findings may be significant since DHA and EPA could modulate impaired systemic microcirculation, ocular blood flow, and optic neuropathy, which are the main changes associated with glaucoma.[92]

Magnesium. 500mg per day. Magnesium improves microcirculation in glaucoma patients and may protect the retinal ganglion cell against oxidative stress and cell death. Some studies conclude that magnesium improves peripheral circulation and improves the visual field in glaucoma patients with blood vessel constriction.[93][94][95]

Helpful

Coleus forskohlii. 350mg–500mg per day. A clinical trial of a glaucoma supplement containing the active ingredient forskolin along with a form of taurine, carnosine, folic acid, B1, B2, B6, and magnesium found that this reduced IOP and improved nerve cell health in the retina.[96]

Green-leafy vegetables, carrots, and beets. Researchers found a 30% percent decline in glaucoma risk in diets that include green leafy vegetables, carrots, and beets. This group of participants also had a 40-50% reduced risk of developing a sub-type of the condition known as early paracentral visual field (VF) loss (peripheral/side vision), which is linked to poor ability to maintain constant blood flow.[97]

Green tea extract. 725mg per day. One study shows that antioxidants from green tea are absorbed in the lens, retina, and other eye tissue, and reduces oxidative stress in the eyes.[98]

Resveratrol. 125mg-175mg daily. The antioxidant resveratrol is able to cross the semi-permeable barriers in the eyes; it is bio-available to eye tissue to help combat oxidative stress in the eye.[99]

Quercetin. 250mg–500mg per day. Research indicates that supplementing with quercetin has direct effects on protecting the loss of retinal ganglion cells in glaucoma patients.[100]

Turmeric (curcumin). 500mg per day. The antioxidant curcumin has possible benefit with respect to oxidative stress in the eyes.[101]

Melatonin. Intraocular pressure is usually lowest at night, which is also when natural levels of melatonin are near their high in the circadian cycle. IOP is highest in the morning when melatonin is low. There seems to be a correlation between IOP and melatonin; supplementing with melatonin may lower IOP.[102]

Note. A clinical study shows that taking glucosamine sulfate, 750mg three times daily for 3 months, can *increase* intraocular pressure (IOP) in some people.[103]

Diet

*Foods Known to **Increase** IOP*

Coffee. Drinking just 1 cup of coffee can increase IOP by 1-4mm Hg for at least 90 minutes.[104] [105] Regular coffee drinkers have a higher average IOP (approximately 3mm Hg).[106]

However, coffee beans also contain antioxidant compounds. These antioxidative effects and their possible neuroprotective implications need further research. One study concluded that oxidative stress can be a causative factor in glaucoma, and targeted nutrients can reduce oxidative stress at the level of mitochondria. This can be achieved by supplementing with ginkgo biloba and liquids that contain polyphenolic compounds (such as tea, red wine, dark chocolate, or coffee), which all have antioxidative properties.[107]

Glutamate. Evidence also exists that glutamate contributes to glaucoma, so it is best to avoid any foods with monosodium glutamate (MSG). Glutamate that is not biochemically bound to other amino acids, causes our inherent glutamate levels to increase rapidly. These "free" forms of glutamate are found in nearly all processed or packaged foods. Currently, genetic predisposition to glutamate sensitivity is being investigated.

Glutamate naturally found in some food is linked to amino acids and is slowly processed by the digestive system. Free glutamate passes through the digestive system rapidly and is quickly absorbed into the bloodstream. In some foods—such as aged or cured cheese or meats, soy sauce, mushrooms, tomatoes, broccoli, peas, walnuts, and gluten—glutamate exists in a free form.[108]

Glutamate is an essential nutrient for proper brain functioning, but excess glutamate results in "excitotoxicity" causing nerve cell death. Normally the brain is protected by the blood-brain barrier but such protection can break down in cases such as head injury, stroke, or high blood pressure and as a by-product of aging. If the blood-brain barrier is compromised, then excess glutamate in the brain and nerve cell death can be the result.[109]

Artificial sweeteners. Avoid artificial sweeteners as studies indicate possible neurotoxicity. Though more research needs to be done on this, we recommend avoiding all artificial sweeteners.

*Foods Known to **Decrease** IOP*

Studies have shown that there are natural ways to reduce intraocular pressure naturally including the following: eating a healthy diet high in fruits and vegetables.[110] People with glaucoma can reduce their eye pressure by five to seven millimeters of mercury (mm/Hg) with an improved diet and supplement program—a reduction that is as good as, or better than, achieved with drugs. In general, a diet high in beta-carotene, vitamin C, vitamin E, and selenium is recommended.

Foods containing those nutrients include garlic, onions, beans, spinach, celery, turnips, yellow and orange vegetables, green leafy vegetables, seaweed, apples, oranges, and tomatoes.

In addition, drinking lots of water helps maintain the flow of nutrients to the eye and drains metabolic wastes and toxins from eye tissues. Optimally, you should drink 16 four-ounce glasses of water per day, every half-hour. Our bloodstream can only handle being diluted by about four ounces at any one time. When you drink more than four ounces at a time, this means more work for the kidneys to filter water that hasn't had a chance to travel through the lymph system and clean body tissues.

Avoid carbonated, caffeinated, and alcoholic beverages since they can actually dehydrate eye tissues. Your optimal water intake depends upon your particular physiology, diet, climate, and physical activity. Too much water intake can reduce blood salt levels (hyponatremia) and cause cells to flood. A good way to gauge if you are properly hydrated is by the color of your urine. If it is dark yellow, then you are dehydrated and need to drink more water. If your urine is as clear as water, then you have over-hydrated and should cut back intake. Green tea is very beneficial for your health and body, but too much is dehydrating.

Lifestyle

Activities Known to Increase IOP

Excessive exercise. Exercise where the heart rate is at 80% maximum increases short-term IOP by 4.7mm Hg.[111] Weight lifting can cause a temporary increase in IOP of approximately 4mm Hg.[112]

Breath control. Playing a high-resistance wind instrument such as an oboe can double IOP during playing.[113] It returns to baseline after playing ceases.

Inverted yoga postures. An inverted posture where the eyes are below the heart can cause a doubling of IOP (returns back to baseline after 5 minutes). Certain yoga exercises such as Shirshasana leads to a two- to three-fold rise in IOP from baseline for a short duration.[114]

Tight neckties. These can increase IOP 2mm Hg (returns to baseline when loosened).[115] [116]

Computer use. In a 2004 study of programmers, software engineers, and gamers with a mean age of 43 years, one third were found to have glaucoma. Even more significant was that heavy computer users who were farsighted (presbyopia) or nearsighted (myopia) seemed to have a higher risk. Nearsightedness was found in 82% of those with glaucoma.[117]

The connection between computer use and glaucoma may be physical. Computer users tend to have a hunched over posture over their keyboard which makes it necessary for them to raise their head to see the screen. The head weighs on average 7-10% of body weight and its effective weight increases for every 1cm (.393 inches) away from the spine. Over a period of time, the weight of keeping the head up causes the muscles of the neck to shorten (side and back), which compresses the nervous, vascular, and lymph systems of the neck, and compromises circulation to the brain (and eyes). This hunched posture eventually becomes habitual, so the person, even when standing, maintains the slouched posture. Additionally, the hunched posture collapses the lungs which reduces the capacity of oxygen.

Note. To help reduce the effect of chronic computer use, take regular breaks, at least every hour, to relax the eyes, and do some eye exercises (seeChapter 10-4, Eye Exercises).

Alcohol and glaucoma. Intake of large quantities of beer or water increases IOP significantly because the kidneys cannot process large quantities of liquid quickly. However, a few studies did not report any association between alcohol intake and IOP.[118] Neuro-protective effects of red wine have also been reported. Although consuming one alcoholic drink per day may have some cardiovascular benefits, it also increases the risk of liver disease.[119]

Both acute and chronic alcohol consumption have severe effects on the structure and function of the entire gastrointestinal tract.[120] The eyes rely on receiving significant amounts of essential nutrients from the food we eat to maintain healthy vision; compromises in absorption and gut health can severely affect eye health.

Activities That Lower IOP

Regular exercise. Studies have shown that people who exercise regularly and are more physically fit have a lower average IOP.[121] [122] [123] Regular exercise means exercise 5 days a week such as a brisk walk.[124] Other studies reinforce exercise as a way to lower eye pressure and reduce the risk of developing glaucoma.[125] [126] [127]

Hormone supplementation. Hormonal use in postmenopausal women reduced IOP and improved blood flow to the optic nerve.[128] The use of estrogen plus progesterone (but not estrogen alone) was associated with a 42% reduced risk of high tension POAG.[129] Women under 45 years of age entering menopause showed a 2.6% increase in risk of glaucoma.[130]

Other health risks however, are associated with hormone supplementation, including increased risks of endometrial cancer in women with an intact uterus, urinary incontinence, dementia, stroke, blood clots, heart attack, and breast cancer.[131]

Breathing. Breathing through the nose, versus breathing through the mouth, and a correctly aligned posture that expands the lung can increase oxygenation by at least 20% and release nitric oxide, a vasodilator.[132] It is the exhale stroke of breathing which pumps the most oxygen into the lungs. Reduced breathing occurs due to a hunched over posture which compresses the lungs. Shallow breathing causes an imbalance in the oxygen and carbon dioxide ratio, reducing the ability of oxygen being transferred into tissues, and this causes stress through activation of the sympathetic nervous system.

Sleep position. One study reported that a low head position elevates IOP compared to lying on one's right side. Proper adjustment of the pillow height may help lessen IOP elevations that result from lying with a low pillow or with no pillow.[133] Another study concluded that asymmetric sleep behavior is common. Right-sided sleep was preferred and correlated with a lower visual field index for those sleeping on their left side.[134]

Manage stress. Above average stress has been shown to increase the risk for high eye pressure by almost three times.[135] [136] We recommend meditation, yoga, tai chi, Qi gong, psychotherapy, or a combination of these to help with life stress.

Recommended eye exercises. The exercises listed below are ones we recommend to do regularly for glaucoma (you can practice other eye exercises as well).

- Hot dog, near-far focus, and palming

See Chapter 10-4 for eye exercises and acupressure points that are good for all eye conditions and overall eye health.

Marijuana. This cannabinoid has been proposed as an IOP-lowering agent for a long time. The active ingredient in marijuana (delta-9-tetrahydrocannabinoid) reduces IOP by reducing aqueous humor production.[137] [138] [139] However, the IOP-lowering effect of marijuana is short term, and one would need to smoke marijuana every 3 hours for 24-hour IOP control. Note: The essential ingredient in marijuana is now available in CBD oil that can be ingested by mouth, without causing any effect of getting "high," or having the negative effects of inhaling smoke. We recommend this over smoking marijuana, though more research is needed in this area.

Other Modalities

Chinese Medicine and Glaucoma

In Chinese medicine, the Liver "opens to the eyes" and is the primary meridian for supporting overall flow of energy and circulation through the eyes. The Kidney meridian nourishes the blood to the eyes. The Spleen meridian also nourishes the blood, while also helping to keep fluids from leaking from blood vessels and reducing dampness (build-up of fluids). Other meridians may be out of balance as well, and that can affect eye health; an evaluation by an acupuncturist can best determine where the out-of-balances are located, and then, offer the optimal treatment strategy.

The following are common patent formulas used for glaucoma:

Xiao yao san. Rambling powder is a classic Liver tonic used in Chinese medicine. The Liver "opens to the eyes" and is the primary meridian (flow energy) that supports healthy circulation and the free flow of energy in the eyes and throughout the body.

Qi ju di huang wan. Rehmannia 6 plus chrysanthemum and lycii nourishes Kidney and Liver blood and yin. Qi ju di huang wan is a classic adaptation of rehmannia 6 (liu wei di huang wan) with a special emphasis on the eyes, in particular dry eyes, redness, and heat caused by yin (fluid) deficiency.

Shu gan tang regulates Liver qi.

Wen dan tang. Warm the Gallbladder decoction nourishes Kidney and Liver yin and brightens the eyes. This is specifically formulated for disharmony between Gallbladder and Stomach meridian systems.

Medicinal mushrooms. Reishi,[140] [141] maitake,[142] [143] bitter tooth,[144] [145] and lion's mane[146] [147] are helpful for glaucoma as they are reported to have neurite outgrowth and neuronal health benefits.

Treatment strategies can vary based on the TCM practitioner's evaluation and intake.

Acupuncture

Combining acupuncture and eye drops is better than eye drops alone for primary open-angle glaucoma,[148] and regular acupuncture treatments improve intraocular pressure (IOP) and retrobulbar circulation (circulation behind the globe of the eye).[149]

Homeopathy

Glaucoma homeopathic pellets. 1–3 pellets dissolved in mouth 2–3 times per day, preferably before meals, or an hour or more after meals. You can keep taking these pellets for as long as you like, keeping in mind that regular check-ups from your eye doctor are essential.

Chelation Therapy

Calcium overload and dysregulation have been found in both trabecular meshwork[150] and lamina cribrosa[151] from human glaucomatous eyes.[152] Ethylenediaminetetraacetic acid (ETDA), particularly combined with MSM,[153] may help reduce excess calcium and zinc, as well as other metals, which in excess, may contribute to eye problems.

Hypnosis

Hypnosis may help lower IOP according to some researchers.[154]

Essential Oils

Laurel leaf for lymph support.

Saffron is an antibacterial, blood purifier, antioxidant, decongestant, and memory enhancer.

Frankincense helps relieve chronic stress and anxiety, reduces pain and inflammation, boosts immunity, and even potentially helps fight cancer.

Spike lavender helps reduce stress, relieves pain, helps with headaches, and has anti-inflammatory properties.

Keep essences away from the mouth, eyes, and mucous membranes; if a few drops get in one of these sensitive areas, it may be uncomfortable for 15–30 minutes, but not harmful. You can lessen discomfort by adding a pure oil like olive or coconut oil to neutralize the irritating effect. For the eye area, dab a few drops around the outside of the eye. Do not put the neutralizing oil in the eye.

Combine ¼ cup of avocado oil with ¼ cup of calendula-infused oil. Slowly add 5 drops each of the essential oils. Then close the bottle and shake well; apply 4 drops of this mixture on your clean face. Massage in gentle circular motions. Leave overnight. See Appendix 9 for more information.

Microcurrent stimulation

Daily use of microcurrent stimulation 100ile helps stimulate circulation in the back of eyes, and helps the eyes eliminate waste (see Chapter 10-3 for more information).[155] This is particularly relevant for those where circulation and nutrition are a factor in maintaining healthy optic nerve.

On the Horizon

Sustained release therapies include contact lenses that slowly release glaucoma medication in place of having to apply eyedrops.[156]

IOP detecting contact lens. An FDA approved contact lens ("Triggerfish," Sensimed AG) detects changes in both visual function and intraocular pressure over the course of a 24-hour period.

Vision training. Researchers report a breakthrough in repairing vision for patients with glaucoma. One clinical trial revealed evidence that visual field loss is in part reversible by behavioral, computer-based, online, controlled-vision training. This comprises a new rehabilitation treatment option in glaucoma.[157]

Gene therapy. Gene therapy may use proteins to help regrow the myelin surrounding nerve cells, which would be a huge step toward reversing nerve damage.[158]

Drug delivery. Envisia is researching a more efficient delivery system of next generation drugs using micro- and nanoparticles for individualized treatment – strategies that could increase safety and efficiency.

Surgical improvements. Medical device companies are developing new surgical techniques in order to reduce complications and side effects of current surgical strategies.

While each of the following techniques have potential advantages, there is limited data supporting long-term efficacy, and even less data that is not derived from studies directly supported by the companies that develop these products.

- **Ex-press mini-shunt** can be used with conventional trabeculectomy techniques to standardize the operation and perhaps reduce the chances of the eye pressure getting too low in the immediate post-operative period. The device shunts fluid from the anterior chamber to a reservoir below the conjunctiva without removing tissue.[159]

- **Trabectome** is a device that removes tissue from the drain inside the eye (the trabecular meshwork) using an electro-surgical hand-piece that disrupts the tissue.[160]

- **Canaloplasty** uses a tiny tube to enlarge the drainage canal (Schlemm's canal) and improve drainage. It has been widely used in patients with open-angle glaucoma and in children with glaucoma at birth.[161]

NCX 125 prostaglandin. This fatty acid compound has been tested with animals and appears to reduce IOP significantly, promoting release of nitric oxide and comparing favorably with latanoprost.[162]

The Schlemm's canal is a component of the eye that plays a fundamental role in draining out the aqueous humor. A new research study has identified certain proteins (growth factors), angiopoietin-1 and 2 (Ang1 and Ang2, respectively), which are proteins important for the growth of new blood vessels. Tie2 is the receptor that binds them. In mice research, these proteins were found to be deficient, resulting in reduced drainage. Once these proteins were increased, drainage improved. More research is needed in this area; it may provide additional treatment strategies in the future.[163]

Eyedrop combinations. Several new formulations are nearing commmercial use. They employ two actions, one to improve outflow, and another to reduce fluid production within the eye. They are latanoprostene, rhopressa, and roclatan. They performed well in clinical trials, better than single action medications, with a side effect of mild red eyes.

Also See

Chapter 7, Vision Diet

Chapter 8, Nutrients

Chapter 10-4, Eye Exercises

Chapter 15-23, Optic Nerve Atrophy

Chapter 15-24, Optic Neuritis

Appendix 5, Recommended Products

Appendix 7, Additional Therapies

---

[1] National Eye Institute. Open-angle glaucoma. Retrieved Dec 15 from https://nei.nih.gov/eyedata/glaucoma.

[2] Crish, S.D., Sappington, R.M., Inman, D.M., Horner, P.J., Calkins, D.J. (2010). Distal axonopathy with structural persistence in glaucomatous neurodegeneration. *Proc Natl Acad Sci U S A*, Mar 16; 107(11):5196-201.

[3] Sachin, J., Aref, A.A. (2015). Senile Dementia and Glaucoma: Evidence for a Common Link. *J Ophthalmic Vis Res*, Apr-Jun; 10(2): 178–183.

[4] Soto, I., Howell, G.R. (2014). The Complex Role of Neuroinflammation in Glaucoma. *Cold Spring Harb Perspect Med*, Jul 3;4(8).

[5] Ibid. Soto. (2014).

[6] Ramirez, A.I., de Hoz, R., Salobrar-Garcia, E., Salazar, J.J., Rojas, B., et al. (2017). The Role of Microglia in Retinal Neurodegeneration: Alzheimer's Disease, Parkinson, and Glaucoma. *Front Aging Neurosci*, Jul 6;9:214.

[7] Kimura, A., Namekata, K., Guo, X., Noro, T., Harada, C., et al. (2017). Targeting Oxidative Stress for Treatment of Glaucoma and Optic Neuritis. *Oxid Med Cell Longev*, 2017:2817252.

[8] Izzotti, A., Bagnis, A., Sacca, S.C. (2006). The role of oxidative stress in glaucoma. *Mutat Res*, Mar;612(2):105-14.

[9] Zhao, J., Wang, S., Zhong, W., Yang, B., Sun, L., et al. (2016). Oxidative stress in the trabecular meshwork. *Int J Mol Med*, Oct;38(4):995-1002.

[10] Encyclopedia Britannica. (2018). Glaucoma. Retrieved Jan 30 2018 from https://www.britannica.com/science/glaucoma

[11] Stephenson, M. (2011). Systemic Drugs with Ocular Side Effects. Review of Ophthalmology. Retrieved Dec 15 2017 from https://www.reviewofophthalmology.com/article/systemic-drugs-with-ocular-side-effects.

[12] Glaucoma Research Foundation. The importance of Corneal Thickness. Retrieved Sep 29 2018 from https://www.glaucoma.org/glaucoma/the-importance-of-corneal-thickness.php.

[13] Majka, C.P., Challa, P. (2006). Diagnosis and Management of Pseudoexfoliation Glaucoma. *EyeNet Mag,* Jun.

[14] Vessani, R.M., Ritch, R., Liebmann, J.M., Jofe, M. (2003). Plasma homocysteine is elevated in patients with exfoliation syndrome. *Am J Ophthalmol,* 136: 41–46.

[15] Leibevitch, I., Kurtz, S., Shemesh, S., Goldstein, M., Sela, B.A., et al. (2003). Hyperhomocysteinemia in pseudoexfoliation glaucoma. *J Glaucoma,* 12: 36–39.

[16] Wang, G., Medeiros, F., Barshop, B.A., Weinreb, R.N. (2004). Total plasma homocysteine and primary open-angle glaucoma. *Am J Ophthalmol,* 137: 401–406.

[17] Tielsch, J.M., Katz, J., Sommer, A., Quigley, H.A., Javitt, J.C. (1994). *Family history and risk of primary open angle glaucoma. The Baltimore Eye Survey.* Arch Ophthalmol, Jan; 112(1):69-73.

[18] Kang, J.H., Willett, W.C., Rosner, B.A., Hankinson, S.E., Pasquale, L.R. (2007). Prospective study of alcohol consumption and the risk of primary open-angle glaucoma. *Ophthalmic Epidemiol,* May-Jun; 14(3):141-7.

[19] Hewitt, A.W., Craig, J.E., Mackey, D.A. (2006*).* Complex genetics of complex traits: the case of primary open-angle glaucoma. *Clin Exp Ophthalmol,* Jul; 34(5):472-84.

[20] Choi, J., Kim, K.H., Jeong J, Cho, H.S., Lee, C.H., et al. (2007). Circadian fluctuation of mean ocular perfusion pressure is a consistent risk factor for normal-tension glaucoma. Invest *Ophthalmol Vis Sci,* 48:104-111.

[21] Hulsman, C.A., Vingerling, J.R., Hofman A, Witteman, J.C., de Jong, P.T. (2007). Blood pressure, arterial stiffness, and open-angle glaucoma: the Rotterdam study. *Arch Ophthalmol,* 125:805-812.

[22] Newman-Casey. (2011). Diabetes and hypertension may increase your risk of glaucoma. To be safe, ask your eye doctor for a yearly glaucoma test. *Heart Advis,* Nov;14(11):5.

[23] He, Y., Leung, K.W., Zhang, Y.H., Duan, S., Zhong, X.E., et al. (2008). Mitochondrial complex I defect induces ROS release and degeneration in trabecular meshwork cells of POAG patients: protection by antioxidants. *Invest Ophthalmol Vis Sci,* 49:1447-58.

[24] Resch, H., Garhofer, G., Fuchsjager-Mayrl, G., Hommer, A., Schmetterer, L. (2009). Endothelial dysfunction in glaucoma. *Acta Ophthalmol,* Feb;87(1):4-12.

[25] Ibid. Hulsman. (2007).

[26] Sonnsjo, B., Krakau, C.E. (1993). Arguments for a vascular glaucoma etiology. *Acta Ophthalmol (Copenh),* Aug;71(4):433-44.

[27] Roedl, J.B., Bleich, S., Schlotzer-Schrehardt, U., von Ansen, N., ., J., et al. (2008). Increased homocysteine levels in tear fluid of patients with primary open-angle glaucoma. *Ophthalmic Res,* 40(5):249-56.

[28] Bleich, S., Roedl, J., von Ahsen, N., Schlotzer-Schrehardt, U., Reulbach, U., et al. (2004). Elevated homocysteine levels in aqueous humor of patients with pseudoexfoliation glaucoma. *Am J Ophthalmol,* Jul;138(1):162-4.

[29] Leibovitch, I., Kurtz, S., Shemesh, G., Goldstein, M., Sela, B.A., et al. (2003). Hyperhomocystinemia in pseudoexfoliation glaucoma. *J Glaucoma,* 12 (1), 36-39.

[30] Ibid. Newman-Casey. (2011).

[31] Cross, J.M., Kirkin, C.A., Owsley, C., McGwin, G. (2008). The Association between Thyroid Problems and Glaucoma. *B J Ophthalmol,* Nov;92(11):1503-5

[32] Ibid. Cross. (2008).

[33] Razeghinejad, M.R., Pro, M.J., Katz, L.J. (2011). Non-steroidal drug-induced glaucoma. *Eye (Lond),* Aug; 25(8): 971–980.

[34] Smith, C.L. (1966). Corticosteroid glaucoma: a summary and review of the literature. *Am J Med Sci,* 252: 239–244.

[35] Rudkin, A.K., Gray, T.L., Awadalia, M., Craig, J.E. (2010). Bilateral simultaneous acute angle closure glaucoma precipitated by non-prescription cold and flu medication. *Emerg Med Australas,* Oct 22(5): 477-9.

[36] Chung, S.D., Lin, H.C., Hung, S.H. (2014). Allergic rhinitis is associated with open-angle glaucoma: a population-based case-control study. *Am J Rhinol Allergy,* Jul-Aug;28(4):e148-51.

[37] Kim, J., Park, D.Y., Bae, H., Park, D.Y., Kim, D. (2017). Impaired angiopoietin/Tie2 signaling compromised Schlemm's canal integrity and induces glaucoma. *J Clin Invest,* Oct 2;27(10):3877-3896.

[38] Gasser, P., Stümpfig, D., Schötzau, A., Ackermann-Liebrich, U., Flammer, J. (1999). Body mass index in glaucoma. *J Glaucoma,* Feb; 8(1):8-11.

[39] Leske, M.C., Connell, A.M., Wu, S.Y., Hyman, L.G. Schachat, A.P. (1995). Risk factors for open-angle glaucoma. The Barbados Eye Study. *Arch Ophthalmol,* Jul; 113(7):918-24.

[40] Zang, E.A., Wynder, E.L. (1994). The association between body mass index and the relative frequencies of diseases in a sample of hospitalized patients. *Nutr Cancer,* 21(3):247-61.

[41] Pescosolido, N., Belcaro, G., Rusciano, D., Steigerwalt, R.D., Nebbioso, M. (2012). Retrospective study of glaucoma and closed-eyelid test: long-term outcomes in an Italian native population. *Panminerva Med,* Nov 9.

[42] Glaucoma Research Foundation. *Preservative-free Glaucoma Medications.* Retrieved Jan 30 2018 from https://www.glaucoma.org/treatment/preservative-free-glaucoma-medications.php.

[43] Stamlans, I., Sunairic, M.G., Cordeiro, M.F., Hommer, A., Rossetti, L., et al. (2013). Preservative-free treatment in glaucoma: who, when, and why. *Eur J Ophthalmol,* Jul-Aug;23(4):518-25.

[44] Takahashi, N., Iwasaka, T., Sugiura, T., Onoyama, H., Kurihara, S., et al. (1989). Effect of coenzyme Q10 on hemodynamic response to ocular timolol. *J Cardiovasc Pharmacol,* Sep;14(3):462-8.

[45] Toris, C.B., (2013). Uveoscleral Outflow: Current understanding and methods of measurement. *Glaucoma Today,* Sep/Oct:36-37.

[46] RXList. Xalatan. Retrieved Nov 27 2017 from https://www.rxlist.com/xalatan-drug.htm#warnings_precautions

[47] Berke, S.J. (2012). PAP: New Concerns for Prostaglandin Use. *Rev Opthalmol,* Oct 4.

[48] International Glaucoma Association. Trabeculectomy. Retrieved Jan 5 2018 from https://www.glaucoma-association.com/about-glaucoma/treatments/surgery/trabeculectomy/

[49] Mayo Clinic. Glaucoma. Retrieved Jan 30 2018 from https://www.mayoclinic.org/diseases-conditions/glaucoma/diagnosis-treatment/drc-20372846

[50] Ibid. Mayo Clinic. (2018).

[51] Ibid. Mayo Clinic. (2018).

[52] Ibid. Mayo Clinic. (2018).

[53] Kumar, D.M., Agarwal. N. (2007). Oxidative stress in glaucoma: a burden of evidence. *J Glaucom,* May; 16(3):334-43.

[54] Rokicki, W., Zalejska-Fiolka, J., Pojda-Wilczek, D., Kabiesz, A., Majewski, W. (2016). Oxidative stress in the red blood cells of patients with primary open-angle glaucoma. *Clin Hemmorheol and Microcir,* Jan 27;62(4):369-78.

[55] Ibid. (2016).

[56] Ibid. Kimura. (2017).

[57] Parekh, N., Voland, R.P., Moeller, S.M., Blodi, B.A., Ritenbaugh, C., et al. (2009). Association between dietary fat intake and age-related macular degeneration in the Carotenoids in Age-Related Eye Disease Study (CAREDS): an ancillary study of the Women's Health Initiative. *Arch Ophthalmol,* Nov;127(11):1483-93.

[58] Flammer, J., Orgül, S., Costa, V.P., Orzalesi, N., Krieglstein, G.K., et al. (2002). The impact of ocular blood flow in glaucoma. *Prog Retin Eye Res,* Jul; 21(4):359-93.

[59] Mozaffarieh, M., Grieshaber, M.C., Orgul, S., Flammer, J. (2008). The potential value of natural antioxidative treatment in glaucoma. *Surv Ophthalmol,* Sep-Oct;53(5):479-505.

[60] Ibid. He. (2008).

[61] Shim, S.H., Kim, J.M., Choi, C.Y., Kim, C.Y., Park, K.H. (2012). Ginkgo biloba extract and bilberry anthocyanins improve visual function in patients with normal tension glaucoma. *J Med Food,* Sep;15(9):818-23.

[62] LifeExtension. Health Protocols: Glaucoma. Retrieved Nov 27 2017 from http://www.lifeextension.com/Protocols/Eye-Ear/Glaucoma/Page-01

[63] Ibid. He. (2008).

[64] Filina, A.A., Davydova, N.G., Endrihovskii, S.N., Shamshinova, A.M. (1995). Lipoic acid as a means of metabolic therapy of open-angle glaucoma. *Vestn Oftalmol,* Oct- Dec;111(4):6-8

[65] Packer, L., Tritschler, H.J., Wessel, K. (1997). Neuroprotection by the metabolic antioxidant alpha-lipoic acid. *Free Radic Biol Med,* 22(1-2):359-78.

[66] Muller, U., Krieglstein, J. (1995). Prolonged pretreatment with alpha-lipoic acid protects cultured neurons against hypoxic, glutamate-, or iron-induced injury. *J Cereb Blood Flow Metab,* Jul;15(4):624-30.

[67] Neufeld, A.H., Sawada, A., Becker, B. (1999). Inhibition of nitric-oxide synthase 2 by aminoguanidine provides neuroprotection of retinal ganglion cells in a rat model of chronic glaucoma. *Proc Natl Acad Sci U S A*, Aug 17;96(17):9944-8.

[68] Steigerwalt, R.D., Belcaro, G., Morazzoni, P., Bombardelli, E., Burki, C. (2010). Mirtogenol potentiates latanoprost in lowering intraocularpressure and improves ocular blood flow in asymptomatic subjects. *Clin Ophthalmol*, 4:471–476.

[69] Quaranta, L., Bettelli, S., Uva, M.G., Semeraro, F., Turano, R., et al. (2003). Effect of Ginkgo biloba extract on preexisting visual field damage in normal tension glaucoma. *Ophthalmology*, 110:359–62.

[70] Ou, H.C., Lee, W.J., Lee, I.T., Chiu, T.H., Tsai, K.L., et al. (1985). Ginkgo biloba extract attenuates oxLDL-induced oxidative functional damages in endothelial cells. *J Appl Physiol*, May;106(5):1674-85.

[71] Abdel-Kader, R., Hauptmann, S., Keil, U., Scherping, I., Leuner, K., et al. (2007). Stabilization of mitochondrial function by Ginkgo biloba extract (EGb 761). *Pharmacol Res*, Dec;56(6):493-502.

[72] Abu-Amero, K.K., Morales, J., Bosley, T.M. (2006). Mitochondrial abnormalities in patients with primary open-angle glaucoma. *Invest Ophthalmol Vis Sci*, Jun; 47(6):2533-41.

[73] Wu, Y., Li, S., Cui, W., Zu, X., Du, J., et al. (2008). Ginkgo biloba extract improves coronary blood flow in healthy elderly adults: role of endothelium-dependent vasodilation. *Phytomedicine*, Mar; 15(3):164-9.

[74] Fennessy, F.M., Moneley, D.S., Wang, J.H., Kelly, C.J., Bouchier-Hayes, D.J. (2003). Taurine and vitamin C modify monocyte and endothelial dysfunction in young smokers. *Circulation*, Jan 28;107(3):410-5.

[75] Froger, N., Moutsimilli, L., Cadetti, L., Jammoul, F., Wang, Q.P., et al. (2014). Taurine: the comeback of a neutraceutical in the prevention of retinal degenerations. *Prog Retin Eye Res*, Jul;41:44-63.

[76] Cole, G.M., Teter, B., Grautschy, S.A. (2007). *Neuroprotective* effects of curcumin. *Adv Exp Med Biol,* 595:197–212.

[77] Asregadoo, E.R. (1979). Blood levels of thiamine and ascorbic acid in chronic open-angle glaucoma. *Ann Ophthalmol*, Jul; 11(7):1095-1100.

[78] Christen, W.G., Glynn, R.J., Chew, E.Y., Manson, J.E. (2007). Folic acid plus B-vitamins and age-related macular degeneration in a randomized trial in women. *Invest Ophthalmol Vis Sci*, 48:1152.

[79] Kang, J.H., Loomis, S.J., Wiggs, J.L., Willett, W.C., Pasquale, L.R. (2014). *A Prospective* Study of Folate, Vitamin B-6, and Vitamin B-12 Intake in Relation to Exfoliation Glaucoma or Suspected Exfoliation Glaucoma. *JAMA Ophthalmol*, May;132(5):549-59

[80] Sakai, T. Murata, M., Amemiya, T. (1992). Effect of long-term treatment of glaucoma with vitamin B12. *Glaucoma*. 14 167-70.

[81] Ibid. Sakai. (1992).

[82] Aleksidze, A.T., Beradze, I.N., Golovachev, O.G. (1989). Effect of the ascorbic acid of the aqueous humor on the lipid peroxidation process in the eye in primary open-angle glaucoma. *Oftalmol Zh*, (2):114-6.

[83] Xu, P., Lin, Y., Porter, K., Liton, P.B. (2014). Ascorbic acid modulation of iron homeostasis and lysosomal function in trabecular meshwork cells. *J Ocul Pharmacol Ther*, Mar-Apr;30(2-3):246-53.

[84] Boyd, H.H. (1995). *Eye* Pressure Lowering Effect of Vitamin C. *J Orthomol Med*, 10(2):165-168

[85] Lien, E.L., Hammond, B.R. (2011). Nutritional influences on visual development and function. *Prog Retin Eye Res*, May; 30(3):188-203.

[86] Engin, K.N., Engin, G., Kucuksahin, H., Oncu, M., Engin, G, et al. (2007). Clinical evaluation of the neuroprotective effect of alpha tocopherol in glaucomatous damage. *Eur J Ophthalmol*, Jul-Aug;17(4):528-33.

[87] Kunisaki, M., Bursell, S.E., Clermont, A.C., Ishii, H., Ballas, L.M., et al. (1995). Vitamin E prevents diabetes-induced abnormal retinal blood flow via the diacylglycerol-protein kinase C pathway. *Am J Physiol*, 269:239-46.

[88] Lee, I.K., Koya, D., Ishi, H., Kanoh, H., King, G.L. (1999). d-alpha tocopherol prevents hyperglycemia induced activation of the diacylglycerol (DAG)-protein kinase C pathwayin vascular smooth muscle cells by an increase in DAG kinase activity. *Diabetes Res Clin Pract*, 45:183-90.

[89] Davis, B.M., Tian, K., Pahlitzsch, M., Brenton, J., Ravidran, N., et al. (2017). Topical Coenzyme Q10 demonstrates mitochondrial-mediated neuroprotection in a rodent model of ocular hypertension. *Mitochondrion*, Sep;36:114-123.

[90] Sim, M.S., Lee, D., Kim, K.Y., Weinreb, R., Ju, W.K. (2013). Effect of coenzyme Q10 on oxidative stress and mitochondrial DNA alteration in a mouse model of glaucoma. *Inves Oph Vis Sci*, Jun;54(15).

[91] Cellini, M. Caramazza, N., Mangiafico, P., Possati, G.L., Caramazza, R. (1998). Fatty acid use in glaucomatous optic neuropathy treatment. *Acta Ophthalmol Scand Suppl*, (227):41.

[92] Ren, H., Magulike, N., Ghebremeskel, K., Crawfrd, M. (2006). Primary open-angle glaucoma patients have reduced levels of blood ocosahexaenoic and eicosapentaenoic acids. *Prostaglandins Leukot Essent Fatty Acids*, 74:157-63.

[93] Gaspar, A.Z., Gasser, P., Flammer, J. (1995). The influence of magnesium on visual field and peripheral vasospasm in glaucoma. *Ophthalmologica*, 209(1):11-3.

[94] Aydin, B., Onol, M., Hondur, A., Kaya, M.G., Ozdemir, H., et al. The effect of oral magnesium therapy on visual field and ocular blood flow in normotensive glaucoma. *Eur J Ophthalmol*, Jan-Feb;20(1):131-5.

[95] Mozaffarieh, M., Flammer, J. (2013). New insights in the pathogenesis and treatment of normal tension glaucoma. *Curr Opin Pharmacol*, Feb;13(1):43-9

[96] Mutolo, M.G., Albanese, G., Rusciano, D., Pescosolido, N. (2016). Oral Administration of Forskolin, Homotaurine, Carnosine, and Folic Acid in Patients with Primary Open Angle Glaucoma: Changes in Intraocular Pressure, Pattern Electroretinogram Amplitude, and Foveal Sensitivity. *J Ocul Pharmacol Ther,* Apr;32(3):178-83.

[97] Kang, J.H., Willett, W.C., Rosner, B.A., Buys, E., Wiggs, J.L. et al. (2016). Association of Dietary Nitrate Intake With Primary Open-Angle Glaucoma: A Prospective Analysis From the Nurses' Health Study and Health Professionals Follow-up Study. *JAMA Ophthalmol*, Mar;134(3):294-303.

[98] Chu, K.O., Chan, K.P., Wang, C.C., Chu, C.Y., Li, W.Y., et al. (2015). Effects of EGCG content in green tea extract on pharmacokinetics, oxidative status and expression of inflammatory and apoptotic genes in the rat ocular tissues. *J Nutr Biochem*, Nov;26(11):1357-67.

[99] Wang, S., Wang, Z., Yang, S., Yin, T., Zhang, Y., et al. (2017). Tissue Distribution of trans-Resveratrol and Its Metabolites after Oral Administration in Human Eyes. *J Ophthalmol*, 2017:4052094.

[100] Gao, F.J., Zhang, S.H., Xu, P., Yang, B.O., Zhang, R., et al. (2017). Quercetin Declines Apoptosis, Ameliorates Mitochondrial Function and Improves Retinal Ganglion Cell Survival and Function in In Vivo Model of Glaucoma in Rat and Retinal Ganglion Cell Culture In Vitro. *Front Mol Neurosci,* 7;10:285.

[101] Cole, G.M., Teter, B., Grautschy, S.A. (2007). Neuroprotective effects of curcumin. *Adv Exp Med Biol,* 595:197–212.

[102] Samples, J.R., Krause, G., Lewy, A.J. (1988). Effect of melatonin on intraocular pressure. *Curr Eye Res*, Jul;7(7):649-53.

[103] Esfandiari, H., Pakravan, M., Zakeri, Z., Ziaie, S. (2017). Effect of glucosamine on intraocular pressure: a randomized clinical trial. *Eye (Lond)* Mar;31(3):389-394

[104] Higginbotham, E.J., Kilimanjaro, H.A., Wilensky, J.T., Batenhorst, R.L., Hermann, D. (1989). *The* effect of caffeine on intraocular pressure in glaucoma patients. *Ophthalmology,* May;96(5):624-6.

[105] Avisar, R., Avisar, E., Weinberger, D. (2002). Effect of coffee consumption on intraocular pressure. *Ann Pharmacother*, Jun; 36(6):992-5.

[106] Chandrasekaran, S., Rochtchina, E., Mitchell, P. (2005). Effects of caffeine on intraocular pressure: the Blue Mountains Eye Study. *J Glaucoma*, Dec; 14(6):504-7.

[107] Mazaffarih, M., Grieshaber, M.C., Orgul, S., Flammer, J. (2008). The potential value of natural antioxidative treatment in glaucoma. *Surv Ophthalmol*, Sep-Oct;53(5):479-505.

[108] Kresser, C. (2014). Beyond MSG: Could Hidden Sources of Glutamate Be Harming Your Health? Retrieved on Jan 4 2018 from https://chriskresser.com/beyond-msg-could-hidden-sources-of-glutamate-be-harming-your-health/

[109] American Nutrition Association. Nutrition Digest. Review of: Excitotoxin: the Taste that Kills. Retrieved Nov 27 1017 from http://americannutritionassociation.org/newsletter/review-excitotoxins-taste-kills.

[110] Coleman, A.L., Stone, K.L., Kodjebacheva, G., Yu, F., Pedula, K.L., et al. (2008). Glaucoma risk and the consumption of fruits and vegetables among older women in the study of osteoporotic fractures. *Am J Ophthalmol*, Jun;145(6):1081-9.

[111] Qureshi, I.A., Xi, X.R., Huang, Y.B., Wu. X.D. (1996). Magnitude of decrease in intraocular pressure depends upon intensity of exercise. *Korean J Ophthalmol*, Dec; 10(2):109-15.

[112] Vieira, G.M., Oliveira, H.B., de Andrade, D.T., Bottaro, M., Ritch, R. (2006). Intraocular pressure variation during weight lifting. *Arch Ophthalmol*, Sep; 124(9):1251-4.

[113] Schuman, J.S., Massicotte, E.C., Connolly, S., Hertzmark, E., Mukherji, B., et al. (2000). Increased intraocular pressure and visual field defects in high resistance wind instrument players. *Ophthalmology*, Jan; 107(1):127-33.

[114] Baskaran, M., Raman, K., Ramani, K.K., Roy, J., Vijaya, L., et al. (2006). Intraocular pressure changes and ocular biometry during Sirsasana (headstand posture) in yoga practitioners. *Ophthalmology*, Aug; 113(8):1327-32.

[115] Teng, C., Gurses-Ozden, R., Liebmann, J.M., Tello, C., Ritch, R. (2003). Effect of a tight necktie on intraocular pressure. *Br J Ophthalmol*, Aug; 87(8):946-8.

[116] Talty, P., O'Brien, P.D. (2005). Does extended wear of a tight necktie cause raised intraocular pressure? *J Glaucoma*, Dec; 14(6):508-10.

[117] Tatemichi, M., Nakano, T., Tanaka, K., Hayashi, T., Nawa, T., et al. (2004). Possible association between heavy computer users & glaucomatous visual field abnormalities: a cross sectional study in Japanese workers. *J Epidemiol Community Health*, Dec; 58(12): 1021–1027.

[118] Wilson, M.R., Hertzmark, E., Walker, A.M., Childs-Shaw, K., Epstein, D.L. (1987). A case-control study of risk factors in open angle glaucoma. *Arch Ophthalmol*, 105:1066–71.

[119] Taylor, B., Rehm, J. (2005). Moderate alcohol consumption and diseases of the gastrointestinal system: A review of pathophysiological processes. *Dig Dis*, 23:177–80.

[120] Ibid. Taylor. (2005).

[121] Qureshi, I.A., Wu, X.D., Xi, X.R., Yang, J., Huang, Y.B. (1997). Resting intraocular pressure of steel factory workers is related to their physical fitness. *Ind Health*, 35:259–63.

[122] Kokkinos, P. (2008). Physical activity and cardiovascular disease prevention: current recommendations. *Angiology*, Apr-May; 59(2 Suppl):26S-9S.

[123] Xu, L., Wang, H., Wang, Y., Jonas, J.B. (2007). Intraocular pressure correlated with arterial blood pressure: the Beijing eye study. *Am J Ophthalmol*, Sep; 144(3):461-2

[124] Williams, P.T. (2009). Relationship of incident glaucoma versus physical activity and fitness in male runners. *Med Sci Sports Exerc*, 41(8):1566-1572.

[125] Natsis, K., Asouhidou, I., Nousios, G., Chatzabalis, T., Vlasis, K., Karabatakis, V. (2009). Aerobic exercise and intraocular pressure in normotensive and glaucoma patients. *BMC Ophthalmol*, 9:6.

[126] Chromiak, J.A., Abadie, B.R., Braswell, R.A., Koh, Y.S., Chilek, D.R. (2003). Resistance training exercises acutely reduce intraocular pressure in physically active men and women. *J Strength Cond Res*, Nov;17(4):715-20.

[127] Passo, M.S. et. al. (2009). Regular exercise lowers intraocular pressure in glaucoma patients. *Investigative Ophthalmology 35. In ARVO Abstracts*, March 15, 1994.

[128] Harris-Yitzhak, M., Harris, A., Ben-Refael, Z., Zarfati, D., Garzozi, H.J., et al. (2000). Estrogen-replacement therapy: effects on retrobulbar hemodynamics. *Am J Ophthalmol*, May; 129(5):623-8.

[129] Pasquale, L.R., Rosner, B.A., Hankinson, S.E., Kang, J.H. (2007). Attributes of female reproductive aging and their relation to primary open-angle glaucoma: a prospective study. *J Glaucoma*, Oct-Nov; 16(7):598-605.

[130] Hulsman, C.A., Westendorp, I.C., Ramrattan, R.S., Wolfs, R.C., Witteman, J.C., et al. (2001). Is open-angle glaucoma associated with early menopause? The Rotterdam Study. *Am J Epidemiol*, Jul 15; 154(2):138-44.

[131] National Cancer Institute. Menopausal Hormone Therapy and Cancer. Retrieved Nov 28, 2017 from https://www.cancer.gov/about-cancer/causes-prevention/risk/hormones/mht-fact-sheet#q3.

[132] Severinsen, S. (2014). Nitrogen Oxide - A pleasant poison! Retrieved Dec 27 2017 from https://www.breatheology.com/nitrogen-oxide-pleasant-poison/.

[133] Seo, H., Yoo, C., Lee, T.E., Lin, S., Kim, Y.Y. (2015). Head position and intraocular pressure in the lateral decubitus position. *Optom Vis Sci*, Jan;92(1):95-101.

[134] Kaplowitz, K., Blizzard, S., Blizzard, D.J., Nwogu, E., Hamil, C.E., et al. (2015). Time Spent in Lateral Sleep Position and Asymmetry in Glaucoma. Invest Ophthalmol Vis Sci, Jun;56(6):3869-74.

[135] Grignolo, F.M., Bongioanni, C., Carenini, B.B. (1977). Variations of intraocular pressure induced by psychological stress. *Klinische Monatsblaten Augenheilkd*, 170 (1977):562-69.

[136] Shily, B.G. (1987). Psychophysiological stress, elevated intraocular pressure, and acute closed-angle glaucoma. *Am J Optom Physiol Opt*, Nov;64(11):866-70.

[137] Porcella, A., Maxia, C., Gessa, G.L., Pani, L. (2000). The human eye expresses high levels of CB1 cannabinoid receptor mRNA and protein. *Eur J Neurosci*, 12:1123–7.

[138] Flach, A.J. (2002). Delta-9-tetrahydrocannabinol (THC) in the treatment of end-stage open-angle glaucoma. *Trans Am Ophthalmol Soc*, 100:215–22.

[139] Green K. (1998). Marijuana smoking vs cannabinoids for glaucoma therapy. *Arch Ophthalmol*, 116:1433–7.

[140] Sun, XZ, Liao, Y., Li, W., Guo, L.M. (2017). Neuroprotective effects of ganoderma lucidum polysaccharides against oxidative stress-induced neuronal apoptosis. *Neural Regen Res*, Jun;12(6):953-958.

[141] Zhang, W., Zhang, Q., Deng, W., Li, Y., Xing, G., et al. (2014). Neuroprotective effect of pretreatment with ganoderma lucidum in cerebram ischemia/reperfusion injury in rat hippocampus. *Neural Regen Res*, Aug 1;9(15):1446-52.

[142] Chen, Z., Tang, Y., Liu, A., Jin, X., Zhu, J., et al. (2017). Oral administration of Grifola fondosa polysaccharides improves memory impairment in aged rats via antioxidant action. *Mol Nutr Food Res,* Nov;61(11).

[143] Phan, C.W., David, P., Naidu, M., Wong, K.H., Sabaratnam, V. (2015). Therapeutic potential of culinary-medicinal mushrooms for the management of neurodegenerative diseases: diversity, metabolite, and mechanism. *Crit Rev Biotechnol,* 35(3):355-68.

[144] Liu, L., Shi, X.W., Zong, S.C., Tang, J.J., Gao, J.M. (2012). Scabrogine M, a novel inhibitor of NGF-induced neurite outgrowth from PC12 cells from the fungus Sacrodon scabrosus. *Bioorg Med Chem Lett,* Apr 1;22(2):2401-6.

[145] Shi, X.W., Liu, L., Gao, J.M., Zhang, A.L. (2011). Cyathane diterpenes from Chinese mushroom Sarcodon scabrosus and their neurite outgrowth-promoting activity. *Eur J Med Chem,* Jul;46(7):3112-7.

[146] Lai, P.L., Naidu, M., Sabaratnam, V., Wong, K.H., David, R.P., et al. (2013). Neurotropic properties of the Lion's mane medicinal mushroom, Hericium erinaceus (Higher Bsidiomycetes) from Malaysia. *Int J Med Mushrooms,* 15(6):539-54.

[147] Mori, K., Obara, Y., Hirota, M., Azumi, Y., Kinugasa, S., et al. (2008). Nerve growth factor-inducing activity of Hericium erinaceus in 1321N1 human astrocytoma cells. *Biol Pharm Bull,* Sep;31(9):1727-32.

[148] Liu, F., Li, B.L., Yang, J.F., Song, L.N., Tang, K., et al. (2013). Clinical observation on combining acupuncture and eye drops for primary open angle glaucoma. *J Acu Tuina Sci,* April(11)2:93-95..

[149] Takayama, S., Seki, T., Nakazawa, T., Aizawa, N., Takahashi, S., et al. (2011). Short-Term Effects of Acupuncture on Open-Angle Glaucoma in Retrobulbar Circulation: Additional Therapy to Standard Medication. *Ev Based Comp Alt Med,* Article ID 157090.

[150] Ibid. He. (2008).

[151] McElnea, E.M., Quill, B., Docherty, N.G., Irnaten, M., Siah, W.F., et al. (2011). Oxidative stress, mitochondrial dysfunction and calcium overload in human lamina cribrosa cells from glaucoma donors. *Mol Vis,* 17:1182–1191.

[152] Ceylan, O.M., Can Demirdöğen, B., Mumcuoğlu, T., Aykut, O. (2013). Evaluation of essential and toxic trace elements in pseudoexfoliation syndrome and pseudoexfoliation glaucoma. *Biol Trace Elem Res,* Jun;153(1-3):28-3.

[153] Zhang, M., Wong, I.G., Gin, J.B., Ansari, N.H. (2009). Assessment of methylsulfonylmethane as a permeability enhancer for regional EDTA chelation therapy. *Drug Deliv,* Jul; 16(5):243-8.

[154] Berger, A.S., Simel, P.J. (1958). Effect of Hypnosis on Intraocular Pressure in Normal and Glaucomatous Subjects. *Psychosomatic Med,* Jul:20(4).

[155] Ibid. Hulsman. (2007).

[156] Carvlho, I.M., Marques, C.S., Oliveira, R.S., Coelho, P.B., Costa, P.C., et al. (2015). Sustained drug release by contact lenses for glaucoma treatment-a review. *J Control Release,* Mar 28;202:76-82.

[157] Sabel, B.A., Gudlin, J. (2014). Vision restoration training for glaucoma: a randomized clinical trial. *JAMA Ophthalmol.* Apr 1;132(4):381-9.

[158] Hoyng, S.A., de Winter, F., Tannemaat, M.R., Blits, B., Malessy, M.J. (2015). Gene therapy and peripheral nerve repair: a perspective. *Front Mol Neurosci,* 8: 32.

[159] Sarkisian, S.R., (2009). The Ex-Press Mini Glaucoma Shunt: Technique and Experience. *Middle East Afr J Ophthalmol,* Jul-Sep; 16(3): 134–137.

[160] Esfandiari, H., Polat, J.K., Loewen, M.D. (2015). Trabectome: Ab Interno Trabeculectomy. EyeWiki. Retrieved Feb 5 2018 from http://eyewiki.aao.org/Trabectome%3A_Ab_Interno_ Trabeculectomy

[161] Glaucoma Research Foundation. Canaloplasty: A surgical alternative for glaucoma. Retrieved Feb 5 2018 from https://www.glaucoma.org/treatment/canaloplasty-a-new-surgical-alternative.php.

[162] Borghi, V., Bastia, E., Guzzetta, M., Chiroli, V., Toris, C.B., et al. (2010). A novel nitric oxide releasing prostaglandin analog, NCX 125, reduces intraocular pressure in rabbit, dog, and primate models of glaucoma. *J Ocul Pharmacol Ther,* Apr;26(2):125-32.

[163] Kim, J., Park, D.Y., Bae, H., Park, D.Y., Kim, D., et al. (2017). Impaired angiopoietin/Tie2 signaling compromises Schlemm's canal integrity and induces glaucoma. *J Clin Invest,* Oct 2;127(10):3877-3896.

15-12. IRITIS

Iritis (also called anterior uveitis) is an immune system related condition affecting the front part of the eye. It is the most common form of uveitis. The iris becomes inflamed and is often experienced as a painful red eye.

Iritis mostly affects people between the ages of 20 and 59 and is uncommon in children. It affects women only slightly more than men, and altogether about 8 in 100,000 people, according to a 1996 study. As of 2013, only three studies had identified the prevalence of iritis in the U.S. within the general population. The three estimates ranged from 58 to 114.5 per 100,000 persons in terms of annual prevalence. Iritis causes 2.8–10% of legal blindness in the US, or nearly 30,000 new cases of blindness each year.[1] [2] [3]

What is Iritis?

There are two types of iritis: acute (nongranulomatous) and chronic (granulomatous).

Acute, traumatic iritis occurs suddenly and is sometimes caused by trauma or injury to the eye. It can be quite painful, but it generally heals on its own within several weeks. This is the most common form of iritis.

Chronic, non-traumatic, and recurring iritis can last for months or years. It responds less readily to treatment than acute iritis and increases the risk of damage to vision. Complications of chronic iritis can include glaucoma, cataracts, cystoid macular edema, corneal calcification, posterior calcification, and possibly blindness. It can be related to a systemic disease or other ocular condition.

Anatomy of the Iris

The front of the eye contains the uvea, a section of the internal eye, which in turn is made up of three parts:

The iris is the circular pigmented membrane, surrounding the pupil of the eye that provides the eye with its color. The iris controls the size of the pupil in reaction to the brightness of light exposure.

The ciliary body is located behind the iris and is responsible for focusing the lens. The ciliary epithelium produces the aqueous humor that circulates within the anterior chamber (space between the iris and cornea).

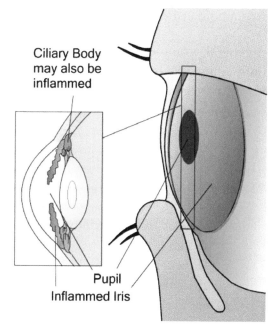

Ciliary Body may also be inflammed

Pupil

Inflammed Iris

The choroid is the vascular layer of the eye that lies between the retina and the sclera.

Pathology

Iritis is more correctly classified as anterior uveitis. When the iris is inflamed, white blood cells (leukocytes) migrate into the anterior chamber of the eye. They can accumulate and adhere between the iris and the lens, causing irritation and inflammation.

Inflammation of the iris region apparently causes the blood-ocular barrier to deteriorate or fail, allowing protein build-up. This condition forces both protein and white blood cells into the aqueous fluid, resulting in the typical iritis symptoms.[4]

Nongranulmatous (acute) iritis

While acute iritis is often caused by trauma to the eye, it is sometimes difficult to determine the cause. Its most common form is linked to the human white blood cell antigen HLA-B27 gene mutation[5] that is associated with psoriasis, ankylosing spondylitis, inflammatory bowel disease, and reactive arthritis. Environmental factors play an important role in HLA-B27's capacity to trigger iritis, and bacterial triggers are most strongly implicated.[6]

Examples of the wide range of hard-to-identify causes include treatment with intense pulsed light,[7] a cosmetic iris implant,[8] and dislocation of a posterior intraocular lens.[9]

Granulmatous (chronic) iritis

Chronic iritis may result from an autoimmune reaction or an immune response to systemic disease such as tuberculosis, Lyme disease, Bechet's disease, sarcoidosis, lupus, juvenile rheumatoid arthritis, or herpes.

In general, granulomatous conditions are autoimmune-related conditions that make the body more vulnerable to bacterial and fungal infections. Granulomas are immune cells that collect at the location of infection. So, in the case of granulomatous iritis, this massing of immune cells takes place at the iris, causing redness and pain.

Signs and Symptoms

The following symptoms are generally the same for both acute and chronic iritis:[10]

- Reddened eye, especially adjacent to the iris
- Eye pain
- Headaches
- Light sensitivity
- The pupil may become smaller in the affected eye
- Blurred or cloudy vision
- Red eye

Causes and Risk Factors

The causes of iritis may vary; they can be connected to problems or diseases occurring in the eye, or they may be a result of an inflammatory disease in other parts of the body, such as Crohn's and ulcerative colitis.[11] Physical trauma, autoimmune disorders, chronic systemic inflammation, and infections[12] are all possible sources. However, it is important to know that iritis is most often a symptom of one or more other disease conditions in the body, and it may be the only symptom that is noticeable. Here is a summary of primary causes:

Blunt trauma to the eye (traumatic or nongranulomatous iritis), such as eye and head injury, problems arising from ocular surgery, or eye treatments and therapies

Association with other diseases or disorders (non-traumatic or granulomatous iritis), such as ankylosing spondylitis, sarcoidosis, Reiter syndrome, inflammatory bowel disease, psoriasis, and collagen vascular diseases such as lupus and cancers

Infectious illnesses (non-traumatic or granulomatous iritis), such as Lyme disease, syphilis, herpes simplex and herpes zoster viruses, tuberculosis, and toxoplasmosis

Conventional Treatment

Since the causes of iritis are not readily known, and potentially multifactorial, an attending physician must take a very careful medical history at the time of diagnosis. Your doctor may recommend chest X-rays, blood tests, stool evaluation, skin tests, and even a spinal tap. You should let your doctor know about exposure to pets, other animals, unusual environmental conditions, recent surgery, illness, or family history of autoimmune conditions as part of the medical history.

The first line of treatment is usually steroid and non-steroidal anti-inflammatory eyedrops. If the inflammation persists or disappears temporarily, and comes back, your doctor may also inject steroids, or prescribe additional oral steroids, antibiotics, antifungals, or antivirals. Unfortunately, the side effects of these medications can be deleterious and can include onset of cataracts, glaucoma, corneal changes, and possibly more inflammation. Therefore, make sure your eye doctor monitors your progress carefully.

In general, traumatic iritis usually goes away within one to two weeks. Non-traumatic iritis may take weeks and occasionally months, or even years to resolve, depending on underlying conditions. Even when the disorder is treated early, it often recurs if the underlying cause has not been successfully identified or addressed. This is why a thorough health evaluation at the time of diagnosis is crucial.

As you might suspect, certain cases of iritis (those associated with systemic or difficult to treat diseases, such as sarcoidosis, ankylosing spondylitis, or Lyme disease) may be chronic or recurrent. Similarly, when iritis is linked to an infection, it will likely only resolve once measures are taken to treat the infection.

Complementary Approach

We believe that eye problems such as chronic iritis reflect the health of the whole body. Where there is inflammation in one part of the body, there is often inflammation in another. Therefore diet, nutrition, and lifestyle choices can play a major role in having and maintaining good vision.

Since non-traumatic iritis is typically a symptom of underlying health conditions involving inflammation, augmenting conventional treatments with targeted antioxidants can be essential in helping preserve vision while managing the symptoms of iritis.

Antioxidants are available through a healthy anti-inflammatory and alkalinizing diet (see Diet, Chapter 7) as well as through nutritional supplements. They help in a number of ways, including:

- Neutralizing the potentially damaging effects of free radicals that are a by-product of inflammation (particularly chronic inflammation)
- Delivering essential nutrients to all parts of the eyes, which are vital for healthy eyes
- Reducing inflammation (through specific supplements that have natural anti-inflammatory properties)

Nutrients

Essential

A high-quality, whole-food, organic eye formula. Follow directions on bottle (see Advanced Eye and Vision Support Formula, Appendix 5).

Essential fatty acids. 2,000mg–3,000mg per day with a meal. The anti-inflammatory benefits of this supplement can be duplicated by eating three or four servings per week of fish, specifically sardines, mackerel, salmon, tuna (especially white tuna, or albacore), cod, or halibut. To help assimilate the oils and prevent them from becoming rancid in the body, make sure you take at least 100 IUs of **vitamin E** each day (fish oil supplements often include vitamin E). Make sure the fish is wild caught, not farm raised. Use caution with canned albacore tuna, which has up to three times the mercury levels as light or skipjack tuna.[13]

Astaxanthin. 6mg–12mg per day. Astaxanthin is a fat-soluble carotenoid that, in its value as an antioxidant, is ten times more powerful than beta-carotene, lutein, or zeaxanthin (and from 60–500 times stronger than vitamin E).[14] After eight weeks of daily use, astaxanthin reduces levels of C-reactive protein, the inflammatory marker.[15]

Trans-resveratrol. 175mg per day. This potent antioxidant helps protect nerve cells from damage,[16] reduce oxidative damage,[17] [18] and support a healthy inflammatory response.[19] It reduces retinal pigment epithelial (RPE) cell degeneration, leading to malfunction of blood-retinal barrier and loss of vision.[20]

Lutein. 10mg–20mg per day. Researchers identify lutein as having therapeutic potential in managing uveitis, inflammatory eye conditions, and dry eye.[21] [22]

MSM capsules. 2,000mg per day. MSM helps nourish and strengthen body tissues and has natural anti-inflammatory properties.[23]

Curcumin. 375mg, 3 times per day. In a study of 53 patients with iritis, a 375mg dose of curcumin (turmeric root extract), 3 times per day for 3 months, showed improvement comparable to the effects seen with a similar corticosteroids dose.[24]

Glutathione reduced (GSH). 500mg–900mg per day. This is taken preferably in an intraoral or sublingual form, as glutathione is not absorbed well through the digestive system. The sublingual form has 5–10 times greater absorption, so the dosage will be smaller. Follow label instructions. Glutathione is one of the super antioxidants that neutralizes the full range of free radicals.[25] GSH levels decline in human eyes with aging.[26] Glutathione is normally present in high levels in the ocular lens, cornea, aqueous humor, and retina, where it performs multiple roles, including maintaining normal tissue hydration, lens transparency, and protecting against oxidative damage. Decreased levels of GSH have been associated with several age-related eye disorders.[27] [28] [29]

Helpful

Serrapeptase. 60,000 IU–120,000 IU per day. Serrapeptase is an enzyme that helps break down excess protein in tissue and blood that may be contributing to chronic inflammation. It is best to split the recommended dosage into two, and take twice a day, away from food.

Green tea supplement. 500mg–750mg per day. Green tea extract has demonstrated potent anti-inflammatory and anti-cancer properties in animal studies. The most abundant catechin (a naturally occurring phenol and antioxidant) in green tea is epigallocatechin-3-gallate, commonly called EGCG. Studies show the beneficial properties of green tea, specifically EGCG, and that it is a potent anti-inflammatory compound with therapeutic potential.[30]

Vitamin E. 400 IU per day, and **Vitamin C (buffered)** 2,000 IU per day. Studies have indicated vitamin E (and vitamin C) have a protective effect on the eyes or those with iritis.[31]

Note 1. Other studies have concluded that the following nutrients (also mentioned above) may help reduce symptoms of anterior uveitis: vitamin C and E, a multivitamin containing antioxidant vitamins A, C, E, and the B vitamins; trace minerals such as magnesium, calcium, zinc, and selenium; omega-3 fatty acids, turmeric, and lutein (for overall eye health).[32]

Note 2. If an underlying health condition is identified to be contributing to, or causing the iritis, additional nutrients may be recommended, depending on the specific diagnosis.

Diet

Alkaline diet. Maintain an alkaline diet with plenty of fresh fruits and vegetables, low in refined carbohydrates. See the Vision diet in Chapter 7. The Vision diet is primarily alkaline (versus acid-forming or acidic), which helps reduce and manage chronic inflammation naturally. However, there are some adjustments to the diet that could be made to enhance alkalinity. You will see a basic chart of alkaline versus acidic foods in Appendix 11.

Anti-inflammatory diet. Anti-inflammatory foods include turmeric (curcumin), mint, cucumber, and green leafy vegetables. Go easy on spicy foods and herbs that are "warming" such as cinnamon, ginger, cloves, and licorice. Determine whether nightshade plants worsen your symptoms such as tomatoes, potatoes, eggplant, most peppers, and tobacco. Generally, these are avoided in anti-inflammatory diets.

Antioxidants. Blueberries and bilberries contain anti-inflammatory, antioxidant anthocyanins that support eye health. These berries can be eaten along with other berries, although it is recommended that blueberries comprise at least 75% of each serving. Eat about ½-cup of blueberries per day on average, or about 1 bag of frozen blueberries per week. These can be fresh, cooked, or frozen, as the pigments are relatively heat and cold resistant.

Antioxidant carotenoids found in leafy greens, non-inflammatory red/orange vegetables such as beets and winter squash are also valuable.

Note. Caution with eating frozen foods if you have a weak digestive system and are prone to gas, bloating, and loose stools.

Juicing of vegetables and fruits is a good way to get absorbable nutrients from foods. Favor these alkalizing fruits and vegetables, preferably organic:

- Green, leafy vegetables, celery, cucumber, carrot, parsley, beets, all types of berries, apple, lemon, leafy greens, ginseng, garlic, and green tea
- Go easy on the fruit, carrots and beets due to their high sugar content.
- Add a squeeze of lemon, which aides in the body's uptake of iron (from the greens) and also results in increased alkalinity in the body.
- Try to use room temperature vegetables and fruit.
- Do not add ice or very cold liquids since cold foods and liquids will eventually extinguish the stomach's digestive fire.
- Do not juice as often during the cooler months of the year, and instead, switch to vegetable soups or stews.

Lifestyle

Eyedrops. Homeopathic eyedrops can help reduce inflammation in the eye. These can sometimes be found in your local health food store. These include Natural Ophthalmics and Similisan who commercially produce these types of eyedrops.

Eye exercises. Include palming and massaging the acupressure points around the eyes on a daily basis (see Chapter 10 for more information).

Exercise. In addition to a healthy diet, get regular, moderate exercise including walking, swimming, moderate jogging, light-weight lifting, yoga, and tai chi. Basically, regular exercise tends to lower markers of systemic inflammation while acute exercise increases markers of acute inflammation.

Reduce stress. Work to keep your daily stress to a minimum. Yoga, meditation, and a daily walk can prove beneficial.

Grounding. Connecting any bare skin to the earth such as touching a rock, tree, walking bare foot, swimming in a natural water source, etc. will allow the flow of negative ions from the earth to enter your body. This has similar benefits to taking antioxidants and will reduce inflammation. Do this daily. See Appendix 7 for more information about grounding.

Other Modalities

Chinese Medicine

In terms of Traditional Chinese Medicine (TCM), inflammation in the eye can be related to yin deficiencies. Since yin (cooling aspect) balances yang (heating aspect), when yin is deficient, "heat" will arise in the body and "rise up" to the eyes. In more serious conditions of severe yin deficiency, a TCM practitioner may diagnose "fire rising," which causes more acute symptoms. For example, symptoms of Liver fire include dizziness, temple headaches, red (or swollen or painful) eyes, ringing in the ears, and fits of anger. In addition to yin deficiency, chronic inflammatory conditions can be related to TCM patterns such as Spleen dampness and/or Liver wind. A skilled TCM practitioner will be able to identify the nuances of your pattern upon intake.

Common patent formulas include:

Qi ju di huang tang (lycium-rehmannia with radix bupleuri, radix angelicae sinensis, and fructus schisandrae chinesis) tonifies Kidney yin, tonifies Blood, and clears the eyes.

Ming mu di huang wan (rehmannia pills to "brighten the eyes") addresses the following patterns: Liver Blood deficiency, Kidney yin deficiency, Liver yin deficiency, all of which are associated with iritis.

A basic formula for chronic uveitis consists of two parts which should total 70-80% of a custom formula:

1. For reduction of inflammation use chrysanthemum flower, turmeric root, buddleia flower, gentiana root, elderberry, eclipta, dandelion root, conch shell, or triphala.
2. To alleviate Blood congestion use tien chi root (high doses), red peony root, bromelain, salvia root (high doses), persica seed (tao ren, or prunus persica), and other herbs from the Blood-moving group.

It is best to consult a qualified acupuncturist or herbalist who can guide you to the best formula rather than self-prescribe. As you can see by these examples, Chinese herbal medicine is complex, and the development of ideal formulas requires thorough training. There are two exceptions to this recommendation:

1. Individuals with chronic health conditions such as high (or low) blood pressure that require medication to control, are advised to work through your health care practitioner (for example, an acupuncturist, herbalist, or naturopathic doctor) to determine which herbal formulas would be best for you.

2. It is okay for a layperson to administer general tonics such as Kidney and Liver patented formulas, which are designed for universal, whole-body benefits; as such, they are safe to take on an ongoing basis.

Also See

[1] Suhler, E.B., Lloyd, M.J., Choi, D., Rosenbaum, J.T., Austin, D.F. (2008). Incidence and prevalence of uveitis in Veterans Affairs Medical Centers of the Pacific Northwest. *Am J Ophthalmol*, 146:890–896.

[2] Acharya, N.R., Tham, V.M., Esterberg, E., Borkar, D.S., Parker, J.V., et al. (2013). Incidence and prevalence of uveitis: results from the Pacific Ocular Inflammation Study. *JAMA Ophthalmol*, 131:1405–1412. .

[3] Gritz, D.C., Wong, I.G. (2004). Incidence and prevalence of uveitis in Northern California: the Northern California Epidemiology of Uveitis Study. *Ophthalmology*, 111:491–500.

[4] Lee, R.W., Nicholson, L.B., Sen, H.N, Chan, C.C., Wei, L., et al. (2014). Autoimmune and autoinflammatory mechanisms in uveitis. *Semin Immunopathol*, May 24;36(5):581-594.

[5] Wakefield, D., Chang, J.H., Amjadi, S., Maconochie, Z., Abu El-Asrar, A., et al. (2011). What is new HLA-B27 acute anterior uveitis? *Ocul Immunol Inflamm*, Apr;19(2):139-44.

[6] Ibid. Wakefield. (2011).

[7] Crabb, M., Chan, W.O., Taranth, D., Huilgol, S.C. (2014). Intense pulsed light therapy (IPL) induced iritis following treatment for a medial canthal capillary malformation. *Australas J Dermatol*, Nov;55(4):289-91.

[8] Kelly, A., Kaufman, S.C. (2015). Corneal Endothelial Cell Loss and Iritis Associated With a New Cosmetic Iris Implant. JAMA Ophthalmol, Jun;133(6):723-4

[9] Handzel, D.M. (2012). Iritis with destabilization of the intraocular pressure due to dislocation of a posterior chamber intraocular lens. *Opthalmologe*, Apr;109(4):385-7.

[10] National Eye Institute. Facts About Uveitis. Retrieved Nov 18 2017 from https://nei.nih.gov/health/uveitis/uveitis.

[11] Isaacs, K.L. (2008). How prevalent are extraintestinal manifestations at the initial diagnosis of IBD. *Inflamm Bowel Dis*, Oct;14 Suppl 2:S198-9.

[12] Ibid. National Eye Institute. Facts About Uveitis.

[13] Environmental Defense Fund. Mercury alert: Is canned tuna safe? Retrieved Nov 18 2017 from https://www.edf.org/oceans/mercury-alert-canned-tuna-safe-eat.

[14] Maher, T.J. (2000) Astaxanthin: Continuing Education Module. *New Hope Institute of Healing*. Aug.

[15] Spiller, G.A., Dewell, A., Chaves, S., Rakiddzich, Z. (2006). Effect of daily use natural astaxanthin on C-reactive protein. Retrieved Dec 18 2017 from https://www.cyanotech.com/pdfs/bioastin/batl43.pdf.

[16] Anekonda, T.S., Adamus, G. (2008). Resveratrol prevents antibody-induced apoptotic death of retinal cells through upregulation of Sirt1 and Ku70. *BMC Res Notes*, Dec 1;1:122

[17] Remsberg, C.M., Yanez, J.A., Ohgami, Y., Vega-Villa, K.R., Rimando, A.M., et al. (2008). Pharmacometrics of pterostilbene: preclinical pharmacokinetics and metabolism, anticancer, antiinflammatory, antioxidant and analgesic activity. *Phytother Res*, Feb;22(2):169-79.

[18] Perecko, T., Jancinova, V., Drabikova, K., Nosal, R., Harmatha, J. (2008). Structure-efficiency relationship in derivatives of stilbene. Comparison of resveratrol, pinosylvin and pterostilbene. *Neuro Endocrinol Lett,* Oct;29(5):802-5.

[19] Currais, A, Prior, M., Dargusch, R., Armando, A., Ehren, J., et al. (2014). Modulation of p25 and inflammatory pathways by fisetin maintains cognitive function in Alzheimer's disease transgenic mice. *Aging Cell,* Apr;13(2):379-90

[20] Antonetti, D.A., Klein, R., Gardner, T.W. (2012). Diabetic retinopathy. *N Engl J Med*, Mar 29; 366(13):1227-39.

[21] Chao, S.C., Vagaggini, T., Nien, C.W., Huang, S.C., Lin, H.Y. (2015). Effects of Lutein and Zeaxanthin on LPS-induced Secretion of IL-8 by Uveal Melanocytes and Relevant Signal Pathways. *J Ophthalmol*, 152854.

[22] Chao, S.C., Nien, C.W., Iacob, C., Hu, D.N., Huang, S.C., et al. (2016). Effects of Lutein on Hyperosmoticity-Induced Upregulation of IL-6 in Cultured Corneal Epithelial Cells and Its Relevant Signal Pathways. *J Ophthalmol*, 2016:8341439.

[23] Butawan, M., Benjamin, R.L., Bloomer, R.J. (2017). Methylsulfonylmethane: Applications and Safety of a Novel Dietary Supplement. *Nutrients*, Mar 16;9(3).

[24] Lal, B., Kapoor, A.K., Asthana, O.P., Agrawal, P.K., Prasad, R., et al. (1999). Efficacy of curcumin in the management of chronic anterior uveitis. *Phytother Res*, Jun;13(4):318-22

[25] Huang, S.Y., Jeng, C., Kao, S.C., Yu, J.J., Liu, D.Z., (2004). Improved haemorrheological properties by Ginkgo biloba extract (Egb 761) in type 2 diabetes mellitus complicated with retinopathy. *Clin Nutr*, Aug;23(4):615-21

[26] Harding, J.J. (1970). Free and protein-bound glutathione in normal and cataractous human lenses. *Biochem J*, May; 117(5):957-60.

[27] Bhat, K.S., John, A., Reddy, P.R., Reddy, P.S., Reddy, V.N. (1991). Effect of pigmentation on glutathione redox cycle antioxidant defense in whole as well as different regions of human cataractous lens. *Exp Eye Res*, Jun; 52(6):715-21.

[28] Moreno, M.C., Campanelli, J., Sande, P., Sánez, D.A., Keller Sarmiento, M.I., et al. (2004). Retinal oxidative stress induced by high intraocular pressure. *Free Radic Biol Med*, Sep 15; 37(6):803-12.

[29] Sternberg, P., Davidson, P.C., Jones, D.P., Hagen, T.M., Reed, R.L., et al. (1993). Protection of retinal pigment epithelium from oxidative injury by glutathione and precursors. *Invest Ophthalmol Vis Sci*, Dec; 34(13):3661-8.

[30] Chatterjee, P., Chandra, S., Dey, P., Bhattacharya, S. (2012). Evaluation of anti-inflammatory effects of green tea and black tea: A comparative in vitro study. *J Adv Pharm Technol Res*, Apr;3(2):136-8.

[31] van Rooij, J., Schwartzenberg, S.G.W.S., Mulder, P.G.H., Baarsma, S.G. (1999). Oral vitamins C and E as additional treatment in patients with acute anterior uveitis: a randomised double masked study in 145 patients. *Br J Ophthalmol*, Nov;83(11):1277-82.

[32] University of Maryland Medical Center. Uveitis. Retrieved Nov 18 2017 from http://www.umm.edu/health/medical/altmed/condition/uveitis

15-13. KERATOCONUS

Keratoconus (bulging of the cornea) is a degenerative condition and is the most common form of corneal dystrophy.[1] Approximately 50–200 of every 100,000 people are afflicted with this condition. In the U.S., a study found that keratoconus prevailed in 54.5 per 100,000 people.[2] It occurs in all races and typically develops in both eyes. It is more prevalent in those who wear contacts and in people who are nearsighted (myopic).

What is Keratoconus?

Keratoconus is characterized by a thinning and protrusion of the cornea, resulting in an irregular conical shape rather than maintaining the normal, gentle, rounded shape. Because the cornea is the first point of focusing light that comes into the eyes, vision is distorted. The condition often starts in puberty, and it is reported by teens who come to their eye doctor because their vision is poor. It then progresses gradually into adulthood and eventually stabilizes. Severe astigmatism can result causing poorer vision. Consequently, keratoconus is often mistaken for astigmatism.[3]

Anatomy of the Cornea

Six layers make up the structure of the cornea.

The outermost layer is a thin layer of protective cells called the **epithelium**.

The **Bowman's layer** contains collagen fibers that help maintain the cornea's shape. It becomes thinner with aging.

The **Dua layer** is a strong, thin, air-proof layer of collagen.

The corneal **stroma** is transparent but very fibrous and tough. It is the thickest layer of the cornea. It is a special tissue (mesenchymal) composed of organized layers of types I and V collagen with fibroblast cells between the layers. These cells secrete a matrix to maintain both strength and transparency.[4]

Cornea thins and bulges outward
Endothelium
Descemet's Membrane
Stroma
Dua's Layer Tears
Bowman's Layer Deteriorates
Epithelium

Descemet's membrane is comprised of type IV and VIII collagen fibers. If this layer is damaged (usually by Fuch's dystrophy, see Chapter 15-10), a corneal transplant may be required. If this membrane fails, then the cornea becomes increasingly cloudy.

Corneal **endothelium** is the "basement" of the cornea on which the other layers and membranes are seated.

The cornea is tightly populated with nerve fibers, making it the most sensitive of all tissues: 20-40 times more sensitive than the root of your tooth.[5]

Types of Keratoconus

The different types of keratoconus are determined where the area of bulging is occurring. A technique known as corneal topography measures the elevation of the cornea. Normal corneal topography displays a regular and uniform surface without strong declivities.

Forme frust. The irregularities are mild, and neither slit-lamp exams nor corneal topography will show abnormalities; but by considering the results of these techniques along with normality and biomechanical status, the doctor can screen for this early form of keratoconus. The patient does not notice symptoms, and the condition is correctable with glasses or soft contact lenses.[6] Forme frust can be seen with using an instrument called a typographer. This essential instrument needs to be used for diagnosis of any keratoconus. The Pentacam typographer can show both anterior and posterior corneal surface, and can even detect posterior keratoconus.[7]

Nipple cone. There is a small isolated area of bulging at, or near, the center of the cornea.[8] Vision can be significantly distorted however, because the area of bulging is very near the pupil.[9]

Oval cone. This is the most common form. With the development of the oval (or sagging) cone, comes more difficulty in fitting contact lenses, along with scarring and corneal hydrops (rupture of the cornea).[10] The bulging is more to the side of the cornea rather than the center, but it continues into the center where it distorts vision.[11] Special types of contact lenses can correct vision.

Globus cone. This condition has significant thinning and bulging, covering 75% of the cornea. It is the most severe form and is also uncommon. It typically requires a corneal transplant.[12]

Pathology

Keratoconus progresses through an increasingly severe breakdown of Bowman's layer, partially or fully due to tears in Dua's layer and Descemet's membrane. These tears result in fluid that, from inside the eye, permeates the cornea.

Dua's layer helps control the flow of fluid from the eye, contributing to the functioning of the sieve-like trabecular meshwork in the periphery of the cornea. A poor functioning trabecular meshwork can lead to glaucoma.[13] Tears developing in the Dua's layer contribute to fluid build-up. Additionally, in cases of severe bulging, a tear in the Descemet's membrane can also develop, allowing fluid from inside the eye to permeate the cornea. These changes result in severe haziness, which is often accompanied by blister like lesions of the superficial cornea, resulting in impairment of vision and discomfort.

Furthermore, researchers have found that the damaged cornea shows signs of oxidation damage to the Bowman's layer caused by free radicals. The cells create a common antigen-related protein (LAR) that is not found in normal corneas. It is felt that if cornea membrane cells are only partially damaged, they can heal, but over time corneal cells can die, causing vision loss.

Signs and Symptoms

Symptomatic abnormalities include deterioration of cornea cells, collagen fibers, membranes, mitochondria swelling, and protein synthesis abnormalities. These alterations take place both within the cells and in the spaces between cells. Signs and symptoms may also include:

- Visual distortion with and without eyeglasses
- Standard contact lenses not fitting well
- Multiple 'ghost' images (monocular polyopia)
- Glare, streaking, flaring from lights
- Light sensitivity
- Poor night vision with distortions worsened

One study showed that patients suffer increased symptoms of dry eye and increased tear instability when mucin content of their tears is reduced.[14]

Causes and Risk Factors

The specific cause of corneal deterioration is unknown, but it is thought to be due to a combination of genetic vulnerability, environmental, and hormonal factors.[15]

- **Oxidative damage** by free radicals is a risk factor.[16] [17]
- **Allergies** are found in approximately 40–50% of keratoconus patients. Allergies may be a contributing factor, perhaps resulting from constant eye rubbing due to itchiness.[18]
- **Magnesium deficiencies** are linked to keratoconus.[19] Alcoholism, pregnancy, diabetes, hyperthyroidism, diuretics, and stress can lead to a magnesium deficiency. Low magnesium can cause a thinning of elastic membranes such as the cornea.
- **Genetic disposition** is a risk factor (when family members have had this condition). Six genes are associated with keratoconus.[20]
- Those with **Downs syndrome** have a 6 times greater risk of keratoconus.[21] Five to 8% of Downs patients have keratoconus.
- **African Americans and Latinos** have a 50% greater rate as compared to the white population.[22]
- Those suffering from **sleep apnea** and **asthma** are at greater risk.[23]
- **Other vision conditions** associated with keratoconus include retinitis pigmentosa and Lebers disease.[24]
- **Other factors** such as chronic eye rubbing and wearing hard contact lenses are associated with keratoconus. [25]

Conventional Treatment

Keratoconus treatment depends on your symptoms. When your symptoms are mild, your vision can be corrected with eyeglasses. Later you may need to wear special hard contact lenses to help keep vision in proper focus.

- **Contact lenses** can be fitted by a specialist who fits contacts for keratoconus.[26] **Soft** lenses can be used in the early stages and help hide the effects of irregularities in the cornea. **Gas permeable** (GP) lenses can be used when soft lenses are not sufficient; they cover a larger area of the cornea needed to provide a good fit. **Piggyback** lenses can be used if the patient is intolerant of the GP lenses. A soft contact lens is first fitted for the patient, then, a gas permeable lens is made to fit over the soft lens. **Scleral contacts** are most often used for treatment compared to gas permeable. Their vaulting effect of the central bulge is important and more comfortable than GP lenses.
- **Surgery** may be recommended when the above options do not work. **Intacs** can be implanted to enhance the stability of the cornea and achieve a more stable fit. **Cross linking** is the only FDA-approved treatment for halting the progression of keratoconus. It involves administering riboflavin (vitamin B2) eye drops and UVA light in carefully selected parameters that strengthen the front layers of the cornea (clear covering of the eye) and avoid damage to the back part of the eye.[27]
- If keratoconus is severe, a **corneal transplant**, (penetrating keratoplasty),[28] is recommended by eye doctors in 25% of cases. With the discovery of the Dua layer, surgeons are more able to pinpoint location and so avoid damage to the corneal stroma. The femtosecond laser technology's accuracy additionally reduces surgical injury.

Complementary Approach

Though there is no cure for keratoconus, there are natural ways to help corneal health.

Nutrients

Very Important

A good whole-food and organic **antioxidant formula** for the eye is recommended, because free radical activity has been implicated in corneal conditions.

Helpful

MSM eyedrops (one drop in each eye, 2–3 times per day or as needed) have natural anti-inflammatory properties and help soften tissue to allow better transport of nutrients.[29]

Homeopathic eyedrops that contain ingredients such as euphrasia and calendula help support corneal health and healing.

Preservative-free lubricating eyedrops help keep the eyes moist, as for some, this condition can be related to dry eyes and poor production of the mucin layer of the tears.

Omega-3 fatty acids (2,000 IU–3,000 IU per day, with a meal) supports eye health and reduces overall inflammation. It also helps with natural tear production.

Whole-food organic multivitamins are recommended for overall eye health and general health.

Diet

Maintain an alkaline diet (see Chapter 7 for the Vision diet). It is possible that your diet can help to at least slow the rate of tissue deterioration. You should include lots of antioxidant-rich foods such as dark leafy greens and brightly colored vegetables and fruits.

Lifestyle

Eye exercises can help relax the eyes and improve circulation (see Chapter 10).

- Palming and massage the acupressure points around the eyes, daily.

Sunglasses with 100% UVA and UVB protection and wraparound sunglasses with a brimmed hat are recommended when you are outdoors. Amber colored lenses are the most effective in neutralizing blue light. Wear blue-light blocking glasses when working on the computer and reading from electronic devices.

Also See

Chapter 8, Nutrients

Chapter 10-4, Eye Exercises

Chapter 15-10, Fuch's Disease

Appendix 5, Recommended Products

1 Eye Health Central. Keratoconus. Retrieved Feb 8 2018 from https://www.contactlenses.co.uk/education/keratoconus.htm

2 Kennedy, R.H., Bourne, W.M., Dyer, J.A. (1986). A 48-year clinical and epidemiologic study of keratoconus. *Am J Ophthalmol*, 1986 Mar 15;101(3):267-73.

3 Ibid. Eye Health Central. Keratoconus.

4 GeneCardsSuite. Corneal Stroma. Retrieved Feb 8 2018 from https://discovery.lifemapsc.com/in-vivo-development/eye/corneal-stroma.

5 Wikipedia. Cornea. Retrieved Feb 8 2018 from https://en.wikipedia.org/wiki/Cornea.

6 Ueki, R., Maeda, N., Fuchihata, M., Koh, S., Kitaoka, T., et al. (2014). Differentiation of forme fruste keratoconus from normal cornea using parameters of corneal tomography, aberration, and biomechanics. *IVOS*, 55(13): 3705.

7 Ibid. Vazirani. (2013).

8 Perry, H.D., Buxton, J., Fine, B.S. (1980). Round and oval cones in keratoconus. *Ophthalmology*, Sep;87(9):905-9.

9 Precision Family Eyecare. Types and Severity of Keratoconus. Retrieved Feb 8 2018 from http://www.precisionfamilyeyecare.com/types-of-keratoconus/.

10 Ibid. Perry. (1980).

11 Ibid. Precision Family Eyecare.

12 Ibid. Precision Family Eyecare

13 H. S. Dua, L. A. Faraj, M. J. Branch, A. M. Yeung, M. S. Elalfy, D. G., et al. (2014). The collagen matrix of the human trabecular meshwork is an extension of the novel pre-Descemet's layer (Dua's layer). *Br J Ophthal*, May;98(5):691-7.

14 Carracedo, G., Recchioni, A., Alejandre-Alba, N., Martin-Gil, A., Crooke, A., et al. (2015). Signs and Symptoms of Dry Eye in Keratoconus Patients: A Pilot Study. *Curr Eye Res*, 40(11):1088-94.

15 Wikipedia. Keratoconus. Retrieved Feb 8 2018 from https://en.wikipedia.org/wiki/Keratoconus

16 Armal, E., Peris-Martinez, C., Menezon, J.L., Johnsen-Soriano, S., Romero, F.J. (2011). Oxidative stress in keratoconus? *Invest Ophthalmol Vis Sci*, Nov 4;52(12):8592-7.

[17] Toprak, I., Kucukatay, V., Yildirim, C., Kilic-Toprak, E., Lilic-Erkek, O. (2014). Increased systemic oxidative stress in patients with keratoconus. *Eye (Lond)*, Mar;28(3):285-9.

18 Sharma, N., Rao, K., Maharana, P.K., Vajpayee, R.B. (2013). Ocular allergy and keratoconus. *Indian J Ophthalmol*, Aug;61(8):407-409.

19 Thalasselis, A. (2005). The possible relationship between keratoconus and magnesium deficiency. *Ophthalmic Physiol Opt*, Jan;25(1):7-12.

20 Ibid. Wikipedia. Keratoconus.

21 Woodward, M.A., Blachley, T.S., Stein, J.D. (2016). The Association Between Sociodemographic Factors, Common Systemic Diseases, and Keratoconus: An Analysis of a Nationwide Health Care Claims Database. *Ophthalmology*, Mar;123(3):457-65.

22 Ibid. Woodward

23 Ibid. Woodward

24 Vazirani, J., Basu, S. (2013). Keratoconus: current perspectives. *Clin Ophthalmol*, 7:2019-2030.

25 Ibid. Vazirani. (2013).

26 Deepak Gupta. (2004). The Steep End: Contact Lenses Fit for Keratoconus Patients. Rev Optom, Nov;14(11).

27 Cornea Research Foundation of America. Corneal Crosslinking. Retrieved Dec 12 2017 from http://www.cornea.org/Learning-Center/Treatment-Options/Corneal-Crosslinking.aspx.

28 Cannella A. Use of contact lenses in the visual correction of keratoconus. Retrieved Feb 10 2018 from https://www.pofce.org/docs/UseOfContactLensesInTheVisualCorrectionOfKeratoconus.pdf.

[29] Kim, Y.H., Kim, D.H., Lim, H., Baek, D.Y., Shin, H.K., et al. (2009). The anti-inflammatory effects of methylsulfonylmethane on lipopolysaccharide-induced inflammatory responses in murine macrophages. *Biol Pharm Bull*, Apr;32(4):651-6.

15-14. LATTICE DEGENERATION

Lattice degeneration gets its name from the crisscrossing, fine, white lines on the surface of the retina, which an eye doctor can see during examination. It occurs in 7–8% of the general population,[1] most often in patients with myopia (nearsightedness) and over the age of 20. It also appears that neither race nor sex is a risk factor. Approximately 45% of those affected have lattice degeneration in both eyes.[2] Patients with lattice degeneration are typically symptom-free.

What is Lattice Degeneration?

Lattice degeneration occurs when the outside edge of the retina (away from the central macula), responsible for peripheral vision, shrinks, thins, develops holes, or otherwise atrophies. Clinical features may include retinal thinning, branching, whitish lines on the retinal surface, and even small holes in the retina. In addition, lesions can form.

Sometimes lesions cause holes or breaks in the retina, which are atrophic in nature. Atrophic means that they are due to the wasting away or diminishing of portions of the retina. Unlike retinal detachment, these breaks and holes are not associated with pulling between the vitreous and retina. They are usually an incidental finding of a dilated ophthalmologic examination that may occur within the lattice (present in 25–35%) and result from progressive retinal thinning.[3] The fine lines seen in lattice degeneration are present in roughly only 10% of all lesions. The other 90% are known as uncomplicated lattice degeneration, with lesions but no tears, holes, or breaks.

Lattice Anatomy

Lattice degeneration occurs between the retinal equator and the vitreous base.

The **retinal equator** is an imaginary boundary midway between the front and the back of the eyeball. The **vitreous base** lies toward the front of the eye where the retina, vitreous membrane, and pigmented layers firmly attach to each other. Lattice degeneration may show up as sharply demarcated areas of thinning. The thinning typically involves the vitreous and the inner layers of the retina. Sometimes thinning also

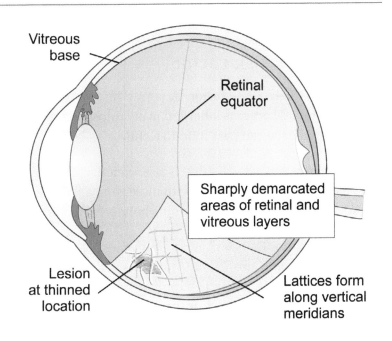

occurs in the retinal pigment layer and rarely along the fine blood capillaries. The lattices usually form along the vertical meridians and perpendicular to the retinal equator.[4]

Pathology of Lattice Degeneration

People with lattice degeneration are more likely to develop tears, breaks, or holes in their retina, which may progress further into retinal detachment (RD), though retinal detachment is extremely rare (1 in 10,000). Approximately one-third of all spontaneous retinal detachments are associated with lattice degeneration.[5] In fact, lattice degeneration is a key cause of retinal detachment in young individuals with myopia. Overall, the lifetime risk of RD in a patient with lattice is less than 1%.[6] In one long-term study, retinal detachments occurred in 1.08% of the lattice cases. Clinical or progressive subclinical RD occurred in 2% of eyes with atrophic holes. Subclinical RD was seen in 6.7% of 150 eyes with atrophic holes.[7]

The presence of uncomplicated lattice degeneration does not interfere with visual function and does not constitute a high risk for future development of retinal detachment.[8] However, it is a compromising factor in overall retinal and eye health, and it needs to be monitored by your eye doctor.

Lattice does not interfere with central vision, and early symptoms are rare. The symptoms go undetected unless a patient undergoes a thorough peripheral retinal exam. More acute development of lattice degeneration, however, can result in a reduction of peripheral vision (side vision) and a significant decrease in overall vision, due to fewer or obstructed peripheral-retinal capillaries.

Signs and Symptoms

Except for the possibility of flashing lights (photopsia), a sudden onset of eye floaters, or a partial loss of peripheral vision, symptoms are rare for this condition.

Causes and Risk Factors

Heredity is likely a risk factor. A family history[9] and certain variants in the COL4A4 gene may be risk factors.[10] Lattice is inherited in an autosomal dominant manner; the affected parent having one mutated gene can pass it on to a child.

Myopia increases risk. Lattice is associated with those who have high myopic eyes, and its prevalence may be associated with increasing axial length, reaching 15% in the longest eyes. This is especially true of axial eye lengths between 29–30mm and 25–27mm.[11]

Poor circulation. Lattice degeneration may also be linked to an insufficient blood supply or a blood supply with insufficient nutrients reaching the retina. From the front of the eye, to the retinal equator, the retina is supplied with nutrients by the posterior ciliary artery. When its circulation is degraded or obstructed, a "watershed zone" develops where there are fewer microcapillaries.[12]

Other conditions. Researchers have also found a high rate of lattice degeneration in patients with full-thickness macular holes.[13]

Conventional Treatment

No standardized treatment exists for lattice degeneration. Clinical studies of interventions to prevent retinal detachment in lattice patients have been evaluated, but reviewers found that controlled trials were lacking, and no conclusions could be drawn.[14] In certain cases where retinal holes or tears are present, a doctor might recommend laser photocoagulation or cryotherapy (extreme cold laser therapy), with the goal of sealing the area surrounding the tear. What mode is chosen depends on the location of the tear and whether there is fluid associated with it.

In most cases of lattice degeneration, no treatment is necessary. Treatment is recommended when a retinal tear occurs, if the other eye has had a retinal detachment, or if there is a strong family history of retinal detachments. Surgical intervention may be required if vitreous fluid is found to be leaking into the retina, which can complicate the lattice and atrophic holes, or if it is found in a patient who has suffered a previous retinal detachment (in an opposite eye).

Preventative or prophylactic treatment is indicated when the following occurs:

- Lattice degeneration complicated by **tractional tears** as the result of an acute, symptomatic, posterior vitreous detachment, which significantly increases the risk for a future retinal detachment
- The presence of **lattice lesions** in the eye of patients who have sustained retinal detachment in the other eye

Complementary Approach

Since poor circulation and nutrient deficiency have been identified as possible contributing causes for lattice degeneration, there may be natural ways to improve these situations, thereby boosting retinal health. Even in the case where lattice degeneration is inherited, the body is still trying to maintain healthy vision. So targeted supplements (antioxidants, in particular) and a healthy lifestyle can help to stop or slow down the progression of the disease and support healthy vision.

Nutrients

See Appendix 5 for products that contain combinations of the following nutrients.

Essential

Lutein. 6mg–20mg per day. This carotenoid is well researched for retinal support and essential for supporting the retinal pigment.[15] Another study showed that taking lutein along with zeaxanthin and astaxanthin resulted in significant improvement in visual acuity (vision sharpness).[16]

Zeaxanthin. 2mg–12mg per day. Along with lutein, zeaxanthin is a potent antioxidant found in the retina. It maintains the retina's health.[17]

Astaxanthin. 6mg–12mg per day. Astaxanthin is effective in protecting against damage from light due to its antioxidant effect.[18]

Omega-3 fatty acids. 2,000mg–3,000mg per day. Omega-3 fatty acids, *along with* **lutein** *and* **zeaxanthin**, helps preserve vision.

Vitamin D3. 2,000 IU–5,000 IU per day. Lower levels of vitamin D are associated with retinal microvascular damage, suggesting that the link with cardiovascular risk may partly run through changes in the microvasculature.[19]

Ginkgo biloba, 120mg per day, *and/or* **vinpocetine**, 10mg–30mg per day. Ginkgo contains many different flavonoids, including polyphenolic flavonoids, which have been proven to exert antioxidative properties by stabilizing free radicals.[20] Ginkgo improves overall circulation.[21]

Bilberry. 120mg–180mg per day. Bilberry is neuroprotective and has been shown to improve microcirculation.[22] [23] [24] [25] It decreases vascular permeability and capillary fragility.

Very important

Taurine. 500mg–750mg per day. Deficiency of taurine, an amino acid, has been shown to lead to retinal degeneration; taurine has been used as a supplement, with some success, to prevent, treat, and stabilize retinal changes.[26] [27] [28] [29]

Resveratrol, 125mg–175mg per day (trans-resveratrol is a well absorbed form), **grapeseed extract** (300mg per day), and **pycnogenol** (100mg–200mg per day). These antioxidants have similar benefits of helping strengthen blood vessels, reducing inflammation, supporting healthy circulation, modulating inflammatory response, and neutralizing free radicals.[30]

Multivitamin. Take a high-quality, whole-food, organic multivitamin

Helpful

Green tea. 500mg–750mg per day. Studies have shown that green tea has excellent capacity to scavenge free radicals such as the superoxide, hydroxyl, and peroxyl radicals.[31] [32] [33] [34]

Saffron. 20mg per day. Saffron generally supports the health of the retina, as evidenced in studies on macular degeneration, by protecting photoreceptor cells from damage and supporting healthy circulation to the retina. Although lattice does not involve the macula, the general protection is valuable.[35] [36] [37] [38]

Lycopene. 3mg per day. Studies show that the antioxidant properties of lycopene make it particularly effective in maintaining healthy LDL oxidation and protecting against free radical activity on the arterial wall.[39] This is of interest because one possible cause of lattice is damage to the blood supply to the retina.

Diet

Follow the same recommendations as for macular degeneration.

Very important

Favor leafy greens and antioxidants, reduce refined sugars, drink lots of water, and don't smoke.

Important

Reduce fats (especially trans-fats), dairy, and refined carbohydrates.

Juicing. Juice daily, and use organic produce, if possible. Our recipe to support retinal health is a combination of the following:

- Spinach, wheatgrass, celery, parsley, leeks, cabbage, carrots, beets, ginger, garlic, apples, grapes, raspberries, and lemon
- Try using at least 4–6 of the nutrients recommended, plus your favorite fruits and vegetables. Avoid using too many carrots or beets or too much fruit, because of their high, natural, sugar content.
- Try to use room temperature vegetables and fruit.
- Do not add ice or very cold liquids since cold foods and liquids will eventually extinguish the stomach's digestive fire.
- Do not juice as often during the cooler months of the year, and instead, switch to vegetable soups or stews.

Lifestyle

The following are additional measures to prevent or treat lattice degeneration:

Eyedrops. No specific eyedrops are recommended for this condition.

Eye exercises. See Eye Exercises, Chapter 10-4. Include "palming" and "figure eights" in your daily routine.

Exercise. Daily exercise, such as a brisk walk, is strongly recommended for vision and general health.

Microcurrent stimulation therapy (MCS). Performed daily at home, this therapy helps support healthy circulation to the retina. It also increases circulation and energy production (ATP) within the retinal cells, which stimulates the overall function of the retina and helps the retina eliminate waste. The recommended use (with an MCS 100ile unit) is five minutes, two to four times a day (for a total of 10–20 minutes daily), or one to two double five-minute sessions (doing a five-minute session and then repeating it) two times per day. See Chapter 10-3 for more information.

> **Note**. Usage may vary depending on the type of microcurrent unit you use, so check with your healthcare practitioner to get proper instructions before using. Also, if you have a

history of retinal bleeding, check first with your eye doctor. Contraindications include having a pacemaker or a history of epilepsy.

Wear sunglasses. To protect your eyes from UV radiation and blue light, amber or brown wrap-around glasses are best.

Other Modalities

Chinese Medicine

In Chinese medicine, the Liver "opens to the eyes" and is the primary meridian for supporting overall flow of energy and circulation through the eyes. The Kidney meridian nourishes the blood to the eyes, and the Spleen meridian also nourishes the blood while helping to keep fluids from leaking from blood vessels. Other meridians that can affect eye health may also be out-of-balance; an evaluation by an acupuncturist can best determine where the out-of-balances are and offer the optimal treatment strategy.

Gui pi tang (restore the Spleen decoction) increases qi, tonifies blood, strengthens the Spleen, nourishes the Heart, and helps the Spleen control the blood.

Ming mu di huang wan (rehmannia pills "to brighten the eyes") addresses the following patterns: Liver blood deficiency, Kidney yin deficiency, and Liver yin deficiency

Xiao yao san is a classic Liver tonic used in Chinese medicine.

Zhu jing wan (preserve vistas pill) tonifies and nourishes the Liver and Kidneys, enriches the yin, and improves vision.

Also See

---

[1] Adrean, S.D., Eliott, D. (2005). Prophylaxis for Retinal Detachment. Retrieved from https://www.reviewofophthalmology.com/article/prophylaxis-for-retinal-detachment

[2] Foos, R.Y., Simons, K.B. (1984). Vitreous in lattice degeneration of retina. *Ophthalmology*, 91:452-7.

[3] Byer, N.E. (1989). *Long*-term natural history of lattice degeneration of the retina. *Ophthalmology*, 96:1396-401.

[4] Semes, L.P. (1992). Lattice degeneration of the retina and retinal detachment. *Optom Clin*, 2(3):71-91.

[5] Silva, R.A., Blumenkrantz, M.S. (2013). Prophylaxis for Retinal Detachments. Retrieved from http://www.aao.org/munnerlyn-laser-surgery-center/prophylaxis-retinal-detachments.

[6] Ibid. Byer.

[7] Ibid. Byer.

[8] Pandya, H.K. (2017). Lattice Degeneration. Retrieved from http://emedicine.medscape.com/ article/1223956.

[9] Edward, A.O., Robertson, J.E. Jr. (2001). Hereditary vitreoretinal degenerations. *Retina*, 3rd ed. St. Louis. Mosby; 482-98.

[10] Meguro, A., Ideta, H., Ota, M., Ito, N., Ideta, R., et al. (2012). Common variants in the COL4A4 gene confer susceptibility to lattice degeneration of the retina. *PLoS One*, 7(6):e39300.

[11] Sanchez, M., Pallares, R.M. (2001). Myopia: frequency of lattice degeneration and axial length. *Arch Soc Esp Oftalmol*, May; 76(5):291-6.

[12] Takahashi, K., Muraoka, K., Kishi, S., Shimizu, K. (1996). Watershed zone in the human peripheral choroid. *Ophthalmology*, Feb;103(2):336-42.

[13] Zhang, J., Li, Y., Zhao, X., Cai, Y., Yu, X., Lu, L. (2015). Relationship between full-thickness macular hole and retinal break/lattice degeneration. *Eye Sci*, 30(4):156-9.

[14] Wilkinson, C.P. (2014). Interventions for asymptomatic retinal breaks and lattice degeneration for preventing retinal detachment. *Cochrane Database Syst Rev*, Sep 5;(9):CD003170

[15] Landrum, J.T., Bone, R.A., Kilburn, M.D., Moore, L.L., et al. (1997). A one year study of the macular pigment: the lutein supplement. *Exp Eye Res*, Jul;65(1):57-62

[16] Piermarocchi, S., Saviano, S., Parisi V, Tedeschi, M., Panozzo, G., et al. (2012.) Carotenoids in age-related maculopathy Italian study, *Eur J Ophthalmol*, Mar-Apr:22(2):216-25.

[17] National Eye Institute. (2013) NIH study provides clarity on supplements for protection against blinding eye disease. Retrieved Feb 18 2018 from https://nei.nih.gov/news/pressreleases/ 050513

[18] Otsuka, T., Shimazawa, M., Nakanishi, T., Ohno, Y., Inoue, Y., et al. (2013). Protective effects of a dietary carotenoid, astaxanthin, against light-induced retinal damage, *J Pharmacol Sci*, 123(3):209-18

[19] Mutlu, U., Ikram, M.A., Hofman, A., de Jong, P.T., Uiterlinden, A.G., et al. (2016). Vitamin D and retinal microvascular damage: The Rotterdam Study. *Medicine (Baltimore)*, Dec; 95(49): e5477.

[20] Ou, H.C., Lee, W.J., Lee, I.T., Chiu, T.H., Tsai, K.L., et al. (2009). Ginkgo biloba extract attenuates oxLDL-induced oxidative functional damages in endothelial cells. *J Appl Physiol*, 106:1674–85.

[21] Chung, H.S., Harris, A., Kristinsson, J.K., Ciulla, T.A., Kagemann, C., et al. (1999). Ginkgo biloba extract increases ocular blood flow velocity. *J Ocul Pharmacol Ther*, 15:233–40.

[22] Matsunaga, N., Imai, S., Inokuchi, Y., Shimazawa, M., Yokota, S., et al. (2009). Bilberry and its main constituents have neuroprotective effects against retinal neuronal damage in vitro and in vivo. *Mol Nutr Food Res*, Jul;53(7):869-77.

23 Zhu, Y., Xia, M., Yang, Y., Liu F., Li, Z. et al. (2011). Purified anthocyanin supplementation improves endothelial function via NO-cGMP activation in hypercholesterolemic individuals. *Clin Chem*, Nov;57(11):1524-33.

24 Cohen-Boulakia, F., Valensi, P.E., Boulahdour, H., Lestrade, R., Dufour-Lamartinie, J.R., et al. (2000). In vivo sequential study of skeletal muscle capillary permeability in diabetic rats: effect of anthocyanosides. *Metabolism*, Jul;49(7):880-5.

25 Yao, Y., Vieira, A., (2007). Protective activities of Vaccinium antioxidants with potential relevance to mitochondrial dysfunction and neurotoxicity. *NeuroToxicology*, 28 (2007) 93–100

26 Birdsall, T.C. (1998). Therapeutic applications of taurine. *Altern Med Rev*, Apr;3(2):128-36.

27 Shpak, N.I., Naritsyna, N.I., Konovalova, N.V. (1989). Taufon and emoksipin in the combined treatment of sclerotic macular dystrophy. *Oftalmol Zh*, 1989;(8):463-5

28 Lombardini, J.B. (1991). Taurine: retinal function. *Brain Res Rev*, May-Aug;16(2):151-69

29 Imaki, H., Maretz, R., Wisniewski, H., Neuringer, M., Sturman, J. (1987). Retinal degeneration in 3-month rhesus monkey infants fed a taurine-free human infant formula. *J Neurosci Res*, 18(4):602-14

30 Wang, Z. Wang S., Yang, S., Yin, T., Zhang, Y., et al. (2017). Tissue Distribution of trans-Resveratrol and Its Metabolites after Oral Administration in Human Eyes, *J Ophthalmol*, Mar. 2017:4052094.

31 Chen, L., Yang, X., Jiao, H., Zhao, B. (2003). Tea catechins protect against lead-induced ROS formation, mitochondrial dysfunction, and calcium dysregulation in PC12 cells. *Chem Res Toxicol*, Sep;16(9):1155-61.

32 Kondo, K., Kurihara, M., Miyata, N., Suzuki, T., Toyoda, M. (1999) Mechanistic studies of catechins as antioxidants against radical oxidation. *Arch Biochem Biophys*, Feb 1;362(1):79-86..

33 Sinha, D., Roy, S., Roy, M. (2010). Antioxidant potential of tea reduces arsenite induced oxidative stress in Swiss albino mice. *Food Chem Toxicol*, Apr;48(4):1032-9.

34 Sun, Y., Hung, W.C., Chen, F.Y., Lee, C.C., Huang, H.W. (2009). Interaction of tea catechin (-)-epigallocatechin gallate with lipid biolayers. *Biophys J,* Feb;96(3):1026-35

35 Falsini, B., Piccardi, M., Minnella, A., Savastano, C., Capoluongo, E., et al. (2010). Influence of saffron supplementation on retinal flicker sensitivity in early age-related macular degeneration. *Invest Opththalmol Vis Sci,* Dec;51(12):6118-24.

36 Marangoni, D., Falsini, B., Piccardi, M., Ambrosio, L., Minnella, A.M., et al. (2013). Functional effect of Saffron supplementation and risk genotypes in early age-related macular degeneration: a preliminary report. *J Transl Med,* Sep;11:228.

[37] Bisti, S., Maccarone, R., Falsini, B. (2014). Saffron and retina: neuroprotection and pharmacokenetics. *Vis Neurosci,* Sep;31(4-5):355-61.

38 Corso, L., Cavallero, A., Baroni, D., Garbati, P., Prestipino, G., et al. (2016). Saffron reduces ATP-induced retinal cytotoxicity by targeting P2X7 receptors. *Purinergic Signal,* Mar;12(1):161-74.

[39] Erdman, J.W., Ford, N.A., Lindshield, B.L. (2009). Are the health attributes of lycopene related to its antioxidant function? *Arch BiochemBiophys,* Mar 15;483(2):229-35..

15-15. LEBER HEREDITARY OPTIC NEUROPATHY

Leber hereditary optic neuropathy (LHON), Leber optic atrophy, is a genetic condition in which retinal nerve cell mitochondria are mutated. These cell energy producers are essential and without them cell death occurs in the retinal nerves.[1] The condition typically arises during one's teens or twenties. Rarely, Leber's may develop in early childhood when it is known as Leber's congenital amaurosis. Men are affected more than women.

Leber's affects about 1 in 50,000 people worldwide. About 1 in 8,500 carry a mutated gene.[2] LHON's prevalence is similar to other inherited neurological disorders.[3] Every year, about 100 Americans lose their central vision and about 4,000 are vision impaired due to LHON. Not all who carry the LHON genetic mutation experience vision problems. More than 50% of men and 85% of women carry the mutation but do not experience vision loss. They do, however, remain at risk, and lifestyle choices that support the health of the mitochondria become very important.

Anatomy of Leber's

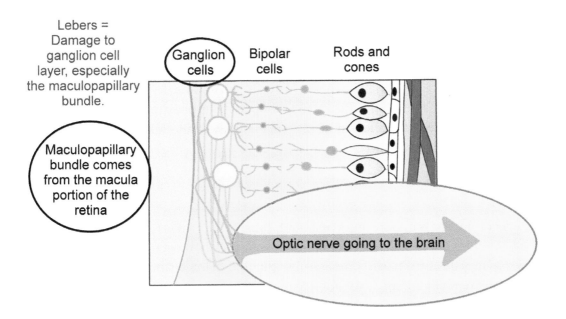

The normal functioning optic nerve requires healthy functioning mitochondria—the energy producers of nerve cells and virtually all cells. The optic disc (the point on the retina where the optic nerve enters) contains high concentrations of mitochondria, which suggests that the presence of properly functioning mitochondria is essential. Leber's involves damage to mitochondria in the ganglion cells, especially those cells that are part of the maculopapillary bundle, which comes from the macula.

Mitochondria are found only in the part of the optic nerve that is not protected by the myelin sheath. Researchers suspect that oxidative stress and/or defective synthesis of ATP may be at the root of mitochondria damage.[4] The enzyme, ATP synthase, creates energy storage molecules within the cell.[5] Nerve cells have unique needs, and the fact that some parts of the nerve axons contain mitochondria while others do not, may be a key to understanding LHON. [6]

The body normally initiates cell death as part of its very specific evolution. The process of programmed cell death is known as apoptosis. Mitochondria play an important part in regulation of apoptosis. Researchers have found some clues as to the connection between LHON and apoptosis. The optic nerve deteriorates, structurally and biochemically, in a manner consistent with apoptosis. Finally, mitochondrial apoptosis appears to take place in the presence of heightened levels of oxidative stress.[7] It is thought that glutamate transport is impaired, contributing to oxidative stress, which in turn leads to retinal ganglion cell death.[8]

Leber's and Genetics

Normal cells in our body contain 23 pairs of chromosomes; each cell contains 46. Each chromosome contains hundreds of thousands of genes, which are short segments of DNA that carry the genetic blueprint of our bodies. Each cell also contains mitochondria, which are the energy producers of the body, and without them, we could not survive. These mitochondria *also* carry genes, but only from the mother. If a mother carries a mutated mitochondria gene, which is linked to LHON, that mutation is passed to all of her children.[9]

The vast majority of LHON cases are associated with one of three primary mitochondrial DNA mutations; these are MT-ND4/G11778A, MT-ND1/G3460A4, and MT-ND6/T14484C. The most common is the G11778A mutation. This gene accounts for approximately 50–70% of all LHON cases.[10] There are some twenty different genes currently known to take part in the development of LHON. Three particular mutations account for 85–90% of all cases of LHON. [11]

Pathology

Typically, Leber's develops in only one eye at first, causing blurriness and cloudiness. During this acute phase, if it does not initially begin in both eyes, typically it occurs in the second eye within a few weeks or month. It primarily damages central and color vision that we need for detailed work like reading or recognizing faces. For a few patients, central vision gradually improves, but usually the deterioration of vision is marked and lasting. Recovery depends upon which gene is mutated. Improvement can also yield small islands of normal vision.

Some patients may have Leber's, combined with other systemic or neurological problems. There may be electrical signaling abnormalities controlling the heartbeat, body tremors, and movement disorders (dystonia). Patients may also experience numbness, muscle weakness, and other symptoms similar to multiple sclerosis. Inflammation of the cerebellum may develop, which impacts gait and muscle coordination.[12]

In the lab, researchers are noting that in some LHON models the ability of some nutrients, such as glutathione, to protect ganglion cells from cell death, may explain why the mutation affects ganglion cells, even though other neurons may also carry the mutation but are not affected. [13]

Signs and Symptoms

- At first, one eye typically and suddenly loses central vision.
- Cloudiness and blurriness are experienced.
- About a month or two later, the other eye also becomes affected.

There are many variations of the pattern.

Causes and Risk Factors

Although young men are most often affected, Leber's may develop at any age in women or men. There may be some protective factor in women's X chromosomes, since women develop the condition more rarely. The female hormones, progesterone and estrogen, are currently suspected to play a role in protecting female carriers.[14]

Many LHON specialists suggest that people who have developed LHON, or are carrying a LHON mutation, should avoid environmental factors that could create additional stress on the mitochondria. These factors include:[15]

- Tobacco smoke
- Alcohol
- Some antibiotics and medications that create additional stress on the body including tetracycline, minocycline, streptomycin, erythromycin, chloramphenicol, ethambutol, and linezolid
- Other drugs causing stress, including drugs treating cancer, viruses, AIDS, malaria, heart arrhythmia, high blood pressure, and epilepsy.
- Possibly cyanogens
  - Cyanogens are chemical compounds that are found in some plant foods, such as peas, beans, and other legumes, almonds and other nuts, and apricots. They serve as a chemical defense against pest and competitive herbivores such as insects.[16] The chemical is usually concentrated in the seeds, kernels, or wilted leaves of the plant, but it is also easily overcome by careful pre-ingestion food processing, such as soaking, sprouting, fermenting, cooking, pulverizing, and drying,[17] or some combination thereof. Cigarette smoke also contains quantities of these substances.
- Fumes from paints, varnishes, hair dyes, and especially fat-soluble chemicals (liquids and vapors) that have benzene rings in their chemical structure, such as toluene
  - The acute and chronic effects of exposure to benzene can involve the central nervous system.[18]
- Stress-related chemicals that are naturally produced and released by the body, such as adrenaline, catecholamines, etc., as well as testosterone, and oxidizing chemicals.

o Oxidation creates free radicals in the body that have to be neutralized by antioxidants. Otherwise, the free radicals not neutralized damage healthy cells and ultimately contribute to, or cause, onset of disease that include chronic and degenerative illness such as cancer, autoimmune disorders, aging, cataracts, rheumatoid arthritis, cardiovascular and neurodegenerative diseases.[19]

- Factors that deplete the number of functional mitochondria and ATP production include:[20]

    o Trans fats and hydrogenated fats that can destroy cell membranes
    o Poorly functioning thyroid that reduces the number of mitochondria in cells
    o Toxins including heavy metals such as lead, mercury, and cadmium
    o Dental infections in teeth and jaw bones

Conventional Treatment

Currently there are no approved conventional treatments or cures for LHON.

Clinical trials of idebenone, a synthetic molecule that performs the same function in the mitochondria as Coenzyme Q10, show modest effectiveness in slowing progression of Leber's cases. [21] [22] Similar drugs with an antioxidant role, such as EPI-743 and Bendavia similarly help to reduce oxidative stress, slowing progression.[23]

There has been inconsistent anecdotal evidence for ubiquinone, a coenzyme Q10-like derivative that was shown to mildly alter progress of the disease, and in some cases, and for some mutations, cause spontaneous recovery.[24] [25] It is thought that inadequate amounts of CoQ10 reaching the mitochondria were the cause for early experimental treatment failures.

Complementary Approach

Researchers report that LHON carriers are at risk for LHON, but might not develop the condition due to incomplete penetrance. This means that the mutation is "necessary but not sufficient" for LHON to develop. Therefore supporting mitochondrial integrity in LHON-impacted families with LHON carriers may be helpful in preventing onset. "… unaffected mutation carriers have a significantly higher mitochondrial DNA copy number and mitochondrial mass compared with their affected relatives and control individuals."[26]

Copy number refers to the number of copies of a particular gene in a person's genotype. Efficient mitochondrial biogenesis, the ability of mitochondria to grow and divide, then, is a possible key to lowering the risk of developing Leber's.[27]

Therefore, we approach LHON from two sides. First, because copy number and mitochondrial mass are factors, we support neuronal health and mitochondria biogenesis. Second, we address environmental factors, such as smoking and excessive alcohol consumption, which may increase the risk of developing Leber's for people who carry the gene mutation. Living a healthy lifestyle, therefore, is highly recommended for those with Leber's, or at risk for developing it. Free radical activity may also be a contributing factor. Eating a healthy diet, exercising regularly, and taking targeted antioxidants for eye health may slow down the progression of the disease and promote healthy vision.

In addition, research suggests that the sense of smell, olfaction, and vision interact at an early, possibly involuntary stage, of perception.[28] Olfactory dysfunction is often linked to neurodegeneration.[29]

Our goal is to help people learn how to preserve healthy vision and introduce natural ways to boost circulation and energy production in the eyes. This supports nourishment of the optic nerve and related mitochondria and other parts of the eye, through the targeted delivery of antioxidants and other nutrients.

Nutrients

Antioxidants have been described as key factors in providing stability to the nerve cells and decreasing the likelihood of oxidative damage caused by free radicals.

Essential

Carnosine. 500mg-1,000mg per day. Carnosine has the ability to react with free radicals that attack protein, forming "protein-carbonyl-carnosine adducts;"[30] this ability, even more than its antioxidant capacity is what makes it effective in protecting nerve cells against premature death.[31] Carnosine also acts as an anti-glycating agent[32] and metal chelating agent. Through these means, carnosine is valuable in reducing DNA damage from environmental causes.[33] Oxidation of lipids produces malondialdehyde (MDA), which is a biomarker for oxidative stress, and its levels markedly increase in many neurological diseases. Carnosine provides excellent protection against MDA-caused cell damage, perhaps far more effectively than other antioxidants.[34] Carnosine's anti-glycating capacity is also important because excessive destructive sugar metabolism (catabolism) results in high levels of a biochemical (methyglyoxal) that is linked to mitochondria dysfunction.[35]

Taurine. 750mg–1,000 mg per day. Taurine protects against retinal ganglion cell degeneration[36] [37] and protects mitochondria from oxidative damage according to a review of the research; among other benefits. It plays an essential role in brain development in the cerebellum, pyramidal cells, and visual cortex.[38] In an animal model, taurine deficiency is linked to mitochondrial birth defects.[39]

D-Ribose. 1–5 grams per day. D-ribose is found in cells and particularly in the mitochondria where it is essential for energy production. It improves cellular processes when there is mitochondria dysfunction. When ATP production is reduced, mitochondrial function declines. D-ribose is associated with ATP production support.[40]

Glutathione. 500mg–900mg if taken in capsule or pill form. The sublingual form has 5–10 times greater absorption, so the dosage will be smaller. Follow label instructions. In experimental models use of external application of glutathione rescues retinal ganglion cells from cell death.[41]

Glutathione in mitochondria is the main line of their defense against oxidative damage, toxic lipid peroxides, mitochondria dysfunction, and cell death.[42]

Pyrroloquinoline quinone (PQQ). 20mg per day. PQQ is an enzyme cofactor in bacteria that behaves like a powerful antioxidant[43] that defends against decay of mitochondria, with the ability to resist oxidation exposure 5,000 times as much as vitamin C. It influences the cell signaling pathways particular to new mitochondria formation.[44] The body does not produce it on its own; it must be taken as a supplement.

Vitamin C (buffered and ascorbated). 2000mg daily. Vitamin C is important to protect mitochondrial respiration and functioning, helps to prevent formation of mitochondrial free radicals, and lessens mitochondrial aging.[45]

Vitamin B complex. As with vitamin C, the B complex protects mitochondrial respiration and energy production, helps to prevent formation of mitochondrial oxidants, and slows mitochondrial aging.[46]

Zinc. 40mg with 2mg–3mg copper, daily. Zinc enhances, mitochondrial biogenesis, with more stable membrane potential and elevated ATP production,[47] and it also does so in a toxic environment.[48]

Magnesium. 500mg, daily. Mitochondria both collect and release magnesium, acting in a storage capacity. Disruption of magnesium balance has a strong effect on mitochondrial functions that determine cell survival.[49]

Acetyl-l-carnitine. 500mg–800mg. Daily acetyl-l-carnitine helps protect neurons,[50] [51] and maintains overall good health by facilitating the transfer of long-chain fatty acids across the mitochondrial membrane for cellular energy production.[52]

Omega-3 fatty acids. 2,000mg–3,000mg per day. DHA from omega-3 fatty acids accounts for approximately 50–60% of the total fatty acid content within the outer segments of photoreceptor rods and tends to be very deficient in today's diet.[53] [54] It is critical for maintaining retinal health.[55]

Saffron. 20mg per day. Studies show that saffron helps protect photoreceptor cells from damage as well as supporting healthy circulation in the retina.[56] [57]

Vitamin D3. 2,000 IU–5,000 IU per day. Studies investigating the link between vitamin D and indices of microvascular disease have shown that vitamin D deficiency is associated with poor coronary microcirculation.[58]

Astaxanthin. 6mg–12mg per day. Astaxanthin is also unique among the antioxidants in that it spans both layers of the cell membrane, allowing it to trap free radicals, outside and inside the cell. Astaxanthin's powerful antioxidant benefits help prevent retinal damage[59] and mitochondria health.[60] [61] [62] [63] [64]

Ginkgo biloba. 120mg per day. Ginkgo biloba improves microcapillary circulation in the eye and slows deterioration of the macula through its antioxidant effects.[65] [66] Studies have shown that it improves overall circulation,[67] [68] stabilizes capillaries, and makes capillaries less fragile.[69] [70] [71]

Bilberry. 180mg–240mg per day. Bilberry extracts have antioxidative properties that not only are neuroprotective but also help suppress photooxidative processes (the breakdown of oxygen molecules that create an unstable environment for healthy cells). Bilberry extracts have also been shown to improve small capillaries. Photooxidation is accelerated by exposure to sunlight. The anthocyanoside content of bilberry may be especially beneficial for nighttime visual acuity.[72] [73] [74] [75] [76] [77] [78] [79] [80]

CoQ10. 200mg per day (ubiquinol form is best absorbed). CoQ10 also has powerful antioxidant properties, protecting important proteins and mitochondrial DNA6 from oxidative damage.[81] CoQ10 is used for cell growth and maintenance and functions as an antioxidant, protecting the body from damage caused by harmful molecules. Cofactors that enable improved use of CoQ10 in the body include:

- Shilajit (which is a rich brown organic material that forms in the thin layer of earth where living roots and microorganisms interact with the rocky core of the planet itself). Shiljit contains fulvic acid that augments CoQ10 with the following: speeding up and facilitating essential electron flow in mitochondria, helping protect mitochondria against oxidative damage, and reducing dangerous lipid peroxidation.[82]
- L-carnitine (500mg per day)
- Alpha-lipoic acid (300mg per day)

CoQ10 is of particular interest because it not only supports the mitochondrial respiratory chain but also acts as a powerful antioxidant in mitochondrial membranes.

 Other compounds such as genistein, hydroxy-tyrosol, and quercetin have been found to improve respiratory control in the mitochondria and stimulate mitochondrial biogenesis. They may be helpful in diseases that involve defective mitochondrial function such as Leber's.[83]

Microcurrent stimulation (MCS). Also see Chapter 10-3 on microcurrent stimulation. Research suggests that daily MCS to support retinal and photoreceptor health by supporting healthy retinal circulation, increasing energy (ATP—the energy produced by mitochondria) within the retinal cells, helping the retina eliminate waste.[84] [85] [86] [87] [88] [89] Daily sessions at home are recommended.

Very Important

Three antioxidants (Take one or all three):

- **Trans-resveratrol**. 50mg–175mg per day. Studies indicate that resveratrol may be the most effective compound for maintaining optimal health and promoting longevity. One study shows that resveratrol may be effective in the microcirculation of the eye.[90]

- **Grapeseed extract**, 300mg per day, *or* **pycnogenol**, 100mg–200mg per day. These antioxidants provide a similar benefit of strengthening blood vessels and reducing inflammation. They have also been found to support healthy circulation and neutralize free radicals.

A high-quality, whole-food, organic multivitamin. Follow dosage directions on the bottle.

Helpful

Green tea extract. 500mg–750mg per day. Green teas and their extracts are potentially neuroprotective in the photoreceptor outer segments and retinal pigment epithelium (RPE).[91]

Diet

Follow the Vision diet described in Chapter 7.

Juicing. Juice daily and use organic produce, if possible. Our recipe, designed to help support overall retinal health, is a combination of the following:

- Ginger, garlic, parsley, leeks, beets, cabbage, carrots, spinach, celery, apples, grapes, raspberries, lemon, and wheatgrass.
- Feel free to add your favorite fruits and vegetables. Avoid using too much fruit or too many carrots or beets because of their high natural sugar content.
- Try to use room temperature vegetables and fruit.
- Do not add ice or very cold liquids since cold foods and liquids will eventually extinguish the stomach's digestive fire.
- Do not juice as often during the cooler months of the year, and instead, switch to vegetable soups or stews.

Lifestyle

Eye exercises. Also see recommended eye exercises in Chapter 10.
- Palming
- Near and far
- Hot dog

Infrared light exposure, for example infrared sauna or low-level light therapy, helps boost mitochondrial energy (ATP) production.[92]

Other exercises. Supporting healthy circulation and movement of the energy through general exercise helps the body maintain healthy vision. Even in cases where there are genetic reasons for vision loss, exercise may help slow down the progression of vision loss. Activities such as speed walking, swimming, gym workouts, and aerobics, at least 4-5 days a week, are helpful for enhancing circulation. Circulation supports the free flow of energy and blood in the body, enabling the better delivery of nutrients to the eyes and to the rest of the body, and it improves elimination of toxins.

Several studies using magnetic resonance spectroscope testing have found that supervised aerobic activity can improve exercise capacity, reduce lactate, and improve ATP recovery kinetics.[93] In more studies, aerobic training was found to efficiently improve oxidative capacity in patients with mitochondrial myopathy, and regular aerobic exercise may be recommended for them.[94]

Manage stress. Additionally, yoga, meditation, Tai chi, and other practices are helpful for reducing stress and regulating the central nervous system, which in turn, helps protect mitochondria.

Other Modalities

Chinese Medicine:

The Liver meridian supports the healthy flow of blood and energy throughout the body and to the eyes, while the Spleen and Kidney meridians support blood production and eye nourishment. Your acupuncturist or herbalist is best able to determine the herbal formulas that would be most relevant to supporting your eyes regarding Leber's; but here are some general eye formula suggestions.

Chinese Medicine Patent Formulas:

Preserve vistas pill (zhu jing wan) tonifies and nourishes the Liver and Kidneys, enriches the yin, and improves vision.

Ming mu di huang wan (rehmannia pills to "brighten the eyes") addresses the following patterns: Liver blood deficiency, Kidney yin deficiency, and Liver yin deficiency.

Regular acupuncture treatments may also be helpful to stimulate energy and blood flow in the eyes. One Chinese study, conducted in 2004, showed positive benefit of acupuncture for Leber's disease.[95]

On the Horizon

A study published in 2012 reported that researchers have been screening drugs that may improve ATP production defects caused by Leber's. Two possibilities, papaverine or zolpidem, appear to require TSPO (mitochondrial translocator protein) mechanisms or address cAMP (phosphodiesterases degrade cyclic AMP) functioning in order to act on the LHON defect.[96]

In 2008, a team of scientists, funded by the National Eye Institute, reported major progress in the treatment of Leber's, using gene therapy. In 2013 however, the team reported that although treatment improved eyesight, cells in the eye that are crucial for vision continued to diminish in number. The new finding suggested the importance of continued research, and that successful treatment protocols may require a combination therapy that both restores vision and protects the eye's cells.[97]

A study with idebenone in patients with chronic-vision loss due to Leber's hereditary optic neuropathy was last updated in 2014. This ongoing study's objective is to determine whether administration of idebenone can shorten the time of visual acuity improvement in patients with chronic vision loss due to LHON. Current results of this study suggest that the technique is safe, and in some cases, can restore night vision.[98]

Currently studied is the gene transfer of a nuclear version of mitochondria ND4 to produce a functioning protein to replace the mutated one.[99]

Also See

Chapter 7, Vision Diet

Chapter 8, Nutrients

Chapter 10-4, Eye Exercises

---

1 Genetics Home Reference. Leber hereditary optic neuropathy. Retrieved Feb 9 2018 from https://ghr.nlm.nih.gov/condition/leber-hereditary-optic-neuropathy.

2 Man, P.Y.W., Griffiths, P.G., Brown, D.T., Howell, N., Turnbill, D.M., et al. (2003). The Epidemiology of Leber Hereditary Optic Neuropathy in the North East of England. *Am J Hum Genet*, Feb; 72(2): 333–339.

3 Ibid. Man. (2003).

4 Abu-Amero, K.K. (2011). Leber's Hereditary Optic Neuropathy: The Mitochondrial Connection Revisited. *Middle East Afr J Ophthalmol,* Jan;18(1):17-23.

5 Wikipedia. ATP synthase. Retrieved Feb 9 2018 from https://en.wikipedia.org/wiki/ATP_synthase.

6 Ibid. Abu-Amero. (2011).

7 Ibid. Abu-Amero. (2011).

8 American Academy of Ophthalmology. Eye Wiki. Leber Hereditary Optic Neuropathy. Retrieved Feb 9 2018 from http://eyewiki.aao.org/Leber_Hereditary_Optic_Neuropathy.

9 LHON Global. LHON Inheritance. Retrieved Feb 9 2018 from https://lhon.global/lhon-inheritance/.

10 Kirches, E. (2011). LHON: Mitochondrial Mutations and More. *Curr Genomics*, Mar; 12(1): 44–54.

11 Melov, S., Hinerfeld, D., Esposito, L., Wallace DC. (1997). Multi-organ characterization of mitochondrial genomic rearrangements in ad libitum and caloric restricted mice show striking somatic mitochondrial DNA rearrangements with age. *Nucleic Acids Res,* Mar 1;25(5):974-82.

12 Ibid. Genetics Home Reference. Leber heriditary optic neuropathy.

13 Ghelli, A., Porcelli, A.M., Zanna, C., Martinuzzi, A., Carelli, V., et al. (2008). Protection against oxidant-induced apoptosis by exogenous glutathione in Leber hereditary optic neuropathy cybrids. *Invest Ophthalmol Vis Sci*, 49(2):671–6.

14 Hudson, G., Keers, S., Yu-Wai-Man, P., Griffiths, P., Huoponen, K., et al. (2005). Identification of an X-chromosomal locus and haplotype modulating the phenotype of a mitochondrial DNA disorder. *Am J Hum Genet,* Dec;77(6):1086-91.

15 Sadun, A.A., Carelli, V., Salomao, S.R., Berezovsky, A., Quiros, P.A., et al. (2003). Extensive investigation of a large Brazilian pedigree of 11778/haplogroup J Leber hereditary optic neuropathy. *Am J Ophthalmol*, Aug;136(2):231-8.

16 Jones, D.A. (1998). Why are so many food plants cyanogenic? *Phytochemistry*, Jan;47(2):155-62.

17 Montagnac, J.A., Davis, C.R., Tanumilhardjo. (2008). Processing Techniques to Reduce Toxicity and Antinutrients of Cassava for Use as a Staple Food. *Comprehensive Reviews*, Jan:17-27.

18 Kanada, M., Miyagawa, M., Sato, M., Hasegawa, H., Honma, T. (1994). Neurochemical profile of effects of 28 neurotoxic chemicals on the central nervous system in rats (1). Effects of oral administration on brain contents of biogenic amines and metabolites. *Ind Health*, 32(3):145-64.

19 Pham-Huy, L.A., He, H., Pham-Huy, C. (2008). Free Radicals, Antioxidants in Disease and Health. *Int J Biomed Sci,* Jun;4(2):89-96.

20 Senergy.us Jones, L. Voltage: The Key to Rebuilding Your Health. Retrieved April 24 2018 from http://senergy.us/Assets/PDFs/Dr. Tennant Articles/Voltage, The Key to Rebuilding You Life.pdf

21 Klopstock, T., Yu-Wai-Man, P., Dimitriadis, K., Rouleau, J., Heck, S., et al. (2011). A randomized placebo-controlled trial of idebenone in Leber's hereditary optic neuropathy. *Brain,* Sep; 134(Pt 9):2677-86

22 Carelli, V., La Morgia, C., Valentino, M.L., Rizzo, G., Carbonelli, M., et al. (2011). Idebenone treatment in Leber's hereditary optic neuropathy. *Brain, Sep; 134(Pt 9):e188.*

[23] Manickam, A.H., Michael, M.J., Ramasamy, S. (2017). Mitochondrial genetics and therapeutic overview of Leber's hereditary optic neuropathy. *Indian J Ophthalmol,* Nov;65(11):1087-1092.

24 Mashima, Y., Kigasawa, K., Wakakura, M., Oguchi, Y. (2000). Do idebenone and vitamin therapy shorten the time to achieve visual recovery in Leber hereditary optic neuropathy? *J Neuroophthalmol,* Sep; 20(3):166-70.

25 Barnils, N., Mesa, E., Muñoz, S., Ferrer-Artola, A., Arruga, J. (2007). Response to idebenone and multivitamin therapy in Leber's hereditary optic neuropathy. *Arch Soc Esp Oftalmol,* Jun; 82(6):377-80.

[26] Giordano, C., Lommarini, L., Giordano, L., Maresca, A., Pisano, A., et al. (2014). Efficient mitochondrial biogenesis drives incomplete penetrance in Leber's hereditary optic neuropathy. *Brain,* Feb;137(2):335-353.

[27] Ibid. Giordano. (2014).

[28] Munoz, L.M.P. (2014). Smell Stimulates Early Visual Processing Women But Not in Men. *Cog Neuro Soc,* Nov 21.

[29] Hipkiss, A.R. (2008). Would carnosine or a carnivorous diet help suppress aging and associated pathologies? *Ann N Y Acad Sci*, May;1067:369-74.

[30] Hipkiss, A.R. (2000). Carnosine and protein carbonyl groups: a possible relationship. *Biochemistry (Mosc).* Jul;65(7):771-8.

[31] Hipkiss, A.R. (2007). Could carnosine or related structures suppress Alzheimer's disease? *J Alzheimers Dis.* May;11(2):229-40.

[32] Brown, B.E., Kim, C.H., Torpy, F.R., Bursill, C.A., McRobb, L.S., et al. (2014). Supplementation with carnosine decreases plasma triglycerides and modulates atherosclerotic plaque composition in diabetic apo E(-/-) mice. Atherosclerosis, Feb;232(2):403-9.

[33] Reddy, V.P., Garrett, M.R., Perry, G., Smith, M.A. (2005). Carnosine: a versatile antioxidant and antiglycating agent. Sci Aging Knowledge Environ, May 4;2005(18):pe12.

[34] Cheng, J., Wang, F., Yu, D.F., Wu, P.F., Chen, J.G. (2011). The cytotoxic mechanism of malondialdehyde and protective effect of carnosine via protein cross-linking/mitochondrial dysfunction/reactive oxygene species/MAPK pathway in neurons. Eur J Pharmacol, Jan 10;650(1):184-94.

[35] Hipkiss, A.R. (2014). Aging risk factors and Parkinson's disease: contrasting roles of common dietary constituents. Neurobiol Aging, 2014 Jun;35(6):1469-72.

36 Froger, N., Cadetti, L., Lorach, H., et al. (2002). Taurine provides neuroprotection against retinal ganglion cell degeneration. *PLoS One,* 7(10):e42017.

These are for taurine
Taurine. 750mg – 1,000mg daily. Supports protects the mitochondria. (Mol Vis. 2012; 18: 2673–2686) from oxidative damage to enhance energy production within cells.
A Neurosci Lett. 2015 Mar 17;590:52-7.
Adv Exp Med Biol. 2015;803:397-405mino Acids. 2015 Apr;47(4):735-44.

[37] Lombardini, J.B. (1991). Taurine: retinal function. *Brain Res Brain Res Rev*, May-Aug;16(2):151-69.

[38] Ripps, H., Shen, W. (2012). Review: Taurine: A "very essential" amino acid. Mol Vis, 18: 2673–2686.

[39] Heller-Stilb, B., van Roeyen, C., Rascher, K., Hartwig, H.G., Huth, A., et al. (2002).

Disruption of the taurine transporter gene (taut) leads to retinal degeneration in mice. Faseb J, Feb; 16(2):231-3.

[40] Mahoney, D.E., Hiebert, J.B., Thimmesch, A., Pierce, J.T., Vacek, J.L., et al. (2018). Understanding D-Ribose and Mitochondrial Function. *Adv Biosci Clin Med,* 6(1):1-5.

[41] Ibid. Ghelli. (2008).

[42] Mari, M., Morales, A., Colell, A., Garcia-Ruiz, C., Fernandez-Checa, J.C. (2009). Mitochondrial glutathione, a key survival antioxidant. *Antioxid Redox Signal,* Nov;11(11):2685-700.

[43] Rucker, R., Chowanadisai, W., Nakano, M. (2009). Potential physiological importance of pyrroloquinoline quinone. *Altern Med Rev,* Sep;14(3):268-77.

[44] Chowanadisai, W., Bauerly, K.A., Tchaparian, E., Wong, A., Cortopassi, G.A., et al. (2010). Pyrroloquinoline quinone stimulates mitochondrial biogenesis through cAMP response element-binding protein phosphorylation and increased PGC-1 alpha expression. *J Biol Chem,* Jan 1;285:142-52.

[45] Kucharská, J. (2008). Vitamins in Mitochondrial Function. In: Gvozdjáková A. (eds) Mitochondrial Medicine. Springer, Dordrecht.

[46] Ibid. Kucharská. (2008).

[47] Rudolf, E., Rudolf, K. (2017). Increases in Intracellular Zinc Enhance Proliferative Signaling as Well as Mitochondrial and Endolysomal Activity in Human Melanocytes. *Cell Physiol Biochem,* 43(1):1-16.

[48] Yang, X., Wang, H., Huang, C., He, X., Xu, W., et al. (2017). Zinc enhances the cellular energy supply to improve cell motility and restore impaired energetic metabolism in a toxic environment induced by OTA. *Sci Rep,* Nov 7;7(1):14669.

[49] Pilchova, I., Klacanova, K., Tatarkova, Z., Kaplan, P., Racay, P. (2017). The Involvement of Mg^{2+} in Regulation of Cellular and Mitochondrial Functions. *Oxid Med Cell Longev,* Jul 5;6797460.

[50] Lau, T., Bigio, B., Zelli, D., McEwen, B.S., Nasca, C. (2017). Stress-induced structural plasticity of medial amygdala stellate neurons and rapid prevention by a candidate antidepressant. *Mol Psychiatry,* Feb;22(2):227-234.

[51] Dhitavat, S., Ortiz, D., Shea, T.B., Rivera, E.R. (2002). Acetyl-L-carnitine protects against amyloid-beta neurotoxicity: roles of oxidative buffering and ATP levels.

[52] National Institutes of Health. Carnitine. Retrieved Sep 6 2018 from https://ods.od.nih.gov/factsheets/Carnitine-HealthProfessional/.

53 Bush, R.A., Malnoe, A., Reme, C.E., Williams, T.P. (1994). Dietary deficiency of N-3 fatty acids alters rhodopsin content and function in the rat retina. *Invest Ophthalmol Vis Sci,* 35(1):91–100.

54 Stillwell, W., Wassall, S.R. (2003). Docosahexaenoic acid: membrane properties of a unique fatty acid. *Chem Phys Lipids,* 126(1):1–27.

55 Elner, V.M. (2002). Retinal pigment epithelial acid lipase activity and lipoprotein receptors: effects of dietary omega-3 fatty acids. *Trans Am Ophthalmol Soc,* 100:301–338.

56 Marangoni, D., Falsini, B., Piccardi, M., Ambrosio, L., Minnella, A.M., et al. (2013). Functional effect of Saffron supplementation and risk genotypes in early age-related macular degeneration: a preliminary report. *J Trans Med,* Sep 25;11:228.

57 Falsini, B., Piccardi, M., Minnella, A., Savastano, C., Capoluongo, E.,et al. (2010). Influence of saffron supplementation on retinal flicker sensitivity in early age-related macular degeneration. *Invest Opththalmol Vis Sci.* Dec;51(12):6118-24.

58 Capitanio, S., Sambuceti, G. Giusti, M., Morbelli, S., Murialdo, G., et al. (2013). 1,25-Dihydroxy vitamin D and coronary microvascular function. *Eur J Nucl Med Mol Imaging,* 40:280–9.

59 Nakajima, Y., Inokuchi,Y., Shimazawa, M., Otsubo, K., Ishibashi, T., et al. (2008). Astaxanthin, a dietary carotenoid, protects retinal cells against oxidative stress in-vitro and in mice in-vivo. *J Pharm Pharmacol.* Oct;60(10):1365-74.

60 BetaForce. Astaxanthin: The Most Powerful Natural Antioxidant Ever Discovered. Retrieved Apr 2 2018 from http://www.beta-glucan-info.com/astaxanthin.htm.

61 Chiro.org. Antioxidants: Relative Singlet Oxygen Quenching Rates. Retrieved Apr 16 2018 from http://www.chiro.org/nutrition/FULL/ Antioxidants_Relative_Singlet_Oxygen_Quenching_Rates.html.

62 Kidd, P. (2011). Astaxanthin, cell membrane nutrient with diverse clinical benefits and anti-aging potential. *Altern Med Rev,* Dec;16(4):355-64.

63 Song, X., Wang, B., Lin, S., Jing, L., Mao, C., et al. (2014). Astaxanthin inhibits apoptosis in alveolar epithelial cells type II in vivo and in vitro through the ROS-dependent mitochondrial signaling pathway. *J Cell Mol Med,* Nov;18(11):2198-212.

64 Kuroki, T., Ikeda, S., Okada, T., Maoka, T., Kitamura, A., et al. (2013). Astaxanthin ameliorates heat stress-induced impairment of blastocyst development in vitro:--astaxanthin colocalization with and action on mitochondria--. *J Assist Reprod Genet*, Jun;30(5):623-31.

65 Droy-Lefaix, M.T., Cluzel, J., Menerath, J.M., Bonhomme, B., Doly, M. (1995) Antioxidant effect of a Ginkgo biloba extract (EGb 761) on the retina. *Int J Tissue React*, 17(3):93-100.

66 Thiagarajan, G., Chandani, S., Harinarayana, R.S., Samuni, A.M., Chandrasekaran, K., et al. (2002). Molecular and cellular assessment of ginkgo biloba extract as a possible ophthalmic drug. *Exp Eye Res,* Oct;75(4):421-30.

67 Wu, Y.Z., Li, S.Q., Zu, X.G., Du, J., Wang, F.F. (2008) Ginkgo biloba extract improves coronary artery circulation in patients with coronary artery disease: contribution of plasma nitric oxide and endothelin-1. *Phytother Res*, Jun;22(6):734-9.

68 Wu, Y.Z., Li, S.Q., Zu, X.G., Du, J., Wang, F.F. (2008). Ginkgo biloba extract improves coronary blood flow in healthy elderly adults: role of endothelium-dependent vasodilation. *Phytomedicine,* Mar;15(3):164-9.

69 Welt, K., Weiss, J., Martin, R., Hermsdorf, T., Drews, S., et al. (2007). Ginkgo biloba extract protects rat kidney from diabetic and hypoxic damage. *Phytomedicine,* Feb;14(2-3):196-203.

70 Qiu, Y., Rui, Y.C., Li, T.J., Zhang, L., Yao, P.Y. (2004). Inhibitory effect of extracts of Ginkgo biloba leaves on VEGF-induced hyperpermeability of bovine coronary endothelial cells in vitro. *Acta Pharmacol Sin,* Oct;25(10):1306-11.

71 Huang, S.Y., Jeng, C., Kao, S.C., Yu, J.J., Liu, D.Z. (2004). Improved haemorrheological properties by Ginkgo biloba extract (Egb 761) in type 2 diabetes mellitus complicated with retinopathy. *Clin Nutr*, Aug;23(4):615-21.

72 Muth, E.R., Laurent, J.M., Jasper, P. (2000). The effect of bilberry nutritional supplementation on night visual acuity and contrast sensitivity. *Altern Med Rev,* Apr;5(2):164-73.

73 Matsunaga, N., Imai, S., Inokuchi, Y., Shimazawa, M., Yokota, S., et al. (2009). Bilberry and its main constituents have neuroprotective effects against retinal neuronal damage in vitro and in vivo. *Mol Nutr Food Res*, Jul;53(7):869-77.

74 Zhu, Y., Xia, M., Yang, Y., Liu, F., Li, Z., et al. (2011). Purified anthocyanin supplementation improves endothelial function via NO-cGMP activation in hypercholesterolemic individuals. *Clin Chem,* Nov;57(11):1524-33.

75 Contestabile, M., Appolloni, R., Suppressa, F. et al, (1991). Prolonged treatment with anthocyanosides of cranberry with high dossage: electrophysiological responses in myopic patients. *Boll Ocul*, 70:1157-1169.

76 Yao, Y., Vieria, A. (2007). Protective activities of Vaccinium antioxidants with potential relevance to mitochondrial dysfunction and neurotoxicity. *Neurotoxicology*, 28 93–100.

77 Fiorini, G., Biancacci, A., Graziano, F.M. (1965). Perimetric and adaptometric modifications after ingestion of myrtillin associated with betacarotene. *Ann Ottalmol Clin Ocul*, 91:371-86.

78 Cohen-Boulakia, F., Valensi, P.E., Boulahdour, H., Lestrade, R., Dufour-Lamarinie, J.F., et al. (2000). In vivo sequential study of skeletal muscle capillary permeability in diabetic rats: effect of anthocyanosides. *Metabolism*, Jul;49(7):880-5.

79 Belleoud, L., Leluan, D., Boyer, Y. (1966). Study on the effects of anthocyanin glycosides on the nocturnal vision of air traffic controllers. *Rev Med Aeronaut Spatiale*, 18:3–7.

80 Zadok, D., Levy, Y., Glovinsky, Y. (1966).The effect of anthocyanosides in a multiple oral dose on night vision. *Rev Med Aeronaut Spatiale,* 18:3-7. 5.

81 Littarru, G.P., Tiano, L. (2007). Bioenergetic and antioxidant properties of coenzyme Q10: recent developments. *Mol Biotechnol*, Sep;37(1):31-7.

82 Piotrowska, D., Długosz, A., Witkiewicz, K., Pajak, J. (2000). The research on antioxidative properties of TOŁPA Peat Preparation and its fractions. *Acta Pol Pharm,* Nov;57 Suppl:127-9.

83 Stratton, R.D., Hauswirth, W.W., Gardner, T.W. (2012). Studies on Retinal and Choroidal Disorders. New York, NY: Springer Science+Business Media.

84 Michael, L.D., Allen, M.J. (1993). Nutritional supplementation, electrical stimulation and age related macular degeneration. *J Orthomol Med*, 8: 168-171.

85 Halloran, G. (1997). Bioelectrical Stimulation in an Integrated Treatment for Macular Degeneration, RP, Glaucoma, CMV-Retinitis, and Diabetic Retinopathy. *Fourth Annual Symposium on Biological Circuits*, Oct. Mankato University, MN.

86 Wallace, L. B. (1997). Treatment for Macular Degeneration Utilizing Micro-Current Stimulation. *J. Opt Photother*, Mar.

87 Paul, E.L. (1997). The Treatment of Retinal Diseases With Micro Current Stimulation And Nutritional Supplementation. Retrieved Apr 23 2018 from http://www.fieldsforlife.org /bibliography_microcurrent_files/paulstudy.pdf

88 O'Clock, G.D., Jarding, J.B. (2009). Electrotherapeutic device/protocol design considerations for visual disease applications. *Conf Proc IEEE Eng Med Biol Soc*, 2009:2133-6.

89 Chaikin, L., Kashiwa, K., Bennet, M., Papastergiou, G., Gregory, W. (2015). Microcurrent stimulation in the treatment of dry and wet macular degeneration. *J Clin Ophthalmol*, Dec 17;9:2345-53.

90 Bola, C., Bartlett, H., Eperjesi, F. (2014). Resveratrol and the eye: activity and molecular mechanisms. *Graefes Arch Clin Exp Ophthalmol*, May;252(5):699-713.

91 Jarrett, S.G., Boulton, M.E. (2012). Consequences of oxidative stress in age-related macular degeneration. *Mol Aspects Med*, Aug;33(4):399–417.

92 Sivapathasuntharam, C., Sivaprasad, S., Hogg, C., Jeffery, G. (2017). Aging retinal function is improved by near infrared light (670 nm) that is associated with corrected mitochondrial decline. *Neurobiol Aging,* Apr; 52: 66–70.

93 Tarnopolsky, M. (2004). Exercise testing as a diagnostic entity in mitochondrial myopathies. *Mitochondrion*, Sep; 4(5-6):529-42.

94 Jeppesen, T.D., Schwartz, M., Olsen, D.B. (2006). Aerobic training is safe and improves exercise capacity in patients with mitochondrial myopathy. *Brain*. 129:3402–3412.

95 Tianjin Journal of Traditional Chinese Medicine. Retrieved Apr 25 2018 from http://en.cnki.com.cn/Journal_en/E-E056-TJZY-2004-02.htm

96 Datta, S., Tomilov, A., Cortopassi, G. (2016). Identification of small molecules that improve ATP synthesis defects conferred by Leber's hereditary optic neuropathy mutations. *Mitochondrion,* Sep;30:177-186.

97 Cideciyan, A.V., Jacobson, S.G., Beltran, W.A., Sumaroka, A., Swider, M., et al. (2013). Human retinal gene therapy for Leber congenital amaurosis shows advancing retinal degeneration despite enduring visual improvement. *PNAS*, 110(6)E517-E525.

98 Klopstock, T., Yu-Wai-Man, P., Dimitriadis, K., Rouleau, J., Heck, S., Bailie, M., et al. (2011). A randomized placebo-controlled trial of idebenone in Leber's hereditary optic neuropathy. *Brain,* Sep; 134(9): 2677–2686.

99 Gardner, T.W., Hauswirth, W.W., Stratton, R.D. (2012). *Studies on Retinal and Choroidal Disorders*. Springer, New York, New York.

15-16. LIGHT SENSITIVITY

Light sensitivity (photophobia) occurs when eyes are overly sensitive to light, sometimes causing pain, tearing, and discomfort. Some eye doctors do not consider it an eye condition in itself, but a common side effect of other conditions, such as migraine headaches and brain or nervous system problems. Despite its prevalence, it is not well understood, and it is difficult to treat.[1]

How Our Eyes Normally Process Light

When light enters the eyes, it causes a chemical reaction in the back of the eyes that stimulates the photoreceptors, allowing us to adapt to various differences in brightness, light, and darkness. The photoreceptors contain visual pigments, which are composed of proteins called opsins and molecules called chromophores. The visual pigment in the rods' outer segment is called rhodopsin (comprised of one type of opsin and a light sensitive vitamin A derivative), and the visual pigment in the cones is one of three different color sensitive opsins (red-, green-, or blue-light sensitive). If there is an imbalance in how the photoreceptors work, then we have difficulty adapting efficiently when going from dark to light and vice versa.

When light reaches the retina, it is absorbed by the photoreceptors' visual pigment, where it is transformed into an electrical signal. The signal travels from the photoreceptor to the optic nerve, and to the visual cortex in the brain where it is interpreted. This processing action causes the photoreceptor cells to shed their outer layer, which becomes a waste product. In a healthy eye, this waste is completely absorbed. The outer shell regenerates in approximately 45 minutes.

Pathology

There are several ways that the visual process can go wrong. Sensitivity to light involves delicate neural pathways which, when imbalanced physically or electro-chemically, cause pain. There is a connection between photosensitivity and migraines: nearly 80% of people who have migraines are photosensitive.[2] Similarly, there is a connection between blepharospasm (eyelid spasm) and light sensitivity, with 80–95% of these patients reporting some level of discomfort.[3]

While scientists are not sure about the causes of migraines, some think they may be triggered by inflammatory substances released in the tissues that surround the circulatory and nerve systems (of the head and brain). Specifically, ocular migraines appear to be tied to blood-vessel spasms in the retina, or in the back of the eye in the vessels that supply blood to the retina.[4] Therefore, inflammation may play a role in increasing sensitivity and pain to light.

Hypersensitivity to light can result from a dysfunction of the cornea, iris, or pupil, the inability of the photoreceptors to adapt, trauma caused by injury or surgery, and/or dysfunction of ocular nerves and the eye-brain connection.

Signs and Symptoms

- Sharp or throbbing pain, a headache (including migraines), and even nausea
- Watering eyes which may sometimes be accompanied by burning sensation
- Discomfort in sunlight, in bright interior light, and/or with glare on a hazy day
- Poor night vision or problems while driving at night due to glare and oncoming light

Causes and Risk Factors

In general, people with light colored eyes and skin are more sensitive to light. Here are some other possible contributors:

- **Headaches,** particularly migraines, are the most common cause of light sensitivity. Up to 80% of people with migraines also experience photophobia.[5] Cluster headaches and tension headaches can also cause photophobia. Doppler studies have revealed cessation of retinal arterial flow during an exercise-induced retinal-migraine episode.[6]
- **Nutrient deficiencies** such as a deficiency of beta-carotene, lutein, or zeaxanthin may contribute to light sensitivity.
- **Other health conditions** may contribute, such as thyroid conditions, pituitary gland tumors, diabetes, rabies, Lyme disease, and certain types of poisoning.
- **Dry eye syndrome**, a deficiency in tears, causes the surface of the cornea to become irritated and more sensitive to light, and in severe cases, this can lead to cornea damage.
- **Computer eyestrain** has been the topic of studies that show that people blink much less and not as completely when looking at a computer screen, which can result in dry eyes.
- **Nervous system problems**[7] may contribute to light sensitivity, including supranuclear palsy, serious or mild traumatic brain injury (MTBI), autism spectrum, dyslexia, meningitis, over-stimulation of photoreceptors, an over-active optic nerve or central nervous system, and damage to oculomotor nerve that disallows pupil dilation.
- **Other eye conditions** that may contribute include severe conjunctivitis, uveitis, keratitis, iritis, cataracts, Sjogren's, blepharospasm, and overstimulation of photoreceptors. Also, eye conditions where too much light enters the eyes, such as: corneal abrasion, albinism (lack of pigment makes irises translucent, decreasing protection from light), and adrenal fatigue where the iris muscles are unable to maintain pupillary constriction in brighter lighting.
- **Some drugs and medications** include antibiotics, acne medications, diuretics used to treat high pressure, nonsteroidal anti-inflammatory drugs (NSAIDs), anti-malarial drugs, antihistamines, blood pressure medications, and Digoxin (used for heart failure or heart irregularity).
- **Eye surgery**, such as Lasik surgery, may contribute to light sensitivity.
- **ADHD** patients have a high prevalence of self-reported light sensitivity.[8]

Conventional Treatment

The first and most important action is to determine if there is an underlying cause for the light sensitivity, such as a thyroid problem or diabetes. Additionally, a thorough eye exam is recommended to evaluate the health of the eye.

The most important conventional treatment is a simple one: Wear sunglasses. Amber or grey lenses that are 100% UVA/UVB protecting are the best. The lens should be polarized to reduce glare. Also, wraparound sunglasses that touch your eyebrow area are helpful.

Complementary Approach

Targeted supplementation can help reduce light sensitivity and support overall eye health.

Nutrients

Carotenoids and Macular Pigment

Research shows that people with higher macular pigment levels tolerate light better.[9] [10] Supplementing with a combination of mesozeaxanthin (10mg), lutein (10mg), and zeaxanthin (2mg); or mesozeaxanthin (17mg), lutein (3mg), and zeaxanthin (2mg) results in the best macular pigment density.[11]

When exposed to both bright, white light and short-wavelength blue light, people with greater macular-pigment optical density have better vision compared to subjects with lower optical density.[12] Supplementation just with lutein and zeaxanthin reduces glare effects.[13] [14] Recovery time for the subject with the lowest macular pigment optical density is twice as long as subjects with the highest macular pigment levels.[15]

Note. In one study, researchers found that a moderate dose of 13.3mg combined carotenoids, comprised of 83% lutin (11mg), 10% zeaxanthin (1.33mg), 7% mesozeaxanthin (.93mg), was more effective than higher doses in enhancing macular pigment, even though higher doses were reflected in serum blood levels.[16]

Essential

Lutein. 6mg–20mg per day. Lutein and zeaxanthin are antioxidants used in both the retina and lens of the eyes and act to filter out sunlight, like a pair of internal eyeglasses. Lutein is an essential antioxidant for maintaining the health of the retina and protecting the retina and lens from sunlight damage.[17] Lutein is helpful in reducing glare.[18]

Zeaxanthin. 2mg–12mg per day. Carotenoid nutrients such as lutein and specific forms of zeaxanthin make up your macular pigment. This part of your retina protects underlying photoreceptor cells from the harmful effects of excess blue and ultraviolet light.[19]

Astaxanthin. 6mg–12mg per day. This powerful carotenoid crosses the blood-eye barrier, supporting vascular and cellular health within the eye.[20] [21] [22] [23] [24] [25]

Bilberry. 180mg–240mg per day. Bilberry extracts have antioxidant properties that are not only neuroprotective, but also help suppress photooxidative processes. Bilberry has been shown to improve small blood vessels, such as capillaries that provide the delivery of blood to the retina. Its anthocyanoside content may also be especially beneficial for nighttime visual acuity.[26] [27] [28] [29] [30]

Very Important

Vitamin A (palmitate). 5,000mg per day. This nutrient helps support the photoreceptor cells.[31]

> **Note**. Vitamin A is contra-indicated for those suffering from Stargardt disease (see Stargardt's chapter for more information). Pregnant women should not take vitamin A.

Helpful

Ginkgo biloba, 120mg per day, *and/or* **vinpocetine,** 10mg–30mg per day. Ginkgo biloba's antioxidant capacity improves circulation within the tiny capillaries in the eye,[32] [33] [34] stabilizing them and making them less fragile.[35]

Vitamin B complex. Preferably a whole-food organic formula, or a whole-food organic multivitamin is recommended, as directed. If not a whole-food formula, we recommend dosages of vitamin B complex as follows: vitamin B6 (100mg), vitamin B12 methylcobalamin (1,000mcg), biotin (400mcg), folate (400mcg), riboflavin/B2 (50mg), and benfotiamine/B1 (400mg). These dosages will be smaller in a whole-food multivitamin, and will vary depending on the B complex formula you purchase.

Essential fatty acids (fish oil or from algae if you are vegetarian). 2,000 IU–3,000 IU per day. DHA from omega-3 fatty acids accounts for about 50–60% of the total fatty acid content in the rods of the photoreceptor cells and tends to be very deficient in today's diet.[36] [37]

Green tea extract. Green teas and their extracts may protect the outer segments of the photoreceptors as well as the retinal pigment epithelium.[38]

Saffron. Studies have shown that saffron helps protect photoreceptor cells from damage and supports healthy circulation in the retina.[39]

Eyedrops

Lubricating eyedrops (preservative free) are helpful for light sensitivity due to dry eyes.

Homeopathic eyedrops with calendula and euphrasia are helpful for light sensitivity due to corneal issues.

For Migraine Headaches

Riboflavin (vitamin B2). 200mg per day. B2 therapy has been shown to reduce migraine symptoms.[40] B2 supports mitochondrial energy production, and researchers have discovered that patients who suffer from migraines have depleted mitochondrial energy reserves between attacks. Riboflavin helps increase neuronal energy production and has been shown to be effective as migraine-preventive therapy.[41] [42]

Butterbur. 50mg-150mg per day. Butterbur can reduce symptoms of migraine headaches up to 50%.[43] [44] [45] It can also help prevent onset of migraines.[46] [47] [48]

Magnesium. 500mg per day. Magnesium reduces peripheral vascular resistance and promotes a healthy cardiovascular system.[49]

Feverfew extract (.5% perthenolide). 50mg, 1–2 times per day. Feverfew is a traditional remedy used for a number of different health issues, including headaches and migraines.[50]

Ginger extract (20% gingerol and shogaol). 300mg per day. Ginger is recognized for its ability to combat inflammation, nausea, and pain.[51]

Diet

Dark leafy greens. Consume lots of dark green vegetables such as spinach and collards, which are high in lutein and zeaxanthin. Maintain an alkaline diet. Avoid chocolate or other foods that you find bring on migraines; such foods might include vegetables in the nightshade family (tomatoes, eggplant, peppers, potatoes, tomatillos, and goji berries).

Juicing. We suggest fresh organic fruits and vegetables for juicing. Choose at least 4-6 items to combine.

- Ginger, garlic, leeks, parsley, beets, orange peppers, cabbage, carrots, celery, spinach, kale, collard greens, apples, grapes, raspberries, lemon, chlorophyll, wheatgrasses
- Add your favorite fruits and vegetables as well. Do not use too many carrots or too much fruit due to their sweetness.
- Try to use room temperature vegetables and fruit.
- Do not add ice or very cold liquids since cold foods and liquids will eventually extinguish the stomach's digestive fire.
- Do not juice as often during the cooler months of the year, and instead, switch to vegetable soups or stews.

Lifestyle

Eye exercises. See Chapter 10 for eye exercises and acupuncture points that are good for all eye conditions and overall eye health. We recommend these exercises:

- Palming
- Eye massage

Sunglasses. Always wear sunglasses outside, especially on bright days. (Blue and green-eyed people are particularly sensitive to potential sun-induced damage, so the use of eye protection is paramount). Amber and grey lenses are the most effective protection against UVA/UVB and blue light. Lenses should be polarized to reduce glare.

Driving. Drive only during the day if possible. Even good lighting conditions at night, such as found in a big city, may be troublesome to someone who suffers from photophobia.

- Increase your driving vision by cleaning your headlights.
- Slow down; that way, you give yourself more time to react to any unexpected hazards.
- Get prescription glasses for driving at night, if needed. See your eye doctor to determine if glasses would be helpful.
- When driving at night, look partially to the right. Look at the roadway's edge to the right (or left) to help you avoid the glare of oncoming headlights.

Other Modalities

Chinese Medicine

Ming mu di huang wan (brighten the eyes). This formula treats what is known as Kidney and Liver yin deficiency. It helps treat symptoms typical of yin deficiency such as sensitivity to light.

Also See

Chapter 8, Nutrients

Chapter 15-21, Poor Night Vision

Chapter 15-22, Ocular Migraine

1 Digre, K.B., Brennan, K.C. (2012). Shedding Light on Photophobia. *J Neuroophthalmol*, Mar; 32(1): 68–81.

2 Doran, M. (2005). Photophobia: Looking for Causes and Solutions. Retrieved Feb 4 2018 from https://www.aao.org/eyenet/article/photophobia-looking-causes-solutions?novemberdecember-2005.

3 Ibid. Doran. (2005).

4 Nakajima, Y., Inokuchi, Y., Shimazawa, M., Otsubo, K., Ishibashi, T., et al. (2008). Astaxanthin, a dietary carotenoid, protects retinal cells against oxidative stress in-vitro and in mice in-vivo. *J Pharm Pharmacol*, Oct;60(10):1365-74.

5 Ibid. WebMD. What is Photophobia.

6 Jehn, A., Dettwiler, B., Fleischhauer, J., Mojon, D.J. (2002). Exercise-induced vasospastic amaurosis fugax. *Arch Ophthalmol*, 120:220–2.

7 Wikipedia. Photophobia. Retrieved Feb 13 2018 from https://en.wikipedia.org/wiki/ Photophobia.

8 Koij, J.J.S., Deijlenga, D. (2014). High Prevalence of Self-Reported Photophobia in Adult ADHD. *Front Neurol*, Dec 10.

9 Stringham, J.M., Fuld, K., Wenzel, A.J. (2004). Spatial properties of photophobia. *Invest Ophthalmol Vis Sci*, Oct; 45(10):3838-48.

10 Wenzel, A. J., Fuld, K., Stringham, J. M., Curran-Celentano, J. (2006). Macular pigment optical density and photophobia light threshold. *Vis Res*, 46(28):4615–4622.

11 Akuffo, K.O., Nolan, J.M., Howard, A.N., Moran, R., Stack, J., et al. (2015). Sustained supplementation and monitored response with differing carotenoid formulations in early age-related macular degeneration. *Eye (Lond)*, Jul; 29(7):902-12.

12 Stringham, J.M., Hammond, B.R. (2007). The glare hypothesis of macular pigment function. *Optom Vis Sci*, Sep; 84(9):859-64.

13 Scripsema, N.K., Hu, D.N., Rosen, R.B. (2015). Lutein, Zeaxanthin, and *meso*-Zeaxanthin in the Clinical Management of Eye Disease. *J Ophthalmol*, 2015:865179

14 Stringham, J.M., Garcia, P.V., Smith, P.A., McLin, L.N., Foutch, B.K. (2011). Macular pigment and visual performance in glare: benefits for photostress recovery, disability glare, and visual discomfort. *Invest Ophthalmol Vis Sci*, Sep 22; 52(10):7406-15.

15 Stringham, J.M., Hammond, B.R. (2008). Macular pigment and visual performance under glare conditions. *Optom Vis Sci*, Feb; 85(2):82-8.

[16] Stringham, J.M., Stringham, N.T. (2016). Serum and retinal response to three different doses of macular carotenoids over 12 weeks of supplementation. *Exp Eye Res*, Oct;151:1-8.

17 Bernstein, P.S., Zhao, D.Y., Wintch, S.W., Ermakov, I.V., McClane, R.W., et al. (2002). Resonance Raman measurement of macular carotenoids in normal subjects and in age-related macular degeneration patients. *Ophthalmology*, Oct;109(10):1780-7.

18 Stringham, J.M., Bovier, E.R., Wong, J.C., Hammond, B.R. (2010). The influence of dietary lutein and zeaxanthin on visual performance. *J Food Sci*, Jan-Feb;75(1):R24-9.

19 Moukarzel, A.A., Bejjani, R.A., Fares, F.N. (2009). Xanthophylls and eye health of infants and adults. *J Med Liban*, Oct-Dec;57(4):261-7.

20 Goto, S., Kogure, K., Abe, K., Kimata, Y., Kitahama, K., et al.(2001). Efficient radical trapping at the surface and inside the phospholipid membrane is responsible for highly potent antiperoxidative activity of the carotenoid astaxanthin. *Biochimica et Biophysica Acta*, 2001;1512 :251-8.

21 Beta Force. Betaxanthin Retrieved April 24 2018 from http://www.beta-glucan-info.com/astaxanthin.htm.

22 Phiro Resources. Pioneering Astaxanthin Retrieved April 25 2018 from http://www.chiro.org/nutrition/FULL/Antioxidants_Relative_Singlet_Oxygen_Quenching_Rates.html .

23 Kidd, P. (2011). Astaxanthin, cell membrane nutrient with diverse clinical benefits and anti-aging potential. *Altern Med Rev*, Dec;16(4):355-64.

24 Song, X., Wang, B., Lin, S., Jing, L., Mao, C., et al.(2014). Astaxanthin inhibits apoptosis in alveolar epithelial cells type II in vivo and in vitro through the ROS-dependent mitochondrial signaling pathway. *J Cell Mol Med*, Nov;18(11):2198-212.

25 Kuroki, T., Ikeda, S., Okada, T., Maoka, T., Kitamura, A., et al. (2013). Astaxanthin ameliorates heat stress-induced impairment of blastocyst development in vitro:--astaxanthin colocalization with and action on mitochondria. *J Assist Reprod Genet*, Jun;30(5):623-31

26 Muth, E.R., Laurent, J.M., Jasper, P. (2000). The effect of bilberry nutritional supplementation on night visual acuity and contrast sensitivity. *Altern Med Rev*, Apr;5(2):164-73.

27 Contestabile, M., Appolloni, R., Suppressa, F. (1991). Prolonged treatment with blueberry anthocyanosides administered in high doses: electrophysiological response in myopic patients. *Boll Ocul*. 70:1157-1169.

28 Matsunaga, N., Imai, S., Inokuchi, Y., Shimazawa, M. Yokota, S., et al. (2009). Bilberry and its main constituents have neuroprotective effects against retinal neuronal damage in vitro and in vivo. *Mol Nutr Food Res*, Jul;53(7):869-77.

29 Yao, Y., Vieira, A. (2007). Protective activities of Vaccinium antioxidants with potential relevance to mitochondrial dysfunction and neurotoxicity. *Neurotoxicology*, Jan;28(1):93-100..

30 Belleoud, L., Leluan, D., Boyer, Y. (1966). Study on the effects of anthocyanin glycosides on the night vision of flight personnel. *Commun Soc Fr Physiol Med Aeronaut Cosmonaut* 17.

31 Zhong, M., Kawaguchi, R., Kassai, M., Sun, H. (2012). Retina, retinol, retinal and the natural history of vitamin A as a light sensor. *Nutrients*, Dec 19;4(12):2069-96.

32 Suter, A., Niemer, W., Klopp, R. (2011). A new ginkgo fresh plant extract increases microcirculation and radical scavenging activity in *elderly* patients. *Adv Ther*, Dec;28(12):1078-88.

33 Droy-Lefaix, M.T., Cluzel, J., Menerath, J.M., Bonhomme, B., Doly, M. (1995). Antioxidant effect of a Ginkgo biloba extract (EGb 761) on the retina. *Int J Tissue React*, 17(3):93-100.

34 Thiagarajan, G., Chandani, S., Harinarayana, R., Ayelet, M. Samuni, D., et al. (2002). Molecular and Cellular Assessment of Ginkgo Biloba Extract as a Possible Ophthalmic Drug. *Exp Eye Res*, Oct;75(4):421-30.

35 Huang, S.Y., Jeng, C., Kao, S.C., Yu, J.J., Liu, D.Z. (2004). Improved haemorrheological properties by Ginkgo biloba extract (Egb 761) in type 2 diabetes mellitus complicated with retinopathy. *Clin Nutr.* Aug;23(4):615-21.

36 Bush, R.A., Malnoe, A., Reme, C.E., Williams, T.P. (1994). Dietary deficiency of N-3 fatty acids alters rhodopsin content and function in the rat retina. *Invest Ophthalmol Vis Sci*, 35(1):91–100.

37 Stillwell, W., Wassall, S.R. (2003). Docosahexaenoic acid: membrane properties of a unique fatty acid. *Chem Phys Lipids*, 126(1):1–27.

38 Zhang, B., Safa, R., Rusciano, D., Osborne, N.N. (2007). Epigallocatechin gallate, an active ingredient from green tea, attenuates damaging influences to the retina caused by ischemia/reperfusion. *Brain Res*, Jul 23;1159:40-53

39 Corso, L, Cavallero, A., Baroni, D., Garbati, P., Prestipino, G., et al. (2016). Saffron reduces ATP-induced retinal cytotoxicity by targeting P2X7 receptors. *Purinergic Signal*, Mar;12(1):161-74.

40 Boehnke, C., Reuter, U., Flach, U., Schuh-Hofer, S., Einhaupl, K.M., et al. (2004). High-dose riboflavin treatment is efficacious in migraine prophylaxis: an open study in a tertiary care centre. *Eur J Neurol*, Jul;11(7):475-7.

41 Sándor, P.S., Afra, J., Ambrosini, A., Schoenen, J. (2000). Prophylactic treatment of migraine with beta-blockers and riboflavin: differential effects on the intensity dependence of auditory evoked cortical potentials. *Headache*, Jan;40(1):30-5.

42 Schoenen, J., Jacquy, J., Lenaerts, M. (1998). Effectiveness of high-dose riboflavin in migraine prophylaxis. A randomized controlled trial. *Neurology*, Feb;50(2):466-70.

43 Lipton, R.B., Gobel, H., Einhaupl, K.M., Wilks, K., Mauskop, A. (2004). Petasites hybridus root (butterbur) is an effective preventive treatment for migraine. *Neurology*, Dec 28;63(12):2240-4.5.

44 Grossmann, M., Schmidramsl, H. (2000). An extract of Petasites hybridus is effective in the prophylaxis of migraine. *Int J Clin Pharmacol Ther.* Sep;38(9):430-5. 6.

45 Diener, H.C., Rahlfs, V.W., Danesch, U. (2004). The first placebo-controlled trial of a special butterbur root extract for the prevention of migraine: reanalysis of efficacy criteria. *Eur Neurol*, 51(2):89-97.

46 Pothmann, R., Danesch, U. (2005). Migraine prevention in children and adolescents: results of an open study with a special butterbur root extract. *Headache*, Mar;45(3):196-203.

47 Ibid. Lipton (2004).

48 Ibid. Grossmann. (2000).

49 Mauskop, A. Varughese. J. (2012). Why all migraine patients should be treated with magnesium. *J Neural Transm (Vienna)*, May;119(5):575-9.

50 Pareek, A., Suthar, M., Rathore, G.S., Bansal, V. (2011). Feverfew (Tanacetum parthenium L.): A systematic review. *Pharmacogn Rev*, Jan;5(9):103-10

51 No authors listed. (2003). Zingiber officinale (ginger). Monograph. *Altern Med Rev* Aug;8(3):331-5.

15-17. LYME DISEASE AND VISION

Lyme disease is the best-known worldwide type of tick-borne disease, in which a tick, infested with a spirochete, bites a human and transmits the bacterium into the bloodstream. A spirochete is a bacterium with a spirally twisted form. The bacterium responsible for Lyme disease is called Borrelia burgdorferi, which burrows its way into various tissues in the body, in particular the collagen tissues. The number of Lyme disease cases in the U.S. has doubled since 1991. Each year, more than 30,000 cases of Lyme disease are reported nationwide, while studies suggest the actual number of people diagnosed with Lyme disease is more likely around 300,000.[1]

How Lyme Disease Spreads

In the northeast, mid-Atlantic, and north-central U.S., Lyme is spread by the blacklegged deer tick (Ixodes scapularis), and on the Pacific coast, by the western-blacklegged tick (Ixodes pacificus).[2] Other tick species not known to transmit Lyme disease include: Dermacentor variabilis (American dog tick), Ambylomma americanum (lone star tick), Dermacentor andersonii (Rocky Mountain wood tick), and Rhipicephalus sanguineous (brown dog tick).[3]

Lyme disease develops into a multi-system inflammatory disease caused by an organism called a spirochete. It may start with skin rashes and/or flu-like symptoms, and then later spread to the joints, central nervous system, and other organ systems. According to recent research, "There are at least 5 subspecies of Borrelia burgdorferi, over 100 strains in the U.S., and 300 strains worldwide. This diversity is thought to contribute to the antigenic variability of the spirochete and its ability to evade the immune system and antibiotic therapy, leading to chronic infection."[4]

Frequent Misdiagnosis

Only 50–60% of patients recall a tick bite; **the rash is reported in only 35–60% of patients**; and joint swelling occurs in only 20–30% of patients. A significant number of people who contract Lyme disease are misdiagnosed during the early stages, leading to a progression of the disease. In one study, 54% of the patients were initially misdiagnosed. Of these, 13% did not present with a rash, and of those with a rash, 23% were not diagnosed correctly, initially.[5]

Symptoms

The symptoms of Lyme disease can mimic many health conditions. Eye conditions related to Lyme disease include:[6] [7]

- **Conjunctivitis**, or redness and discharge due to inflammation of the conjunctiva, can occur in the early phase of Lyme disease.
- **Uveitis** is an inflammation of the uvea. The uvea is made up of the iris, the colored part of the eye; the ciliary body, which makes the fluid that fills the eye and flexes the eye lens; and the choroid, the layer beneath the retina.
- **Optic neuritis** is an inflammation of the fibers that cover the optic nerve. Symptoms include pain in the eye, inability to see color, and vision loss.

- **Keratitis** is inflammation of the cornea. Symptoms may include pain in the eye, light sensitivity, tearing, and blurred vision.
- **Retinal vasculitis** is an inflammation of the blood vessels of the retina. Though painless, symptoms could include gradual vision loss.
- **Branch retinal vein occlusion** (BRVO) is a blockage in the veins of the retina. There is no pain associated with a BRVO, but vision loss occurs if the blockage causes swelling in the macula and is not treated.
- **Diplopia** or blurred vision or changes in vision
- **Strabismus** and eye tracking conditions
- **Sensitivity to light** and glare and eye pain.
- **Swelling around the eyes**
- **Eye floaters**

Stages of Lyme Disease

There are 3 stages of Lyme disease.

- Stage 1 is characterized by a skin lesion or rash, which has a "bull's eye" appearance only 20% of the time; other rashes can also manifest.[8] The rash is usually accompanied by chills and pain in the neck muscles and extremities.
- Stage 2 includes multi-organ involvement with a predilection for affecting the cardiovascular and central nervous systems.
- Stage 3 is the chronic stage affecting the joints, peripheral nervous system, central nervous system, and subcutaneous tissues. This can occur months after the initial tick bite.

Bull's Eye Rash

The bull's-eye rash is not the most common rash.

One of the first symptoms of Lyme disease might be a bulls-eye rash, called erythema chronicum migrans, appearing in only 20% of cases. This rash usually radiates from the bite site as a red blotch or a central spot with a bull's-eye ring around it. The rash usually appears from one to two weeks after transmission of the disease and can be accompanied by joint pain (particularly in the knees), chills, fever, fatigue, and "brain fog."

Seventy-five percent of Lyme disease patients will have a skin discoloration that lasts from several days to several weeks, and it gets larger. The bulls-eye rash, not the most common manifestation of Lyme, occurs only 20% of the time. **"Rather, a uniformly red or reddish-blue rash, round or oval in shape, with sharply demarcated borders is most common."**[9] The rash commonly occurs in places that are moist and where clothing is snug: knee, groin, or armpit, occurring at prime tick season, such as the late spring and early summer. The multiple ways in which the immune system responds may explain the variety of outcomes.[10] The spirochete that causes Lyme disease has the ability to avoid immune cell attacks by creating a "biofilm" around itself. This takes time to do, which may account for why Lyme disease can develop slowly.

As the disease progresses, the symptoms can include severe fatigue, stiff neck, persistent headaches, and often tingling or numbness of the extremities and face. The central nervous system is invaded. If the disease progresses, the symptoms do as well, which can include cardiac abnormalities as well as cognitive and mental problems.

Because the spirochetes causing Lyme disease can invade almost every organ system of the body, symptoms such as nausea or vomiting, and a change in bowel functions such as constipation, diarrhea, or cramping can sometimes occur. If the urinary system is infected, it can create cystitis, or irritable bladder syndrome. Other neurological symptoms often include Bell's palsy (facial paralysis), poor balance, tremor, difficult speech, blurry vision, and neuropathies.

Prevention

Cover up. When in wooded or grassy areas, wear shoes, long pants tucked into your socks, a long-sleeved shirt, a hat, and gloves. Try to stick to trails and avoid walking through low bushes and long grass. Keep your dog on a leash.

Use insect repellents. Apply insect repellent with a 20% or higher concentration of DEET to your skin. Avoid getting onto hands, eyes, and mouth as chemicals can be toxic, so follow directions carefully. Apply products with permethrin to clothing or buy pretreated clothing.

Check yourself, your children, and your pets for ticks. Ticks can be very tiny (the size of a pinhead), so be sure to check yourself and your children carefully after being in areas where ticks are prevalent such as wooded or grassy areas.

Tick removal. Remove a tick as soon as possible with tweezers. Gently grasp the tick near its head or mouth. Don't squeeze or crush the tick but pull carefully and steadily. Once you've removed the entire tick, dispose of it, and apply antiseptic to the bite area.

Shower. Ticks can remain on the skin for hours before attaching themselves, so taking a shower after hiking or being in areas with a higher tick population is recommended. Use a washcloth to fully wipe down.

Remove habitat. Do your best to tick-proof your yard. Clear brush and leaves where ticks live. Keep woodpiles in sunny areas.

Conventional Treatment

Most people with Lyme disease recover completely with appropriate antibiotic treatment. For those who develop syndromes after their infection is treated, pain medications may provide symptomatic relief. Common antibiotics used include: Doxycycline, Ceftriaxone, Amoxicillin, and Penicillin, along with NSAIDS (nonsteroidal anti-inflammatory drugs) such as Ibuprofen to treat fever and mild to severe pain. But note that Lyme disease can recur.

Complementary Approach

Targeted nutrients, exercise, and lifestyle considerations can help reduce the symptoms of Lyme disease and help support the immune system (see Appendix 5 for recommended products).

Nutrients[11]

Essential

Vitamin C (buffered and preferably ascorbated). 1,000mg–2,000mg per day, split up with meals. This powerful antioxidant and immune supporter also has antihistamine actions that make this a powerful ally to support the body's ability to deal with Lyme disease. Vitamin C also has significant antioxidant actions, fighting free radicals, soothing inflamed tissues, and helping to maintain healthy connective tissue that is often ravaged with Lyme disease.[12] [13] [14] [15]

Important

Vitamin D3. 2000 IU–5,000 IU per day. Recent research shows how important this vitamin is in promoting bone health, modulating cell growth and proliferation, supporting immune and neuromuscular functions, and reducing inflammation.[16]

Essential fatty acids. 2,000 IU per day. EFAs support coronary health and also have strong anti-inflammatory actions, supporting the system as a whole, but particularly the joints.[17] [18]

Helpful

Probiotics. Probiotics are the beneficial bacteria that support all of the mucous linings of the body. These friendly bacteria support a healthy digestion as well as urinary function, and they act to control yeast in our systems. Poor digestion and yeast overgrowth (such as Candida albicans) deplete the immune function, leaving us more vulnerable to invasion by foreign pathogens, like Lyme spirochetes. Antibiotic treatments for Lyme disease do not discriminate between good or bad bacteria; they often kill them all, leaving yeast to proliferate. An effective probiotic will re-establish a healthy gut environment.[19] [20]

Coenzyme Q10. 50mg–100mg per day. CoQ10 is a powerful antioxidant that supports circulation and general coronary artery functioning, which makes it a significant player in the prevention and treatment of coronary artery disease. Its other main function is equally as important, that is, its vital role in the production of the body's energy on a cellular level.[21]

Magnesium. 500mg per day. Lyme disease and other tick-borne diseases have been shown to deplete magnesium from our body. Besides supporting the functioning of bone and the central nervous system, magnesium plays an important role in the repair of all body cells.

Herbal combinations can help boost the immune system. These can include: Astragalus membranaceus, cat's claw (Uncaria tomentosa), wormwood (Artemisia absinthium and Artemesia annual), nettle (Urtica dioica), olive leaf (Olea europaea), sarsparilla (Smilax ornata), barberry (Berberis vulgaris), clivers (Galium aparine), and eleuthero (Eleuthercoccus senticosus). Also see LymeOut Formula in Appendix 5 and other related Lyme formulas.

Glutathione (reduced form). 500mg–900mg per day, preferably in an intraoral or sublingual form where the dosage (5–10 times higher absorption rate than capsules) would be lower, as glutathione (GSH) is not well absorbed through the digestive system. Supplementing with amino acids, which are GSH precursors, supports GSH synthesis in the liver and reduces oxidative damage and inflammation.[22] [23]

Castor oil eyedrops (hexane free) help lubricate the eyes and help heal redness and irritation in the eyes and eyelids.

Tear stimulation homeopathic eyedrops help lubricate the eyes and support tear production.

Diet

Avoid sugar, refined carbohydrates, and processed foods. Sugar feeds the spirochetes! For example, white flour instantly metabolizes as sugar in the body after eating and affects us in the same way as sweets do, increasing inflammation and negatively impacting our immune response.

Eat fiber-rich foods, including vegetables, fruits, and whole grains.

Drink plenty of fresh water, up to twelve 4 oz. glasses every day. Since most of the bottled water we buy has been shown to be no better than tap water, it is best to drink filtered water. Proper hydration serves many essential functions that support the body's effectiveness in dealing with Lyme disease. Sufficient hydration supports the natural detoxification of the body's waste by making the kidneys work more effectively.

Lifestyle

Regular movement and exercise promote the circulation of energy and blood throughout the body. Many Lyme-literate doctors prescribe regular exercise to their patients because exercise supports the immune functions and helps to regulate the body's inflammation response.

Also See

Appendix 5, Recommended Products (for immune support and Lyme support)

[1] Center for Disease Control and Prevention. Lyme and other tickborne diseases. Retrieved Nov 22 2017 from https://www.cdc.gov/media/dpk/diseases-and-conditions/lyme-disease/index.html.

[2] Center for Disease Control and Prevention. Lyme Disease Transmission. Retrieved Feb 10 2018 from https://www.cdc.gov/lyme/transmission/index.html

[3] Ibid. Center for Disease Control and Prevention. Lyme Disease Transmission

[4] ILADS About Lyme. Basic Information about Lyme Disease. Retrieved Dec 20 2017 from http://www.ilads.org/lyme/about-lyme.php.

[5] Aucott, J., Morrison, C., Munoz, B., Rowe, P.C., Schwarzwalder, A., et al. Diagnostic challenges of early Lyme disease: lessons from a community case series.
BMC Infect Dis. 9: 79.

[6] Lesser, R.L. (1995). Ocular manifestations of Lyme disease. *Am J Med,* Apr 24;98(4A):60S-62S.

[7] Canadian Lyme Disease Foundation. Symptoms. Retrieved Mar 10 2018 from https://canlyme.com/lyme-basics/symptoms/.

[8] Columbia University Medical Center. Lyme and Tick-Borne Disease Research Center. 2011 Lyme and Tick Borne Diseases National Conference. Retrieved Feb 10 2018 from http://columbia-lyme.org/research/scientific.html.

[9] Ibid. Columbia. Lyme and Tick-Borne Disease Research Center. (2011).

[10] Ibid. Columbia. Lyme and Tick-Borne Disease Research Center. (2011).

[11] Five Element Healing. In Depth Healing Strategies for Lyme Disease. Retrieved Apr 4 2017 from https://fiveelementhealing.net/in-depth-healing-strategies-for-lyme-disease-new/

[12] Du, J., Cullen, J.J., Buettner, G.R. (2012). Ascorbic acid: chemistry, biology and the treatment of cancer. *Biochem Biophys Acta,* Dec;1826(2):443-57.

[13] Kaida, S., Ohta, Y., Imai, Y., Kawanishi, M. (2010). Protective effect of L-ascorbic acid against oxidative damage in the liver of rats with water-immersion restraint stress. *Redox Rep,* 15(1):11-9.

[14] Levine, M., Padayatty, S.J., Espey, M.G. (2011). Vitamin C: a concentration-function approach yields pharmacology and therapeutic discoveries. *Adv Nutr,* Mar;2(2):78-88.

[15] Cangemi, R., Angelico, F., Loffredo, L., Del Ben, M., Pitnatelli, P. (2007). Oxidative stress-mediated arterial dysfunction in patients with metabolic syndrome: Effect of ascorbic acid. *Free Radic Biol Med,* Sep 1;43(5):853-9.

[16] National Institutes of Health, Office of Dietary Supplements, Dietary Supplement Fact Sheets. Retrieved Dec 20 2017 from https://ods.od.nih.gov.

[17] Udell, I.J., Abelson, M.B. (1983). Chemical mediators of inflammation. *Int Ophthalmol Clin,* 23:1:15-26.

[18] Abelson, M.B., Butrus, S.I., Kliman, G.H., Larson, D.L., Corey, E.J., et al. (1987). Topical arachidonic acid: A model for screening anti-inflammatory agents. *J Ocul Pharmacol,* 3:63-75.

[19] Khanna, S., Tosh, P.K. (2014). A clinician's primer on the role of the microbiome in human health and disease. *Mayo Clin Proc,* Jan;89(1):107-14.

[20] National Institutes of Health. National Center for Complementary and Integrative Health. Probiotics: In Depth. Retrieved Dec 20 2017 fromhttps://nccih.nih.gov/health/probiotics/introduction.htm.

[21] Littarru, G.P., Tiano, L. (2007). Bioenergetic and antioxidant properties of coenzyme Q10: recent developments. *Mol Biotechnol.* Sep;37(1):31-7.

[22] Gurler, B., Vural, H., Yilmaz, N., Oguz, H., Satici, A., et al. (2000). The role of oxidative stress in diabetic retinopathy. *Eye (Lond),* Oct;14 Pt 5:730-5.

[23] Sekhar, R.V., McKay, S.V., Patel, S.G., Guthikonda, A.P. Reddy, V.T., et al. (2011). Glutathione Synthesis Is Diminished in Patients With Uncontrolled Diabetes and Restored by Dietary Supplementation With Cysteine and Glycine. *Diabetes Care,* Jan; 34(1): 162–167.

15-18. MACULAR DEGENERATION

Macular degeneration (AMD) is the leading cause of irreversible blindness, and it is the leading cause of vision loss among people over 60.[1] It is also known as age-related macular degeneration (ARMD). By the year 2020, an estimated 7.5 million Americans will suffer significant vision loss due to this disease. In 2010, 2.5% of white adults, age 50 and older, had AMD. By comparison, AMD affected 0.9% each of Blacks, Hispanics, and people of other races. The risk of AMD increases with age. The disease is most common among older white Americans, affecting more than 14% of white Americans age 80 and older.[2] Although there is no effective conventional treatment yet, natural remedies can go a long way to help prevent this disorder from progressing to the point of vision loss.

What is Macular Degeneration?

Macular degeneration is the slow deterioration of cells in the macula, a tiny yellowish area near the center of the retina where vision is most acute. This deterioration affects central vision, the vision used for reading, writing, driving, and identifying faces. With macular degeneration, straight lines become crooked, distinct shapes are blurry, lines become wavy, and a fog forms in the center of vision. Peripheral vision, however, is not typically affected.

If AMD is found first in one eye, the other eye tends to follow the same progression. This is because the nutrient deficiencies and other system-wide problems would exist in both eyes but manifest in one eye before the other.

The two most common types of macular degeneration are the dry and wet type. Most people with macular degeneration have the **dry type**, in which small yellow spots called "drusen" form underneath the macula. The drusen slowly break down the cells in the macula, causing distorted vision. In approximately 10–15% of cases, dry macular degeneration can progress to the second, more severe type called wet macular degeneration. In the **wet type** of macular degeneration, choroidal neovascularization occurs. This is a process in which abnormal blood vessels begin to grow toward the macula. These new vessels often leak blood, further deteriorating the macula, and causing rapid and severe vision loss if not treated.

There is a great deal of peer review research showing that the likelihood of the onset of AMD can be significantly reduced through healthy lifestyle choices such as diet,[3] [4] [5] regular exercise,[6] no smoking,[7] [8] avoidance of heavy drinking[9] (moderate drinking of wine may have a beneficial effect),[10] management of chronic stress,[11] avoidance of excess weight,[12] control of blood pressure[13] and high cholesterol,[14] and supplementation with targeted nutrients such as lutein, zeaxanthin, and omega-3 fatty acids (such as fish oil or DHA from algae).

Even when advanced AMD has developed, healthy lifestyle choices and targeted supplementation can still play a major role in slowing down and stabilizing the AMD. But lost vision, due to retinal cells no longer living, cannot at this time be regenerated, though excellent research such as with stem cells and the regeneration of lost retinal cells is underway. Keep in mind that patients can sometimes experience improved vision as retinal cells that are not active may still be living, but are low functioning. These cells can be stimulated and helped to be more active through diet, exercise, and targeted supplementation.

The Retina

Retinal Layers

The retina consists of four different layers:

1. Outer neural layer that contains nerve cells and blood vessels
2. Photoreceptor layer, a single layer containing the light sensing rods and cones
3. Pigmented retinal epithelium (RPE), with the Bruch's membrane separating the RPE from the 4th (choroid) layer
4. Choroid layer, consisting of connective tissue and very fine capillaries (choriocapillaries), that carry nutrients and oxygen to the cellular layers above them

The RPE's role is to nourish the fragile nerve tissue of the retina and maintain its health by providing blood and nutrients to the photoreceptor cells, getting rid of dead cells, secreting hormones, and modulating immune factors. It closely interacts with photoreceptors in the maintenance of visual function.

The choroid layer contains most of the eyeball's blood vessels. It is also the layer prone to bacterial and secondary infections. If not treated, abnormal blood vessel growth can readily develop, resulting in sight impairment or eventually, total vision loss.

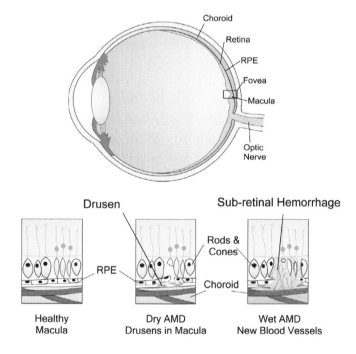

The Macula

The macula is located at the center of the retina where focused vision takes place. The remainder of the retina, at the margins or periphery, is more responsible for low light vision.

The macula contains two areas of unusually high concentrations of cones, which are the photoreceptors responsible for color vision, fine detail, and central vision. There is a slightly depressed area in the center of the macula called the fovea where there are no retinal cells, only photoreceptors, approximately 199,000–300,000 cones per square millimeter. At the center of the fovea is the foveola. Here too there are only cones, no rods.

The gradual breakdown of these cells in the macula results in damage to, or loss of, your central vision. Because the macula provides focus in the center of vision, where your vision sharpness is most acute, such deterioration reduces the ability to read and to recognize faces, two important tasks that require central vision.

Types of Macular Degeneration

Dry Macular Degeneration

Dry AMD, about 90% of cases, is also known as geographic atrophy. The atrophy results from the inability of the retina to reabsorb natural waste created in the retina in the process of passing light from the photoreceptor cells to the optic nerve (and other normal physiological activity). This further results in a slow deposit of the waste (drusen) onto the retina, which over time, can result in loss of healthy vision.

Drusen

Drusen are thought to be comprised of waste proteins and lipids (oily material) that begin to accumulate due to poor circulation and waste flushing in the eye. Antioxidants are important for the normal waste-clearing process and have the potential for reducing drusen in the eyes.[15][16][17][18] The drusen slowly crowd, distort, or break the cells in the macula, leading to deterioration, and resulting in blurred vision. Because drusen also include immune-system regulating molecules, it is thought that they are part of the immune system.[19]

Early Diagnosis

AMD has few symptoms in the early stages, so it is important to have your eyes examined regularly. If there are drusen on the retina, the initial diagnosis may not be dry AMD until the eye doctor determines that the number of drusen is increasing. For people who have early (dry) AMD in both eyes, about 10–15% will develop wet AMD in at least one eye after 10 years.

Wet Macular Degeneration

Untreated dry macular degeneration can worsen to "wet" macular degeneration. New blood vessels begin to form near the macula (choroidal neovascularization). These new vessels can leak fluid and blood, which may lead to swelling and damage of the macula. Unlike the more gradual course of dry AMD, wet AMD damage can be rapid and severe. It is possible to have both geographic atrophy (dry) and neovascular (wet) AMD in the same eye, and either condition can appear first. A retinal exam can identify whether there is leakage or bleeding in the retina or only drusen. Research shows that a healthy diet and taking targeted supplements can significantly reduce the onset of neovascularization.[20][21][22]

Stargardt Disease

Stargardt disease affects about 1 in 10,000 children in the U.S. Although the disease starts before age 20, you may not notice vision loss until age 30–40. It is a genetic form of macular degeneration where patients need to avoid supplements with vitamins that contain vitamin A and beta-carotene, foods high in vitamin A and beta-carotene, and certain carotenoids that can be converted to vitamin A in the body.[23] See more details in the Stargardt Chapter, 15-29.

Myopic Macular Degeneration

Myopic macular degeneration typically occurs in those people who are very nearsighted. In these cases, there is an extreme elongation of the eyeball, which causes stretching of the retina and can result in tears in the macula and bleeding beneath the retina. Over time, this can cause cells in the macula at the center of the retina to atrophy or die, causing a blind spot in the center of the visual field. In some cases, this form of macular degeneration can turn into wet AMD. People who are very nearsighted who generally require glasses of -6 diopters or more, are at risk for myopic macular degeneration. The risk is higher as myopia becomes worse than -10 diopters.

Pathology of Macular Degeneration

The development and progression of macular degeneration rests upon the occurrence of the following pathological changes in the eye:

Oxidative stress is the imbalance between free radicals and protective antioxidants. The retina is especially vulnerable to stress from free radicals. Inability of the retina tissue to have enough oxygen leads to deterioration of the pigmented layer, which protects the retina from UV and blue-light damage.[24] Antioxidants can significantly reduce the effects of oxidation stress.[25]

Angiogenesis, the development of new and extra blood vessels, is caused by insufficient oxygen in the retina. The tightly-packed retinal formation gets crowded by these additional blood vessels, and the retina becomes distorted. Targeted nutrients can inhibit such new and unwanted blood-vessel growth.[26]

Apoptosis, cell death, is a natural phenomenon in the body, by which worn and damaged tissue is removed and replaced. However, in the retina, excessive cell death is closely tied to oxidative stress.[27] Reducing oxidative stress through nutrients such as antioxidants and enzymes can reduce apoptosis.[28]

Inflammatory response is a process where the body rushes nutrients and oxygen-carrying blood to an injured location. The body always attempts to rescue tissue from cell injury due to oxidative stress through this response. However, this natural response can also result in vision damage over time, due to scar tissue and bleeding in the retina (angiogenesis).[29]

Signs and Symptoms

- Lines look distorted or wavy. Try the Amsler test (see Appendix 6 for both dry and wet AMD). In more developed AMD, the Amsler grid can look quite distorted.
- Shapes look blurred, fuzzy, or hazy in central vision.
- Colors appear dimmer and less distinct.
- Words are hard to read because they are blurred.

- Blank or dark areas hide the center area of your vision.
- The center of vision looks foggy or cloudy.

Causes and Risk Factors

AMD that is diagnosed from childhood into adulthood but before the age of 50 is typically considered to be the result of genetics.

One study determined that there was a 12-fold increase in the risk of getting macular degeneration if you have a sibling with AMD.[30] The risk factor was considered high if you have a parent with AMD.[31]

Heredity is a risk factor. People who have a family history of AMD are more at risk to develop it. The field of epigenetics shows that, even though one may have a genetic disposition for AMD (or any other health condition), environmental factors, including early childhood nurturing and lifestyle choices, can play a significant role in whether these genes become active or not.[32]

Free radicals can damage the eyes. They are formed when the blue and ultraviolet sunlight passes through the crystalline lens of the eye. Free radicals are also byproducts of our bodies' natural metabolic processes. These chemicals are highly reactive and cause oxidation; the result is destabilization of healthy macula cells.[33]

Phototoxicity is caused by exposure to blue and ultraviolet (UV) radiation, both of which adversely affect the functioning of retinal pigment epithelium (RPE) cells. RPE cells are susceptible to cell death induced by ultraviolet B (UVB) radiation. Exposure to sunlight without protective sunglasses is a risk factor for AMD.

Nutrition and diet can play an important role. Research has proven that elder people with poor diets are more prone to developing AMD. Micronutrient supplementation enhances antioxidant defense and healthy eyes, and it might prevent, retard, and modify vision loss.[34] People with AMD are often deficient in a number of nutrients that are essential to eye health: antioxidants, carotenoids, essential fatty acids, enzymes, minerals, and amino acids.[35]

Hypertension. People with high blood pressure are more likely to develop AMD than those with normal blood pressure.[36]

Smoking increases the risk of AMD by 200–300%. Smoking, chronic fatigue, and a weakened immune system hasten damage from free radicals.[37] [38]

Systemic inflammation, indicated by high levels of C-reactive protein, has been tied to increased macular degeneration risk.[39]

High homocysteine levels may contribute to AMD.[40] [41]

Women[42] and **diabetics**[43] are more at risk to develop AMD.

Prescription and over-the-counter drugs can damage the retina.[44] These include:

- Plaquenil (hydroxychloroquine sulfate), often prescribed for rheumatoid arthritis and found to cause permanent damage to the retina
- Catapres (clonidine hydrochloride is the generic name) for high blood pressure
- Chloridine (Catapres) for high blood pressure
- NSAIDS (non-steroidal, anti-inflammatory drugs) include ibuprofen, aspirin, ketoprofen, flurbiprofen, and naproxen sodium; side effects from regular use include retinal hemorrhages

Related Conditions

Poor circulation in the eye is a contributing factor to many eye conditions and is a side effect of diabetes.[45] Elevated homocysteine levels have been associated not only with macular degeneration but also glaucoma, diabetic retinopathy, optic neuropathy, and ocular complications from Behcet disease.[46] Also related are macular pucker or epiretinal membrane (where a thin layer of tissue grows over the retina), and retinitis pigmentosa (a degenerative disorder of the photoreceptor cells of the retina).

Conventional Treatment

No effective conventional treatment currently exists for dry macular degeneration. However, since the AREDS studies in 2001, 2003, and clarification in 2013, some eye doctors are beginning to recognize the value of nutritional supplementation.

Injections

Wet macular degeneration is typically treated with injections of Lucentis, Avestin, or Eylea. These drugs have antiangiogenic properties, meaning they help prevent the growth of new blood vessels, while drying up existing blood vessels that leak. The injections are typically necessary on an ongoing basis, depending on the severity and history of bleeding. Over the long run, they do not necessarily prevent vision loss; however, they can be essential for helping to slow down the progression of wet AMD. Moreover, these drugs are not designed to address the underlying problem, which in most cases is the inability of the body to deliver essential nutrients to the retina, and/or lack of critical nutrients, and/or inability of the eyes to naturally eliminate waste materials that are generated on an ongoing basis in the retina. Ultimately, our short-term goal is to stabilize the AMD, and the long-term goal is to maintain healthy vision and prevent additional vision loss. Drugs can have potentially serious side effects, so the benefits of using them should be evaluated with your eye doctor and your family.

Surgery

Laser surgery (photodynamic therapy) may be an alternative option to injections if the eye doctor determines that the injections may be ineffective or contraindicated for the patient. Your eye doctor will be able to provide guidance on the best therapy for you. Laser surgery accurately targets and seals leaking blood vessels through the injection of a form of ink into the blood stream, which gets absorbed at a much higher rate by leaking blood vessels than healthy ones. Then a non-thermal or "cold" laser is directed at the abnormal blood vessels in the eye for approximately 90 seconds. The laser activates the dye, which destroys the abnormal blood vessels and spares the normal retina and normal blood vessels.

Genetic Testing

For AMD Risk

Though genetic testing is available now to help determine one's risk of getting AMD, there has been some controversy among eye-care professionals as to whether genetic testing should be done for at-risk patients with certain genetic polymorphisms that have discrete genetic variations: CFH and ARMS2.

For Zinc Hyper-Immune Response

Sometimes certain supplements can cause problems for specific genetic variations of AMD. It has been suggested that certain patients actually do worse with zinc supplementation. In 2015, the recommendations from Bascom Palmer stated that there was not enough evidence to recommend routine genetic testing when considering supplementation. Dr. Stuart Richer, lead researcher in the last lutein antioxidant supplementation trial, recommends that the use of lower amounts of zinc (less than 50mg daily) is as effective as higher doses. He also recommends that genetic testing be offered to monocular-vision patients (where our two eyes have two views; we see near and far distance differently) to avoid the possibility of a zinc hyper-immune response, which is a possibility for 1 out of 7 high-risk AMD patients.

Complementary Approach

As always, prevention is the best medicine. Since less than 1% of people with macular degeneration have progressed to the point of legal blindness, most are in a position to benefit greatly from preventive measures, particularly at the earlier stages of the disease.

Taking targeted supplements and establishing healthy lifestyle habits are still helpful at any stage of AMD, keeping in mind that the preservation of vision and potential level of vision improvement is based on the vision level the patient has at the time of incorporating complementary approaches.

Proper diet, nutritional supplementation, and lifestyle improvements, including regular exercise and stress management, are fundamental to any prevention program, or adjunct to treatment for macular degeneration. Macular degeneration is a difficult disease to control, and we need to incorporate the best of current knowledge in nutritional support and supplementation.

Nutrients

Essential

Lutein. 6mg–20mg per day. Lutein and zeaxanthin are two similarly structured carotenoids that make up the macular pigment in the retina and help protect against damaging blue light (visible), as well as acting as powerful antioxidants. These carotenoids are also used in the lens of the eyes, and they act as a sort of internal pair of sunglasses that protect the eyes against damage from sunlight.[47] [48] [49] [50] [51]

Zeaxanthin. 2mg–12mg per day.[52] Lutein and zeaxanthin supplements are best taken separately from beta-carotene supplements because of competition for absorption. Lutein and zeaxanthin need fat to absorb well, so take them with food or a small amount of oil.

> Researchers found that a **moderate dose of 13.3mg combined carotenoids**, comprised of 83% lutein (11mg), 10% zeaxanthin (1.33mg), and 7% mesozeaxanthin (.93mg), was more effective than higher doses in enhancing **macular pigment**, even though higher doses were reflected in serum blood levels.[1]

What do lutein and zeaxanthin do for our eyes? The macular pigment is composed of lutein and zeaxanthin; this pigment functions as a color filter to protect the light-sensitive photoreceptor cells (the cones) from light-originated free-radical damage.

Omega-3 fatty acids. 2,000mg–3,000mg per day. Omega-3 fatty acids, found in fish, is a primary component of retinal photoreceptors and of the myelin sheath that surrounds nerve fibers in the eye. DHA (a component of omega-3 fatty acid) has been found to have antioxidative, anti-inflammatory, antiapoptotic, and anti-angiogenic (limiting growth of new blood vessels) effects.[53] [54] [55] [56] [57] [58] [59] [60]

Vitamin D3. 2,000 IU–5,000 IU per day. Numerous studies have found that low levels of vitamin D3 in the body can be connected to an increase in the presence of macular degeneration.[61]

Astaxanthin. 6mg–12mg per day. Shown to be effective in protecting against damage from light due to its antioxidant effect.[62] [63]

Mesozeaxanthin. 10mg. This carotenoid of the lutein family is found to help central vision in the retina. Studies show that supplementing with mesozeaxanthin helps protect central vision for those with AMD. One 2007 study found that levels of all three carotenoids (lutein, zeaxanthin, and mesozeaxanthin), when increased in the blood, increased macular pigment density.[64] [65]

Resveratrol. 150mg–175mg per day, (trans-resveratrol is a well absorbed form). It helps strengthen blood vessels and reduce inflammation.[66] [67]

Grapeseed extract. 300mg per day. Grapeseed extract has benefits similar to resveratrol,[68] helping to strengthen blood vessels, maintaining healthy platelet function and other aspects of platelet responses, and protecting the central nervous system from reactive oxygen species (free radicals).[69] [70]

Vitamin C (buffered and ascorbated). 2,000mg–3,000mg per day. As an antioxidant, vitamin C scavenges free radicals in the body and protects tissues from oxidative stress.[71 72 73 74 75]

Saffron. Studies have shown that saffron helps protect photoreceptor cells from damage and supports healthy circulation in the retina.[76 77 78 79 80 81]

Very Important

Bilberry. 120mg–180mg per day. Bilberry extracts have been shown to help nighttime vision, and it has potent antioxidative properties that are not only neuroprotective but also help suppress photooxidative processes. They have been shown to improve microcapillary circulation.[82 83 84 85]

Ginkgo biloba. 120mg per day. Ginkgo helps support healthy circulation to the eyes and body and helps maintain the normal function and tone of blood vessels.[86 87 88]

Glutathione (GSH), reduced. 500mg–900mg per day. This potent antioxidant has been shown to help protect retinal cells from damage. Best to take sublingually, as it is not well absorbed through capsules or tablets.[89 90] Sublingual doses are typically lower, as they are absorbed 5–10 times more efficiently than capsules or tablets.

Taurine. 750mg–1,000mg per day. Taurine is another potent antioxidant found in the retina. It is essential in helping the eyes eliminate waste and enhancing the rods and cones within the retina, which serve as visual receptors.[91 92 93]

Lycopene. 3mg per day. People with the lowest serum levels of lycopene, the most abundant carotenoid in the serum, were twice as likely to have macular degeneration when compared to those with the highest levels.[94]

Melatonin. A research study showed that a combination of melatonin (3mg), zinc (8.7mg), and selenium (50 mcg), taken before bedtime, helped stabilize AMD with some remarkable improvement in the fundus of the eye after taking the combination for 6 months.[95 96]

Helpful

Green tea. 500mg–750mg per day. The epicatechins (a natural plant phenolic antioxidant) have been found to inhibit ocular neovascularization and protect the microcapillaries of the retinal pigment epithelium.[97 98 99]

CoQ10. 100mg–200mg per day. Study findings strongly suggest that an appropriate combination of acetyl-L-carnitine, omega-3 fatty acids, and coenzyme Q10, which affect mitochondrial lipid metabolism, may improve and subsequently stabilize visual functions; it may also improve fundus alterations in patients affected by early AMD and helps reduce drusen.[100 101]

Selenium. 200mcg per day. AMD patients have low blood plasma levels of selenium.[102 103]

Dietary enzymes. These increase glutathione synthesis that can prevent free-radical induced apoptosis (cell suicide), which may help prevent or treat AMD.

Goji berries. A study found that daily supplementation with a milk and goji formulation increased the levels of zeaxanthin in the blood and increased protection from additional drusen formulation or loss of pigmentation.[104]

Diet

We recommend the Vision diet; see Chapter 7. Follow a strong alkaline diet to reduce overall inflammation in the body, as chronic inflammation has been identified as a contributing factor to macular degeneration.[105] Both local and systemic inflammatory processes contribute to the development and progression of AMD.[106] For some people, chronic inflammation may be related to leaky gut syndrome, so if applicable, an anti-inflammatory diet should be adopted.

Many research studies have shown that diet has a significant effect on health of the macula. Unfortunately, once a person has macular degeneration, a healthy diet is not enough to prevent this disease from worsening, so other interventions are needed, which may include conventional as well as targeted supplementation, diet, exercise, and lifestyle changes.

Very Important

Leafy greens. Make sure your diet includes plenty of fresh, preferably organic, dark leafy greens. These vegetables are rich in carotenoids, which help plants absorb light energy for use in photosynthesis, and they deactivate free radicals, meaning they have antioxidant properties and are helpful for the entire body. Two of these carotenoids, lutein and zeaxanthin, are of particular importance to eye health. So, even if you don't like vegetables such as collard greens, kale, Swiss chard, and spinach, you can add them to soups, puree them in green drinks, juice them with other fruits and vegetables, or add them to other greens in salads. The nutrients found in these healthy vegetables lower the risk of developing macular degeneration.[107]

Antioxidants. Diets high in antioxidants help protect AMD patients from vision loss and play two critical roles: first, they significantly reduce the risk of AMD onset, and second, they help protect AMD patients from vision loss.[108] [109] [110] [111] A diet high in antioxidants includes fruits, particularly colored fruit such as berries that are lower in sugar, and vegetables, particularly leafy-green vegetables and colored vegetables such as red, green, and yellow peppers.

Reduce sugars. Reduce or eliminate all types of refined sugars (particularly white sugar, but also fructose, sucrose, fruit juice concentrates, maltose, dextrose, glucose, and refined carbohydrates). This includes "natural" drinks that contain a lot of sugar, including all fruit juices. Even milk sugar, lactose, found in all dairy products, can contribute to macular degeneration. Sugar contributes to overall body inflammation and poor circulation throughout the body and eyes. In one study, those in the highest one-fifth of the dietary glycemic index, (a system that ranks foods, based on their blood-sugar effect on a scale from 1 to 100), had more than a 40% increased risk of significant macular degeneration than those in the lowest one-fifth.[112]

Water. Drink 8 eight-ounce glasses of water per day (preferably filtered or purified). This is optimally taken as a four-ounce glass of water every half-hour, to equal 16 four-ounce glasses. Our bloodstream can only effectively handle about four ounces at any one time. When you drink more than four ounces at a time, it means more work for the kidneys to filter water that hasn't had a chance to travel through the lymph system and clean body tissues. Adequate water intake helps maintain the flow of nutrients to the lens and release wastes and toxins from tissues.

Spring water without chlorine or fluoride is the best. Sip water throughout the day, and do not rely on feeling thirsty before drinking.[113] At the point you feel thirsty, your body is already dehydrated. Neurological changes start occurring when there is a 2% drop in total body water. Also, certain eye diseases, as well as general health diseases, have been associated with dehydration.[114]

Important

Reduce fats. Favor a diet moderate in fats, as high levels can disturb the proper balance of gut bacteria essential for proper digestion and overall health.[115] [116] Keep polyunsaturated fats to a minimum,[117] and eliminate any trans-fatty acids in your diet, which can increase cholesterol levels, free-radical activity, and inflammation, all of which affect the eyes' blood vessels.[118] [119]

Take **omega-3 fatty acids** from oily fish, such as wild caught salmon and sardines. These reduce the risk of developing AMD.[120] [121] [122] [123] [124] [125]

Limit refined carbohydrates.[126]

Dairy. Limit or eliminate dairy products. For some people, regular consumption of dairy products can exacerbate eye problems by causing sinus congestion, which can impair lymph and blood drainage from the area around the eyes. When lymph and blood cannot flow in and out of the eyes, nutrients cannot efficiently reach the eyes, and toxins and metabolic wastes are not eliminated as well.

Many people are lactose intolerant to some degree, so you may want to avoid dairy for at least one month to experience the effects and observe the differences in your body and eyes. As a general rule, reducing or eliminating dairy from your diet has many benefits.

Regular milk contains two types of beta-casein protein: A1 and A2. A2 milk, marketed under that brand name, contains no A1 protein. There is controversy as to whether A1 milk is more harmful than A2, but the evidence is not conclusive. It may be that the type of feed, chemicals, antibiotics, and pasteurization/homogenization cause problems rather than casein type.

If you want to consume dairy, you can try organic products from A2 cows. Alternatively, you can switch to goat milk since milk from goats does not carry the A1 gene, or at the very least, obtain fresh, raw milk from local farmers for the freshest product. In general, changes in lifestyle related to healthier vision and the taking of targeted supplements will start making a difference right away, though it may take 3–6 months before maximum benefits begin.

Juicing. Fresh vegetable and fruit juices are a great way to deliver nutrients to your body. Use at least four of the recommended foods below to make juice. We suggest as many organic products as possible.

- Broccoli, green and red bell pepper, raspberries, apples, copious amounts of dark leafy greens, and carrots
- You can add favorite fruits and vegetables. Don't use a lot of carrots, beets, and fruits because of their natural high-sugar content.
- Try to use room temperature vegetables and fruit.
- Do not add ice or very cold liquids since cold foods and liquids will eventually extinguish the stomach's digestive fire.
- Do not juice as often during the cooler months of the year, and instead, switch to vegetable soups or stews.

Lifestyle

The following are additional measures for the prevention or treatment of macular degeneration:

Microcurrent stimulation. Daily sessions at home. The MCS 100ile unit is the most researched unit used for retinal health related to AMD. The modality is both effective and safe according to researchers, and it has a positive benefit for AMD patients.[127] [128] [129] [130] [131] [132] [133] [134] For more information, see Chapter 10-3 about MCS.

> **Note**. Usage may vary depending on the type of microcurrent unit you use, so check with your healthcare practitioner to get proper instructions. Also, if you have a history of retinal bleeding, do not use MCS without checking with your eye doctor. Contraindications include having a pacemaker or a history of epilepsy.

Sunglasses. Wear outside in bright sunlight. They should be 100% UVA and UVB blocking lenses with wrap-around sides. Amber or brown lenses are the most effective colors for neutralizing the blue-light spectrum, which is as potentially damaging as UVA and UVB light. Wear sunglasses along with a three-inch brimmed hat.

Exercise regularly. Exercise positively affects the health of our bodies in many ways, including increased circulation.

Avoid aspirin. Aspirin thins the blood, so some doctors recommend it for improving blood flow to the retina; but several studies have shown that aspirin actually can cause macular degeneration through retinal hemorrhages.[135] Therefore, try to avoid aspirin, particularly if you have a family history of macular degeneration.

Do not smoke. Smoking increases the risk of AMD onset by 2–3 times.[136]

Avoid EMF. Avoid, or severely restrict, sources of non-native electromagnetic frequencies (nn-EMF). Higher EMF exposure leads to hypoxia, dehydration, and inflammation.[137] [138] [139] [140] Turn off all wi-fi signals at night such as the internet modem, wireless printers, cell phones, computers, etc.

Avoid blue light. Reduce exposure to artificial blue light from computer screens, cell phones, LED, and fluorescent lighting. Even low levels of blue-light exposure (400-470nm) may induce photoreceptor and retinal-pigment-epithelial cell damage.[141] Light-induced damage also increases with age, due to a decrease in protective enzymes such as superoxide dismutase (SOD). Artificial blue-light exposure appears to be more damaging at night than during the day.[142] Blue light permanently damages retinal cells, and once lost, they cannot regenerate. Replace all fluorescent and LED lighting with incandescent bulbs. Other lighting options include beeswax candles and Himalayan salt lamps. There are blue-light-blocking glasses (ex: Blutech lenses or complete protection BP1550 tints) that can be worn while on the computer, as well as blue-light-blocking programs that can be downloaded to your computer and phone.

Touch the earth. Ground yourself as much as possible by allowing any part of your body (bare skin) to directly touch the ground (by walking barefooted or by gardening without gloves). This allows you access to the earth's abundant negative ions that can protect us from free-radical induced inflammation and cellular damage. Grounding connects you to the earth's magnetic field and can protect your body from man-made EMF, UV light, and cosmic radiation.[143] See Appendix 7 for more information about grounding.

Eye Exercises. We recommend the following eye exercises:

- Palming
- Eye massage
- Near and far
- Hot dog

See Chapter 10 for how to do these eye exercises and where to find acupuncture points that are good for all eye conditions and overall eye health.

Other Modalities

Chinese Medicine

In Chinese medicine, the Liver "opens to the eyes" and is the primary meridian for supporting overall flow of energy and circulation through the eyes. The Kidney meridian nourishes the blood to the eyes, and the Spleen meridian also nourishes the blood while helping to prevent fluids from leaking from blood vessels. Other meridians may also be out of balance that can affect eye health, so an evaluation by an acupuncturist can best determine where the out-of-balances are and offer the optimal treatment strategy.

Chinese Medicine Patent Formulas

Xiao yao san is a classic Liver tonic used in Chinese medicine that supports healthy circulation and the free flow of energy in the eyes as well as throughout the body.

Ming mu di juang wan is another classic formula used in Chinese medicine for eye health. It helps nourish the Kidneys and Liver. It is known to help with blurriness of vision, tearing against wind, and conjunctive congestion with pain and swelling.

Celosia 10 was designed for retinal disorders on the basis of formulas described in Chinese research reports.

Homeopathic Formulas

Homeopathic preparations, such as macula homeopathic pellets (by Natural Ophthalmics), support macula health. Follow directions on the bottle.

Essential Oils

Carrot seed improves the eyes by protecting against macular degeneration, detoxifying blood vessels, toning the liver, relieving stress and anxiety, and providing many nourishing vitamins and minerals.

Frankincense has been around since antiquity, a sacred plant that can be helpful in showing us our visual blind spots. Frankincense tells us to "open up that third eye."

Keep essences away from the mouth, eyes, and mucous membranes; if a few drops get in one of these sensitive areas it may be uncomfortable for 15–30 minutes, but not harmful. You can lessen discomfort by adding a pure oil like olive or coconut oil to neutralize the irritating effect. For the eye area, dab a few drops around the outside of the eye. Do not put the neutralizing oil in the eye.

Combine ¼ cup of avocado oil with ¼ cup of calendula-infused oil. Slowly add 5 drops each of the essential oils. Then close the bottle and shake well; apply 4 drops of this mixture on your clean face. Massage in gentle circular motions. Leave overnight.

For more information, see Appendix 9.

Chelation Therapy

At least one case study has been published where chelation therapy was helpful for macular degeneration caused by blockage in the choroid capillaries.[144]

EDTA, a synthetic amino acid, is commonly used as part of chelation therapy, as it may directly remove calcium found in fatty plaques that block arteries, thus breaking up the plaques. In one study, the researchers found a clinically modest, but statistically significant, benefit of chelation therapy for cardiovascular events.[145] In another study, calcification in coronary artery disease was reversed by EDTA-tetracycline long-term chemotherapy.[146]

Caution. Chelation therapy removes minerals from the body, resulting in deficiencies. Your doctor will need to monitor mineral and kidney function.

Hyperbaric Oxygen Therapy

Hyperbaric oxygen therapy may be effective in the treatment of both wet and dry macular degeneration. The treatment involves inhalation of 100% total oxygen in a chamber where atmospheric pressure is increased and controlled, according to the Hyperbaric Medical Society.[147] [148] There was one report of exacerbation of macular edema linked to this therapy.[149]

Ozonetherapy

Two small clinical studies suggest that ozonetherapy triggers defenses against damage to photoreceptors by improving blood flow and various biomarkers indicative of dry AMD resulting in improved vision sharpness.[150]

Intravenous (IV) Nutrient Therapy

IV nutrient therapy is a technique in which vitamins and other nutrients are delivered directly into the bloodstream in an IV solution, flooding the body's cells with higher levels of the nutrients than they would get from ingesting them. IV nutrient therapy can help both wet and dry AMD by delivering essential nutrients needed by the retina to help maintain healthy vision.

In his August 2010 issue of *Bottom Line Natural Healing*, Mark Stengler, licensed naturopathic medical doctor, discusses intravenous nutrient therapy for macular degeneration. Although no clinical studies have been done, some anecdotal results have been impressive, for example, seeing more clearly after one 90-minute treatment.[151]

On the Horizon

Ultra-fast lasers deliver gene therapy to macular degeneration patients. By using ultrafast near-infrared lasers, researchers at the University of Texas at Arlington (UTA) provide hope for eye patients suffering from photo-degenerative ailments. The platform is an improvement from current therapies that mostly slow down, or stop, degeneration, but they do not repair damaged parts of the retina.

Epigenetic therapy integrates genetic based therapy, bio-identical hormones, and nutrition to help the body naturally repair itself at the cellular level, and it may reduce the number of injections currently needed for many with wet AMD.[152] [153]

Stem cell research has found that the cells comprising both dental pulp and the retina develop from certain stem cells. It may be possible to "re-program" these cells and coax them into becoming retina cells. There are many safety concerns, but it is a promising avenue of exploration.[154]

Implantation of a tiny telescope for end stage AMD patients involves using micro-optical technology to magnify images, which would normally be seen in one's "straight ahead" or central vision. The telescope is smaller than a pea and uses micro-optical technology to magnify images, which are projected onto the healthy portion of the retina not affected by the disease, making it possible for patients to see or discern the central vision object of interest. This procedure is performed on an outpatient basis.

Early diagnosis. There is a simple test, currently being researched, called AdaptDx, that may be available to assess retinal function and diagnose early macular degeneration.

Vitamin E. A study published in 2018 found that blue light changes and damages a signaling biochemical, phosphatidylinositol 4,5 bisphosphate (PIP2), causing cell death; alpha-tocopherol appears to reduce that change.[155]

Also See

Chapter 7, Vision Diet

Chapter 8, Nutrients

Chapter 10-4, Eye Exercises

Chapter 15-29, Stargardt Disease

Appendix 5, Recommended Products

Appendix 6, Amsler Test

[1] Macular Degeneration Partnership. AMD is the leading cause of vision loss of people over 60. Retrieved Oct 15 2016 from http://www.amd.org/what-is-amd.html.

[2] National Eye Institute. Age-Related Macular Degeneration (AMD). Retrieved Oct 31 2017 from https://nei.nih.gov/eyedata/amd.

[3] (2014). Micronutrient supplementation enhances antioxidant defense and healthy eyes and might prevent/retard/modify AMD. *J Ophthalmol*, 2014;2014:901686.

[4] Cooper, D.A., Eldridge, A.L, Peters, J.C. (1999). Dietary carotenoids and certain cancers, heart disease, and age-related macular degeneration: a review of recent research. *Nutr Rev*, 57(7):201-214.

[5] Chiu, C.J., Milton, R.C., Gensler, G,, Taylor, A. (2007). Association between dietary glycemic index and age-related macular degeneration in nondiabetic participants in the Age-Related Eye Disease Study. *Am J Clin Nutr*, 86(1):180-8.

[6] McGinness, M.B., Karahalios, A., Simpson, J.A., Guymer, R.H., Robman, L.D. (2016). Past physical activity and age-related macular degeneration: the Melbourne Collaborative Cohort Study. *Brit J Ophthalmol*, Oct;100(10):1353-8.

[7] Stanislovaitiene, D., Zaliuniene, D., Krisiukaitis, A., Petrolis, R., Smalinskiene, A. (2017). SCARB1 rs5888 is associated with the risk of age-related macular degeneration susceptibility and an impaired macular area. *Ophthalmic Genet*, May-Jun;38(3):233-237.

[8] Seddon, J.M., Willett, W.C., Speizer, F.E. (1996). A Prospective Study of Cigarette Smoking and Age-Related Macular Degeneration in Women. *JAMA*, Oct 9;276(14):1141-6.

[9] Cederbaum, A. (1989). Role of lipid peroxidation and oxidative stress in alcohol toxicity. *Free Radic Biol Med*, 7:537–5394. Biologically, heavy drinking may cause oxidative damage to the retina leading to the development of AMD.

[10] Obisesan, T.O., Hirsch, R., Kosoko, O., Carlson, L., Parrott, M. (1998). Moderate wine consumption is associated with decreased odds of developing age-related macular degeneration in NHANES-1. *J Am Geriatr Soc*, 46:1–7.

[11] Dougherty, B.E. Cooley, S. L.., Davidorf, F.H. (2017). Measurement of Perceived Stress in Age-Related Macular Degeneration. *Optom Vis Sci*, Mar;94(3):290-296.

[12] Zhang, Q.Y., Tie, L.J., Wu, S.S., Lv, P.L., Huang, H.W., et al. (2016). Overweight, Obesity, and Risk of Age-Related Macular Degeneration. *Invest Ophthalmol Vis Sci* Mar,57(3):1276-83.

[13] Hyman, L., Schachat, A.P., He, Q., Leske, M.C. (2000). Hypertension, cardiovascular disease, and age-related macular degeneration. Age-Related Macular Degeneration Risk Factors Study Group. *Arch Ophthalmol*, Mar;118(3):351-8.

[14] Sene A, and Khan A. et al. (2013). Impaired cholesterol efflux in senescent macrophages promotes age-related macular degeneration. *Cell Metab*, Apr 2;17(4):549-61.

[15] Feher, J., Kovasc, B., Kovacs, I., Schvoller, M., Papale, A., et al. (2005). Improvement of visual functions and fundus alterations in early age-related macular degeneration treated with a combination of acetyl-L-carnitine, n-3 fatty acids, and coenzyme Q10. *Ophthalmologica*, May-Jun;219(3):154-66.

[16] Ibid. Feher. (2005).

[17] Bucheli, P., Vidal, K., Shen, L., Gu, Z., Zhang, C., et al. (2011). Goji berry effects on macular characteristics and plasma antioxidant levels, *Optom Vis Sci*, Feb;88(2):257-62.

[18] VandenLangenberg, G.M., Mares-Perlman, J.A., Klein, R., Klein, B.., Brady, W.E., et al. (1998). Associations between antioxidant and zinc intake and the 5-year incidence of early age-related maculopathy in the Beaver Dam Eye Study. *Am J Epidemiol*, Jul 15;148(2):204-14.

[19] Seddon, J.M., George, S., Rosner, B., Rifai, N. (2005). Progression of age-related macular degeneration: prospective assessment of C-reactive protein, interleukin 6, and other cardiovascular biomarkers. *Arch Ophthalmol*, Jun;123(6):774-82.

[20] Seddon, J.M., Ajani, U.A., Sperduto, R.D., Hiller, R., Blair, N., et al. (1994). Dietary carotenoids, vitamins A, C, and E, and advanced age-related macular degeneration. Eye Disease Case-Control Study Group. *JAMA*, 272(18):1413-1420.

[21] Augood, C., Chakravarthy, U., Young, I., Vioque, J., de Jong, P.T., et al. (2008). Oily fish consumption, dietary docosahexaenoic acid and eicosapentaenoic acid intakes, and associations with neovascular age-related macular degeneration. *Am J Clin Nutr*, 88(2): 398–406.

[22] Seddon, J.M., Rosner, B., Sperduto, R.D., Yannuzzi, L., Haller, J.A., et al. (2001). *Dietary fat and risk for advanced age-related macular degeneration.* Arch Ophthalmol. 119(8): 1191–1199.

[23] Sofi, F., Sodi, A., Franco, F., Murro, V., Biagini, D., et al. (2016). Dietary profile of patients with Stargardt's disease and Retinitis Pigmentosa: is there a role for a nutritional approach? *BMC Ophthalmol*, Jan 22;16:13.

[24] Mares-Perlman, J.A., Millen, A. E., Ficek, T.L., Hankinson, S.E. (2002). The body of evidence to support a protective role for lutein and zeaxanthin in delaying chronic disease. *J Nutr*, 132(3):518S-524S.

[25] Vives-Bauza, C., Anand, M., Shiraz, A.K., Magrane, J., Vollmer-Snarr, H. et al. (2008). The age lipid A2E and mitochondrial dysfunction synergistically impair phagocytosis by retinal pigment epithelial cells, *J Bio Chem,* Sep 5;283(36):24770-80.

[26] Ibid. Seddon. (2005).

[27] Ibid. Vives-Bauza. (2008).

[28] Cai, J., Nelson, K.C., Wu, M., Sternberg, P., Jones, D.P. (2000). Oxidative damage and protection of the RPE. *Prog Ret Eye Res*, 19(2), 205-22.

[29] Boekhoorn, S.S., Vingerling, J.R., Witteman, J.C.M., et al. (2007). C-reactive Protein Level and Risk of Aging Macula DisorderThe Rotterdam Study. *Arch Opthalmol*, 125(10):1396-1401.

[30] Shahid, H., Khan, J.C., Cipriani, V., Sepp, T., Baljinder, K., et al. (2012). Age-related macular degeneration: the importance of family history as a risk factor. *Br J Ophthalmol*, 96(3):427-431.

[31] Ibid. Shahid. (2012).

[32] Ibid. Shahid. (2012).

[33] Ibid. VandenLangenberg. (1998).

[34] Ibid. VandenLangenberg. (1998).

[35] Buschini, E., Fea, A.M., Lavia, C.A., Nassasi, M., Pignata, G., et al. (2015). Recent developments in the management of dry age-related macular degeneration. *Clin Ophthalmol*, Apr 1;9:563-74

[36] Hyman, L., Schachat, A.P., He, Q., Leske, M.C. (2000). Hypertension, cardiovascular disease, and age-related macular degeneration. Age-Related Macular Degeneration Risk Factors Study Group. *Arch Ophthalmol,* Mar;118(3):351-8.

[37] Ibid. Stanislovaitiene. (2017).

[38] Ibid. Seddon. (1996).

[39] Mitta, V.P., Chisten, W.G., Glynn, R.J., Semba, R.D., Ridker, P.M., et al. (2013). C-reactive protein and the incidence of macular degeneration: pooled analysis of 5 cohorts. Ophthalmol, Apr;131(4):507-13.

[40] Coral, K., Raman, R., Rathi, S., Rajesh, M., Sulochana, K.N., et al. (2005). Plasma homocysteine and total thiol content in patients with exudative age-related macular degeneration. *Eye (Lond),* Feb;20(2):203-7

[41] Huang, P., Wang, F., Sah, B.K., Jiang, J., Ni, Z., et al. (2015). Homocysteine and the risk of age-related macular degeneration: a systematic review and meta-analysis. *Sci Rep*, Jul 21;5:10585.

[42] Feskanich, D., Cho, E., Schaumberg, D.A., Colditz, G.A., Hankinson, S.E. (2008). Menopausal and Reproductive Factors and Risk of Age-Related Macular Degeneration. *Arch Ophthalmol*, Apr;126(4):519-24

[43] Mares-Perlman JA, Millen AE, Ficek TL, Hankinson SE. The body of evidence to support a protective role for lutein and zeaxanthin in delaying chronic disease. Overview. *J Nutr*, 2002;132(3):518S-524S.

[44] American Macular Degeneration Foundation. Medication Cautions in Macular Degeneration. Retrieved Sep 21 2017 from https://www.macular.org/medications-use-caution.

[45] Wu, J., Uchino, M., Sastry, S.M., Schumberg, D. (2014). Age-Related Macular Degeneration and the Incidence of Cardiovascular Disease: A Systematic Review and Meta-Analysis. *PLoS One*, 2014; 9(3): e89600.

[46] Bleich, S., Roedl, J., Von Ahsen, N., Schlotzer-Schrehardt, U., Reulbach, U., et al. (2004). Elevated homocysteine levels in aqueous humor of patients with pseudoexfoliation glaucoma. *Am J Ophthalmol*, Jul;138(1):162-4.

[47] Snellen, E.L., Verbeek, A.L., Van Den Hoogen, G.W., Crysberg, J.R., Hoyng, C.B. (2002). Neovascular age-related macular degeneration and its relationship to antioxidant intake. *Acta Ophthalmol Scand*, Aug;80(4):368-71.

[48] Richer, S., Stiles, W., Statkute, L., Pulido, J., Frankowski, J., et al. (2004). Double-masked, placebo-controlled, randomized trial of lutein and antioxidant supplementation in the intervention of atrophic age-related macular degeneration: the Veterans LAST study (Lutein Antioxidant Supplementation Trial). *Optometry*, Apr;75(4):216-30.

[49] Souied, E.H., Delcourt, C., Querques, G., Bassols, A., Merle, B., et al. (2013). Oral docosahexaenoic acid in the prevention of exudative age-related macular degeneration: The Nutritional AMD Treatment 2 Study. *Ophthalmology*, Aug;120(8):1619-31.

[50] Landrum, J.T., Bone, R.A., Joa, H., Kilburn, M.D., Moore, L.L., et al. (1997). A one year study of the macular pigment: the effect of 140 days of a lutein supplement. *Exp Eye Res*, Jul;65(1):57-62.

[51] Bernstein, P.S., Zhao, D.Y., Winch, S.W., Ermakov, I.V., McClane, R.W., et al. (2002). Resonance Raman measurement of macular carotenoids in normal subjects and in age-related macular degeneration patients. *Ophthalmology*, Oct;109(10):1780-7.

[52] Delcourt, C., Carriere, I., Delage, M., Barberger-Gateau, P., Schalch, W. (2006). Plasma Lutein and Zeaxanthin and Other Carotenoids as Modifiable Risk Factors for Age-Related Maculopathy and Cataract: The POLA Study. *Inves Ophthal Vis Sci*, Jun:47:2329-35.

[53] Ibid. Delcourt. (2006).

[54] Ibid. Merle. (2001).

[55] Ibid. Smith. (2000).

[56] Ibid. Seddon. (2001).

[57] Ibid. SanGiovanni. (2005).

[58] Ibid. Cho. (2001).

[59] C. Delcourt, I. Carriere, Cristol, J.P., Lacroux, A. Gerber, M. (2007). Dietary fat and the risk of age-related maculopathy: the POLANUT Study. *Euro J Clin Nutr*, Nov;61(11):1341-4.

[60] Ibid. Chong. (2008).

[61] Millen, A.E., Meyers, K.J., Liu, Z., Engelman, C.D., Wallace, R.B., et al. (2015). Association between vitamin D status and age-related macular degeneration by genetic risk. *JAMA Ophthalmol*, Oct: 133(10: 1171-79.

[62] Piermarocchi, S., Saviano, S., Parisi, V., Tedeschi, M., Panozzo, G., et al. (2012). Carotenoids in Age-related Maculopathy Italian Study (CARMIS): two-year results of a randomized study. *Eur J Ophthalmol*, Mar-Apr;22(2):216-25.

[63] Otsuka, T., Shimazawa, M., Nakanishi, T., Ohno, Y., Inoue, Y., et al. (2013). Protective effects of a dietary carotenoid, astaxanthin, against light-induced retinal damage. *J Pharmacol Sci*, 123(3):209-18.

[64] Bone, R.A., Landrum, J.T., Cao, Y., Howard, A.N., Alvarez-Calderon, F. (2007). Macular pigment response to a supplement containing meso-zeaxanthin, lutein and zeaxanthin. *Nutr Metab (Lond)*, Pub. online May 11.

[65] Ma, L., Liu, R., Du, J.H., Liu, T., Wu, S.S. (2016). Lutein, Zeaxanthin and Meso-zeaxanthin Supplementation Associated with Macular Pigment Optical Density. *Nutrients*, Jul 12;8(7):E426.

[66] Ibid. Wang. (2014).

[67] Wang, S., Wang, Z., Yang, S., Yin, T., Zhang, Y. (2017). Tissue Distribution of trans-Resveratrol and Its Metabolites after Oral Administration in Human Eyes, *J Ophthalmol*, 4052094, 12 pp.

[68] Ibid. Wang. (2017).

[69] Vitseva, O., Varghese, S., Chakrabarti, S., Folts, J.D., Freedman, J.E. (2005). Grape seed and skin extracts inhibit platelet function and release of reactive oxygen intermediates. *J Cardiovasc Pharmacol*, Oct;46(4):445-51

[70] Balu, M., Sangeetha, P., Murali, G., Panneerselvam, C. (2005). Age-related oxidative protein damages in central nervous system of rats: modulatory role of grape seed extract. *Int J Dev Neurosci*, Oct;23(6):501-7.

[71] Chew, E.Y., Clemons, T.E., Agron, E., Sperduto, R.E., Sangiovanni, J.P., et al. (2013). Long-term effects of vitamins C and E, β-carotene, and zinc on age-related macular degeneration: AREDS report no. 35. *Opthalmology*, Aug;120(8):1604-11.

[72] Du, J., Cullen, J.J., Buettner, G.R. (2012). Ascorbic acid: chemistry, biology and the treatment of cancer. *Biochem Biophys Acta*, Dec;1826(2):443-57.

[73] Ibid. AREDS Research Group. (2001).

[74] Cangemi, R., Angelico, F., Loffredo, L., Del Ben, M., Pignatelli, P., et al. (2007). Oxidative stress-mediated arterial dysfunction in patients with metabolic syndrome: Effect of ascorbic acid. *Free Radic Biol Med*, Sep 1;43(5):853-9.

[75] Ibid. Cho. (2004).

[76] Falsini, B., Piccardi, M., Minnella, A., Savastano, C., Capoluongo, E., et al. (2010). Influence of saffron supplementation on retinal flicker sensitivity in early age-related macular degeneration. *Invest Opththalmol Vis Sci*, Dec;51(12):6118-24.

[77] Marangoni, D., Falsini, B., Piccardi, M., Ambrosio, L., Minnella, A.M., et al. (2013). Functional effect of Saffron supplementation and risk genotypes in early age-related macular degeneration: a preliminary report. *J Transl Med*, Sep;11:228.

[78] Alavizadeh, S.H., Hosseinzadeh, H. (2014). Bioactivity assessment and toxicity of crocin: a comprehensive review. *Food Chem Toxicol*, Feb;64:65-80.

[79] Broadhead, G.K., Grigg, J.R., Chang, A.A., McCluskey, P. (2015). Dietary modification and supplementation for the treatment of age-related macular degeneration. *Nutr Rev*, Jul;73(7):448-62.

[80] Broadhead, G.K., Chang, A., Grigg, J., McCluskey, P. (2016). Efficacy and Safety of Saffron Supplementation: Current Clinical Findings. *Cril Rev Food Sci Nutr*, Dec 9;56(16):2767-76.

[81] Corso, L., Cavallero, A., Baroni, D., Garbati, P., Prestipino, G., et al. (2016). Saffron reduces ATP-induced retinal cytotoxicity by targeting P2X7 receptors. *Purinergic Signal*, Mar;12(1):161-74.

[82] Muth, E.R., Laurent, J.M., Jasper, P. (2000). The effect of bilberry nutritional supplementation on night visual acuity and contrast sensitivity. *Altern Med Rev*, Apr;5(2):164-73.

[83] Matsunaga, N., Imai, S., Inokuchi, Y., Shimazawa, M., Yokota, S., et al. (2009). Bilberry and its main constituents have neuroprotective effectsagainst retinal neuronal damage in vitro and in vivo. *Mol Nutr Food Res*, Jul;53(7):869-77.

[84] Zhu, Y., Xia, M., Yang, Y., Liu, F., Li, Z., et al. (2011). Purified anthocyanin supplementation improves endothelial function via NO-cGMP activation in hypercholesterolemic individuals. *Clin Chem*, Nov;57(11):1524-33.

[85] Yao, Y., Vieria, A. (2007). Protective activities of Vaccinium antioxidants with potential relevance to mitochondrial dysfunction and neurotoxicity. *Neurotoxicology*, 28 93–100.

[86] Lebuisson, D.A., Leroy, L., Rigal, G. (1986). Treatment of senile macular degeneration with Ginkgo biloba extract. A preliminary double-blind drug vs. placebo study. *Presse Med*, Sep 25;15(31):1556-8.

[87] Fies, P., Dienal, A. (2002). Ginkgo extract in impaired vision--treatment with special extract EGb 761 of impaired vision due to dry senile macular degeneration. *Wien Med Wochenschr*, 152(15-16):423-6.

[88] Diamond, B.J., Shiflett, S.C., Feiwel, N., Matheis, R.J., Noskin, O., et al. (2000). Ginkgo biloba extract: mechanisms and clinical indications. *Arch Phys Med Rehabil*, May;81(5):668-78.

[89] Ayalaxomayajula, S.P., Kompella, U.B. (2002). Induction of vascular endothelial growth factor by 4-hydroxynonenal and its prevention by glutathione precursors in retinal pigment epithelial cells. *Eur J Pharmacol*, Aug 9;449(3):213-20.

[90] Sternberg, P., Davidson, P.C., Jones, D.P., Hagen, T.M., Reed, R.L.,et al. (1993). Protection of retinal pigment epithelium from oxidative injury by glutathione and precursors. *Invest Ophthalmol Vis Sci*, Dec;34(13):3661-8

[91] Birdsall, T.C. (1998). Therapeutic applications of taurine. *Altern Med Rev*, Apr;3(2):128-36.

[92] Shpak, N.I., Naritsyna, N.I., Konovalova, N.V. (1989). Taufon and emoksipin in the combined treatment of sclerotic macular dystrophies. *Oftalmol Zh*, (8):463-5.

[93] Lombardini, J.B. (1991). Taurine: retinal function. *Brain Res Brain Res Rev*, May-Aug;16(2):151-69.

[94] Mares-Perlman, J.A., Brady, W.E., Klein, R., Klein, B.E., Bowen, P., et al. (1995). Serum antioxidants and age-related macular degeneration in a population-based case-control study. *Arch Ophthalmol*, Dec;113(12):1518

[95] Stefanova, N.A., ZHdankina, A.A., Fursova, A.Z., Kolosova, N.G. (2013). Potential of melatonin for prevention of age-related macular degeneration: experimental study. *Adv Gerontol*, 26(1):122-9.

[96] Yi, C., Pan, X., Yan, H., Guo, M., Pierpaoli, W. (2005). Effects of melatonin in age-related macular degeneration. *Ann N Y Acad Sci,* Dec;1057:384-92.

[97] Lee, H.S., Jun, J.H., Jung, E.H., Koo, B.A., Kim, Y.S. (2014). Epigalloccatechin-3-gallate inhibits ocular neovascularization and vascular permeability in human retinal pigment epithelial and human retinal microvascular endothelial cells via suppression of MMP-9 and VEGF activation. *Molecules*, Aug 13;19(8):12150-72.

[98] Cia, D., Vergnaud-Gauduchon, J., Jacquemot, N., Doly, M. (2014). Epigallocatechin gallate (EGCG) prevents H2O2-induced oxidative stress in primary rat retinal pigment epithelial cells. *Curr Eye Res*, Sep;39(9):944-52.

[99] Li, C.P., Yao, J., Tao, Z.F., Li, X.M., Jiang, Q., Yan, B. (2013). Epigallocatechin-gallate (EGCG) regulates autophagy in human retinal pigment epithelial cells: a potential role for reducing UVB light-induced retinal damage. *Biochem Biophys Res Commun*, Sep 6;438(4):739-45.

[100] Ibid. Feher. (2005).

[101] Zhang, X., Tohari, A.M., Marcheggiani, F., Zhou, X., Reilly, J., et al. (2017). Therapeutic potential of co-enzyme Q10 in retinal diseases. *Curr Med Chem*, Aug 1.

[102] Tsang, N.C., Penfold, P.L., Snitch, P.J., Billson, F. (1992). Serum levels of antioxidants and age-related maculardegeneration. *Doc Ophthalmol*, 81(4):387-400.

[103] Mayer, M.J., van Kuijk, F.J., Ward, B., Glucs, A. (1998). Whole blood selenium in exudative age-related maculopathy. *Acta Ophthalmol Scand*, Feb;76(1):62-7.

[104] Ibid. Bucheli. (2011).

[105] Tan, P.L., Rickman, C.B., Katsanis, N. (2016). AMD and the alternative complement pathway: genetics and functional implications. *Hum Genomics*, 10: 23

[106] Kauppinen, A., Paterno, J.J., Blasiak, J., Salminen, A., Kaarniranta, K. (2016). Inflammation and its role in age-related macular degeneration, *Cell Mol Life Sci*, 1765–1786.

[107] Cho, E., Seddon, J.M., Rosner, B., Willett, W.C., Hankinson, S.E. (2004). Prospective study of intake of fruits, vegetables, vitamins, and carotenoids and risk of age-related maculopathy. *Arch Ophthalmol*, 122(6):883-892

[108] Wang, J.J., Buitendijk, G.H., Rochtchina, E., Lee, K.E., Klein, B.E., et al. (2014). Genetic susceptibility, dietary antioxidants, and long-term incidence of age-related macular degeneration in two populations. *Ophthalmology*, Mar;121(3):667-75.

[109] Hogg, R., Chakravarthy, U. (2004). AMD and micronutrient antioxidants. *Curr Eye Res*, Dec;29(6):387-401.

[110] Ibid. Vives-Bauza. (2008).

[111] Ibid. Cho. (2004).

[112] Ibid. Chiu. (2007).

[113] Kruse, J. (2012). Quantum Biology 5: Coherent Water=EZ Water. Retrieved Nov 26 2017 from https://www.jackkruse.com/quantum-biology-5-coherent-water/.

[114] Sherwin, J.C., Kokavec, J., Thornton, S.N. (2015). Hydration, fluid regulation and the eye: in health and disease. *Clin Exp Ophthalmol*, Nov;43(8):749-64

[115] Andriessen, E.M., Wilson, A.M., Mawambo, G., Dejda, A., Miloudi, K. et al. (2016). Gut microbiota influences pathological angiogenesis in obesity-driven choroidal neovascularization. *EMBO Mol Med*, Dec 1;8(12):1366-1379.

[116] Rowan, S., Jiang, S., Korem, T., Szymanski, J., Chang, M.L., et al.(2017). Involvement of a gut-retina axis in protection against dietary glycemia-induced age-related macular degeneration. *Proceedings of the National Academy of Science, USA*, May:114(22)4472-81.

[117] Age-Related Eye Disease Study Research Group. (2001). A randomized, placebo-controlled, clinical trial of high-dose supplementation with vitamins C and E, beta carotene, and zinc for age-related macular degeneration and vision loss: AREDS report no. 8. *Arch Ophthalmol*, 119(10):1417–1436.

[118] Cho, E., Hung, S., Willett, W.C., Spiegelman, D., Rimm, E.B., et al. (2001). Prospective study of dietary fat and the risk of age-related macular degeneration. *Am J Clin Nutr*, 73(2): 209–218.

[119] Ibid. Cho. (2001).

[120] Smith, W., Mitchell, P., Leeder, S.R. (2000). Dietary fat and fish intake and age-related maculopathy. *Arch Ophthalmol*, 118(3): 401–404.

[121] SanGiovanni, J.P., Chew, E.Y. (2005). The role of omega-3 long-chain polyunsaturated fatty acids in health and disease of the retina. *Prog Retin Eye Res*, 2005;24(1): 87–138.

[122] Merle, B., Delyfer, M.N., Korobelnik, J.F., Rougier, M.B., Colin, J., et al. (2001). Dietary omega-3 fatty acids and the risk for age-related maculopathy: the Alienor Study. *Invest Ophthalmol Vis Sci*, 2001;52(8): 6004–6011.

[123] Augood, C., Chakravarthy, U., Young, I., Vioque, J., de Jong PT, Bentham G, et al. (2008). Oily fish consumption, dietary docosahexaenoic acid and eicosapentaenoic acid intakes, and associations with neovascular age-related macular degeneration. *Am J Clin Nutr*, 88(2): 398–406.

[124] Merle, B.M., Delyfer, M.N., Korobelnik, J.F., Rougier, M.B., Malet, F., et al. (2013). High concentrations of plasma n3 fatty acids are associated with decreased risk for late age-related macular degeneration. *J Nutr*, 143(4): 505–511.

[125] Chong, E.W., Kreis, A.J., Wong, T.Y., Simpson, J.A., Guymer, R.H. (2008). Dietary omega-3 fatty acid and fish intake in the primary prevention of age-related macular degeneration: a systematic review and meta-analysis. *Arch Ophthalmol*, 126(6): 826–833

[126] Chiu, C.J., Milton, R.C., Klein, R., Gensler, G., Taylor, A. (2007). Dietary carbohydrate and the progression of age-related macular degeneration: A prospective study from the Age-Related Eye Disease Study. *Am J Clin Nutr*, 86(4):1210-8.

[127] Allen, M.J., Jarding, J.B., Zelner, R. (1998). Macular Degeneration Treatment with Nutrients and Micro Current Electricity. *J. Orthomol Med*, 13:10-12.

[128] Leland, D.M., Allen, M.J. (1993). Nutritional supplementation, electrical stimulation and age related macular degeneration. *J Orthomol Med*, 8:168-171.

[129] Shinoda, K., Imamura, Y., Matsuda, S., Seki, M., Uchida, A., et al. (2008). Transcutaneous Electrical Retinal Stimulation Therapy for Age-Related Macular Degeneration. *Open Ophthalmol J*, 2: 132–136.

[130] Reader, A,L., Halloran, G. (1997). Bioelectrical Stimulation in an Integrated Treatment for Macular Degeneration, RP, Glaucoma, CMV, and DR. *Fourth Annual Symposium on Biological Circuits*, Oct. Mankato University, MN.

[131]. Wallace, L.B. (1997). Treatment for Macular Degeneration Utilizing Micro-Current Stimulation, Journal of Optometric Phototherapy. *J Optom Photo*, March.

[132] Paul, E. (2002). The Treatment of Retinal Disease With MCS and Nutritional Supplementation. *International Society for Low-Vision Research and rehabilitation* at the Low Vision Congress in Gothenberg, Sweden

[133] O'Clock, G.D., Jarding, J.B. (2009). Electrotherapeutic device/protocol design considerations for visual disease applications. *Engineering in Medicine and Biology Society*, EMBC 2009. Annual International Conference of the IEEE. 2009:2133-6.

[134] Chaikin, L., Kashiwa, K., Bennet, M., Papastergious, G., Gregory, W. (2015). Microcurrent stimulation in the treatment of dry and wet macular degeneration. *Clin Ophthalmol*, 9: 2345–2353.

[135] Liew, G., Mitchell, P., Wong, T.Y., Rochtchina, E., Wang, J.J. (2013). The association of aspirin use with age-related macular degeneration. *JAMA Intern Med*, Feb 25;173(4):258-64.

[136] Myers, C.E., Klein, B.E., Gangnon, R., Sivakamaran, T.A., Iyengar, S.K., et al. (2014). Cigarette smoking and the natural history of age-related macular degeneration: the Beaver Dam Eye Study. *Ophthalmology*, Oct;121(10):1949-55

[137] Kruse, J. (2013). EMF 5: What are the Effects of EMF? Retrieved Oct 20 2017 from https://www.jackkruse.com/emf-5-what-are-the-biologic-effects-of-emf.

[138] Kim, J.H., Yu, D.H., Kim, H.J., Huh, Y.H., Cho, S.W., et al. (2017). Exposure to 835 MHz radiofrequency electromagnetic field induces autophagy in hippocampus but not in brain stem of mice. *Toxicol Ind Health*, Jan 1:748233717740066.

[139] D'Angelo, C., Costantini, E., Karnal, M.A., Reale, M. (2015). Experimental model for ELF-EMF exposure: Concern for human health. *Saudi J Biol Sci*, Jan;22(1):75-84.

[140] Patruno, A., Tabrez, S., Pesce, M., Shakil, S., Kamal, M.A., et al. (2015). Effects of extremely low frequency electromagnetic field (ELF-EMF) on catalase, cytochrome P450 and nitric oxide synthase in erythro-leukemic cells. *Life Sci*, Jan 15;121:117-23.

[141] Feng, J., Chen, X., Sun, X., Wang, F., Sun, X. (2014). Expression of endoplasmic reticulum stress markers GRP78 and CHOP induced by oxidative stress in blue light-mediated damage of A2E-containing retinal pigment epithelium cells. *Ophthalmic Res*, 52(4):224-33.

[142] Tosini, G., Ferguson, I, Tsubota, K. (2016). Effects of blue light on the circadian system and eye physiology. *Mol Vis*, PMC4734149.

[143] Kruse, J. (2012). EMF 1: Does Your Rolex Work? Retrieved Nov 28 2017 from www.jackkruse.com/emf-1.

[144] Kondrot, E.C. Macular Degeneration and Chelation. Retrieved Nov 28 2017 from http://www.fmpug.com/images/upload_files/Macular%20Degeneration%20and%20Chelation_Kondrot.pdf.

[145] NIH Research News. (2013). Chelation Therapy May Help Reduce Cardiovascular Events. Retrieved Nov 20 2017 from https://www.nih.gov/news-events/nih-research-matters/chelation-therapy-may-help-reduce-cardiovascular-events.

[146] Maniscalco, B.S., Taylor, K.A. (2004). Calcification in coronary artery disease can be reversed by EDTA-tetracycline long-term chemotherapy. *Pathophysiology*Oct;11(2):95-101.

[147] Undersea & Hyperbaric Medical Society. Retrieved Nov 28 2017 from http://www.uhms.org.

[148] Malerbi, F.K., Novais, E.A., Emmerson, B., Bonomo, P.P., Pereira, A.J. (2015). Hyperbaric oxygen therapy for choroidal neovascularization: a pilot study. *Undersea Hyperb Med,* Mar-Apr;42(2):125-31.

[149] Yonekawa, Y., Hypes, S.M., Abbey, A.M., Williams, G.A., Wolfe, J.D. (2016). Exacerbation of macular oedema associated with hyperbaric oxygen therapy. *Clin Exp Oppthalmol,* Sep;44(7):625-626.

[150] Borrelli, E., Bocci, V. (2013). Visual improvement following ozonetherapy in dry age related macular degeneration; a review. *Med Hypothesis Discov Innov Ophthalmol,* Summer;2(2):47-51.

[151] BottomLineInc. Slow Down Macular Degeneration with IV Nutrient Therapy. Retrieved 8/10/2017 from https://bottomlineinc.com/health/macular-degeneration/slow-down-macular-degeneration-with-iv-nutrient-therapy.

[152] Gemenetzi, M., Lotery, A.J. (2014). The role of epigenetics in age-related macular degeneration. Eye,Dec; 28(12): 1407–1417

[153] Wei, L., Chen, P., Lee, J.H., Nussenblatt. (2014). Genetic and Epigenetic Regulation in Age-related Macular Degeneration. *Asia Pac J Ophthalmol (Phila),* July-August; 2(4): 269–274.

[154] Levin, D. (2015). New Approach to Treating Macular Degeneration. Retrieved May 2 2018 from http://now.tufts.edu/articles/new-approach-treating-macular-degeneration.

[155] Ratnayake, K., Payton, J.L., Lakmal, O.H., Karunarathne, A. (2018). Blue light excited retinal intercepts cellular signaling. *Sci Rep,* Jul 5;8:10207

15-19. MACULAR EDEMA

Macular edema is the swelling of the macula, the small area of the retina responsible for central vision. It is the leading cause of vision loss for diabetics, and it is common in patients with retinitis pigmentosa. It is found in patients with retinal vein occlusion, central serous chorioretinopathy,[1] advanced macular degeneration,[2] inflammation in the eye, uveitis,[3] retinitis pigmentosa,[4] epiretinal membrane formation, vitreous detachment, and other vision conditions.

In other words, swelling of the macula, which causes distortion and potential vision loss, is a component or side effect of many other vision conditions.

What is Macular Edema?

The central 5% of the retina is responsible for our most detailed vision, enabling us to perform close-up activities such as reading, sewing, and seeing facial details. This very small area of the macula is rich in cones and nerve endings that detect color; it is also the area of the eye entirely responsible for daytime vision.

Macular edema is typically painless, although serious vision loss can occur if it is left untreated. The amount of vision loss and the time frame over which the vision loss may occur, depends on the severity of the edema and the time it has gone untreated. Macular edema rarely causes a permanent loss of vision, but recovery is often a slow, gradual improvement over two to 15 months.

With macular edema, blurring occurs in the middle, or just to the side, of the central visual field. It can appear as if you are looking through cellophane. Loss of vision may progress over a period of months, which can be very annoying because of the inability to focus clearly. It is ideal to seek out treatment the moment you notice symptoms.

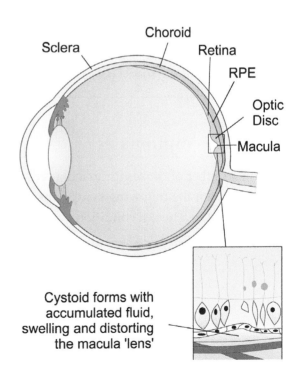

Cystoid forms with accumulated fluid, swelling and distorting the macula 'lens'

Types of Macular Edema

Macular edema is found as a primary or secondary result of many vision conditions including age related macular degeneration, retinal vein occlusion, diabetes, uveitis, a side effect of medications, genetic disorders such as retinoschisis or retinitis pigmentosa, rheumatoid arthritis, multiple sclerosis, or other chronic inflammatory conditions.

Cystoid macular edema (CME). This form of macular edema is characterized by the presence of cyst-like areas of fluid that accumulate in the macula and cause swelling and distortion. Researchers found that 44% of patients with moderately advanced retinitis pigmentosa have bilateral cystoid macular edema.[5] CME is one of several characteristics of central retinal vein occlusion where there is obstruction of the major vein that returns blood from the eye to the circulatory system.[6] It can develop after an occlusion, after eye surgery, in serious uveitis cases,[7] and in other conditions.

Diabetic macular edema (DME). About 3.8% of diabetic patients have been identified as having diabetic macular edema. Focal DME develops due to blood vessel abnormalities in the fovea of the eye (center of the macula); generally, diffuse DME is the widening or swelling of capillaries.[8] DME includes clinically significant macular edema (CSME) in which treatment is required.

Microcystic macular edema (MME). This variant is characterized by microcysts that are limited to the inner nuclear layer of the retina, and it is typically associated with optic neuropathy as well as other nervous system conditions such as multiple sclerosis. It apparently is caused by deterioration in the inner retinal layers.[9]

Pathology

Edema occurs when fluid, such as blood or other fluids, leaks from weakened retinal blood vessels into various layers of the macula. It is common for those with health conditions such as diabetes, rheumatoid arthritis, age-related macular degeneration, chronic uveitis, and central retinal vein occlusion. It can develop in response to cataract surgery, high blood pressure, atherosclerosis, and the use of prescription drugs. It also could be idiopathic, meaning there is no specific cause determined.

Signs and Symptoms

Due to the number of causes for macular edema and their complexity, there is no particular time frame as to when the following symptoms may occur, and not everyone who develops macular edema has a related health condition.

- Central vision seems blurry or cloudy.
- Vision is distorted; for example, straight lines may look wavy, especially when viewing the Amsler grid (see Appendix 6), a graphic that can help you test your central vision.
- Vision has a pinkish hue or colors might appear faded.
- Sensitivity to bright light and glare increases.

Causes and Risk Factors

Because many tiny capillaries surround the macula, *any* condition affecting blood circulation in the body (diabetes, atherosclerosis, etc.) affects the eye; the result may be macular edema. The reason this is important is that macular edema is usually a symptom of a more serious health problem that needs to be addressed. In the case of the latter, macular edema typically occurs within 1-2 months post-surgery; though it can even happen many months, and even years, afterward.

Important. Anyone with diabetes should have their eyes checked annually, at the least, as there are a number of eye concerns linked to this disorder.

Here is a list of the possible key causes of macula edema:

- **Oxidative stress.** The imbalance between the antioxidant defense system, production of free radicals (reactive oxygen species, ROS), cause oxidative stress in the body and in the tissues of the eye. Damage from ROS causes a host of problems, including inflammation and fluid leakage in the macula and other parts of the eye.

- **Other eye conditions**. Macular edema is caused by many diseases, including retinal vein occlusion, idiopathic central serous chorioretinopathy, macular degeneration, inflammation in the eye, diabetic retinopathy, anterior or posterior uveitis, pars planitis, retinitis pigmentosa,[10] retinopathy arising from radiation, epiretinal membrane formation, or posterior vitreous detachment. These disorders can be due to circulatory problems associated with hypertension, high cholesterol, etc.

- **Other health conditions**. The disorder can be related to general circulatory problems linked to hypertension, high cholesterol, and to nervous system-related conditions such as multiple sclerosis.

- **Diabetes**. A 2006 study of diabetics determined that 9% had macular edema; more recent evaluations find 3.8% in diabetics over 40. High levels of hemoglobin A1c, a biomarker for diabetes, are associated with higher diabetic macular edema risk.[11] Having diabetes for 10 years or longer increases the risk.[12]

- **Medicines**. A history of use of topical epinephrine or prostaglandin analogs for glaucoma is a factor.

- **Eye surgery**. Surgery for cataracts, glaucoma, or other retinal disease[13] can result in macular edema, sometimes months after the surgery. Edema can occur due to post-operative lesions.[14]

- **Ethnicity**. Non-Hispanic Blacks are at greater risk of developing diabetic macular edema.[15]

- **Injury**. If you injure your eye and notice fuzziness in your central vision, be sure to see your eye doctor immediately.

- **Inflammation**. Inflammatory disease disorders such as cytomegalovirus infection, retinal necrosis, sarcoidosis, Behçet's syndrome, toxoplasmosis, Eales' disease, and Vogt-Koyanagi-Harada syndrome[16] are often accompanied by macular edema.

Conventional Treatment

The first line of treatment for macular edema is usually anti-inflammatory eyedrops. In certain cases, medication is injected into the back of the eye for a more concentrated effect, possibly along with an injection of steroids. Injections may include: Anti-VEGF (vascular endothelial growth factor) such as (Lucentis, Avestin, Regeneron, and/or Eylea). Steroids can also be implanted into the retina that slowly release medication overtime, including Ozurdex, Retisert, or Iluvien. Oral medications such as nonsteroidal anti-inflammatory drugs (NSAIDs) or steroids such as Prednisone may be prescribed to reduce the swelling.

In some cases, a vitrectomy may be recommended when blood has leaked in the vitreous (the gel that fills the area between the lens and the retina), due to pulling on the retina. This surgery is typically done on an outpatient basis.

Complementary Approach

Taking targeted supplements and establishing healthy lifestyle habits are important, both for long-term help in reducing inflammation and for neutralizing free radicals that are produced in excess due to ongoing inflammation (which can destroy healthy cells and affect vision).

Nutrients

Essential

Astaxanthin. 6mg–12mg per day. Astaxanthin is a fat-soluble carotenoid that, in its value as an antioxidant, is 10 times more powerful than beta-carotene, lutein, or zeaxanthin, and is from 60–500 times stronger than vitamin E. Astaxanthin destroys the unstable molecules called reactive-oxygen species (ROS), commonly known as free radicals, and wards off their constant attack towards all parts of the body.[17]

Lutein. 6mg–20mg per day. Lutein is well researched in its ability to support the retina, reduce eye inflammation, and support the retinal pigment. Taking lutein along with zeaxanthin and astaxanthin results in significant improvement in visual acuity (vision sharpness).[18] Supplementing with lutein protects against retinal neural damage caused by inflammation due to uveitis (EIU).[19] [20]

Zeaxanthin. 2mg–4mg per day. Along with lutein, zeaxanthin is a potent antioxidant found in the retina that helps maintain the health of the retina and reduce the risk of macular degeneration.[21]

Bilberry. 180mg–240mg per day. Bilberry is neuroprotective and has been shown to improve microcirculation.[22] [23] [24] [25]

Omega-3 fatty acids. 2,000mg–3,000mg per day. This nutrient is essential for retinal health. Research also shows it has anti-inflammatory properties.[26]

Trans-resveratrol. 175mg per day. This potent antioxidant helps protect nerve cells from damage,[27] reduces oxidative damage,[28] and supports a healthy inflammatory response.[29] It also maintains the health of existing blood vessels while suppressing the growth of new ones (angiogenesis), similar to the neovascularization that can affect those with diabetic retinopathy. It also reduces retinal pigment epithelial (RPE) cell degeneration that leads to malfunction of blood-retinal barrier and loss of vision.[30]

Very Important

Alpha-lipoic acid. 300mg–600mg per day. This antioxidant compound improves insulin sensitivity in individuals with type 2 diabetes, and may prevent diabetic retinopathy.[31] One study showed that alpha-lipoic acid has beneficial effects on the development of diabetic retinopathy, and reduces oxidative stress in the retina.[32]

Curcumin (as highly absorbed phospholipid blend). 630mg per day. Curcumin is the active chemical component of the Indian herb turmeric, commonly used in Indian food preparations; it is also what gives turmeric its bright yellow color. Curcumin has been found to have blood-sugar-lowering properties related to diabetes,[33] anti-inflammatory properties,[34] and antioxidant properties.[35] It also has been shown to help protect retinal pigment epithelial cells against oxidative stress, which can be increased by chronic inflammation. Curcumin supports pancreatic function by encouraging pancreatic islet health.[36] A 2016 study found that curcumin stops blood vessel leakage.[37]

Ginkgo biloba. 120mg per day. Flavonoids such as quercetin and kaempferol derived from ginkgo biloba are potent antioxidants and scavengers of many species of free radicals, protecting against oxidative cell damage.[38] It stabilizes capillaries and makes them less fragile.[39] [40] [41] It also helps improve circulation by inhibiting blood clots, enabling better transport of red blood cells,[42] [43] and helps prevent damage in the eye due to low oxygen conditions or the formation of abnormal blood vessels.[44]

Glutathione (GSH), reduced. 500mg–900mg per day. Preferably taken in an intraoral or sublingual form (in which case dosage will be smaller, follow label instructions), as glutathione is not absorbed well through the digestive system. Glutathione is one of the super antioxidants that neutralize the full range of free radicals.[45] GSH is normally present in high levels in the ocular lens, cornea, aqueous humor, and retina where it performs multiple roles, including maintaining normal tissue hydration, lens transparency, and protects against oxidative damage that may increase through chronic inflammation often associated with macula edema. With age, GSH levels decline in human eyes.[46]

MSM capsules. 2,000mg per day, split up with meals or with water. MSM helps nourish and strengthen body tissues and has natural anti-inflammatory properties.[47]

Taurine. 750mg–1,000mg per day. Taurine is found naturally in high concentrations in the heart and retina; smaller amounts are found in the brain, kidneys, intestine, and skeletal muscle.

Taurine has also been reported to protect diabetics' visual function,[48] while helping to prevent damage due to oxidative stress. Deficiency of taurine has been shown to lead to retinal degeneration, and it has been used as a supplement with some success to prevent, treat, and stabilize retinal changes that may be caused by chronic inflammation.[49] [50] [51] [52]

Helpful

Serrapeptase. 500mg–800mg, 1–2 times per day, on an empty stomach. Serrapeptase has been found to help reduce inflammation for a number of conditions.[53] [54] [55] In use in Europe for over 25 years, it is believed to dissolve fibrin and other dead or damaged tissue without harming living tissue, thereby helping to reduce related inflammation and support cardiovascular health. Excess debris in the body can stimulate an ongoing immune response. The result is chronic inflammation in the body and the eyes, as well as circulatory problems due to scar tissue buildup in the blood vessels. Circulatory issues are directly linked to macular edema and numerous other eye problems, including macular degeneration, glaucoma, and cataracts.

Diet

Maintain a healthy diet with plenty of vegetables, fruits, and grains. We recommend the Vision diet and the Mediterranean diet[56] on which the Vision diet is based. We also recommend that you favor an alkaline diet. See Chapter 7 for more information.

Supplement your diet with a good daily multivitamin and/or a good organic green drink (typically 1 scoop in an 8oz. glass of water, fruit juice, rice milk, or almond milk).

Go organic. Organic products are more nutritious than conventional produce and do not carry the high levels of added synthetic hormones, pesticides, herbicides, antibiotics, and other toxins that conventional produce maintains.

Juicing. Juice daily and use organic produce, if possible. Our recipe to support retinal health is a combination of the following:

- Green, leafy vegetables, celery, cucumber, carrot, parsley, beets, all types of berries, apple, lemon, ginseng, green tea, and garlic
- Try using at least 4–6 of the above nutrients, plus your favorite fruits and vegetables. Avoid using too many carrots, beets, or too much fruit because of their sugar content.
- Try to use room temperature vegetables and fruit. Do not add ice or very cold liquids since cold foods and liquids will eventually extinguish the stomach's digestive fire.
- Do not juice as often during the cooler months of the year, and instead, switch to vegetable soups or stews.

Limit refined products. Lessen sugar intake (particularly white or refined sugar) and refined carbohydrates. Try stevia herb as a sweetener rather than sugar. Stevia does not affect blood sugar levels; it is far more concentrated, so you only need a small amount.

Avoid aspartame and other artificial sweeteners and foods labeled "diet." Aspartame is potentially cancer causing and is known to cause a wide range of symptoms, including headaches, heart palpitations, memory loss, insomnia, anxiety attacks, skin problems, loss of hearing and taste, seizures, diabetes, vision problems, and much more.

Avoid man-made fats such as corn oil, safflower oil, hydrogenated vegetable oils, trans-fatty acids (TFAs), including canola oil and most margarines, also trans fats foods (made with shortening or partially hydrogenated vegetable oils), such as doughnuts, biscuits, pies, cookies, crackers, muffins, and cakes. Consumption of TFAs increases total and low-density lipoprotein (LDL) cholesterol and decreases the "good" high-density lipoprotein (HDL) cholesterol.[57][58] Many other studies have also found an increase in the risk of coronary heart disease associated with intake of TFAs.[59][60][61]

Cut down on caffeine, coffee, and soft drinks. Watch your intake of soft drinks (three tablespoons of sugar per can!) and processed foods that contain sugar. Sugary sodas are linked to a 23% greater risk of heart failure.

Avoid monosodium glutamate (MSG), a flavor enhancer that is a potential retinal toxin.[62]

Avoid fat blockers like Olestra, which impair the absorption of carotenoids.

Eliminate or significantly reduce fast foods and fried foods.

Read the labels when you buy processed foods and avoid artificial flavorings and colorings. Foods that contain hydrogenated fats and trans-fatty acids disrupt the digestive process and contribute to an increased risk of cardiovascular disease.

Limit alcohol consumption to one glass of red wine daily. Alcohol potentially reduces protective glutathione levels because it interferes with liver functioning.

Lifestyle

Wear wrap-around sunglasses with 100% UVA and UVB protection whenever out in the sun. The best lens color is amber, which neutralizes blue light. Brown is the next best color.

Note: Cheaper glasses may have a coating to block out UV light that, over time, can rub off. Many people think it is the tint that helps protect one's eyes, but it is actually the UV filter on, or in, the lens that is helpful. A dark lens without UV protection increases pupil dilation allowing more light to enter the eyes.

Eliminate smoking. Smoking produces cyanide, a retinal toxin. A 2005 review of 17 research studies determined that the risk of macular degeneration in smokers is two to three times higher than in non-smokers. A 2015 study looked at this issue again, this time investigating specific damage to the macula as a result of smoking, and finding significant damage to many tissue layers of the macula.[63]

Limit the amount of medications. Talk to your doctor or get a second opinion to make sure that 1). you are not taking more medications (both prescription and non-prescription) than you need, and 2). your medications do not conflict.

Exercise every day. Get at least 20 minutes of aerobic exercise daily by walking, swimming, or engaging in other sports or activities that you enjoy.

Avoid microwaves. Steaming and slow cooking is the best option for retaining the maximum amount of nutrients in food. High temperature cooking and microwaving both cause greater nutritional deterioration. We feel that if you are going to use a microwave, then warming up foods in the microwave is preferable to cooking in the microwave.

Manage your mental health. Emotional well-being is very important to good physical health. Fear, anger, stress, etc., are important factors in many diseases. You can help balance your emotions through meditation, prayer, exercise, martial arts, etc.

Do yoga. One study found that 12 minutes a day of yoga brought about measurable changes in 68 genes, resulting not only in reduced stress, but reduced inflammation—an issue in diabetic retinopathy, optic neuritis, macular edema, heart disease, depression, rheumatoid arthritis, and diabetes.

Eye exercise. We recommend the following for macular edema.

- Palming
- Eye massage
- Acupressure points massaged daily

See Chapter 10 for eye exercises and acupuncture points that are helpful for eye conditions, as well as overall eye health.

Other Modalities

Chinese Medicine

In Traditional Chinese Medicine, edema is generally believed to originate in the following organ systems: Lung, Spleen, and Kidney. The basic principle is that when these organs fail to transport and transform body fluids, water is stored throughout the body, and edema results.

Patients generally respond to herbal treatment within 3–4 weeks, with a significant reduction in blood glucose levels and little fluctuation throughout the day. However, some patients may require up to 6–8 weeks.

Chinese Medicine Patent Formulas for Macular Edema

Ming mu di huang wan. Nourish the blood, Liver blood, and yin

Qi ju di huang wan. Nourish Kidney, Liver blood, and yin

Tien ma gou teng yin. Nourish yin and clear inflammation (Liver wind)

Shi hu ye guang wan. Nourish yin and clear inflammation (Liver wind)

Celosia 10 was designed for retinal disorder treatment based on formulas described in Chinese research reports.

Herbal formulas and treatment strategies can vary significantly based on the Chinese Medicine practitioners' evaluation and intake.

On the Horizon

Oxygen Therapy

A study on supplemental oxygen therapy for patients with diabetic macula edema showed an average of a 44% reduction in thickness of the center of the macula in three months.[64] Lack of oxygen to the retina apparently causes the macula to thicken. The increase of macular thickness that occurs due to DME can often result in a loss of visual acuity rather than the inflammation than the edema itself.[65]

Also See

Chapter 7, Diet and Vision

Chapter 9, Traditional Chinese Medicine

Chapter 10, Self Help and More

Chapter 15-6, Diabetic Retinopathy

Chapter 15-18, Macular Degeneration

Appendix 6, Amsler Test

[1] Schuler, K., Mruthyunjaya, P. (2006). Diagnosing and Managing Central Serous Chorioretinopathy.

[2] National Eye Institute. Facts About Macular Edema. Retrieved Feb 19 2018 from https://nei.nih.gov/health/macular-edema/fact_sheet.

[3] Goldhardt, R., Rosen, B.S. (2016). Uveitic Macular Edema: Treatment Update. *Curr Ophthalmol Rep*, Mar; 4(1): 30–37.

[4] Adakapara, C.A., Sunness, J.S., Dibernardo, C.W., Melia, B.M., Dagnelie, G. (2008). Prevalence of cystoid macular edema and stability in oct retinal thickness in eyes with retinitis pigmentosa during a 48-week lutein trial. *Retina*, Jan;28(1):103-10.

[5] Ibid. Adakapara. (2008).

[6] Channa, R., Smith, M., Campochairo, P.A. (2011). Treatment of macular edema due to retinal vein occlusions. *Clin Ophthalmol*, 5: 705–713.

[7] Ibid. Goldhardt. (2016).

[8] VSP. Diabetic Macular Edema. Retrieved Feb 19 2018 from https://www.vsp.com/diabetic-macular-edema.html

[9] Burggraff, M.C., Trieu, J., de Vries-Knoppert, W.A., Balk, L., Petzoid, A. (2014). The clinical spectrum of microcystic macular edema. *Invest Ophthalmol Vis Sci*. Feb 18;55(2):952-61.

[10] Ibid. Adakapara. (2008).

[11] Varma, R., Bressler, N.M., Doan, Q.V., Gleeson, M., Danese, M., et al. (2014). Prevalence of and Risk Factors for Diabetic Macular Edema in the United States. *JAMA Ophthalmol*, 2014 Nov;132(11):1334-40.

[12] Ibid. Varma. (2014).

[13] Ibid. National Eye Institute. Facts About Macular Edema.

[14] Ibid. Burggraff. (2014).

[15] Ibid. Varma. (2014).

[16] Ibid. National Eye Institute. Facts About Macular Edema.

[17] Maher, T.J., PhD (2000), Astaxanthin, Continuing Education Module, New Hope Institute of Healing.

[18] Piermarocchi, S., Saviano, S., Parisi, V., Tedeschi, M., Panozzo, G., et al. (2012). Carotenoids in Age-related Maculopathy Italian Study (CARMIS): two-year results of a randomized study. Eur J Ophthalmol, Mar-Apr;22(2):216-25

[19] Sasaki, M., Ozawa, Y., Kurihara, T., Noda, K., Imamura, Y., et al. (2009). Neuroprotective effect of an antioxidant, lutein, during retinal inflammation. Invest Ophthalmol Vis Sci, 2009 Mar; 50(3):1433-9.

[20] Jin, X.H., Ohgami, K., Shiratori, K., Suzuki, Y., Hirano, T., et al. (2006). Inhibitory effects of lutein on endotoxin-induced uveitis in Lewis rats. Invest Ophthalmol Vis Sci, Jun; 47(6):2562-8.

[21] National Eye Institute. (2013) NIH study provides clarity on supplements for protection against blinding eye disease. Retrieved Feb 18 2018 from https://nei.nih.gov/news/ pressreleases/050513

[22] Matsunaga, N., Imai, S., Inokuchi, Y., Shimazawa, M., Yokota, S., et al. (2009). Bilberry and its main constituents have neuroprotective effects against retinal neuronal damage in vitro and in vivo. Mol Nutr Food Res, Jul;53(7):869-77.

[23] Yao, Y., Vieria, A. (2007). Protective activities of Vaccinium antioxidants with potential relevance to mitochondrial dysfunction and neurotoxicity. Neurotoxicology, 28 93–100.

[24] Zhu, Y., Xia, M., Yang, Y., Liu, F., Li, Z., et al. (2011). Purified anthocyanin supplementation improves endothelial function via NO-cGMP activation in hypercholesterolemic individuals. Clin Chem, Nov;57(11):1524-33.

[25] Cohen-Boulakia, F., Valensi, P.E., Boulahdour, H., Lestrade, R. Dufour-Lamarinie, J.F., et al. (2000). In vivo sequential study of skeletal muscle capillary permeability in diabetic rats: effect of anthocyanosides. Metabolism, Jul;49(7):880-5.

[26] Udell, I.J., Abelson, M.B.(1983). Chemical mediators of inflammation. Int Ophthalmol Clin, 23:1:15-26.

 Abelson, M.B., Butrus, S.I., Kliman, G.H., Larson, D.L., Corey, E.J., et al. (1987). Topical arachidonic acid: A model for screening anti-inflammatory agents. J Ocul Pharmacol, 3:63-75.

[27] Anekonda, T.S., Adamus, G. (2008). Resveratrol prevents antibody-induced apoptotic death of retinal cells through upregulation of Sirt1 and Ku70. BMC Res Notes, Dec 1;1:122

[28] Perecko, T., Jancinova, V., Drabikova, K., Nosal, R., Harmatha, J. (2008). Structure-efficiency relationship in derivatives of stilbene. Comparison of resveratrol, pinosylvin and pterostilbene. Neuro Endocrinol Lett, Oct;29(5):802-5.

[29] Currais, A, Prior, M., Dargusch, R., Armando, A., Ehren, J., et al. (2014). Modulation of p25 and inflammatory pathways by fisetin maintains cognitive function in Alzheimer's disease transgenic mice. Aging Cell, Apr;13(2):379-90.

[30] Antonetti, D.A., Klein, R., Gardner, T.W. (2012). Diabetic retinopathy. N Engl J Med, Mar 29; 366(13):1227-39.

[31] Nebbioso, M., Pranno, F., Pescosolido, N. (2013). Lipoic acid in animal models and clinical use in diabetic retinopathy. Expert Opin Pharmacother, Sep;14(13):1829-38.

[32] Kowluru, R.A., Odenbach, S. (2004). Effect of long-term administration of alpha-lipoic acid on retinal capillary cell death and the development of retinopathy in diabetic rats. Diabetes, 2004 Dec;53(12):3233-8.

[33] Srinivasan, M. (1972). Effect of curcumin on blood sugar as seen in a diabetic subject. Indian J Med Sci, Apr; 26(4):269-70.

[34] Srimal, R.C., Dhawan, B.N. (1972). Pharmacology of diferuloyl methane (curcumin), a non-steroidal anti-inflammatory agent. J Pharm Pharmacol, Jun; 25(6):447-52.

[35] Sharma, O.P. (1976). Antioxidant activity of curcumin and related compounds. Biochem Pharmaco, Aug 1; 25(15):1811-2.

[36] Woo, J.M., Shin, D.Y., Lee, S.J., Joe, Y., Zheng, M., et al. (2012). Curcumin protects retinal pigment epithelial cells against oxidative stress via induction of heme oxygenase-1 expression and reduction of reactive oxygen. Mol Vis, 18: 901–908.

[37] Li, J., Wang, P., Ying, J., Chen, Z., Yu, S. (2016). Curcumin Attenuates Retinal Vascular Leakage by Inhibiting Calcium/Calmodulin-Dependent Protein Kinase II Activity in Streptozotocin-Induced Diabetes. Cell Physiol Biochem, 39(3):1196-208.

[38] Feng, X., Zhang, L., Zhu, H. (2009). Comparative anticancer and antioxidant activities of different ingredients of Ginkgo biloba extract (EGb 761). Planta Med, Jun;75(8):792-6.

[39] Welt, K., Weiss, J., Martin, R., Hermsdorf, T., Drews, S., et al. (2007). Ginkgo biloba extract protects rat kidney from diabetic and hypoxic damage. Phytomedicine, Feb;14(2-3):196-203.

[40] Ibid. Qiu. (2004).

[41] Huang, S.Y., Jeng, C., Kao, S.C., Yu, J.J., Liu, D.Z., (2004). Improved haemorrheological properties by Ginkgo biloba extract (Egb 761) in type 2 diabetes mellitus complicated with retinopathy. Clin Nutr. Aug;23(4):615-21.

[42] Ibid. Oh. (2013).

[43] Lanthony, P., Cosson, J.P., (1988). Evolution of color vision in diabetic retinopathy treated by extract of Ginkgo biloba. *J Ophthalmol*, 11:671–74.

[44] Ibid. Oh. (2013).

[45] Ibid. Huang. (2004).

[46] Harding, J.J. (1970). Free and protein-bound glutathione in normal and cataractous human lenses. *Biochem J*, May; 117(5):957-60.

[47] Butawan, M., Benjamin, R.L., Bloomer, R.J. (2017). Methylsulfonylmethane: Applications and Safety of a Novel Dietary Supplement. *Nutrients*, Mar 16;9(3).

[48] Yu, X., Xu, Z., Mi, M., Xu, H., Zhu, J., et al. (2008). Dietary taurine supplementation ameliorates diabetic retinopathy via anti-excitotoxicity of glutamate in streptozotocin-induced Sprague-Dawley rats. *Neurochem Res*, 33:500–7.

[49] Birdsall, T.C. (1998). Therapeutic applications of taurine. *Altern Med Rev*, Apr;3(2):128-36.

[50] Shpak, N.I., Naritsyna, N.I., Konovalova, N.V. (1989). Taufon and emoksipin in the combined treatment of sclerotic macular dystrophies. *Oftalmol Zh*, (8):463-5.

[51] Lombardini, J.B. (1991). Taurine: retinal function. *Brain Res Brain Res Rev*, May-Aug;16(2):151-69.

[52] Imaki, H., Moretz, R., Wisniewski, H., Neuringer, M., Sturman, J. (1987). Retinal degeneration in 3-month-old rhesus monkey infants fed a taurine-free human infant formula. *J Neurosci Res*, 18(4):602-14.

[53] Mazzone, A., Catalani, M., Costanzo, M., Drusian, A. Mandoli, A., et al. (1990). Evaluation of serratia peptidase in acute or chronic inflammation of otorhinolaryngology pathology: a multicentre, double-blind, randomized trial versus placebo. *J Int Med Res*, 18 (5); 379-88.

[54] Tachibana, M, Mizukoshi, O., Harada, Y., Kawamoto, K., Nakai, Y. (1984). A muti-centre, double-blind study of serrapeptase versus placebo in post-antrotomy buccal swelling. *Pharmatherapeutica*, 3(8); 526-30.

[55] Panagariya A, Sharma AK. (1999). A preliminary trial of serratiopeptidase in patients with carpal tunnel syndrome. *J Assoc Physicians India*, 47 (12); 1170-1172.

[56] Ibid. National Eye Institute. (2013).

[57] Mensink, R.P., Katan, M.B. (1990). Effect of dietary trans fatty acids on high-density and low-density lipoprotein cholesterol levels in healthy subjects. *N Engl J Med*, Aug 16; 323(7):439-45.

[58] Willett, W.C., Stampfer, M.J., Manson, J.E., Colditz, G.A., Speizer, F.E., et al, Intake of trans fatty acids and risk of coronary heart disease among women. *Lancet*, Mar 6; 341(8845):581-5.

[59] Mozaffarian, D., Katan, M.B., Ascherio, A., Stampfer, M.J., Willett, W.C. (2006). Review Trans fatty acids and cardiovascular disease. *N Engl J Med*, Apr 13; 354(15):1601-13.

[60] Hu, F.B., Stampfer, M.J., Manson, J.E., Rimm, E., Colditz, G.A., et al. (1997). Dietary fat intake and the risk of coronary heart disease in women. *N Engl J Med*, Nov 20; 337(21):1491-9.

[61] Ascherio, A., Willett, W.C. (1997). (1997). Review Health effects of trans fatty acids. *Am J Clin Nutr*, Oct; 66(4 Suppl):1006S-1010S.

[62] Agarwal, R., Gupta, S.K., Agarwal, P., Saxena, R., Agrawal, S.S. (2009). Current concepts in the pathology of glaucoma. *Inv Oph*, 37: 1618-24).

[63] Thornton, J., Edwards, R., Mitchell, P., Harrison, R.A., Buchan, I., Kelly, S.P. (2005). Smoking and age-related macular degeneration: a review of association. *Eye (Lond)*, Sep;19(9):935-44.

[64] Nguyen, Q.D., Shah, S.M., Van Anden, E., Sung, J.U., Vitale, S., et al. (2004). Supplemental oxygen improves diabetic macular edema: a pilot study. *Invest Ophthalmol Vis Sci*, Feb;45(2):617-24.

[65] Nussenblatt, R.B., Kaufman, S.C., Palestine, A.G., Davis, M.D., Ferris, F.L. (1987). Macular thickening and visual acuity. Measurement in patients with cystoid macular edema. *Ophthalmology*, Sep; 94(9):1134-9.

15-20. MACULAR HOLE

The macula is located at the center of the retina and provides the sharp, central vision we need for reading, driving, and seeing fine detail. When a hole develops in the macula, central vision can become distorted or darkened and potentially, over time, lost if not treated. In the U.S., for those over 55 years, the prevalence is about .33%, with most macular holes arising when the patient enters their 70s. Women are generally affected more than men. Internationally, the rate is lower, .16% in China and .17% in India.[1]

What is a Macular Hole?

A macular hole is a small hole in the macula that is at the center of the retina. The eye contains a jelly-like substance called the vitreous. With age, the vitreous contracts and pulls away from the retina surface. Usually, this separation occurs without noticeable negative effect. The patient might notice floaters and possibly flashes but there is no significant visual change.

For some people, however, in areas where the vitreous is firmly attached to the retina surface, pulling can occur on the retina, and a small hole may eventually form in the macula. In addition, as we age, the vitreous fluid becomes more liquid and less gel-like. At times it can seep through the resulting defect and cause a dark spot or defect in the patient's central vision, noticed through distortion and loss of central vision.

Pathology

Trauma-Related Macular Hole

Trauma-caused macular holes are thought to be linked to a concussive blow delivered from the opposite site of the head. As a result, the macula ruptures at its thinnest point.[2]

Idiopathic-Related Macular Hole

The retina is connected tightly to the vitreous, a layer surrounding the interior of the eye that is filled with vitreous gel. The vitreous is constructed of millions of very fine intertwined fibers. As we age, the vitreous gel begins to liquefy and/or clump and shrink.

Idiopathic macular holes are caused by pulling of the vitreous to the side (at a tangent) as the gel and vitreous sac contracts. The retina is attached to the vitreous, and when the vitreous shrinks, it pulls the retina and creates a hole at the thinnest part of the macula. Both retinal and vitreous detachments are aggravated by the contracting vitreous. There are four stages of idiopathic macular holes.[3] Each stage has distinct visual characteristics that allow an eye doctor to identify the severity in an eye exam.

Stage 1a. Foveal elevation. The fovea is a slight depression in the retina where the center of vision is focused. It is colored yellow, due to the concentration of carotenoid pigments located there. This first stage is, therefore, often called the yellow-dot stage, because the yellow color becomes more prominent.[4]

Stage 1b. Foveal detachment. The foveal part of the retina raises to the level of surrounding tissue, and the yellow dot changes to a yellow doughnut shaped ring around the fovea. Continued pulling leads to rupture of the deeper layers of the retina at the raised fovea.[5]

Fifty percent of cases may improve without treatment in stages 1a and 1b.

Stage 2. Partial-thickness hole. The hole is less than 400 microns in size. This is actually a full thickness hole, but there may be a thin cap or top layer that is raised but still partly attached. In stage 2 macular holes, about 70% of cases will worsen without treatment.

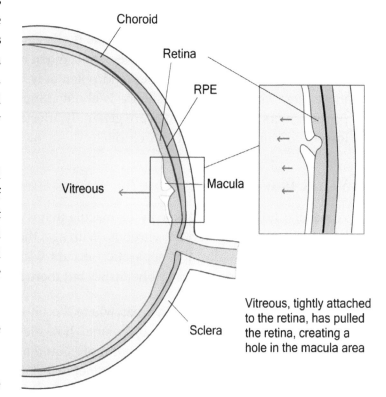

Vitreous, tightly attached to the retina, has pulled the retina, creating a hole in the macula area

Stage 3. Full-thickness hole. A full thickness hole exists, the top cap (pseudo-operculum) has fallen away. The hole is greater than 400 microns in size, and it is still being pulled by the contracted vitreous.[6] This phase causes severe central vision loss.

Stage 4. Full-thickness hole and **complete vitreous detachment.** A thin shell of vitreous may remain to contribute to the enlargement of the hole.[7]

Signs and Symptoms

The severity of the symptoms is dependent upon whether the hole is partial or full-thickness. Signs and symptoms include:

- Distorted, wavy vision
- Blurred central vision
- Difficulty in detail tasks, such as reading
- Central blind spot or gray area

Causes and Risk Factors

There have been a few studies to determine the causes and distribution of macular holes, and a few risk factors have been suggested, such as cardiovascular disease, hypertension, and hysterectomy, but none of these risks were statistically significant.[8] Trauma or injury to the eye causes a macular hole less than 10% of the time.[9] Usually these holes seem to develop spontaneously. The medical term describing this type of development is *idiopathic*, which means the cause is unknown. There may be other factors. Researchers have reported cases of macular hole formation after complete posterior vitreous detachment and vitrectomy. Other theories have been proposed such as a fluid-flow theory. Despite the prevalence of this condition in women, no clear associations have been made.[10]

Conventional Treatment

Surgery is often used to treat severe macular holes. A surgical procedure called *vitrectomy* is often used to treat holes that go all the way through the macula. The vitreous is removed to prevent it from pulling on the retina. It is replaced with a gas bubble that eventually fills with natural fluids. Following surgery, usually patients must keep their faces down for about a week. This position allows the bubble to press against the macula and seal the hole. The air bubble itself, however, may take anywhere from 6-8 weeks to be gradually reabsorbed by the body, and the vitreous cavity is then filled with liquid that is produced by cells in the front of the eye.

Recovery of vision varies. Vitrectomy can lead to complications; the most common reaction is an increased risk of cataract development. Other less common complications include infection and retinal detachment either during surgery or afterward.

Complementary Approach

While surgery is generally considered necessary at a certain stage of macular hole progress, with good nutrition we may prevent connective tissue impairments. About 50% of "stage 1" macular holes can heal by themselves. Targeted supplements, along with a healthy diet and regular exercise, can nourish the retina, and support the body's natural healing process. For those that may be prone to macular holes, especially nearsighted seniors, targeted supplements can help keep the retina strong and healthy.

Nutrients

Essential

Lutein. 6mg–20mg per day. This carotenoid is well researched for retinal support and essential for supporting the retinal pigment.[11] Another study showed that taking lutein along with zeaxanthin and astaxanthin resulted in significant improvement in visual acuity.[12]

Zeaxanthin. 2mg–12mg per day. Along with lutein, zeaxanthin is a potent antioxidant found in the retina to help maintain its health; it also reduces the risk of macular degeneration.[13]

Mesozeaxanthin. 10mg per day. This carotenoid is found in the center of the macula, supporting healthy central vision. A 2015 study showed that supplementing daily with mesozeaxantin significantly increased macular pigment (found to be compromised in those with macular degeneration).[14]

Omega-3 fatty acids. 2,000mg–3,000mg per day. Fifty percent of the retina is comprised of essential fatty acids; it is an essential nutrient for retinal health. Research shows that it has anti-inflammatory properties as well.[15] [16]

Ginkgo biloba. 120mg per day. Ginkgo contains many different flavonoids, including polyphenolic flavonoids, which have been proven to exert antioxidative properties by delivering electrons to free radicals.[17] Numerous studies have shown that ginkgo biloba improves overall circulation[18] and microcirculation.[19] [20] [21] [22]

Hyaluronic acid. 100mg–200mg per day. Found in the vitreous, it is believed to help support the integrity of the vitreous and related connective tissue.[23] [24]

Vitamin C (buffered and ascorbated). 2,000mg–3,000mg per day, split up with meals. Vitamin C helps support the vitreous and connective tissue.[25] Tests have shown ascorbic acid is found at a high concentration in the human eye, and it has been postulated to react with oxygen in ocular fluids.[26] [27] [28]

Helpful

Silica. 40mg–120mg per day. Silica helps support connective tissue, as well as bone health.[29]

Resveratrol. 150mg–300mg per day, preferably trans-resveratrol, as this is a more highly absorbable form. Researchers in one study noted that resveratrol had potent antioxidant and anti-inflammatory properties, along with its capacity to inhibit formation of extra blood vessels, making it valuable as a nutrient for wet macular degeneration and for diabetic retinopathy.[30]

Vitamin D3. 2,000 IU–5,000 IU per day. Lower levels of vitamin D are associated with retinal microvascular damage.[31]

Astaxanthin. 6mg–12mg per day. Researchers concluded that astaxanthin was effective in protecting against damage from light, due to its antioxidant effect.[32] [33] It is a potent antioxidant and a critical nutrient for eye support. This powerful carotenoid crosses the blood-eye barrier, supports vascular health within the eye, and protects the eyes' sensitive cells.[34]

Multivitamin. Take a good whole-food, organic multivitamin.

Diet

Follow the Vision diet described in Chapter 7.

Juicing. Juice daily with organic produce if possible. Ingredients include some combination of:

- Ginger, leeks, garlic, parsley, cabbage, beets, carrots, spinach, apples, celery, grapes, lemon, raspberries, wheatgrasses, and chlorophyll
- You can add your favorite fruits and vegetables. Avoid too many carrots, beets, or too much fruit because of their high, natural-sugar content. Try to use room temperature vegetables and fruit.
- Do not add ice or very cold liquids since cold foods and liquids will eventually extinguish the stomach's digestive fire.
- Do not juice as often during the cooler months of the year, and instead, switch to vegetable soups or stews.

Other Modalities

Chinese Medicine

In Chinese medicine, the Liver "opens to the eyes" and is the primary meridian for supporting overall flow of energy and circulation through the eyes. The Kidney meridian nourishes the blood to the eyes. The Spleen meridian also nourishes the blood, while helping to keep fluids from leaking from blood vessels and reducing dampness (build-up of fluids). Other meridians that affect eye health may also be out of balance, so an evaluation by an acupuncturist can best determine where the out-of-balances are, and offer the optimal treatment strategy.

Hu jing wan. Preserve vistas pill tonifies and nourishes the Liver and Kidneys, enriches the yin, and improves vision.

Ming mu di huang wan. Rehmannia pills "to brighten the eyes" is related to the following patterns: Liver blood deficiency, Kidney yin deficiency, and Liver yin deficiency

Gui pi tang. Restore the Spleen decoction increases qi, tonifies blood, strengthens the Spleen, nourishes the Heart, and helps the Spleen control the blood.

Also See

Chapter 7, Vision Diet

Chapter 8, Nutrients

Chapter 15-32, Vitreous Detachment

---

[1] Medscape. Macular Hole. Retrieved Feb 20 2018 from https://emedicine.medscape.com/article/1224320-overview

[2] Ibid. Medscape. Macular Hole.

[3] Johnson, R.N., Gass, J.R. (1988). Idiopathic macular holes. Observations, stages of formation, and implications for surgical intervention. *Opthalmology*, Jul 95(7):917-24.

[4] Ibid. Medscape. Macular Hole

[5] Ibid. Medscape. Macular Hole.

[6] Ibid. Medscape. Macular Hole.

[7] Ibid. Medscape. Macular Hole.

[8] Ibid. Medscape. Macular Hole.

[9] Ibid. Medscape. Macular Hole.

[10] Wender, J., Jumper, J.M. (2007). Revisiting Macular Holes. *Rev Ophthalmol*, 15 Feb.

[11] Landrum, et al. Exp Eye Res 1997 Jul;65(1):57-62

[12] Piermarocchi, S., Saviano, S., Parisi, V., Tedeschi, M., Panozzo, G., et al. (2012). Carotenoids in Age-related Maculopathy Italian Study: two-year results of a randomized study. *Eur J Ophthalmol*, Mar-Apr;22(2):216-25

[13] National Eye Institute. (2013) NIH study provides clarity on supplements for protection against blinding eye disease. Retrieved Feb 18 2018 from https://nei.nih.gov/news/ pressreleases/050513

[14] Ma, L., Liu, R., Du, J.H., Liu, T., Wu, S.S. (2016). Lutein, Zeaxanthin and Meso-zeaxanthin Supplementation Associated with Macular Pigment Optical Density. *Nutrients*, Jul 12;8(7):E426.

[15] Udell, I.J., Abelson, M.B.(1983). Chemical mediators of inflammation. *Int Ophthalmol Clin*, 23:1:15-26.

[16] Abelson, M.B., Butrus, S.I., Kliman, G.H., Larson, D.L., Corey, E.J., et al. (1987). Topical arachidonic acid: A model for screening anti-inflammatory agents. *J Ocul Pharmacol*, 3:63-75.

[17] Ou, H.C., Lee, W.J., Lee, I.T., Chiu, T.H., Tsai, K.L., et al. (2009). Ginkgo biloba extract attenuates oxLDL-induced oxidative functional damages in endothelial cells. *J Appl Physiol*, 106:1674–85.

[18] Chung, H.S., Harris, A., Kristinsson, J.K., Ciulla, T.A., Kagemann, C., Ritch, R. (1999). Ginkgo biloba extract increases ocular blood flow velocity. *J Ocul Pharmacol Ther*, 15:233–40.

[19] Matsunaga, N., Imai, S., Inokuchi, Y., Shimazawa, M., Yokota, S., et al. (2009). Bilberry and its main constituents have neuroprotective effects against retinal neuronal damage in vitro and in vivo. *Mol Nutr Food Res*, Jul;53(7):869-77.

[20] Zhu, Y., Xia, M., Yang, Y., Liu, F., Li, Z., et al. (2011). Purified anthocyanin supplementation improves endothelial function via NO-cGMP activation in hypercholesterolemic individuals. *Clin Chem*, Nov;57(11):152433.

[21] Cohen-Boulakia, F., Valensi, P.E., Boulahdour, H., Lestrade, R. Dufour-Lamarinie, J.F., et al. (2000). In vivo sequential study of skeletal muscle capillary permeability in diabetic rats: effect of anthocyanosides. *Metabolism*, Jul;49(7):880-5.

[22] Yao, Y., Vieria, A. (2007). Protective activities of Vaccinium antioxidants with potential relevance to mitochondrial dysfunction and neurotoxicity. *Neurotoxicology*, 28 93–100.

[23] Stolyszewski, I., Niemcunowicz-Janica, A., Pepinski, W., Spolnicka, M., Zbiec, R., et al. (2007). Vitreous humour as a potential DNA source for postmortem human identification, *Fola Histochem Cytobiol*, 45(2):135-6.

[24] Thimons, J.J. (1992). Posterior vitreous detachment. *Optom Clin*, 2(3):1-24.

[25] Ibid. Stolyzewski. (1992).

[26] Pirie A. (1965). A light-catalysed reaction in the aqueous humor of the eye. *Nature*, 205:500–501.

[27] Takano S, Ishiwata S, Nakazawa M, Mizugaki M, Tamai M. (1997). Determination of ascorbic acid in human vitreous humor by high-performance liquid chromatography with UV detection. *Curr Eye Res*, 16(6):589–594.

[28] Eaton JW. (1991). Is the lens canned? *Free Radic Biol Med*, 11(2):207–213.

[29] Jugdaohsingh, R. (2007). Silicon and Bone Health. *J Nutr Health Aging*, Mar-Apr; 11(2): 99–110.

[30] Wang, Z. Wang S, Yang, S., Yin, T., Zhang, Y., et al, (2017): Tissue Distribution of trans-Resveratrol and Its Metabolites after Oral Administration in Human Eyes, *J Ophthalmol*, 4052094.

[31] Mutlu, U., Ikram, M.A., Hofman, A., de Jong, P.T., Uitterlinden, A.G., et al. (2016). Vitamin D and retinal microvascular damage: The Rotterdam Study. *Medicine (Baltimore)*, Dec; 95(49): e5477.

[32] Parisi, V., Tedeschi, M., Gallianaro, G., Varano, M., Saviano, S., et al. (2008). Carotenoids and antioxidants in age-related maculopathy, *Ophthalmology*, Feb;115(2):324-333.e2.

[33] Otsuka, T., Shimazawa, M., Nakanishi, T., Ohno, Y., Inoue, Y., et al. (2013). Protective effects of a dietary carotenoid, astaxanthin, against light-induced retinal damage, *J Pharmacol Sci*, 123(3):209-18.

[34] Goto, S., Kogure, K., Abe, K., Kimata, Y., Kitahama, K., et al. (2001). Efficient radical trapping at the surface and inside the phospholipid membrane is responsible for highly potent antiperoxidative activity of the carotenoid astaxanthin. *Biochimica Biophysica Acta*, 1512 :251-8.

15-21. NIGHT VISION (POOR)

Poor night vision disorders (night blindness, impaired dark adaptation, etc.) include the experience of reduced vision in dimly lit environments, including at night. They include partial or complete impairment in ability of the eyes to adapt from brightness to darkness. It is not a disease in itself, but rather a symptom of an underlying problem, usually located in the retina. It is common for patients who are myopic (nearsighted) to have some difficulties with night vision, but this is due to optical issues rather than to a retinal condition.

Poor night vision affects more people in other areas of the world than the U.S. because of wide-ranging vitamin A deficiencies in undeveloped nations. Almost one third of children (2015) in developing countries are deficient in vitamin A,[1] which is a significant improvement from ten years prior. According to the World Health Organization, during the period 1995-2005 nearly ten million pregnant women and five million children, in countries affected by vitamin A deficiency (VAD), are affected by poor night vision. The incidence of VAD-related poor night vision is significantly lower in the developed world.[2] In America, it is a rare disease that affects less than 200,000 people.[3]

What is Poor Night Vision?

People with poor night vision typically are not able to see well in the dark. They are, however, able to see perfectly well during the day, even though transitions from bright environments to dim ones, such as when entering a darkened hall from the sunny outdoors, may be challenging.

One key to seeing at night is a healthy amount of rhodopsin, which is an eye pigment in the retina responsible for night vision. It is used specifically by the photoreceptor cone cells to perceive light, while the rods, on the other hand, are highly sensitive to darkness. Rhodopsin enables us to quickly adapt our vision from a dark room to a light room. Vitamin A is an essential component of rhodopsin, so a deficiency in vitamin A can result in poor night vision.[4] Though vitamin A deficiency is rare in industrial nations, there are other reasons vitamin A intake may be compromised, including:

- Iron deficiency can affect vitamin A uptake.
- Small-bowel bypass surgery may reduce vitamin A absorption.[5]
- Excess alcohol consumption impairs absorption.
- Medications can affect fat absorption (Xenical) or cholesterol (statins).
- Low fat diets may be low in vitamin A.
- Zinc deficiency is associated with decreased release of vitamin A from the liver.
- Other conditions such as fibrosis, pancreatic insufficiency, and inflammatory bowel disease affect how vitamin A is utilized in the body.

Worldwide, poor night vision affects 5.2 million preschool-aged children and 9.8 million pregnant women, which corresponds to 0.9% and 7.8% of the population, respectively.[6]

The Photoreceptors

Photoreceptors in the retina are unique types of nerve cells that convert light into electrical signals, which pass through the optic nerve to be interpreted by the brain. The rods and cones work both by themselves, and together, to allow you to adjust to changes in brightness and darkness.[7] There are actually three types of photoreceptor cells that process light and give us vision.

- Cone cells are responsible for the absorption of light and color vision in bright light. They are located in the central portion of the retina for fine visual color and detail.[8] Cones adjust to changes in brightness very quickly and in very bright light.[9]
- Rod cells predominate in the periphery of the retina, away from the central macula. They permit dim and dark light vision and also detect motion. They are responsible for night vision. Rods are more sensitive to light than cones; they can detect single photons of light and isolate that information from other fluctuations.[10] Rods transmit their information to rod bipolar cells that interpret these single photons, in summary, to generate usable information.[11]
- The third group is photosensitive retinal ganglion cells, which were first identified in rod-less and cone-less lab animals and later in rod-less and cone-less humans who could still perceive light. They do not record pattern or image, but instead interpret ambient light intensity.[12] They are modulated by melatonin[13] and contain melanopsin, which affects pupil dilation and dark adaption,[14] so they may be involved in poor night vision, to some extent. Additionally, they appear to be resistant to photoreceptor loss in retinal degeneration conditions.[15]

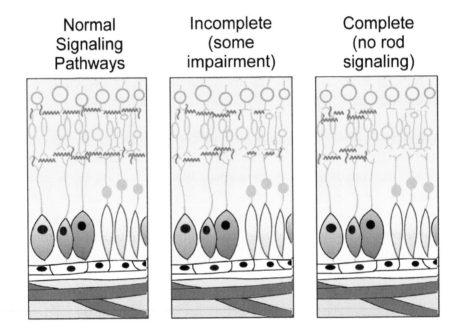

| Normal Signaling Pathways | Incomplete (some impairment) | Complete (no rod signaling) |

At night, melatonin is secreted by rod and cone photoreceptors, functioning as a dark-adaptive signal. In turn, melatonin modulates these ganglion-cell photoreceptors.[16] The photoreceptors transmit messages to bipolar cells that, in turn, transmit the messages to ganglion cells, which send the information to the brain.

Types of Poor Night Vision and Pathology

Presently, medical professionals categorize poor night vision in two different ways: as genetically based or as a symptom of several different diseases or conditions.

Congenital Stationary Night Blindness (CSNB)

CSNB is the genetic form of night blindness and there are two types: the complete form and the incomplete form. Some types of genetic night blindness are X-linked (associated with myopia), but others arise due to dominant and recessive gene mutations.[17]

- The complete form (CSNB1) is characterized by total *absence of* rod pathway function, which means that the rods in the retina do not respond to light, making it impossible to see in dim light conditions. This form of X-linked CSNB is linked to mutations in the NYX gene that encodes a protein with an unknown function.
- The incomplete form (CSNB2) is due to an *impaired* rod and cone pathway function,[18] which tends to allow for some vision in dim conditions. This form is caused by CACNA1F gene mutations. This gene allows a slow rate of deactivation that is important in light adaption.

To summarize, everyone with the complete form has night blindness, while not all people with the incomplete form have night blindness.

Signs and Symptoms

For people whose night vision begins worsening due to other related eye conditions, the vision loss can occur very slowly over time. It can also occur quickly, depending on how acute the eye condition is, such as with untreated retinal bleeding. Cataracts, for example, tend to develop slowly, but for a smaller percentage of the population, they can evolve rapidly.

Symptoms vary (based on the individual) and can include any or all of the following:

- Weak vision in dim light
- Difficulty seeing during night driving
- Slow vision adaption between bright and dim light conditions (such as taking a longer time than other people to adjust to indoor lighting when coming from the bright outdoors)
- Fifty to seventy percent of people with night blindness also have nystagmus and strabismus,[19] [20] as well as low vision and myopia.[21]

Only your doctor can provide an adequate diagnosis of any signs or symptoms, and whether they are night blindness symptoms, or symptoms of another disorder. The determination of the cause of night blindness should be fairly easy with a full, dilated exam and targeted tests, such as an optical coherence tomography scan (commonly known an OCT scan). This is particularly important so that the eye doctor has a history of test results with the patient.

If the night blindness is genetic, your doctor may administer a test called an electroretinogram, which determines the function of the retina and therefore its proper classification.[22]

Causes and Risk Factors

Genetic causes. The rods and cones in the retina pass information via the bipolar cells and the optic nerve to the brain for interpretation. In other words, the photoreceptors are receivers of light energy, but the actual perception of vision is at the occipital cortex at the back of the brain. Genetic defects cause a breakdown in this process.

Photoreceptor dysfunction. In terms of risks and causes related to other eye disorders, retinitis pigmentosa and cone-rod dystrophy are especially associated with cone and rod problems, and therefore, night blindness.

Other vision conditions. Other conditions that may result in poor night vision include cataracts, diabetic retinopathy, effects after LASIK eye surgery, Fuch's dystrophy, keratoconus, myopia, glaucoma, macular degeneration, cone rod dystrophy, retinal detachment, and vitreous detachment.

In terms of poor night vision that occurs as a result of other diseases and conditions, this form can be progressive and potentially debilitating, depending on the cause and the success of treatment for it. However, in some cases, the problem may be reversed as the underlying condition is healed or brought under control, such as with glaucoma, cataracts, and other retinal conditions, particularly in their early stages. In later stages of these eye conditions, however, permanent damage to the photoreceptor cells may have already set in. At this point, the cells cannot be regenerated; therefore, a portion of lost vision will not be restored.

Other health conditions. Side effects of celiac disease, cystic fibrosis, bile duct obstruction, cirrhosis of the liver, Crohn's disease, gastric bypass surgery for obesity, or cystic fibrosis can cause night blindness and/or vitamin A deficiency. Diabetes, which develops due to elevated blood-sugar levels, can also damage the retina. Poor night vision is an early indicator of damage due to diabetes, but keep in mind that this is just one of a number of eye related symptoms that can result from diabetes.

Almost any progressive vision condition can result in poor vision, which tends to be especially problematic at night and also when shifting from dark-to-light or light-to-dark environments (such as when you are driving at night and another car approaches, or when stepping inside after being outside in very bright sunlight). If you are having difficulty seeing at night, in poorly lit environments, or when switching between different levels of lighting, then you should ask your doctor about your symptoms.

Medications. Glaucoma medications and other eye medications may be a cause of night blindness by restricting the opening of the pupil.

Vitamin A deficiency. An early indicator of a deficiency in vitamin A may be night blindness. A primary source of vitamin A is from animal sources, so diets such as a vegan diet without eggs, dairy, fish, and/or organ meats may result in a deficiency of vitamin A, unless vegetables containing beta-carotene (sweet potato, carrots, dark leafy greens, and winter squash), which the liver and small intestines convert to vitamin A, are regularly consumed. The body makes vitamin A from beta-carotene found predominantly in yellow/orange vegetables and fruits, so if those are missing from the diet, the risk is greater. One sign of a vitamin A deficiency is the appearance of small bumps on the backs of your upper arms or legs.

Malabsorption (if it affects vitamin A absorption). Research of trace element deficiencies in night-blinded children aged 3 to 12 found that the children had low levels of zinc, copper, and iron, along with higher-than-normal levels of lead, arsenic, cadmium, and sodium.

Taurine deficiency. Taurine is essential for healthy vision, reducing the impact of oxidative stress on photoreceptors in the retina. There are several possible causes of taurine deficiency, including aging, diseases related to the liver and kidneys, heart failure, diabetes, and cancer.[23]

Deficiency in other vitamins and amino acids, such as zinc, cysteine, and methionine can all slow the body's production of taurine. Certain diets, such as vegetarian and vegan, can lack adequate taurine.[24] Best sources of taurine are eggs, meat, and seafood. Those who do not eat enough eggs, meat, nuts, and seeds often lack the necessary components for the production of appropriate levels of taurine, which to some extent can be produced by the body from a combination of the amino acids methionine and cysteine. Additionally, monosodium glutamate (MSG) degrades taurine.

Zinc deficiency. While zinc alone does not improve night vision, researchers have determined that its role in night vision seems especially important. Zinc is needed for the enzyme that converts retinol (vitamin A) to retinal. This latter form of vitamin A is necessary for the synthesis of rhodopsin, a protein in the eye that absorbs light and thus is involved in dark and light adaptation. If the body is deficient in zinc, vitamin A will not be utilized as efficiently, as zinc supports several aspects of vitamin A metabolism, including its absorption, transport, and utilization.[25] Good food sources of zinc include seafood (oysters), beef and lamb, toasted wheat germ, spinach, pumpkin and squash seeds, cashews, chocolate, chickpeas, and cooked mushrooms. Zinc and protein are important to liberate vitamin A stores in the liver.

Lack of healthy fats. Since vitamin A is a fat-soluble vitamin, lack of good fats and/or bile interfere with optimal absorption. Similarly, lipid-reducing medications such as statins or those that reduce intestinal fat absorption, or foods that contain a fat replacement such as Olestra, can interfere with the absorption of vitamin A.

Conventional Treatment

Although there is no current cure for poor night vision or night blindness, treating the underlying cause, if there is a health condition identified such as diabetes or glaucoma, is essential.

Complementary Approach

A healthy diet combined with targeted supplements help support photoreceptor cells and retinal health, and they can maintain and even improve night vision, as long as the rods still exist in the retina. Sometimes retinal cells are still alive but functioning poorly. These cells can potentially improve function through appropriate nutrients, resulting in vision improvement.

Nutrients

Vitamin A is the most clearly researched deficiency associated with night blindness. Certain other nutrients such as bilberry, lutein, ginkgo biloba, taurine, zeaxanthin, and other vitamins and minerals may help reduce night blindness and preserve vision. The following is a rundown of the most important nutrients:

Essential

Lutein. 6mg–20mg per day. People given lutein, zeaxanthin, and astaxanthin, together with other nutrients, are likely to report significant improvements in vision sharpness.[26]

Zeaxanthin. 2mg–12mg per day. Lutein and zeaxanthin filter harmful high-energy blue wavelengths of light and help protect and maintain healthy cells in the eyes. Of the 600 carotenoids found in nature, only these two are deposited in high quantities in the retina (macula) of the eye.[27] In a 2-year study, an 8mg dosage was linked to improved night driving skills.[28]

Vitamin A (palmitate). 10,000 IU–15,000 IU per day, to overcome deficiency. Vitamin A helps support the photoreceptor cells.[29] Beta-carotene can also be taken to reverse a deficiency, but it is not as effective as taking vitamin A directly; this is because beta-carotene is absorbed slowly by the body, and then slowly converted to vitamin A. 15,000 IU is often the recommended daily dosage (check with your doctor or nutritionist).

> **Note**. Vitamin A is contra-indicated for those suffering from Stargardt disease (see Stargardt chapter for more information). Pregnant women should not supplement with vitamin A.

Bilberry. 180mg–240mg per day. Along with supporting night vision, bilberry is neuroprotective and has been shown to improve microcirculation.[30] [31] [32] [33] Bilberry (a blueberry relative) grows in the wild in northern Europe and North America. It is rich in flavonoids, specifically in anthocyanins, the elements in plants that provide color. These natural chemicals are potent antioxidants that, among other benefits, enhance the creation of the purple pigment, rhodopsin, that is used by the rods in the back of the eye to assist with night vision. Early research has shown that bilberry supplementation improves the speed of adapting to darkness for people who have poor night vision.[34]

Taurine. 750mg–1000mg per day. Taurine is essential for healthy night vision. Taurine supports a process known as rhodopsin regeneration. Rhodopsin is the primary pigment in photoreceptor rods and makes vision in low-light conditions possible. It also helps protect cell membranes from free radical damage while aiding in the removal of toxins and debris. Taurine is found in the photoreceptors at levels ten times greater than other amino acids.[35] [36] [37]

Omega-3 fatty acids. 2,000mg–3,000mg per day. DHA from omega-3 fatty acids accounts for approximately 50–60% of the total fatty acid content within rod outer segments of photoreceptors, and it tends to be very deficient in today's diet.[38] [39]

Very Important

Green tea extract. 500mg–750mg per day. Green teas and their extracts are potentially neuroprotective in the photoreceptor's outer segment and retinal pigment epithelium (RPE) by helping prevent apoptosis (cell death).[40]

Zinc, 40mg–60mg per day, *plus* **copper**, 2mg–4mg per day.[41] Zinc deficiency reduces the activity of an enzyme that helps the body produce vitamin A (retinol dehydrogenase). Research has shown that taking a zinc supplement is helpful. Healthcare providers often recommend 15mg–30mg of zinc daily for vision. At the same time, long-term supplementation with zinc may lower copper levels, so 1mg of copper daily is recommended with 15mg of zinc during extended use. In general, the recommended supplement ratio is 15:1 zinc to copper. If you are supplementing with zinc, consult your medical professional for correct dosages of both zinc and copper.

Helpful

Ginkgo biloba. 120mg per day. Ginkgo helps support healthy circulation,[42] [43] stabilizes capillaries, and makes the capillaries less fragile.[44] [45] [46] Check with your doctor if you are on blood thinners before supplementing with gingko.

Vitamin B complex. Take preferably in a whole-food organic formula or a whole-food organic multivitamin, as directed. If not within a whole-food formula, recommended dosages of the vitamin B complex are as follows: vitamin B6 (100mg), vitamin B12 (1,000mcg), biotin (400mcg), folate (400mcg), riboflavin/B2 (50mg), and thiamine/B1 (100mg). These dosages will be smaller in a whole-food multivitamin.

Diet

Follow the Vision diet described in Chapter 7.

Vegetables. To avoid night blindness or to help heal it after a diagnosis, it is crucial to consume beta-carotene rich vegetables, such as dark green leafy vegetables like spinach, collards, and kale, as well as orange and yellow vegetables, such as carrots, sweet potatoes, and winter squash. Carrots are also rich in vitamin A.

Nuts and seeds. These are rich in the amino acids cysteine and methionine, which help with production of taurine, an important amino acid that promotes cardiovascular health, insulin sensitivity, electrolyte balance, hearing function, and immune modulation.[47] Nuts and seeds should be soaked to reduce phytates which bind to and eliminate minerals such as calcium, zinc, magnesium, iron, and copper from our body. Another way to mitigate the effects of phytic acid, is to ensure a healthy gut microbiome (healthy intestinal bacteria), which can help break down the phytic acid.

Fruits. A diet high in dark fruits such as blackberries, black currants, and blueberries, approximately a cup a day, has been shown to be very beneficial. These fruits contain high levels of cyanidin-3-glucoside (or C3G), a powerful antioxidant seen as a purple pigment in the anthocyanin family of flavonoid molecules. Based on one study, just 50mg per day improved the participants' ability to see in darkness after just 30 minutes.[48] [49] C3G also upregulates the activity of endothelial nitric oxide synthase (eNOS), which helps maintain normal vascular function.[50]

Juicing. The following fruits and vegetables are recommended for this condition. Choose at least 4-6 items to combine, and use organic whenever possible.

- Ginger, garlic, parsley, turnips, spinach, blueberries, beets, carrots, watercress, and wheatgrass
- Add your favorite fruits and vegetables as well. Do not use too many carrots or sweet fruits due to their natural high-sugar content.
- Try to use room temperature vegetables and fruit.
- Do not add ice or very cold liquids since cold foods and liquids will eventually extinguish the stomach's digestive fire.
- Do not juice as often during the cooler months of the year, and instead, switch to vegetable soups or stews.

Lifestyle

Microcurrent stimulation. Daily sessions at home help support photoreceptor and retinal health by assisting healthy circulation to the retina, increasing energy production in the retinal cells, and helping the retina eliminate waste. See Chapter 10-3 for more information.

Eyeglasses. Make sure your eyeglass prescription is up to date and that your lenses are clean. Get prescription glasses for night driving, if they are needed. See your eye doctor to determine if they would be helpful.

- Always wear sunglasses outside, especially on bright days. Blue and green-eyed people are particularly sensitive to potential sun-induced damage, so the use of eye protection is paramount. Amber lenses are the most effective protection against UVA/UVB and blue light. Additionally, you can get eyeglasses treated with a non-glare coating that have reflective properties.
- If you wear prescription glasses at night for driving, have your eyeglasses treated with an anti-reflective coating, which is beneficial in two ways: it minimizes internal reflections

within the lenses, reducing halo problems; and it increases the transmittance of light through the lens to the eye. We do not recommend using any tinted glasses at night, because they reduce visibility by lessening the amount of light that enters the eyes. While yellow lenses can be effective for foggy or hazy daylight conditions, they are not effective against headlight glare, and they should not be worn at dusk or night.

Eye Exercises. See Chapter 10 for eye exercises and acupuncture points that are good for all eye conditions and overall eye health. We recommend the following to perform regularly for night blindness.

- Palming
- Eye massage

Specific tips for driving.

- Increase your visibility. Make sure that your windshield is clean, and that your headlights are clean and properly aligned.
- Slow down. This way, you give yourself more time to react to any unexpected hazards.
- At night, look to the right, to the roadway's edge, to help you avoid the glare of oncoming headlights.
- Leave the driving till tomorrow. Drive only during the day. Even good lighting conditions at night, such as found in a big city, can be troublesome to someone with night blindness.
- Consider driving a car with a built-in infrared scanner. These scanners illuminate the road ahead with light that is invisible to humans, and can improve safety. Also, the auto dimming feature in the rear-view mirrors greatly improve comfort and safety while driving at night.

Other Modalities

Chinese Medicine

Although there are a number of reasons for night blindness, as long as there are rods active in the eyes, these can be supported and nourished through acupuncture and specific herbs. In Chinese medicine, the Liver "opens to the eyes" and is the primary meridian for supporting overall flow of energy and circulation through the eyes. The Kidney meridian nourishes the blood to the eyes, and the Spleen meridian also nourishes the blood while helping to prevent fluids from leaking from blood vessels. Other meridians may also be out of balance that can affect eye health, so an evaluation by an acupuncturist can best determine where the out-of-balances are and offer the optimal treatment strategy. Acupuncture treatments are typically done by inserting needles below the knees and elbows, then in specific points along the orbit of the eye and under the eye.

Chinese Medicine Patent Formulas

Xiao yao san is a classic Liver tonic used in Chinese medicine that supports healthy circulation and the free flow of energy in the eyes and throughout the body.

Ming mu di huang wan is another classic formula that contains a blend of herbs specifically designed to improve eyesight by nourishing two main organs that are energetically responsible for vision: the Liver and Kidney. This formula is known to improve the availability of blood to the eyes and to increase circulation.

On the Horizon

Stem cell therapy. Researchers have discovered a gene that is related to Leber's congenital amaurosis (LCA) that could be responsible for some cases of human night blindness.[51][52]

Also See

Chapter 7, Vision Diet

Chapter 15-5, Cone-Rod Dystrophy

Chapter 15-27, Retinitis Pigmentosa

Chapter 15-29, Stargardt Disease

Appendix 5, Recommended Products

[1] Stevens, G.A., Bennett, J.E., Hennocq, Q., Lu, Y., De-Regil, L.M., et al. (2015).Trends and mortality effects of vitamin A deficiency in children in 138 low-income and middle-income countries between 1991 and 2013: A pooled analysis of population-based surveys. *Lancet Glob. Health*, 3:e528–e536

[2] World Health Organization. Global prevalence of night blindness and number of individuals affected in populations of countries at risk of vitamin A deficiency 1995-2005. Retrieved Nov 14 2017 from http://www.who.int/vmnis/database/vitamina/table1/en/.

[3] Right Diagnosis. Prevalence and Incidence of Night Blindness. Retrieved Nov 15 from http://www.rightdiagnosis.com/n/night_blindness/prevalence.htm.

[4] Unicef. Vitamin A Deficiency and Supplementation UNICEF Data". Retrieved April 4 2017.

[5] Wechsler, H.L. (1979). Vitamin A deficiency following small-bowel bypass surgery for obesity. *Arch Dermatol*, Jan;115(1):73-5.

[6] World Health Organization. Vitamin and Mineral Nutrition Information System. Retrieved Oct 14 2017 from http://www.who.int/vmnis/database/vitamina/table1/en/

[7] Wikipedia, Adaptation (eye). Retrieved Feb 21 2018 from https://en.wikipedia.org/wiki/Adaptation_(eye).

[8] PubMedHealth. Cone Cells. Retrieved Feb 22 2018 from https://www.ncbi.nlm.nih.gov/pubmedhealth/PMHT0024259/.

[9] Lamb, T.D. (2016). Why rods and cones? *Eye (Lond)*, 30(2).

[10] Ibid. Lamb. (2016).

[11] Ibid. Lamb. (2016).

[12] Wikipedia, Intrinsically photosensitive retinal ganglion cells. Retrieved Feb 21 2018 from https://en.wikipedia.org/wiki/Intrinsically_photosensitive_retinal_ganglion_cells.

[13] Pack, W., Hill, D.D., Wong, K.Y., (2015). Melatonin modulates M4-type ganglion-cell photoreceptors. *Neuroscience*, Sep 10;303:178-88.

[14] Cao, D., Nicandro, N., Barrionuevo, P.A. (2015). A five-primary photostimulator suitable for studying intrinsically photosensitive retinal ganglion cell functions in humans. *J Vis*, Jan 26;15(1):15.1.27.

[15] Lin, B., Peng, E.B. (2013). Retinal ganglion cells are resistant to photoreceptor loss in retinal degeneration. *Plos One,* Jun 28;8(6):e68084.

[16] Ibid. Pack. (2015).

[17] Wikipedia. X-linked congenital stationary night blindness. Retrieved Feb 22 2018 from https://en.wikipedia.org/wiki/X-linked_congenital_stationary_night_blindness.

[18] van Genderen, M. M., Bijveld, M. M. C., Claassen, Y. B., Florijn, R. J., Pearring, J. N., et al. (2009). Mutations in TRPM1 are a common cause of complete congenital stationary night blindness. *Am. J. Hum. Genet*, 85: 730-736.

[19] Boycott, K.M., Pearce, W.G., Bech-Hansen, N.T. (2000). Clinical variability among patients with incomplete X-linked congenital stationary night blindness and a founder mutation in CACNA1F. *Can J Ophthalmol*, 35:204–13.

[20] Allen LE, Zito I, Bradshaw K, Patel RJ, Bird AC, et al. (2003). Genotype-phenotype correlation in British families with X linked congenital stationary night blindness. *Br J Ophthalmol*, 87:1413–20.

[21] Ibid. Wikipedia. X-Linked Congenital Stationary Night Blindness.

[22] U.S. National Library of Medicine. X-linked congenital stationary night blindness. Retrieved Dec 10 2017 from https://ghr.nlm.nih.gov/condition/x-linked-congenital-stationary-night-blindness.

[23] Macleavy, I. (2013). The Forgotten Longevity Benefits of Taurine. Retrieved Dec 10 2017 from http://www.lifeextension.com/magazine/2013/6/the-forgotten-longevity-benefits-of-taurine/page-01

[24] Ibid. Macleavy. (2013).

[25] Christian, P., West, K.P. (1998) Interactions between zinc and vitamin A: an update. *Am J Clin Nutr*, Aug;68(2 Suppl):435S-441S.

[26] Parisi, V., Tedeschi, M., Gallianaro, G., Varano, M., Saviano, S., et al. (2008). Carotenoids and antioxidants in age-related maculopathy, *Ophthalmology*, Feb;115(2):324-333.e2.

[27] American Optometric Association Lutein & Zeaxanthin. Retrieved Dec 11 2017 from https://www.aoa.org/patients-and-public/caring-for-your-vision/diet-and-nutrition/lutein.

[28] Richer, S.P., Stiles, W., Graham-Hoffman, K., Levin, M., Ruskin, D., et al. (2011). Randomized, double-blind, placebo-controlled study of zeaxanthin and visual function in patients with atrophic age-related macular degeneration: the Zeaxanthin and Visual Function Study (ZVF) FDA IND #78, 973. *Optometry*, Nov;82(11):667-680.e6.

[29] Berson, E.L., Rosner, B., Sandberg, M.A. (1993). A Randomized Trial of Vitamin A and Vitamin E Supplementation for Retinitis Pigmentosa. *JAMA Ophthalmol*. 111(6):761-772.

[30] Matsunaga, N., Imai, S., Inokuchi, Y., Shimazawa, M., Yokota, S., et al. (2009). Bilberry and its main constituents have neuroprotective effects against retinal neuronal damage in vitro and in vivo. *Mol Nutr Food Res*, Jul;53(7):869-77.

[31] Cohen-Boulakia, F., Valensi, P.E., Boulahdour, H., Lestrade, R. Dufour-Lamarinie, J.F., et al. (2000). In vivo sequential study of skeletal muscle capillary permeability in diabetic rats: effect of anthocyanosides. *Metabolism*, Jul;49(7):880-5.

[32] Zhu, Y., Xia, M., Yang, Y., Liu, F., Li, Z., et al. (2011). Purified anthocyanin supplementation improves endothelial function via NO-cGMP activation in hypercholesterolemic individuals. *Clin Chem*, Nov;57(11):1524-33.

[33] Yao, Y., Vieria, A. (2007). Protective activities of Vaccinium antioxidants with potential relevance to mitochondrial dysfunction and neurotoxicity. *Neurotoxicology*, 28 93–100.

[34] Chu, W.C., Cheung, S.C.M., Lau, R.A.W., Benzie, I.F.F. (2011).*Herbal Medicine: Biomolecular and Clinical Aspects. 2nd edition.* Chapter 4 Bilberry (Vaccinium myrtillus L.). Boca Raton, FL: CRC Press/Taylor & Francis.

[35] Petrosian, A.M., Haroutounian, J.E. (1998). The role of taurine in osmotic, mechanical, and chemical protection of the retinal rod outer segments, *Adv Exp Med Biol*, 442:407-13.

[36] Lopez-Colome, A.M., Pasantes-Morales, H. (1980). Taurine interactions with chick retinal membranes. J *Neurochem*. May;34(5):1047-52

[37] Wright, C.E., Tallan, H.H., Lin, Y.Y., Gaull, G.E. (1986). Taurine: Biological Update. *Ann Rev Biochem*, 55:427-53

[38] Bush RA, Malnoe A, Reme CE, Williams TP. (1994). Dietary deficiency of N-3 fatty acids alters rhodopsin content and function in the rat retina. *Inv Ophthalmol Vis Sci,* 35(1):91–100.

[39] Stillwell W, Wassall SR.(2003). Docosahexaenoic acid: membrane properties of a unique fatty acid. *Chem Phys Lipids*, 126(1):1–27.

[40] Emoto, Y., Yoshizawa, K., Kinoshita, Y, Yuki, M., Yuri, T., et al. (2016). Green tea extract attenuates MNU-induced photoreceptor cell apoptosis via suppression of heme oxygenase-1. *J Toxicol Pathol*, Jan;29(1):61-5.

[41] Christian, P., Khatry, S.K., Yamini, S., Stallings, R., LeClerq, S.C., et al. (2001). Zinc supplementation might potentiate the effect of vitamin A in restoring night vision in pregnant Nepalese women. *Am J Clin Nutr*, Jun;73(6):1045-51.

[42] Wu, Y.Z., Li, S.Q., Zu, X.G., Du, J., Wang, F.F. (2008). Ginkgo biloba extract improves coronary artery circulation in patients with coronary artery disease: contribution of plasma nitric oxide and endothelin-1. *Phytother Res*, Jun;22(6):734-9.

[43] Wu, Y., Li, S., Cui, W., Zu, X., Du, J., Wang, F. (2008). Ginkgo biloba extract improves coronary blood flow in healthy elderly adults: role of endothelium-dependent vasodilation. *Phytomedicine*, Mar;15(3):164-9..

[44] Welt, K., Weiss, J., Martin, R., Hermsdorf, T., Drews, S., et al. (2007). Ginkgo biloba extract protects rat kidney from diabetic and hypoxic damage. *Phytomedicine*, Feb;14(2-3):196-203..

[45] Qiu, Y., Rui, Y.C., Li, T.J., Zhang, L., Yao, P.Y. (2004). Inhibitory effect of extracts of Ginkgo biloba leaves on VEGF-induced hyperpermeability of bovine coronary endothelial cells in vitro. *Adv Ther*, Jan-Feb;15(1):54-65.

[46] Huang, S.Y., Jeng, C., Kao, S.C., Yu, J.J., Liu, D.Z., (2004). Improved haemorrheological properties by Ginkgo biloba extract (Egb 761) in type 2 diabetes mellitus complicated with retinopathy. *Clin Nutr*, Aug;23(4):615-21.

[47] Ibid. Macleavy. (2013).

[48] Nakaishi, H., Matsumoto, H., Tominaga, S., Hirayama, M. (2000). Effects of black currant anthocyanoside intake on dark adaptation and VDT work-induced transient refractive alteration in healthy humans. *Alt Med Rev*, Dec;5(6):553-62.

[49] Yanamala, N., Tirupula, K.C., Balem, F., Klein-Seetharaman, J. (2009). pH-dependent interaction of rhodopsin with cyanidin-3-glucoside. 1. Structural aspects. *Photochem Photobiol*, Mar-Apr;85(2):454-62.

[50] Xu, J.W., Ikeda, K., Yamori, Y. (2004). Cyanidin-3-glucoside regulates phosphorylation of endothelial nitric oxide synthase. *FEBS Lett*, Sep 10;574(1-3):176-80.

[51] Lotery, A.J., Jacobson, S.G., Fishman, G.A. (2001). Mutations in the CRB1 Gene Cause Leber Congenital Amaurosis. *Arch Ophthalmol*. 119(3):415-420.

[52] Levey, S., Weiss, J.N. (2017) (Announcement of Trial) Stem Cell Ophthalmology Treatment Study II (SCOTS2). Retrieved Feb 5 2018 from https://clinicaltrials.gov/ct2/show/NCT03011541.

15-22. OCULAR MIGRAINE

Ocular migraines can be described as a related group of conditions, all affecting vision, usually temporary, and sometimes without pain. The causes of these migraines are still under debate. Ocular migraines are more common in women of childbearing years who have a history of migraines with auras, and for whom the diagnosis is one of exclusion (a diagnosis reached by process of elimination). There are two types of ocular migraine: ophthalmic (migraine with aura) and retinal migraines.

- **Ophthalmic**, or visual, migraines are thought to result from abnormal electrical activity slowly spreading across certain regions of the outer brain cortex. They affect both eyes. This is responsible for the development of the slowly progressing visual changes, usually over 20 to 60 minutes. These migraines are also known as scintillating scotomas.
- In **retinal migraines**, the visual symptoms take place in the retina rather than across the outer brain cortex. They occur in only one eye, before or during the headache phase. The disturbance in retinal migraine may also result from abnormal spreading of electrical activity, except it occurs in the retina. The disturbance may also be due to reduced retinal blood flow.[1]

Migraines with aura cause no permanent visual or brain damage and do not require treatment. Retinal migraines, on the other hand, have more potential for long-term vision loss. Either way, getting evaluated and monitored by your eye doctor is highly recommended to rule out other concerns.

Types of Ocular Migraines

Ophthalmic Migraine Occurs in the Visual Cortex

Ophthalmic migraine is a vision-loss symptom that occurs due to the aura phase of the common migraine headache. It can occur with or without a headache. An ophthalmic migraine takes place in the brain, which affects vision in both eyes, and is generally believed to originate at the occipital (visual) cortex[2] rather than in the eye itself. For this reason it is experienced in both eyes, not just one eye. It is also known as a scintillating scotoma.[3]

Scintillating Scotoma

A scintillating scotoma can occur with or without a migraine headache. Scintillating means sparkling or shining, and a scotoma is a partial loss of vision or a blind spot in an otherwise normal visual field.

This condition is marked by a spasm, or spreading wave of spasms that arise in the occipital area of the brain (visual cortex). Related blood vessel spasm and redilation is likely linked to these electrical charges. The experience of a person suffering from this condition is a sparkling or flickering of lights, as well as dots, wavy lines, zigzags, arcs, camouflage patterns, or blurry areas toward the periphery of vision (or in some cases, off to one side). Typically, the scotoma starts as a small visual disturbance that slowly starts growing over much of the visual field over about 15-20 minutes before disappearing completely.

A headache might follow the visual effect, ranging from mild to severe, or accompanied by feeling tired, depressed, or washed-out. Sometimes a sensory aura (for example, tingling or numbness in a limb, or problems speaking) will occur at the same time or just after the visual aura.

Retinal Migraine Occurs in One Eye

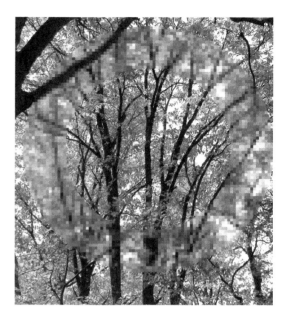

Retinal migraine usually occurs in one eye, and there may be an abnormal spread of electrical activity in the retina. The migraine may also be caused by the sudden constriction (spasm) or blockage behind, or in, an eye. It may occur with, or without, a throbbing headache at the side of the head. The patient may also simultaneously experience sensitivity to light or nausea. The temporary loss or distortion of vision in one eye makes it difficult to conduct close visual work and makes it dangerous to drive. This type of migraine is generally of short duration, an hour or less, and then vision returns to normal. However, some researchers have found that irreversible vision loss is also possible.[4]

Retinal migraine, as defined by the International Headache Society, is actually fairly uncommon. Most cases are diagnosed as ophthalmic migraine.[5]

Ophthalmoplegic Migraine

This rare condition was once thought to be a type of migraine, but instead, it appears to be an inflammation (of cranial nerves) or neuralgia. It is usually accompanied by long-lasting neuropathy of the eye-movement nerve (oculomotor) or of the nerve associated with outward gaze (trochlear), with double vision, pupil abnormalities, and eyelid droop. Symptoms usually resolve fairly quickly.[6]

Migraine Headache

A standard migraine headache is defined by a moderate to severe headache that lasts for 4–72 hours, with a number of connected symptoms. It may be tied to family genetic traits and triggered by certain foods, stress, or environmental factors that affect the proper functioning of the cerebral cortex. Migraine headaches result primarily from changes in the small blood vessels in the head or eyes, either in the form of vasodilation or spasms.

Approximately 20% of migraine headaches are preceded by an aura, usually occurring 20–60 minutes before the headache starts. Visual disturbances may include blind spots, the appearance of flashing lights, spots of light, or wavy lines in the field of vision.

Signs and Symptoms

Symptoms for all types of ocular migraines can be quite varied and related to underlying problems.

Ophthalmic Migraine Symptoms

- Visual changes in both eyes
- A blank spot in the visual field
- Flickering of light, shimmering white light, colored lights in the periphery of vision, or bright colored streaks
- Zigzag lines in the visual field
- Blurred area of vision, mostly around the periphery, as though you were looking at heat waves rising off hot pavement
- Sometimes, allodynia, which includes a hypersensitive area on the face or head during migraine or before or afterward (interictally).

Retinal Migraine Symptoms

- Vision loss in one eye, lasting less than one hour
- Possible migraine headache
- Sensitivity to light
- Throbbing or pulsing feeling
- Feeling worse when you move around

Migraine Headache

"Regular" migraines appear to occur due to constriction and dilation of fine arteries in the head; they can be intensely painful. The pain often stays on one side of the head and might be accompanied by nausea and vomiting. An ocular migraine can appear simultaneously with a migraine headache, in which case the symptoms can be greater, including pulsating and throbbing pain.

Acute Angle-Closure Glaucoma

Ocular emergency. Acute angle-closure (closed-angle or narrow-angle) glaucoma can produce migraine-like symptoms, such as eye pain, intense headache (usually over one brow), halos around lights, dilated pupils, vision loss, red eyes, nausea, and vomiting. If these symptoms are new and unrecognized then you should see your doctor immediately, or go to the emergency room. Narrow-angle issues are typically identified through a comprehensive eye exam.

Causes and Risk Factors

Causes include:

- Spasms in retinal blood vessels (the lining in the back of the eye)
- Electrical changes that spread across the nerve cells in the retina

Risk factors include:

- Being female
- Age under 40 years old
- Personal or family history of migraines or other headaches
- People with diseases such as lupus, hardening of the arteries, sickle cell disease, epilepsy, or depression

Conventional Treatment

Scientists are not sure exactly what causes ocular migraines, but some think that inflammatory substances released in the tissues that surround the circulatory and nerve systems of the head and brain can trigger them. Specifically, ocular migraines do appear to be tied to blood-vessel spasms in the retina or in the back of the eye in the vessels that supply the retina with blood. Doppler studies have revealed cessation of retinal arterial flow during an exercise-induced retinal-migraine episode.[7]

From a broader perspective, ocular migraines may also be caused by stress and fatigue, particularly related to eyestrain. Improper eyeglass prescriptions can certainly add to eye stress or fatigue, as can computer eyestrain. Other related causes include conditions such as hypertension, sinus issues, tumors, hormonal changes, certain foods (alcohol, aged cheese, MSG, or chocolate), or other allergies and sensitivities.

Your eye doctor may recommend medication in certain situations, such as the following:

- Drugs that treat epilepsy, such as divalproex sodium (Depakote) or topiramate (Topamax)
- Tricyclic antidepressants, such as amitriptyline (Elavil) or nortriptyline (Pamelor)
- Blood pressure medicines called beta blockers

Both visual and retinal migraines are generally of short duration. However, if you have these repeatedly, it is a good idea to have an exam. Normal practice is for a medical doctor to get your complete medical history and give you a thorough physical exam. This way, causes of the headache can be ruled out, from other physical conditions. An ophthalmologist or optometrist can verify that eye-related problems are, or are not, contributing to the condition.

Avoid potential triggers, which include the following:

- Chronic stress and anxiety
- High blood pressure
- Smoking
- Dehydration
- Low blood sugar (skipping meals)
- Hormonal birth control pills
- Bending over
- High altitude

- Food triggers, such as chocolate, alcohol (particularly red wine and beer), caffeine, MSG, sugar substitutes, aged cheeses, citrus fruits, cured meats (such as hot dogs and ham), and onions

Similarly, if you have frequent ocular migraines, you should talk to your eye doctor. S/he may also refer you to a neurologist.

Complementary Treatment

Spasms and constriction of tiny blood vessels that cause ocular migraines can be lessened through targeted supplementation, healing modalities such as massage to reduce tension in the neck and shoulder muscles, craniosacral therapy (a gentle, noninvasive form of bodywork that addresses the bones of the head, spinal column, and sacrum), chiropractic (to relieve tension along the spinal column), and acupuncture or shiatsu to balance out meridians that can contribute to, or result in, onset of ocular migraine headaches.

Nutrients

The following nutrients target migraine headaches, but since ocular and visual migraines are also associated with blood vessel constriction, they may be helpful.

Evidence is beginning to support the idea that migraine headaches are associated with mitochondria dysfunction. Supplements such as riboflavin (B2), coenzyme Q10, magnesium, niacin, carnitine, and lipoic acid, which support mitochondrial function, have been shown to help alleviate migraine headaches.[8]

Essential

Magnesium. 500mg per day. Magnesium relaxes the smooth muscles within the blood vessels, thereby reducing peripheral vascular resistance and promoting a healthy cardiovascular system.[9] [10] [11]

Important

Butterbur. 50mg–100mg per day. Butterbur (*Petasites hypridus*) is an herb used mainly to treat headaches and seasonal allergies by reducing smooth muscle spasms and helping to relax the constriction of cerebral blood vessels. In clinical trials in both Germany and the U.S., butterbur reduced the incidence of head cavity discomforts by approximately 61%.[12] [13]

Caution. Butterbur should not contain pyrrolizidine alkaloids; be sure to take only butterbur that is certified as "PA Free." Pyrrolizidine alkaloids can cause liver damage. In addition, butterbur should not be taken by pregnant and breastfeeding women or by people with an ongoing liver condition.

Feverfew. 50mg–100mg per day. Feverfew is used for the prevention of migraines, headaches, arthritis, fevers, muscle tension, and pain. A 2011 study showed that combining feverfew with ginger was effective and safe in reducing the onset of, and providing pain relief during, a migraine attack.[14]

Caution. Feverfew should not be given to children or to pregnant or breastfeeding women.

Helpful

5 HTP (hydroxy tryptophan). 100mg–200mg per day. This naturally occurring amino acid increases serotonin, a mood regulator, and is commonly used to help with obesity (dieting), PMS, migraines, depression, anxiety, insomnia, and addictive behaviors. A 2000 study showed that use of 5 HTP for headaches, significantly reduced the number of days with a headache, as well as lessened the need for use of analgesics.[15]

Riboflavin (vitamin B2). 100mg–400mg per day. Research shows it can help reduce the frequency of migraine attacks.[16]

CoQ10. 100mg–200mg per day. Studies show that CoQ10 along with magnesium may offer a good alternative treatment to medications for migraine headaches.[17] [18]

Diet

Follow the Vision diet in Chapter 7 of this book. Although migraine headaches are not the same as ocular or visual migraines, it might be helpful to reduce foods that are known to cause migraine headaches, such as aged cheeses, dairy, chocolate, caffeine, alcohol (especially red wine), apples, bananas, beans (like broad or fava), corn, citrus fruits, nuts and nut butters, onions, and possible allergens such as tomato sauces, and spicy foods. Gluten sensitivity, MSG, nitrates and nitrites, aspartame, and deficiencies such as with vitamin B2, B12, magnesium, or CoQ10 may also be contributing factors. [19]

Juicing. Below are suggested foods for your juicing recipe. You can select from any combination of these, plus add your favorite fruits and vegetables.

- Celery, carrot, leafy-green vegetables, blueberry, cherries, other berries, parsley, watermelon, lemons, bananas, avocado, melon, coconut, and lemon
- Be careful not to add too much fruit with high natural-sugar content. Try to use room temperature vegetables and fruit.
- Do not add ice or very cold liquids since cold foods and liquids will eventually extinguish the stomach's digestive fire.
- Do not juice as often during the cooler months of the year, and instead, switch to vegetable soups or stews.

Lifestyle

Eye exercises may be helpful for retinal migraines and possibly visual migraines to improve circulation. See the eye exercises and acupressure points in Chapter 10-4, particularly:

- Acupressure points to regularly massage through the day

- Palming, to relax your eyes.

Alternative healing practices can help prevent and even relieve an active migraine. These therapies include acupuncture, shiatsu, chiropractic, homeopathy, aromatherapy, craniosacral therapy, biofeedback therapy, and massage. Other aids include:

- Ice packs. Place directly over your eyes, with cloth between eye pack and eyes.
- Relax in a warm, dark room.

Acupressure. You may include the following acupressure points to massage: in the middle of the eyebrow (Yuyao), the temples (GB1), 1/2 inch above the middle/top part of the ears (GB5 area), in the indentation under the cranium (GB20), trapezius muscles along the top of the shoulders and up the side of the neck (GB41), LV3 (in the web between the 1st and 2nd toes), and LI4 (web between thumb and forefinger).

Manage stress. Meditate, take cool walks in the morning, practice yoga, whatever works well.

Drink plenty of water.

Exercise regularly, at least 3 times per week. Exercise reduces the amount of pain from migraines, although it does not directly stop migraines.

Grounding regularly for migraines. Grounding, which is touching bare skin to the earth, allows an unending supply of electrons to enter the body. These are the same electrons needed by mitochondria to produce ATP fuel for creating energy in the cell.[20] The practice of grounding, or earthing, may help reduce the occurrence or severity of migraines. See Appendix 7 for more information about grounding.

Other Modalities

Essential Oils

Lavender essential oil benefits include its ability to eliminate nervous tension, relieve pain, disinfect the scalp and skin, enhance blood circulation, and treat respiratory problems.

Frankincense helps relieve chronic stress and anxiety, reduces pain and inflammation, and boosts immunity.

Spike lavender helps reduce stress, relieve pain, helps with headaches, and has anti-inflammatory properties. It is similar to lavender, but it contains a much higher level of camphor, which helps reduce nervousness and inflammation.

Keep essences away from the mouth, eyes, and mucous membranes; if a few drops get in one of these sensitive areas it may be uncomfortable for 15–30 minutes, but not harmful. You can lessen discomfort by adding a pure oil like olive or coconut oil to neutralize the irritating effect. For the eye area, dab a few drops around the outside of the eye. Do not put the neutralizing oil in the eye.

Combine ¼ cup of avocado oil with ¼ cup of calendula-infused oil. Slowly add 5 drops each of the essential oils. Then close the bottle and shake well; apply 4 drops of this mixture on your clean face. Massage in gentle circular motions. Leave overnight.

For more information on essential oils, go to Appendix 9.

Chinese Medicine

The most common meridian (when out of balance) related to migraines and ocular migraines is the Liver meridian. The most common pattern related to these headaches is 'Liver yang rising," resulting in excess heat rising to the head, causing the inability of energy to properly redistribute back through the rest of the body. In TCM, one function of the Liver is to move qi energy and blood throughout the body. Emotions such as anger, frustration, or repressed emotions can harm the functioning of the Liver and its partner the Gallbladder. Keep in mind that other meridians out of balance can also contribute to headaches.

Xiao yao san (rambling powder) is a Liver tonic that supports the free flow of energy and blood to the eyes and throughout the body.

Preserve vistas pill (zhu jing wan) tonifies and nourishes the Liver and Kidneys, enriches the yin, and improves vision.

Ming mu di huang wan (rehmannia pills "to brighten the eyes") is related to the following patterns: Liver blood deficiency, Kidney yin deficiency, and Liver yin deficiency.

Tien ma gou teng yin is related to the following patterns: nourishes yin and Liver wind (clears inflammation) used for optic neuritis and migraine headaches.

Food in Chinese Medicine

Foods that have a bitter or sour flavor are decongesting and cleansing for the Liver and Gallbladder. Raw vegetables such as cucumbers, celery, kale, asparagus, leek, artichokes, cabbage, carrots, beets, endive, fennel, kale, parsley, radish, radicchio, mustard greens, green beans, nettles, and fruit such as lemons, limes, green apple, sour cherry, avocado, plums, and quince support the liver. If digestion is weak (gas, bloating, stomach aches, loose stools), then lightly steamed vegetables, soups, and stewed fruit will be more beneficial. Spirulina, dandelion root tea, burdock root, milk thistle, and apple-cider vinegar are very beneficial for liver cleansing and support.

If you are considering doing an intensive Liver/Gallbladder cleanse, it is best done during the spring, which is the "season of the Liver." During the cooler, winter months, our bodies need to keep its energy and warmth. A cleanse during fall and winter is generally too cooling and draining for the body.

Also See

Chapter 7, Vision Diet

Chapter 8, Nutrients

Chapter 10-4, Eye Exercises

Chapter 15-16, Light Sensitivity

Appendix 9, Essential Oils

[1] American Migraine Foundation. Understanding Ocular Migraine. Retrieved Apr 30 2018 from https://americanmigrainefoundation.org/understanding-migraine/understanding-ocular-migraine.

[2] Gupta, V.K. (2006). Migrainous scintillating scotoma and headache is ocular in origin: A new hypothesis. *Med Hypotheses,* 66(3):454-60.

[3] Wikipedia. Retinal Migraine. Retrieved Feb 22 2018 from https://en.wikipedia.org/wiki/Retinal_migraine

[4] Grosberg, B.M., Solomon, S., Lipton, R.B. (2005). Retinal migraine. *Curr Pain Headache Rep,* Aug;9(4):268-71.

[5] Hills, D.L., Daroff, R.B., Ducros, A., Newman, N.J., Biousse, V. (2007). Most cases labeled as "retinal migraine" are not migraine. *J Neurophthalmol,* Mar; 27(1).3-8.

[6] Levin, M., Ward, T.N. (2004). Ophthalmoplegic migraine. *Curr Pain Headache Rep,* Aug;8(4):306-9.

[7] Jehn A, Dettwiler B, Fleischhauer J, Sturzenegger, M., Mojon, D.S. (2002). Exercise-induced vasospastic amaurosis fugax. *Arch Ophthalmol,* 2002;120:220–2.

[8] Yorns, W.R. (2013). Mitochondrial Dysfunction in Migraine. *Sci Dir,* 20(3):188-193.

[9] Houston, M. (2011). The role of magnesium in hypertension and cardiovascular disease. *J Clin Hypertens (Greenwich),* Nov;13(11):843-7.

Magnes Res. 2010 Jun;23(2):60-72.

[10] Flammer, J., Pache, M., Resink, T. (2001). Vasospasm, its role in the pathogenesis of diseases with particular reference to the eye. *Prog Retin Eye Res,* May;20(3):319-49.

[11] Schecter, M. (2010). Magnesium and cardiovascular system. *Magnes Res,* Jun;23(2):60-72

[12] Lipton, R.B., Gobel, H., Einhaupl, K.M., Mauskop, A. (2004). Petasites hybridus root (butterbur) is an effective preventive treatment for migraine. *Neurology,* Dec 28;63(12):2240-4.

[13] Grossmann, M., Schmidramsl, H. (2000). An extract of Petasites hybridus is effective in the prophylaxis of migraine. *Int J Clin Pharmacol Ther,* Sep;38(9):430-5.

[14] Cady, R.K., Goldstein, J., Nett, R., Mitchell, R., Beach, M.E., Browning, R. (2011). A double-blind placebo-controlled pilot study of sublingual feverfew and ginger (LipiGesic™ M) in the treatment of migraine. *Headache,* Jul-Aug;51(7):1078-86.

[15] Ribeiro, C.A. (2000). L-5-Hydroxytryptophan in the prophylaxis of chronic tension-type headache: a double-blind, randomized, placebo-controlled study. *Headache,* 40:451-6

[16] Schoenen, J., Jacquy, J., Lenaerts, M. (1998). Effectiveness of high-dose riboflavin in migraine prophylaxis. A randomized controlled trial. *Neurology,* Feb; 50(2):466-70.

[17] Sândor, P. S., Di Clemente, L., Coppolam G., Saenger, U., Fumal, A., et al. (2005). Efficacy of coenzyme Q10 in migraine prophylaxis: a randomized controlled trial. *Neurology,* 64(4):713–715.

[18] Ibid. Sandor. (2005).

[19] WebMD. Food Triggers for Migraines. Retrieved Feb 18 2018 from https://www.webmd.com/migraines-headaches/migraine-smart-17/migraine-trigger-foods.

[20] Graveline, D. (2010). Earthing - Dr. Duane Graveline, M.D. Retrieved Apr 14 2018 from https://spacedoc.com/articles/earthing-dr-duane-graveline.

15-23. OPTIC NERVE ATROPHY

Optic nerve atrophy, also known as optic neuropathy, simply defined, is the end result of any disease that damages nerve cells anywhere between the retina and a part of the thalamus that links the eye to the brain.[1] Optic nerve atrophy is the condition wherein the optic nerve is limited in its capacity to transmit information accurately. While there are different causes associated with this disorder, the end result is the same, which is a degeneration, or "wasting away," of the nerve. Onset can occur from birth through adulthood.

If the condition is long-standing, then the doctor sees the optic nerve as pale or visibly withered in an eye exam. Whether the nerve is partially or seriously wasted away, determines the degree of loss or change in vision.

The Optic Nerve

The optic nerve is responsible for carrying electrical impulses from the retina to our brain. Impulses that contain the information about what we see. The optic nerve is made up of ganglion nerve cells in the retina and glial cells.

- Retinal ganglion cells receive information from the photoreceptors, and they transmit that information to different parts of the brain in the thalamus, hypothalamus, and midbrain.[2]
- Glial cells are not nerve cells, but they are essential to optic nerve health because they protect and insulate the optic nerve and supply it with nutrients.[3]

Types of Optic Neuropathy

In practice, optic neuropathy is not considered a disease, but rather a sign or symptom of potentially many disease processes. It is closely associated to a group of conditions, some of which are genetically based, while others are due to lifestyle considerations, such as chronic systemic inflammation, trauma, toxins, poor blood flow, and/or a lack of essential nutrients getting to the optic nerve. Thus, the prevalence of optic nerve atrophy depends on the prevalence of an underlying cause.

Ischemic optic neuropathy is caused by insufficient blood flow with an occlusion in blood supply vessels. It occurs in adults and is described as a "stroke" of the optic nerve. One type, arteritic anterior ischemic optic neuropathy, is an ophthalmic emergency.[4] The other non-arteritic type involves swelling, which typically lessens over time, but vision does not improve.[5]

Optic neuritis is caused by an inflamed optic nerve.

In **compressive optic neuropathy,** lesions cause the optic nerve to become compressed. A similar condition in appearance is glaucomatous optic neuropathy.[6]

Infiltrative optic neuropathy occurs when the tumors or an inflammatory process invades the nerve or the space around it.[7]

Traumatic optic neuropathy develops after direct or indirect injury to the eye or sometimes to the back of the head.

Mitochondria optic neuropathy involves failure in mitochondria functioning.

Nutritional optic neuropathy occurs when nutritional deficiencies cause severe problems.

Toxic optic neuropathy arises due to damage from various poisons, toxins, and some drugs.[8]

Hereditary optic neuropathy is caused by genetic mutations, including Leber's hereditary optic neuropathy.

Optic nerve atrophy type 1 appears in childhood, or during puberty, with visual loss that progresses during puberty until adulthood. The subsequent progression is chronic and very slow. This is a complete and permanent breakdown of optic nerve fibers.

Signs and Symptoms

The symptoms described here may not necessarily mean that you have optic nerve atrophy. However, if you experience one or more of these symptoms, contact your eye doctor for a complete exam.

- **Blurred vision**
- **Decrease in visual function**, such as a decrease in sharpness, clarity of vision (visual acuity), or decrease in side (peripheral) vision
- **Color vision and contrast sensitivity** can also be affected
- **Poor constriction of the pupil in light** and eventually its inability to react to light
- **A decrease in observed brightness** (the amount of light one would typically see through a healthy eye) in one eye relative to the other
    - For example, vision in a bright room would appear dimmer through an eye with optic nerve atrophy than through a healthy eye. This would make it more difficult, for instance, to see colors clearly, or it would appear as if there is a cloud in the visual field.
- **Change in the optic disc**, which would be observed by your eye doctor during a dilated eye exam

Causes and Risk Factors

Most commonly, optic nerve atrophy is diagnosed without a known or proven cause. Possible leading causes range from eye injury or trauma to systemic eye conditions and diseases, that include the following:

Optic neuritis, which occurs when the optic nerve is inflamed due to autoimmune conditions, infections (viral, fungal, and bacterial), parasitic diseases, toxins, allergies, digestive problems, diabetes, and/or simply poor circulation. The inflammation essentially attacks the myelin covering, and the optic nerve becomes swollen, and over time, damaged. The person might notice eye pain, which is more severe when they move their eye. Optic neuritis is most commonly found in young to middle-aged women, and some people with this condition can develop multiple sclerosis later in life. See Chapter 15-24.

Leber's hereditary optic neuropathy, an inborn (genetic) condition that generally manifests in young men in their late teens to early 20s, is characterized by the development of painless, serious central visual loss in one eye, over the course of a few weeks, followed by the same process weeks or months later in the other eye. In the beginning, there might be slight swelling, but eventually the optic nerve atrophies, usually resulting in permanent vision loss. See Chapter 15-15.

Toxic optic neuropathy (TON) is the condition where known toxins damage the optic nerve, causing gradual or sudden vision loss. The most common optic neuropathy from poisons and toxins is called tobacco-alcohol amblyopia, thought to be caused by exposure to cyanide from tobacco smoking and low vitamin B12 levels. Other toxins known to contribute to TON include methyl alcohol (moonshine), ethylene glycol (antifreeze), cyanide, lead, and carbon monoxide. Certain medications should also be avoided because of their known toxicity to the optic nerve. These medications include ethambutol and isoniazid, drugs used to prevent tuberculosis; amiodarone, a drug very useful in the treatment of life-threatening cardiac arrhythmias; tamoxifen (Nolvadex), used for both prevention and treatment of breast cancer; and isotretinoin (Accutane), used in the treatment of severe acne vulgaris. Other drugs that have been implicated in the toxic optic neuropathies include chloramphenicol, sulfonamides, linezolid, chloroquine, quinine, streptomycin, digitalis, vincristine, and methotrexate. If you are taking any of these drugs and suffer from optic nerve atrophy, you should review these with your eye doctor and specialist.

Certain drugs are optic nerve toxins, including ethambutol, topiramate (Topamax) that can cause narrow angle glaucoma, and amiodarone that can cause blurred vision and ischemic optic neuropathy.[9] Ethambutol is considered an optic nerve toxin.[10]

Nutritional optic neuropathy may be caused by deficiencies in protein, B vitamins (particularly vitamin B12), and folic acid, which result from poor nutrition, starvation, poor absorption of nutrients, or alcoholism. Vitamin B12 deficiency damages the nerves, and consuming alcohol contributes to poor absorption of vitamin B12. Treatment with B12 injections as well as oral B12 supplementation has been found to result in dramatic vision improvement.[11]

Untreated glaucoma, specifically the characteristic eye pressure associated with it, increases the potential for damage of the optic nerve. See Chapter 15-11.

Compressive optic neuropathy results from a tumor or other lesion pressing on the optic nerve, from elevated intraocular pressure, or from enlargement of eye movement muscles (which is seen in hyperthyroidism and Graves' disease patients).

Syphilis, untreated, can also result in damage to the optic nerve.

Brain tumor or **stroke** may cause optic nerve atrophy.

Conventional Treatment

There is no treatment to reverse atrophy of the optic nerve. However, limiting further optic nerve damage, if possible, is the goal. One possible way to reduce vision loss is through the reduction of increased fluid pressure around the brain and spinal cord (a condition called hydrocephalus). Once the nerve fibers in the optic nerve are lost, they never heal or grow back. If the cause can be found, corrected, or managed, sometimes further damage can be reduced or prevented. This is especially true for identified causes such as system inflammation, glaucoma, and multiple sclerosis.

Complementary Approach

Because some types of optic nerve damage may result from nutritional deficiencies, good nutrition is critical for healthy optic nerves. Vitamin B12 and folic acid deficiencies are at the foundation of nutritional optic neuropathy. Certain nutrients such as ginkgo biloba, bilberry, alpha-lipoic acid, taurine, magnesium, a number of other vitamins and enzymes, and omega-3 fatty acids in the form of fish oil or algae-based supplements (for vegetarians), support optic nerve health. Daily juicing is a very good way to maximize the nutritional value of your diet and to stave off deficiencies. Nutrients from juices are easier to absorb, which is helpful for anyone with digestive difficulties.

Additionally, many of the recommended supplements listed below are antioxidants. Since a number of studies indicate that oxidative stress is a crucial factor in optic nerve problems, antioxidants may play an important role in preventing and treating the condition. As a general rule, make sure to supplement daily with antioxidants, and get as many as possible through a healthy diet. Plant foods, by far, contain more antioxidants than animal products. In Chapter 5, read more about antioxidants and the plant-based foods highest in them.

Nutrients

Essential

Alpha-lipoic acid. 300mg per day. Alpha-lipoic acid is the only antioxidant that is both fat and water-soluble. Studies have shown that its benefits to people with glaucoma include enhanced color vision, enhanced general vision sensitivity, and it helps protect nerve cells from damage.[12] Alpha-lipoic acid also enhances glutathione, vitamins E and C, and essential antioxidants in the eye. R-alpha-lipoic acid (found in nature) has been found to be the most well absorbed form, versus the synthetic S form.[13] If supplementing in the R form alone, the recommended dosage is 150mg daily.

Aminoguarnadine. 75mg tablets, take 3 times per day, split up over the day with or without food. This anti-glycating agent inhibits the "cross-linking" (or glycosylation) of proteins, which may cause, or at least contribute to, many optic nerve and related problems.[14] Aminoguarnadine has been shown in animal studies to have neuroprotective qualities and may help preserve the vision of refractory-glaucoma patients by inhibiting the build-up of nitric oxide synthase-2 (NOS-2), a substance believed to cause nerve cell damage. NOS-2 stimulates the emission of nitric oxide, a compound implicated in diseases such as glaucoma.[15] [16] [17]

Omega-3 fatty acids. 2,000mg–3,000mg per day. DHA from omega-3 fatty acids accounts for approximately 50–60% of the total fatty acid content within rod outer segments of photoreceptors, and it tends to be very deficient in today's diet.[18] [19] Proper amounts are critical for maintaining the health of the retina.[20]

Vitamin D3. 2,000 IU–5,000 IU per day. Vitamin D rejuvenates aging eyes, reduces inflammation that is often associated with optic nerve atrophy, and improves overall vision functionality.[21] Studies that investigate the link between vitamin D and indices of microvascular disease have shown that vitamin D deficiency is associated with poor coronary microcirculation, which is essential for necessary delivery of oxygen and nutrients to the optic nerve.[22]

Ginkgo biloba. 120mg per day. Ginkgo biloba improves microcapillary circulation in the eye and slows deterioration of the macula through its antioxidant effects, which again, are essential for delivery of oxygen and nutrients to the optic nerve.[23] Studies have shown that it improves overall circulation,[24] [25] stabilizes capillaries, and makes capillaries less fragile.[26] [27] [28] [29] Ginkgo has also been shown to have potent antioxidant properties.[30]

Bilberry. 180mg–240mg per day. Bilberry extracts have antioxidative properties that are not only neuroprotective, but they also help suppress photooxidative processes (the breakdown of oxygen molecules that create an unstable environment for healthy cells). Bilberry has been shown to improve small blood vessels, such as capillaries that provide the delivery of blood to the retina and optic nerve. Photooxidation is accelerated by exposure to sunlight. The anthocyanoside content of bilberry may be especially beneficial for nighttime visual acuity.[31] [32] [33]

Vitamin B12 (as methylcobalamin). 1000mcg per day. Research has shown that supplementing with vitamin B12 helps protect vision for those with glaucoma.[34] Deficiency in vitamin B12 has been associated with optic neuritis.[35] [36]

Taurine. 750mg–1,000mg per day. When taurine levels are deficient, a variety of vision problems can occur, including retinal ganglion cell degeneration.[37] Taurine is an amino acid that protects the eyes against neurotoxins. These include excessive levels of glutamate, which is possibly responsible for the loss of ganglion cells and optic nerve damage seen in open-angle glaucoma.[38]

CoQ10. 100mg–200mg per day. CoQ10 also has powerful antioxidant properties, protecting important proteins and mitochondrial DNA6 from oxidative damage.[39] One well-absorbed form of CoQ10 is the ubiquinol form, and it is used for cell growth and maintenance. It also functions as an antioxidant, which protects the body from damage caused by harmful molecules. Cofactors that enable improved use in CoQ10 in the body include shilajit, an adaptogen (helps the body adapt to internal and external stressors). Shilajit is found to augment CoQ10 with the speed and facilitation of essential electron flow in mitochondria, with helping to protect mitochondria against oxidative damage, and with reducing dangerous lipid peroxidation.[40] [41] Other cofactors include **l-carnitine**, 500mg per day, *and* **alpha-lipoic acid**, 300mg per day. CoQ10 is of particular interest because it not only supports the mitochondrial respiratory chain, but it also acts as a powerful antioxidant in mitochondrial membranes.

PQQ (Coenzyme pyrroloquinoline quinone). 20mg per day. Like CoQ10, this acts as an antioxidant and protects against mitochondrial damage, but it also stimulates the production of new mitochondria. Current recommendations are to take PQQ and CoQ10 together, daily.[42]

Very Important

Astaxanthin. 6mg–12mg per day. Astaxanthin's powerful antioxidant benefits help prevent retinal damage[43] and help protect against sun damage.[44] Astaxanthin can cross both layers of the cell membrane, allowing it to trap free radicals, outside and inside the cell. Astaxanthin also protects mitochondria health.[45] [46] [47] [48] [49]

Trans-resveratrol. 50mg–175mg per day. Studies indicate that resveratrol may be the most effective compound for maintaining optimal health and promoting longevity. Research also shows that resveratrol may be effective in the microcirculation of the eye.[50] Also **grapeseed extract**, 300mg per day, *or* **pycnogenol**, 100mg–200mg per day. All of these antioxidants provide a similar benefit of strengthening blood vessels and reducing inflammation (again, often associated with optic nerve atrophy). They have also been found to support healthy circulation and to neutralize free radicals. Take one or all three of these.

Glutathione (GSH), reduced. 500mg-900mg, daily, if taken in capsule or pill form. The sublingual form has 5–10 times greater absorption so the dosage will be smaller. Follow label instructions. GSH is a major non-enzymatic antioxidant present in both intracellular and extracellular spaces.[51] [52] It is a potent antioxidant known as the anti-aging antioxidant, as it can neutralize the full spectrum of free radicals and help prevent damage to the retina and optic nerve due to oxidation.[53] Patients with primary open-angle glaucoma exhibit low levels of circulating glutathione.[54]

Vitamin E (d-alpha-tocopherol). 400 IU's per day. This helps prevent the formation of free radicals, while it also functions as a scavenger in vivo. It effectively alleviates ischemic injury after optic nerve injury, reduces damage, and promotes optic nerve repair. There is also an indication that there is a low level of vitamin E available after optic nerve injury.[55] D-alpha-tocopherol is one form of vitamin E and is best taken in a synergistic blend with the other vitamin E compounds (tocopherols and tocotrienols).

A high-quality, whole-food, organic multivitamin. Follow dosage directions on the bottle.

Helpful

Green tea extract. 500mg–750mg per day. Green teas and their extracts are potentially neuroprotective in the photoreceptor outer segment and retinal pigment epithelium (RPE).[56]

Lycopene. 3mg per day. Lycopene is effective in maintaining healthy LDL oxidation and protecting against free radical activity on the arterial wall.[57][58][59][60][61][62][63][64]

Diet

Follow the Vision diet in Chapter 7 of this guide. Take care to add the following on a regular basis:

Juicing. Juice daily and use organic produce, if possible. Our recipe is designed to help support overall retinal and eye health. Use a combination of the following:

- Ginger, garlic, parsley, leeks, beets, cabbage, carrots, spinach, celery, apples, grapes, raspberries, lemon, and wheatgrass*
- Feel free to add your favorite fruits and vegetables. Avoid using too much fruit or too many carrots or beets because of their high, natural sugar content.
- Try to use room temperature vegetables and fruit.
- Do not add ice or very cold liquids since cold foods and liquids will eventually extinguish the stomach's digestive fire.
- Do not juice as often during the cooler months of the year, and instead, switch to vegetable soups or stews.

*Wheatgrass contains high levels of nutrients, including vitamins A, C, and E, iron, calcium, magnesium, and amino acids. It is used for increasing production of hemoglobin, the chemical in red blood cells that carries oxygen.

Avoid artificial sweeteners, flavorings, and seasonings (such as MSG) that can cause damage to retina cells and subsequently cause optic nerve damage.[65]

Lifestyle

Eye exercises. See our eye exercises in Chapter 10. Any common eye exercise done daily helps improve circulation and the flow of energy through the eyes. Select a few eye exercises to do each day for at least 10 minutes total, or longer if you like, and include daily palming and massage of the acupressure points around the eyes.

Stop smoking. Smoking significantly increases the risk of severe development of optic nerve atrophy.

Exercise frequently. Exercise is the single most important thing you can do for most health conditions, including virtually all vision conditions.

Liver detoxification. Since the eyes are closely related to the liver in Traditional Chinese Medicine, consider a yearly spring liver detoxification under the guidance of a qualified health practitioner.

Microcurrent Stimulation (MCS). A number of research studies show MCS as a method to daily support retinal and photoreceptor health in the following three ways:[66][67][68][69][70] See Chapter 10-3 for more information.

1. It supports healthy circulation to the retina.
2. It increases energy (ATP) production within the retinal cells.
3. It helps the retina eliminate waste.

The recommended usage is 5–10 minutes, two times per day, for a total of 10–20 minutes per day (for the MCS 100ile unit).

Although the MCS research studies focused primarily on retinal diseases, we believe its application may help with optic nerve atrophy. Daily MCS at home also helps improve circulation to the back of the eyes, which in turn helps the body deliver oxygen and essential nutrients.

Note. Usage may vary depending on the type of microcurrent unit you use, so check with your healthcare practitioner before, to get proper instructions. Also, if you have a history of retinal bleeding, do not use MCS without checking with your eye doctor. Contraindications include having a pacemaker or a history of epilepsy. See more about MCS in Chapter 10-3.

Other Modalities

Chinese Medicine

From a Traditional Chinese Medicine (TCM) perspective, there are a number of patterns and imbalances that are related to optic nerve atrophy. Diagnosis from a TCM standpoint depends on the identified underlying cause(s), but a common pattern to investigate is the exhaustion of qi, and blood that denies nourishment to the eyes. Treatment is directed toward nourishing and strengthening the Liver and Kidney systems.

Common patent formulas used in Chinese medicine and suggested for optic nerve atrophy include the following:

Ming mu di huang wan (rehmannia pills to "brighten the eyes") addresses the following patterns: Liver blood deficiency, Kidney yin deficiency, and Liver yin deficiency.

Xiao yao san (rambling powder) supports and tonifies the Liver (meridian), which "opens to the eyes."

Medicinal mushrooms. Reishi,[71][72] maitake,[73][74] bitter tooth,[75][76] and lion's mane[77][78] are essential for optic nerve atrophy as they have neurite outgrowth and neuronal health benefits.

Your acupuncturist may choose to go with these formulas, or others, depending on the intake and diagnosis.

Also See

Chapter 7, Vision Diet

Chapter 8, Nutrients

Chapter 15-5, Cone-Rod Dystrophy

Chapter 15-11, Glaucoma

Chapter 15-15, Leber's Hereditary Optic Neuropathy

Chapter 15-24, Optic Neuritis

[1] Wikipedia. Optic Neuropathy. Retrieved Mar 5 2018 from https://en.wikipedia.org/wiki/Optic_neuropathy

[2] Wikipedia. Retinal ganglion cell. Retrieved March 5 2018 from https://en.wikipedia.org/wiki/Retinal_ganglion_cell

[3] Wikipedia. Neuroglia. Retrieved Mar 5 2018 from https://en.wikipedia.org/wiki/Neuroglia

[4] Hayreh, S.S. (2011). Management of ischemic optic neuropathies. *Indian J Ophthalmol*, Mar-Apr;59(2):123-36.

[5] Wilhelm, H., Beisse, F., Ruther, K. (2015). Non-Arteritic Ischemic Optic Neuropathy (NAION). *Klin Monbl Augenheilkd*, Nov;232(11):1260-9.

[6] Hata, M., Miyamoto, K., Oishi, A., Makiyama, Y., Gotoh, N., et al. (2014). Comparison of optic disc morphology of optic nerve atrophy between compressive optic neuropathy and glaucomatous optic neuropathy. *PloS One*, Nov 6;9(11):e112403

[7] Baloh, R.W., Jen, J. (2012). Neuro-Ophthalmology. Retrieved from https://www.sciencedirect.com/topics/medicine-and-dentistry/optic-neuropathy.

[8] Sharma, P., Sharma, R. (2011). Toxic optic neuropathy. *Indian J Ophthalmol*, Mar-Apr; 59(2): 137–141.

[9] Stephenson, M. (2011). System Drugs with Ocular Side Effects. Retrieved Jan 13 2018 from https://www.reviewofophthalmology.com/article/systemic-drugs-with-ocular-side-effects

[10] Talbert Estin, K.A., Sadun, A.A. (2010). Risk factors for ethambutol optic toxicity. *Int Ophthalmol*, 30:63-72.

[11] Woon, C., Tang, R.A., Pardo, G. (1995). Nutrition and optic nerve disease. *Semin Ophthalmol*, Sep;10(3):195-202.

[12] Packer, L, Tritschler, H.J., Wessel, K. (1997). Neuroprotection by the metabolic antioxidant alpha-lipoic acid, *Free Radical Biol Med*, 22(1-2):359-78.

[13] Unknown. (2006). Alpha-lipoic acid. Monograph. *Altern Med Rev*, Sept;11(3):232-7.

[14] Piercy, V., Toseland, C.D., Tuner, N.C. (1998). Potential benefit of inhibitors of advanced glycation end products in the progression of type II diabetes: a study with aminoguanidine in C57/BLKsJ diabetic mice *Metabolism*, Dec;47(12):1477-80.

[15] Tsai, D.C., Hsu, W.M., Chou, C.K., Chen, S.J., Peng, C.H., et al. (2002). Significant variation of the elevated nitric oxide levels in aqueous humor from patients with different types of glaucoma. *Ophthalmologica*, Sep-Oct; 216(5):346-50.

[16] Neufeldman, A.H., Das, S., Vora, S., Gachie, E., Kawai, S., et al. (2002). A prodrug of a selective inhibitor of inducible nitric oxide synthase is neuroprotective in the rat model of glaucoma. *J Glaucoma*, Jun;11(3):221-5.

[17] Yang, C.W., Yu, C.C., Ko, Y.C., Huang, C.C. (1998). Aminoguanidine reduces glomerular inducible nitric oxide synthase (iNOS) and transforming growth factor-beta 1 (TGF-β1) mRNA expression and diminishes glomerulosclerosis in NZB/W F1 mice. *Clin Exp Immunol*, Aug;113(2):258-264.

[18] Bush, R.A., Malnoe, A., Reme, C.E., Williams, T.P. (1994). Dietary deficiency of N-3 fatty acids alters rhodopsin content and function in the rat retina. *Invest Ophthalmol Vis Sci*, 35(1):91–100.

[19] Stillwell, W., Wassall, S.R. (2003). Docosahexaenoic acid: membrane properties of a unique fatty acid. Chem Phys Lipids, 126(1):1–27.

[20] Elner, V.M. (2002). Retinal pigment epithelial acid lipase activity and lipoprotein receptors: effects of dietary omega-3 fatty acids. *Trans Am Ophthalmol Soc*, 100:301–338.

[21] Lee, V., Rekhi, E., Hoh Kam, J., Jeffery, G. (2012). Vitamin D rejuvenates aging eyes by reducing inflammation, clearing amyloid beta and improving visual function. *Neurobiol Aging,* Oct;33(10):2382.

[22] Capitanio, S., Sambuceti, G., Giusti, M., Morbelli, S., Murialdo, G., et al. (2013). 1,25-Dihydroxy vitamin D and coronary microvascular function. *Eur J Nucl Med Mol Imaging,* 40:280–9.

[23] Droy-Lefaix, M.T., Cluzel, J., Menerath, J.M., Bonhomme, B., Doly, M. (1995). Antioxidant effect of a Ginkgo biloba extract (EGb 761) on the retina. *Antint J Tissue React,* 17(3):93-100.

[24] Wu, Y.Z., Li, S.Q., Zu, X.G., Du, J., Wang, F.F. (2007). Ginkgo biloba extract improves coronary artery circulation in patients with coronary artery disease: contribution of plasma nitric oxide and endothelin-1. *Phytother Res,* Jun;22(6):734-9.

[25] Wu, Y., Li., S., Cui, W., Zu, X., Du, J., et al. (2008). Ginkgo biloba extract improves coronary blood flow in healthy elderly adults: role of endothelium-dependent vasodilation. *Phytomedicine,* Mar;15(3):164-9.

[26] Welt, K., Weiss, J., Martin, R., Hermsdorf, T., Drews, S., et al. (2007). Ginkgo biloba extract protects rat kidney from diabetic and hypoxic damage. *Phytomedicine,* Feb;14(2-3):196-203.

[27] Qui, Y., Rui, Y.C., Li, T.J., Zhang, L., Yao, P.Y. (2004). Inhibitory effect of extracts of Ginkgo biloba leaves on VEGF-induced hyperpermeability of bovine coronary endothelial cells in vitro. *Acta Pharmacol Sin,* Oct;25(10):1306-11.

[28] Huang, S.Y., Jeng, C., Kao, S.C., Yu, J.J., Liu, D.Z. (2004). Improved haemorrheological properties by Ginkgo biloba extract (Egb 761) in type 2 diabetes mellitus complicated with retinopathy. *Clin Nutr,* Aug;23(4):615-21.

[29] Quaranta, L., Bettelli, S., Uva, M.G., Semeraro, F., Turano, R., et al. (2003). Effect of Ginkgo biloba extract on preexisting visual field damage in normal tension glaucoma. *Ophthalmology,* 110: 359-36

[30] Ou, H.C., Lee, W.J., Lee, I.T., Chiu, T.H., Tsai, K.L., et al. (1985). Ginkgo biloba extract attenuates oxLDL-induced oxidative functional damages in endothelial cells. *J Appl Physiol,* May;106(5):1674-85.

[31] Muth, E.R., Laurent, J.M., Jasper, P. (2000). The effect of bilberry nutritional supplementation on night visual acuity and contrast sensitivity. *Altern Med Rev,* Apr;5(2):164-73.

[32] Matsunaga, N., Imai, S., Inokuchi, Y., Shimazawa, M., Yokota, S., et al. (2009). Bilberry and its main constituents have neuroprotective effects against retinal neuronal damage in vitro and in vivo. *Mol Nutr Food Res,* Jul;53(7):869-77

[33] Yao, Y., Vieria, A. (2007). Protective activities of Vaccinium antioxidants with potential relevance to mitochondrial dysfunction and neurotoxicity. Neurotoxicology, 28 93–100

[34] Sakai, T. Murata, M., and Amemiya, T. Effect of long-term treatment of glaucoma with vitamin B12. *Glaucoma,* 14 167-70).

[35] Chavala, S.H., Kosmorsky, G.S., Lee, M.K., Lee, M.S. (2005). Optic neuropathy in vitamin B12 deficiency. *Eur J Intern Med,* Oct;16(6):447-8.

[36] Moschos, M. (1998). Optic neuropathy in vitamin B12 deficiency. *The Lancet,* Jul;352(9122):146-147.

[37] Froger, N., Cadetti, L., Lorach, H., Martins, J., Bemelmans, A.P., et al. (2012) Taurine provides neuroprotection against retinal ganglion cell degeneration. *PLoS One,* 7(10):e42017.

[38] Fennessy, F.M., Moneley, D.S., Wang, J.H., Kelly, C.J., Boucher-Hayes, D.J. (2003). Taurine and vitamin C modify monocyte and endothelial dysfunction in young smokers. *Circulation,* 107:410-15, 2003.

[39] Littarru, G.P., Tiano, L. (2007). Bioenergetic and antioxidant properties of coenzyme Q10: recent developments. *Mol Biotechnol,* Sep;37(1):31-7.

[40] Bhattacharyya, S., Pal, D., Banerjee, D., Ghosal, S. (2009). Shilajit dibenzo—pyrones: mitochondria targeted antioxidants. *Pharmacology online,* Jan;2:690-8.

[41] Bhattacharya, S.K., Bhattacharya, A., Chakrabarti, A. (2000). Adaptogenic activity of Siotone, a polyherbal formulation of Ayurvedic rasayanas. *Indian J Exp Biol,* Feb;38(2):119-28.

[42] Chowanadisai, W., Bauerly, K.A., Tchaparian, E., Wong, A., Cortopassi, G.A., et al. (2010). Pyrroloquinoline quinone stimulates mitochondrial biogenesis through cAMP response element-binding protein phosphorylation and increased PGC-1alpha expression. *J Biol Chem,* Jan 1;285(1):142-52.

[43] Nakajima, Y., Inokuchi, Y., Shimazawa, M., Otsubo, K., Ishibashi, T., et al. (2008). Astaxanthin, a dietary carotenoid, protects retinal cells against oxidative stress in-vitro and in mice in-vivo. *J Pharm Pharmacol,* Oct;60(10):1365-74.

44 Piermarocchi, S., Saviano, S., Parisi, V., Tedeschi, M., Panozzo, G., et al. (2012). Carotenoids in Age-related Maculopathy Italian Study (CARMIS): two-year results of a randomized study. *Eur J Ophthalmol*, Mar-Apr;22(2):216-25.

45 BetaForce. Astaxanthin: The Most Powerful Natural Antioxidant Ever Discovered. Retrieved Apr 2 2018 from http://www.beta-glucan-info.com/astaxanthin.htm.

46 Chiro.org. Antioxidants: Relative Singlet Oxygen Quenching Rates. Retrieved Apr 16 2018 from http://www.chiro.org/nutrition/FULL/ Antioxidants_Relative_Singlet_Oxygen_Quenching_Rates.html.

47 Kidd, P. (2011). Astaxanthin, cell membrane nutrient with diverse clinical benefits and anti-aging potential. *Altern Med Rev*, Dec;16(4):355-64.

48 Song, X., Wang, B., Lin, S., Jing, L., Mao, C., et al. (2014). Astaxanthin inhibits apoptosis in alveolar epithelial cells type II in vivo and in vitro through the ROS-dependent mitochondrial signaling pathway. *J Cell Mol Med*, Nov;18(11):2198-212.

49 Kuroki, T., Ikeda, S., Okada, T., Maoka, T., Kitamura, A., et al. (2013). Astaxanthin ameliorates heat stress-induced impairment of blastocyst development in vitro:--astaxanthin colocalization with and action on mitochondria--. *J Assist Reprod Genet*, Jun;30(5):623-31.

50 Bola, C., Bartlett, H., Eperjesi, F. (2014). Resveratrol and the eye: activity and molecular mechanisms. *Graefes Arch Clin Exp Ophthalmol*, May;252(5):699-713.

51 Dringen, R. (2000). Glutathione metabolism and oxidative stress in neurodegeneration. *Eur J Biochem*, Aug; 267(16):4903.

52 Hall, A.G. (1999). The role of glutathione in the regulation of apoptosis. *Eur J Clin Invest*, Mar; 29(3):238-45.

53 Hanashima, C., Namiki, H. (1999). Reduced viability of vascular endothelial cells by high concentration of ascorbic acid in vitreous humor. *Cell Biol Int*, 23(4):287-98.

54 Gherghel, D., Griffiths, H.R., Hilton, E.J., Cunliffe, I.A., Hosking, S.L. (2005). Systemic reduction in glutathione levels occurs in patients with primary open-angle glaucoma. *Invest Ophthalmol Vis Sci*, Mar; 46(3):877-83.

55Jiang, Y., Xu, H., Liu, J., Li, P, Wu, Y. (2012). Biomechanical analysis of optic nerve injury treated by compound light granules and ciliary neurotrophic factor. *Neural Regen Res*, Dec 25; 7(36): 2889–2900.

56Jarrett, S.G., Boulton, M.E. (2012). Consequences of oxidative stress in age-related macular degeneration. *Mol Aspects Med*, Aug;33(4):399–417.

57 Erdman, J.W., Ford, N.A., Lindshield, B.L. (2009). Are the health attributes of lycopene related to its antioxidant function? *Arc Biochem Biophys*, Mar 15;483(2):229-35.

58 Jian, L., Lee, A.H., Binns, C.W. (2007). Tea and lycopene protect against prostate cancer. *AsiaPac J Clin Nutr*, 16 Suppl 1:453-7.

59 Balestrieri, M.L., De Prisco, R., Nicolaus, B., Pari, P., Moriello, V.S., et al. (2004). Lycopene in association with alpha-tocopherol or tomato lipophilic extracts enhances acyl-platelet-activating factor biosynthesis in endothelial cells during oxidative stress. *Free Radic Biol Med*, Apr 15;36(8):1058-67.

60 Dutta-Roy, A.K., Crosbie, L., Gordon, M.J. (2001). Effects of tomato extract on human platelet aggregation in vitro. *Platelets*, Jun;12(4):218-27.

61 Agarwal, S., Rao, A.V. (1998). Tomato lycopene and low density lipoprotein oxidation: a human dietary intervention study. *Lipids*, Oct;33(10):981-4.

62 Hadley, C.W., Clinton, S.K., Schwartz, S.J. (2003). The consumption of processed tomato products enhances plasma lycopene concentrations in association with a reduced lipoprotein sensitivity to oxidative damage. *J Nutr*, Mar;133(3):727-32.

63 Hsiao, G., Wang, Y., Tzu, N.H., Fong, T.H., Shen, M.Y., et al. (2005). Inhibitory effects of lycopene on in vitro platelet activation and in vivo prevention of thrombus formation. *J Lab Clin Med*, Oct;146(4):216-26.

64 Xu, X., Zhu, M., Hu, M. (2011). Effects of lycopene on blood cells and fibrinolytic activity in hyperlipidemic rats. *Wei Sheng Yan Jiu*, Sep;40(5):620-3.

65 Van Rijn, C.M., Marani, E., Rietveld, W.J. (1986). The neurotoxic effect of monosodium glutamate (MSG) on the retinal ganglion cells of the albino rat. *Histol Histopath*, 1:291-295.

66 Leland, D., Allen, M.J. (1993) Nutritional supplementation, electrical stimulation and age related macular degeneration. *J Orthomol Med*, 18: 168-171)

67 Halloran, G. (1997). Bioelectrical Stimulation in an Integrated Treatment for Macular Degeneration, RP, Glaucoma, CMV-Retinitis, and Diabetic Retinopathy; Fourth Annual Symposium on Biological Circuits, Oct. Mankato University, MN.

[68] American Academy of Ophthalmology. (2004). Microcurrent Stimulation for Macular Degeneration CTA - 2004. Retrieved Mar 7 2018 from https://www.aao.org/complimentary-therapy-assessment/microcurrent-stimulation-macular-degeneration-cta-

[69] O'Clock, G.D., Jarding, J.B. (2009). Electrotherapeutic device/protocol design considerations for visual disease applications. *Conf Proc IEEE Eng Med Biol Soc*, 2009:2133-6.

[70] Chaikin, L., Kashiwa, K., Bennet, M., Papastergiou, G., Gregory, W. (2015). Microcurrent stimulation in the treatment of dry and wet macular degeneration. *Clin Ophthalmol*, Dec 17;9:2345-53.

[71] Sun, XZ, Liao, Y., Li, W., Guo, L.M. (2017). Neuroprotective effects of ganoderma lucidum polysaccharides against oxidative stress-induced neuronal apoptosis. *Neural Regen Res*, Jun;12(6):953-958.

[72] Zhang, W., Zhang, Q., Deng, W., Li, Y., Xing, G., et al. (2014). Neuroprotective effect of pretreatment with ganoderma lucidum in cerebram ischemia/reperfusion injury in rat hippocampus. *Neural Regen Res*, Aug 1;9(15):1446-52.

[73] Chen, Z., Tang, Y., Liu, A., Jin, X., Zhu, J., et al. (2017). Oral administration of Grifola fondosa polysaccharides improves memory impairment in aged rats via antioxidant action. *Mol Nutr Food Res*, Nov;61(11).

[74] Phan, C.W., David, P., Naidu, M., Wong, K.H., Sabaratnam, V. (2015). Therapeutic potential of culinary-medicinal mushrooms for the management of neurodegenerative diseases: diversity, metabolite, and mechanism. *Crit Rev Biotechnol*, 35(3):355-68.

[75] Liu, L., Shi, X.W., Zong, S.C., Tang, J.J., Gao, J.M. (2012). Scabrogine M, a novel inhibitor of NGF-induced neurite outgrowth from PC12 cells from the fungus Sacrodon scabrosus. *Bioorg Med Chem Lett*, Apr 1;22(2):2401-6.

[76] Shi, X.W., Liu, L., Gao, J.M., Zhang, A.L. (2011). Cyathane diterpenes from Chinese mushroom Sarcodon scabrosus and their neurite outgrowth-promoting activity. *Eur J Med Chem*, Jul;46(7):3112-7.

[77] Lai, P.L., Naidu, M., Sabaratnam, V., Wong, K.H., David, R.P., et al. (2013). Neurotropic properties of the Lion's mane medicinal mushroom, Hericium erinaceus (Higher Bsidiomycetes) from Malaysia. *Int J Med Mushrooms*, 15(6):539-54.

[78] Mori, K., Obara, Y., Hirota, M., Azumi, Y., Kinugasa, S., et al. (2008). Nerve growth factor-inducing activity of Hericium erinaceus in 1321N1 human astrocytoma cells. *Biol Pharm Bull*, Sep;31(9):1727-32.

15-24. OPTIC NEURITIS

Optic neuritis is a condition that occurs when the protective myelin sheath that surrounds nerve fibers and the optic nerve becomes inflamed and deteriorates, resulting in pain and loss of vision, usually in one eye. However, in 30% of cases, both eyes are affected.[1] Optic neuritis is treatable, and it may resolve within months. The nerve fibers are capable of repairing themselves, and 60% of cases improve within two months.[2] Although most cases are of unknown origin, it is commonly seen in multiple sclerosis and is considered an early symptom of that condition.[3]

Optic neuritis is most often seen in young adults, especially in young women (75% of cases) between ages 18 and 45, although it may be found in both children and older patients. It affects about .05% of the U.S. and English population.[4] [5] It has been reported all over the world, but mostly in northern Europe, southern Australia, and the middle of North America—the higher the latitude, the more common the condition.[6] [7] [8]

The Optic Nerve

The optic nerve fibers' chief responsibility is to transmit visual impulses from each eye to the visual cortex in the brain. This interprets the information to help us know what we are seeing. The optic nerves are made up of more than a million tiny nerve fibers, each conveying information from each of the photoreceptors in the retina.

As a result of damage to the optic nerve that can take the form of swelling, compression, trauma, lesions, inflammation, etc., the brain receives incomplete information that we experience as vision loss. Central visual acuity needed for sharp, detail work, peripheral vision, color vision, perception of movement, vision in low light, and dark adaption can all be affected.

Types of Optic Neuritis

Optic neuritis is a kind of optic neuropathy (optic nerve atrophy) resulting in damage to the optic nerve due to any number of causes.

Retrobulbar neuritis is the more common form of optic neuritis. It occurs when the part of the nerve in the orbit or socket of the eye is involved. Pain is felt with eye movement or when there is pressure on the eyeball. In an eye exam, the optic disc has a normal pink appearance.

Optic papillitis refers to optic neuritis affecting the head of the optic nerve. It is also called intraocular optic neuritis. At the head of the optic nerve is the optic disc where the optic nerve connects to the retina and where there are no photoreceptors (therefore, the blind spot). In an eye exam, the color of the optic disc of papillitis appears pale. Vision impairment can range from slight to severe. Color perception is often affected. Recovery is sometimes spontaneous, but without treatment of the underlying problem, the damage may be permanent.[9]

Neuroretinitis is the term used when the nerve fibers in the macula are involved.[10]

Neuromyelitis optica, with a less favorable probable outcome, is also known as Devic's syndrome. This condition is characterized by inflammation and demyelination of both the optic nerve and the spinal cord.[11]

Symptoms

Most patients notice the onset of symptoms on a specific date, contrary to some other optic nerve conditions.[12]

- Sudden pain occurs and worsening of vision.
- Pain occurs on eye movement.
- An object swinging back and forth appears to be moving in a circle (Pulfich phenomenon).
- Vision becomes worse with an increase in body temperature, due to, for example, a hot shower (Uhthoff phenomenon).
- Pupils adjust slowly to bright light.

The following symptoms may not be related to optic neuritis; however, if you experience one or more of these symptoms, contact your eye doctor for a complete exam as soon as possible.

- Blurred vision
- Decrease in visual function. This may include a decrease in sharpness and clarity of vision (visual acuity), reduced depth perception, or decrease in side (peripheral) vision. Color vision and contrast sensitivity may also be affected. These may last anywhere from a few minutes, to a few weeks, or much longer.
- Poor constriction of the pupil in light
- Decrease in the perception of brightness, or decrease in color in one eye versus the other
- Flashing or flickering lights

Causes and Risk Factors

Depending on what region of the world the patient lives, the causes vary. In parts of the world where multiple sclerosis is prevalent, the cause of optic neuritis is most often MS. In other places where autoimmune diseases or diseases caused by infections predominate, the cause seems to be associated with those conditions.[13]

- **Multiple sclerosis**, causing 43% of cases[14]
- **Diabetes**, causing 15% of cases with varying prognosis depending on severity[15]
- **Dysfunction of liver**, 7% or **kidney,** 11% with varying prognosis depending on severity[16]
- **Autoimmune reactions** against the optic nerve[17] such as lupus
- **Ocular blood clot,** causing 5% of cases[18]
- **Compressive neuropathy**, such as certain types of brain tumors

- **Inflammatory conditions**, such as sarcoidosis or colitis
- **Infections**, such as infected sinuses or tooth infection
- **Other conditions**, including Lyme disease, syphilis, and herpes
- **Optic nerve injury** or pinched optic nerve, causing 4% of cases[19]
- **Vitamin B12 deficiency**, essential for a healthy nervous system
- **Toxins,** including methanol and certain medications

Conventional Treatment

One third of patients have a mildly swollen optic disc, and 95% of those cases resolve naturally. If diagnosed with neuromyelitis optica or neuroretinitis, a less favorable outcome, a high-dosed methylprednisolone (a corticosteroid) will be administered that can decrease swelling but does not reverse all damage.[20]

Because optic neuritis is often a first sign or precursor of MS, doctors can evaluate MS risk with an MRI scan of the brain. If MS is diagnosed, medications like beta-interferon or glatiramer acetate are prescribed. These drugs are intended to balance or influence anti-inflammatory and proinflammatory biochemicals in the brain and reduce inflammatory cell ability to cross the blood-brain barrier.[21]

Complementary Approach

Free radical activity and oxidative stress are contributing factors to optic neurological conditions. Researchers report that although steroids are commonly used in treatment, reducing oxidative stress has proven effective in preclinical studies.[22]

In addition, environmental factors such as smoking, excessive alcohol consumption, poor diet, medications, stress, and toxins may be linked to your risk of developing optic neuritis, as well as the recovery prognosis. Living a healthy lifestyle, therefore, is highly recommended for those with optic neuritis, or for those at risk for developing it. Eating a healthy diet, exercising regularly, and taking targeted antioxidants for eye health may slow down the progression of the disease and promote healthy vision.

In acute optic neuritis, the outer layer nerve synapses in the retina (known as the outer plexiform layer), as well as photoreceptors, can also become swollen. Therefore, the recommendations listed below include nutrients to support the health of the retina nerve cells, myelin sheath, and the photoreceptors, with the goal of limiting further damage to vision.[23]

Nutrients

Essential

Alpha-lipoic acid (ALA). 150mg–300mg per day. Alpha-lipoic acid is the only antioxidant that is both fat and water soluble, which means that it works in the extra-cellular fluid and also within the cell. It is effective in treating autoimmune conditions, offers neuroprotection, and decreases inflammation in lab animals with an autoimmune-caused optic neuritis.[24] Its benefits to people with related optic nerve damage, such as glaucoma, include enhanced color vision and general vision sensitivity.[25]

Alpha-lipoic acid is an ideal substance in the treatment of oxidative brain and neural disorders involving free radical processes, as it is a potent antioxidant and enhances the benefits of other antioxidants, including vitamin C, CoQ10, and vitamin E. In addition, it raises intracellular glutathione levels in the body.[26] [27] [28] [29] ALA also plays a key role in boosting energy production within the cells (mitochondria).[30] [31]

When supplementing with alpha-lipoic acid, look for R-alpha-lipoic acid that is the form found in nature and not the synthetic S form, although the two may be mixed in formulas.

Aminoguarnadine. This is an anti-glycating agent, meaning that it inhibits the "cross-linking" (or glycosylation) of proteins that may cause, or at least contribute to, many of the problems of old age, including eye problems such as cataracts, glaucoma, and macular degeneration.[32]

Omega-3 fatty acids. 2,000mg–3,000mg per day. Essential fatty acids can help reduce the chronic inflammatory processes associated with optic nerve conditions. The best sources of omega-3 fatty acids are cold-water fish, such as salmon, mackerel, sardines, anchovies and codfish. Black currant seed oil and flaxseed oil are also good sources of essential fatty acids.

One study showed patients with primary open-angle glaucoma had reduced levels of plasma DHA and EPA (O3FAs) compared with healthy siblings. These findings may be significant since DHA and EPA could modulate impaired systemic microcirculation, ocular blood flow, and optic neuropathy, which are the main changes associated with optic nerve problems.[33]

Bilberry. 180mg–240mg per day. Bilberry extracts have antioxidative properties that are not only neuroprotective, but they also help suppress photooxidative processes (the breakdown of oxygen molecules that creates an unstable environment for healthy cells). Bilberry extracts have been shown to improve small blood vessels, for example, capillaries that provide the delivery of blood to the retina. Photooxidation is accelerated by exposure to sunlight. The anthocyanoside content of bilberry may be especially beneficial for nighttime visual acuity.[34] [35] [36]

Taurine. 750mg–1,000mg per day. When taurine levels are deficient, a variety of vision problems can occur, including retinal ganglion cell degeneration.[37] The amino acids act as biomarkers in optic nerve conditions, and their deficiency is noted as a characteristic of optic neuropathies.[38] Taurine is an amino acid that protects the eyes against neurotoxins. These include excessive levels of glutamate, possibly responsible for the loss of ganglion cells and optic nerve damage seen in other optic nerve conditions, such as open-angle glaucoma.

Ginkgo biloba. 120mg per day. Ginkgo biloba appears to prevent damage to cells in the retina from toxic chemicals that can damage neurons.[39] Flavonoids such as quercetin and kaempferol, derived from ginkgo biloba, are potent antioxidants and scavengers of many species of free radicals, protecting against oxidative cell damage.[40]

Trans-resveratrol. 175mg per day. Studies indicate that resveratrol may be the most effective compound for maintaining optimal health and promoting longevity. The flavonol compound in resveratrol can "switch on" the cell-signaling molecules for youthful expression, DNA protection, and healthy cellular function.[41] It has neuroprotective action.[42]

In lieu of trans-resveratrol, **grapeseed extract,** 300mg per day, *or* **pycnogenol,** 100mg–200mg per day would be effective as well. All of these antioxidants provide a similar benefit of strengthening blood vessels and reducing inflammation. They have also been found to support healthy circulation and to neutralize free radicals. Take one of these, or all three.

Vitamin B12 (as methylcobalamin). 1000mcg per day. One cause of optic neuritis is vitamin B12 deficiency, and B12 has been found to be an effective therapy.[43] [44] Low levels of B12 have been detected in patients with the more severe neuromyelitis optica range of disorders.[45]

Vitamin C (from whole fruit such as Camu, not sourced from corn). 2,000mg per day. In one study, patients with optic neuritis (and low levels of vitamin C) were treated intravenously with high-dose vitamin C. Other similarly sized groups received corticosterone intravenously, oral corticosterone, and oral vitamin B12. Improvement was noted in all groups, but the intravenous vitamin C was the most effective.

Vitamin E. 300 IU–600 IU. Patients with optic nerve damage from glaucoma who supplemented with vitamin E, had improved blood flow and reduced vision loss compared to controls.[46]

Very Important

Glutathione (GSH), reduced. 500mg–900mg per day. Preferably take in an intraoral or sublingual form, as glutathione does not get absorbed well through the digestive system. If taken sublingually take as lower dose according to the label. Glutathione is one of the super antioxidants that neutralize the full range of free radicals. GSH is normally present in high levels in the retina where it performs multiple roles, including protection against oxidative damage. Decreased levels of GSH have been associated with several optic nerve or retinal nerve-cell eye disorders, including glaucoma[47] and macular degeneration.[48]

Magnesium. 500mg per day. This has been shown to improve the ocular blood flow in patients with glaucoma, and it may protect the retinal ganglion cell against oxidative stress and apoptosis.[49]

Curcumin (as highly absorbed phospholipid blend). 630mg per day. Curcumin may prevent corneal-epithelial-barrier-function disruption related with ocular inflammation,[50] as well as inhibit proinflammatory cytokines.[51] When curcumin is combined with phosphatidylcholine, plasma levels are fivefold higher than curcumin alone.

Helpful

Green tea extract. 725mg per day. Green teas and their extracts are potentially neuroprotective in the photoreceptor outer segment and retinal pigment epithelium (RPE).[52]

Serrapeptase. 500mg–800mg, 1-2 times per day, taken on an empty stomach. Serrapeptase helps reduce inflammation for a number of conditions.[53] [54] [55] In use in Europe for over 25 years, it is believed to be able to dissolve the fibrin and other dead or damaged tissue without harming living tissue, thereby helping to reduce related inflammation. Excess debris in the body can stimulate an ongoing immune response. The result is chronic inflammation.

Diet

Follow the Vision diet described in Chapter 7.

Avoid excitotoxins. Especially for those with, or at risk for, eye disease, it is important to eliminate all sources of excitotoxins (chemicals that over-excite nerve cells and can result in cell death, aptosis), such as MSG and/or aspartame found in packaged products, even "healthy" products.[56]

Limit alcohol. Alcohol consumption is discouraged for those with eye disease. Alcohol that must be detoxified by the liver, decreases glutathione levels.[57]

Favor foods that help glutathione synthesis. Glutathione is synthesized in the body with three amino acids: L-glutamic acid, L-cysteine, and glycine. Since the body's cells can make glutathione, some foods can be helpful. These include adequate protein-containing foods, such as meats, legumes, whey protein (without casein), foods high in sulfur (garlic, ginger, onion, brassica family / cruciferous vegetables, and eggs), and foods containing ascorbate (vitamin C), which recycles and recovers glutathione, magnesium, and potassium.[58]

Juicing. Choose at least 4-6 items to combine.

- Ginger, parsley, beets, cabbage, carrots, endive, green leafy vegetables, chlorophyll, wheatgrasses, and berries (preferably all organic). Add your favorites.
- Do not use too many carrots or fruit because of their high sugar content.
- Try to use room temperature vegetables and fruit.
- Do not add ice or very cold liquids since cold foods and liquids will eventually extinguish the stomach's digestive fire.
- Do not juice as often during the cooler months of the year, and instead, switch to vegetable soups or stews.

Lifestyle

Stop smoking. Because damage to the optic nerve can result from toxins and from some medications, we recommend avoiding smoking; it exposes the body and optic nerve to cyanide.[59]

Check medications. In general, consult carefully with your doctor about medications and possible side effects. Specific medications and supplements to be aware of include mega-dose vitamin A (only take under doctor's supervision), some heart medications, selected medications for malaria, diabetes, tuberculosis, certain antibiotics, and all oral contraceptives.

Get exercise. As with all other eye conditions, exercise is an important factor in your vision health protocol. Another way of increasing glutathione level is regular, moderate exercise.[60]

Eye exercises. See Chapter 10 for eye exercises and acupuncture points that are good for all eye conditions and overall eye health. We recommend the following:

- Palming
- Eye massage of acupressure points around the eyes

Other Modalities

Chinese Medicine

Optic nerve atrophy can be related to a number of different imbalances in the body, including poor circulation and storage of blood (often related to Liver imbalances), poor absorption and distribution of essential nutrients (often related to Spleen deficiency), and poor production of blood (commonly related to Kidney and Spleen deficiencies). Follow dosages on bottle or as prescribed by your health care specialist.

Dan zhi xiao yao san (moutan and gardenia free wanderer powder). Chronic and long-term emotional depression will cause the stagnation of Liver qi and deprive the eyes of this energy that can result in optic nerve damage.[61]

Ming mu di huang wan (bright eyes pill). This formula treats what is known as Kidney and Liver yin deficiency. It helps treat symptoms typical of yin deficiency, such as dryness, dizziness, night sweats, insomnia, constipation, dry eyes, blurry vision, sensitivity to light, photophobia, excessive tearing (specifically with exposure to wind), and eye pain and/or swelling.

Zhu jing wan (preserve vistas pill). This tonifies and nourishes the Liver and Kidneys, enriches the yin, and improves vision.

Gui pi tang (restore the Spleen decoction). This increases qi, tonifies blood, strengthens the Spleen, nourishes the Heart, and helps the Spleen control the blood. Shen ling bai zhu san (ginseng, poria, and atractylodes macrocephalae powder) strengthens the spleen and dispels dampness.

Ren shen yang rong tang (ginseng supporting and nourishing decoction). This strengthens qi and blood.

Shen qi wan (Kidney qi pill). This strengthens Spleen and Kidney yang.

Bu yang huan wu tang (yang-supplementing and five-returning decoction). This strengthens qi and moves blood.

Medicinal mushrooms. Reishi,[62] [63] maitake,[64] [65] bitter tooth,[66] [67] and lion's mane[68] [69] are very important for optic neuritis because they have neurite outgrowth and neuronal health benefits.

These are general formulas to consider, though your acupuncturist or herbalist may recommend changes to these formulas or other formulas, depending on their intake and evaluation.

Also See

Chapter 7, Vision Diet

Chapter 8, Nutrients

Chapter 10-4, Eye Exercises

Chapter 15-11, Glaucoma

Chapter 15-23, Optic Nerve Atrophy

[1] Medical Dictionary. Optic Neuritis. Retrieved Feb 25 2018 from https://medical-dictionary.thefreedictionary.com/retrobulbar+optic+neuritis.

[2] Langer-Gould A, Brara SM, Beaber BE, Zhang JL (2014). The incidence of clinically isolated syndrome in a multi-ethnic cohort. *J Neurol*, Jul; 261(7):1349-55.

[3] Memon, V., Saxena, R., Misra, R., Phuljhele, S. (2011). Management of optic neuritis. *Indian J Ophthalmol*, Mar-Apr; 59(2):117-122.

[4] Dahl, A.A. Optic Neuritis. Retrieved Feb 25 2018 from https://www.medicinenet.com/optic_neuritis/article.htm#optic_neuritis_facts

[5] Ibid. Menon. (2011).

[6] Rodriguez M, Siva A, Cross SA, O'Brien PC, Kurland LT. (1995). Optic neuritis: A population-based study in Olmsted County, Minnesota. *Neurology*, 45:244–50

[7] Jin YP, de Pedro-Cuesta J, Söderström M, Stawiarz L, Link H. (1998). Incidence of optic neuritis in Stockholm, Sweden 1990-1995: I. Age, sex, birth and ethnic-group related patterns. *J Neurol Sci*, 159:107–14

[8] MacDonald BK, Cockerell OC, Sander JW, Shorvon SD. (2000). The incidence and lifetime prevalence of neurological disorders in a prospective community-based study in the UK. *Brain*, 123:665–76

[9] National Organization for Rare Disorders. Papillitis. Retrieved Feb 26 2018 from https://rarediseases.org/rare-diseases/papillitis/

[10] Wilhelm, H., Schabet, M. (2015). The Diagnosis and Treatment of Optic Neuritis. *Dtsch Arztebl Int*, Sep; 112(37):616–626

[11] Ibid. Wilhelm. (2015).

[12] Ibid. Langer-Gold. (2014).

[13] Ibid. Menon. (2011).

[14] Ibid. Langer-Gould. (2014).

[15] Ibid. Wikipedia. Optic Neuritis.

[16] Ibid. Wikipedia. Optic Neuritis.

[17] Ibid. Wilhelm. (2015).

[18] Wikipedia. Optic Neuritis. Retrieved Feb 26 2018 from https://en.wikipedia.org/wiki/Optic_neuritis.

[19] Ibid. Wikipedia. Optic Neuritis.

[20] Ibid. Wilhelm. (2015).

[21] Wikipedia. Interferon beta-1a. Retrieved Feb 26 2018 from https://en.wikipedia.org/wiki/Interferon_beta-1a

[22] Kimura, A., Namekata, K., Guo, X., Noro, T., Harada, C. et al. (2017). Targeting Oxidative Stress for Treatment of Glaucoma and Optic Neuritis. *Oxid Med Cell Longev*, 2017:2817252

[23] Al-Louzi, O.A., Bhargava, P, Newsome, S.D., Balcer, L.J., Frohman, E.M., et al. (2016). Outer retinal changes following acute optic neuritis. *Mult Scler*, Mar; 22(3):362-372.

[24] Chaudhary, P., Marracci, G., Yu, X., Galipeau, D., Morris, B., Bourdette, D. (2011). Lipoic acid decreases inflammation and confers neuroprotection in experimental autoimmune optic neuritis. *J Neuroimmunol*, Apr;233(1-2):90-6.

[25] Filina, A.A., Davydova, N.G., Endrikovskii, S.N., Shamshinova, A.M. (1995). Lipoic acid as a means of metabolic therapy of open-angle glaucoma. *Vestn Oftalmol*, Oct-Dec;111(4):6-8.

[26] Packer, L., Tritschler, H.J., Wessel, K. (1997). Neuroprotection by the metabolic antioxidant alpha-lipoic acid. *Free Radic Biol Med*, 1997;22(1-2):359-78.

[27] Chen, J.L., Wei, L., Bereczki, D., Hans, F.J., Otsuka, T., et al. (1995). Nicotine raises the influx of permeable solutes across the rat blood-brain barrier with little or no capillary recruitment. *J Cereb Blood Flow Metab*, Jul;15(4):624-30

[28] Hultberg, M., Hultberg, B. (2006). The effect of different antioxidants on glutathione turnover in human cell lines and their interaction with hydrogen peroxide. *Chem Biol Interact,* Nov 7;163(3):192-8.

[29] Guimaraes, S.B., Santos, J.M., Aragao, A.A., de Sandes, K.O., Barbosa, P.H., et al. (2007). Protective effect of alpha-lipoic acid in experimental spermatic cord torsion. *Nutrition*, Jan;23(1):76-80.

[30] Arivazhagen, P., Ramanathan, K., Panneerselvam, C. (2001). Effect of DL-alpha-lipoic acid on mitochondrial enzymes in aged rats. Chem Biol Interact, Nov 28;138(2):189-98.

[31] Hagen, T.M., Moreau, R., Suh, J.H., Visioli, F. (2002). Mitochondrial decay in the aging rat heart: evidence for improvement by dietary supplementation with acetyl-L-carnitine and/or lipoic acid. *Ann N Y Acad Sci*, Apr;959:491-507.

[32] Neufeld, A.H., Sawada, A., Becker, B. (1999). Inhibition of nitric-oxide synthase 2 by aminoguanidine provides neuroprotection of retinal ganglion cells in a rat model of chronic glaucoma. *Proc Nat Acad Sci U S A.*, Aug 17;96(17):9944-8.

[33] Ren, H., Magulike, N., Ghebremeskel, K., Crawford, M. (2006). Primary open-angle glaucoma patients have reduced levels of blood docosahexaenoic and eicosapentaenoic acids. *Prostaglandins Leukol Essent Fatty Acids*, Mar;74(3):157-63.

[34] Muth, E.R., Laurent, J.M., Jasper, P. (2000). The effect of bilberry nutritional supplementation on night visual acuity and contrast sensitivity. *Altern Med Rev*, Apr;5(2):164-73.

[35] Matsunaga, N., Imai, S., Inokuchi, Y., Shimazawa, M., Yokota, S., et al. (2009). Bilberry and its main constituents have neuroprotective effects against retinal neuronal damage in vitro and in vivo. *Mol Nutr Food Res,* Jul;53(7):869-77.

[36] Kemper, K.J. (1965). Bilberry (Vaccinium myrtillus). *Ann Ottalmol Clin Ocul*, 91:371-86.

[37] Froger N, Cadetti L, Lorach H, Bemelmans, A.P., Degardin, D.E., et al. (2012). Taurine provides neuroprotection against retinal ganglion cell degeneration. *PLoS One*, 7(10):e42017.

[38] Gonzalez-Quevedo, A., Obregon, F., Santiesteban, F.R., Fernandez, R., Lima, L. (1998). Amino acids as biochemical markers in epidemic and endemic optic neuropathies. *Rev Cubana Med Trop*, 50 Suppl:241-4.

[39] Zaghlool, S.S., Hanafy, L.K. et al. (2012). Histological and immunohistochemical study on the protective effect of Ginkgo biloba extract against glutamate-induced neurotoxicity in male albino rat retinal cells. *Egypt J Histology*, 2012; 35: 176-188.

[40] Feng, X., Zhang, L., Zhu, H. (2009). Comparative anticancer and antioxidant activities of different ingredients of Ginkgo biloba extract (EGb 761). *Planta Med*. Jun;75(8):792-6.

[41] Maher, P. (2009). Modulation of multiple pathways involved in the maintenance of neuronal function during aging by fisetin. *Genes Nutr*, Dec;4(4):297-307.

[42] Bastianetto, S., Menard, C., Quirion, R. (2015). Neuroprotective action of resveratrol. *Biochem Biophys Acta,* Jun;1852(6):1195-201.

[43] Chavala, S.H., Kosmorsky, G.S., Lee, M.K., Lee, M.S. (2005). Optic neuropathy in vitamin B12 deficiency. *Eur J Inter Med,* Oct; 16(6):447-8.

[44] Moschos (1998). Optic neuropathy in vitamin B12 deficiency. Lancet, 352; Jul (9122):146-147.

[45] Jarius, S., Paul, F., Ruprecht, K., Wildemann, B. (2012). Low vitamin B12 levels and gastric parietal cell antibodies in patients with aquaporin-4 antibody-positive neuromyelitis optica spectrum disorders. *J Neurol,* Dec;259(12):2743-5

[46] Engin, K.N., Engin, G., Kuckusahin, H., Oncu, M., Engin, G., et al. (2007). Clinical evaluation of the neuroptective effect of alpha-tocopherol against glaucomatous damage. *Eur J Ophthalmol*, Jul-Aug;17(4):528-33.

[47] Morenom M.C., Campanelli, J., Sande, P., Sánez, D.A., Keller Sarmiento, M.I., et al. (2004). Retinal oxidative stress induced by high intraocular pressure. *Free Radic Biol Med*. Sep 15; 37(6):803-12.

[48] Sternberg, P., Davidson, P.C., Jones, D.P., Hagen, T.M., Reed, R.L., et al. (1993). Protection of retinal pigment epithelium from oxidative injury by glutathione and precursors. *Invest Ophthalmol Vis Sci*, Dec;34(13):3661-8.

[49] Nakajima, M., Kawamura, T., Tokui, R., Furuta, K., Sugino, M., et al. (2013). Enhanced accumulation of Kir4.1 protein, but not mRNA, in a murine model of cuprizone-induced demyelination. *Brain Res*, Nov 6;1537:340-9.

[50] Kimura, K. (2010). Molecular mechanism of the disruption of barrier function in cultured human corneal epithelial cells induced by tumor necrosis factor-alpha, a proinflammatory cytokine. *Nippon Ganka Gakkai Zasshi*. Nov; 114(11):935-43.

[51] Solomon, A., Dursun, D., Liu, Z., Xie, Y., Macri, A., et al. (2001). Pro- and anti-inflammatory forms of interleukin-1 in the tear fluid and conjunctiva of patients with dry-eye disease. *Invest Ophthalmol Vis Sci*, Sep; 42(10):2283-92.

[52] Jarrett, S.G., Boulton, M.E. (2012). Consequences of oxidative stress in age-related macular degeneration. *Mol Aspects Med,* Aug;33(4):399–417.

[53] Mazzone, A., Catalani, M., Costanzo, M., Drusian, A. Mandoli, A., et al. (1990). Evaluation of serratia peptidase in acute or chronic inflammation of otorhinolaryngology pathology: a multicentre, double-blind, randomized trial versus placebo. *J Int Med Res,* 18 (5); 379-88.

[54] Tachibana, M, Mizukoshi, O., Harada, Y., Kawamoto, K., Nakai, Y. (1984). A muti-centre, double-blind study of serrapeptase versus placebo in post-antrotomy buccal swelling. *Pharmatherapeutica,* 3(8); 526-30.

[55] Panagariya A, Sharma AK. (1999). A preliminary trial of serratiopeptidase in patients with carpal tunnel syndrome. *J Assoc Physicians India*, 47 (12); 1170-1172.

[56] Drance, S.M., Anderson, D.R. (1995). *Optic Nerve in Glaucoma. (p. 224).* Amsterdam/New York. Kugler Publications.

[57] Vogt, B.L., Richie, J.P. (2007). Glutathione Depletion and Recovery After Acute Ethanol Administration in the Aging Mouse. *Bio Chem Pharmacol,* May 15; 73(10): 1613–1621.

[58] Jaffe, R. Top Foods that Increase Glutathione. Retrieved May 1 2018 from https://highintensityhealth.com/russell-jaffe-glutathione-metallothionein-vitamin-c-detox-molecules.

[59] Dhas, P.K., Chitra, P., Jayakumar, S., Mary, A.R. (2011). Study of the effects of hydrogen cyanide exposure in casava workers. *Indian J Occup Environ Med*, 2011 Sep-Dec; 15(3): 133–136.

[60] Elokda, A.S., Nielsen, D.H. (2007). Effects of exercise training on the glutathione antioxidant system. *Eur J Cardiovasc Prev Rehabil,* Oct; 14(5):630-7.

[61] Peng, Q., Frank, C.O. (2014). *TCM Case Studies: Eye, Ear, Nose and Throat Disorders.* Beijing, P.R., China. People's Medical Publishing House.

[62] Sun, XZ, Liao, Y., Li, W., Guo, L.M. (2017). Neuroprotective effects of ganoderma lucidum polysaccharides against oxidative stress-induced neuronal apoptosis. *Neural Regen Res,* Jun;12(6):953-958.

[63] Zhang, W., Zhang, Q., Deng, W., Li, Y., Xing, G., et al. (2014). Neuroprotective effect of pretreatment with ganoderma lucidum in cerebram ischemia/reperfusion injury in rat hippocampus. *Neural Regen Res,* Aug 1;9(15):1446-52.

[64] Chen, Z., Tang, Y., Liu, A., Jin, X., Zhu, J., et al. (2017). Oral administration of Grifola fondosa polysaccharides improves memory impairment in aged rats via antioxidant action. *Mol Nutr Food Res,* Nov;61(11).

[65] Phan, C.W., David, P., Naidu, M., Wong, K.H., Sabaratnam, V. (2015). Therapeutic potential of culinary-medicinal mushrooms for the management of neurodegenerative diseases: diversity, metabolite, and mechanism. *Crit Rev Biotechnol,* 35(3):355-68.

[66] Liu, L., Shi, X.W., Zong, S.C., Tang, J.J., Gao, J.M. (2012). Scabrogine M, a novel inhibitor of NGF-induced neurite outgrowth from PC12 cells from the fungus Sacrodon scabrosus. *Bioorg Med Chem Lett,* Apr 1;22(2):2401-6.

[67] Shi, X.W., Liu, L., Gao, J.M., Zhang, A.L. (2011). Cyathane diterpenes from Chinese mushroom Sarcodon scabrosus and their neurite outgrowth-promoting activity. *Eur J Med Chem,* Jul;46(7):3112-7.

[68] Lai, P.L., Naidu, M., Sabaratnam, V., Wong, K.H., David, R.P., et al. (2013). Neurotropic properties of the Lion's mane medicinal mushroom, Hericium erinaceus (Higher Bsidiomycetes) from Malaysia. *Int J Med Mushrooms,* 15(6):539-54.

[69] Mori, K., Obara, Y., Hirota, M., Azumi, Y., Kinugasa, S., et al. (2008). Nerve growth factor-inducing activity of Hericium erinaceus in 1321N1 human astrocytoma cells. *Biol Pharm Bull,* Sep;31(9):1727-32.

15-25. RETINAL DETACHMENT

Retinal detachment (RD) is one of the most common causes for emergency room visits for critical eye issues. The retina is a thin layer of tissue in the back of the eye. When the retina detaches, it is lifted or pulled from its normal position. With a full detachment, the retinal cells no longer are being nourished by blood and essential nutrients. Total retinal detachments require surgery for repair, and within 24 hours, or there will be permanent vision loss. The sooner the surgery, the better. The next highest categories of visits to the emergency room related to eye issues are central retinal artery occlusion, chemical burns to the eye, and endophthalmitis that require immediate attention. About 10–15 people in 100,000 have a retinal detachment, with a lifetime risk of 3% by age 85.[1]

Retinal Layers

The retina is built of a number of layers, broadly divided:

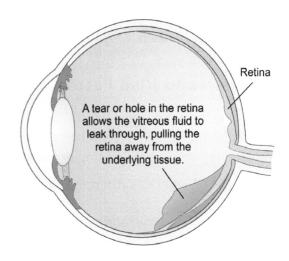

- Inner neurons and photoreceptors
- Outer retinal pigment epithelium (RPE) (epithelium is a thin lining tissue), Bruch's membrane, and the choroid (fine blood vessels)

The retina can detach when **vitreous fluid** from within the eye leaks through a **retinal tear,** resulting in separation of the retina from its underlying tissue. The detachment may be small and not dangerous, or it could involve the entire retina, resulting in blindness if not treated quickly and properly.

Types of Retinal Detachment

Retinal detachments can also proceed "unnoticed" until a large section of the retina is detached. At this time, you may notice that part of your sight is missing (it could be vision loss from above, below, or off-to-one side). Sometimes patients describe this as if a veil, curtain, or shade has been drawn on that part of their visual field.

Rhegmatogenous. This type results from fluid leaking out from a tear or break in the retinal tissue, causing it to separate from the pigment epithelium (RPE), which provides the essential blood and nutrients to the retina.

Tractional. Though this type is less common, it is due to existing scar tissue in the retina causing stress on the retinal layers, resulting in a detachment from the RPE. Existing scar tissue may be the result of chronic inflammation, past leakages, bleeding, etc.

Exudative. This type results from fluid leakage in the retina that builds up pressure, often due to such eye conditions as wet macular degeneration, diabetic retinopathy, macula edema, or possibly eye trauma.

Signs and Symptoms

Sudden awareness of light flashes or floaters. A sudden awareness of bright light spots, streaks, or dark moving specks due to the vitreous pulling retina, often resulting in new eye floaters

Blurred vision. A fairly sudden onset of blurred vision

Peripheral vision, decreasing gradually or a **curtain-like shadow** over your vision

Important. Since a partial retinal detachment may or may not be dangerous, you should always see an eye doctor immediately after becoming aware of sudden bright spots, or streaks, or a partial loss of vision.

Causes and Risk Factors

People who are nearsighted (myopic) are at a greater risk for retinal tears and detachments due to the shape of their eyeball being more oval than round. This causes more stress on the retina, including a potential thinning of the retinal wall.

You are at higher risk of a retinal detachment if you are:

- Severely nearsighted (greater than -6 diopters)
- Have had an eye injury or cataract surgery
- Have a family history of retinal detachment
- Take glaucoma medications that decrease pupil size or cause eye muscle spasms
- Are over age 50 or have had age-related retinal tears
- Experience a blow to the head
- Have diabetic retinopathy or chronic eye infections that cause scarring
- Have other eye disorders, such as retinoschisis, uveitis, degenerative myopia, or lattice degeneration

Conventional Treatment

While retinal tears usually do not cause vision loss and can be repaired effectively, full retinal detachments cause vision loss if not re-attached within 24 hours, and they usually involve in-hospital surgical repair in an operating room.

Retinal tears are typically treated with **laser surgery** (photocoagulation) or **freezing** (cryopexy), usually performed in the doctor's office. For a partial retinal detachment, a procedure may be recommended called pneumatic retinopexy where the eye doctor injects a bubble of air or gas into the center part of the eye (the vitreous cavity). Your head is positioned so that the bubble floats to the detached area and presses against the detachment. The eye doctor then seals the tear in the retina using a freezing probe or laser beam. The fluid that collected in the retina, prior to this procedure, gets reabsorbed by the body.[2]

In another common procedure called **scleral buckling,** doctors "indent" the sclera that is causing a ridge or buckle in the back of the eyes, reducing the pressure from the fluid underneath. This relieves some of the force caused by the vitreous tugging on the retina.

In a **vitrectomy,** the surgeon drains the vitreous fluid that maintains the shape of the back of the eye and replaces it with gas or silicone gel to help flatten the retina and allow healing.

Complementary Approach

Targeted supplementation, along with a healthy diet and regular exercise, can help maintain a healthy retina and vitreous. For people who are prone to retinal tears or otherwise are more at risk of retinal detachments, proper nutrition can help keep the retina strong and healthy. Regular checkups are highly recommended to monitor your progress.

Nutrients

Essential

Lutein. 6mg–20mg per day. Lutein (and zeaxanthin) provide strong antioxidant capacity that is linked to the overall health and integrity of the retinal structure.[3] In an animal retinal-detachment model, lutein protected neuroreceptors from cell death. It is a valuable adjunct to surgery for patients with retinal detachment.[4]

Zeaxanthin. 2mg–12mg per day. Along with lutein, zeaxanthin is a potent antioxidant found in the retina that helps maintain the health of the retina.

Omega-3 fatty acids. 2,000mg–3,000mg per day. Fifty percent of the retina is comprised of essential fatty acids. Supplementary and/or dietary fatty acids are essential nutrients for retinal health. Research also shows that they have anti-inflammatory properties.[5] The photoreceptor cells process light, and they require essential fatty acids for rebuilding. A deficiency of DHA in the membranes of photoreceptors disturbs membrane fluidity and function, and it can alter the process of outer segment renewal.[6] There is a deterioration of visual cells when DHA is deficient.[7]

Hyaluronic acid. 100mg–200mg per day. This nutrient helps strengthen connective tissue and is found in the vitreous, along with ascorbic acid (believed to help support the integrity of the vitreous and related connective tissue to the retina).[8]

Vitamin C (buffered and ascorbated). 2,000mg–3,000mg per day, split up with meals. Vitamin C helps support the vitreous and connective tissue. Vitamin C is found in the vitreous gel, and it is thought to help support the integrity of the vitreous and related connective tissue to the retina, which we believe may reduce the risk of RD.

Very Important

Astaxanthin. 6mg–12mg per day. Astaxanthin is a potent antioxidant and a critical nutrient for eye support. Astaxanthin is able to cross the blood-eye barrier, supporting vascular health within the eye, and protecting the eyes' photoreceptor cells.[9] Long-term damage to the retina, due to sun exposure and free radicals, weakens the retina and poses risks to maintaining healthy vision.

Helpful

The retina is replete with tiny blood vessels that are necessary for providing the blood, nutrients, and oxygen necessary for a healthy retina and related tissue integrity. Strong circulation to the retina can help reduce the risk of retinal detachment and keep vision strong.

Bilberry. 120mg–180mg per day. Along with supporting night vision, bilberry is neuroprotective[10] [11] and has been shown to improve microcirculation.[12] [13]

Resveratrol. 125mg–175mg per day. Trans-resveratrol is a well-absorbed form of resveratrol. **Grapeseed extract**, 200mg per day, and **pycnogenol**, 150mg per day, have similar benefits of helping strengthen blood vessels and reducing inflammation.

Ginkgo biloba. 120mg per day. Ginkgo contains many different flavonoids, including polyphenolic flavonoids that have been proven to exert antioxidative properties by delivering electrons to free radicals.[14] Numerous studies have shown that ginkgo biloba improves overall circulation.[15]

Vitamin D3. 2,000 IU–5,000 IU per day. Lower levels of vitamin D are associated with retinal microvascular damage.[16]

A good whole-food, organic multivitamin. Follow directions on bottle.

Diet

Follow the Vision diet outlined in Chapter 7.

Juicing. Daily juicing of vegetables and fruits is very helpful. Use some combination of the following, and other favorites:

- Ginger, leeks, garlic, parsley, cabbage, beets, carrots, spinach, apples, celery, grapes, lemon, and raspberries
- Use organic produce whenever possible, and limit carrot, beet, and fruit because of the higher natural-sugar content.
- Try to use room temperature vegetables and fruit.
- Do not add ice or very cold liquids since cold foods and liquids will eventually extinguish the stomach's digestive fire.
- Do not juice as often during the cooler months of the year, and instead, switch to vegetable soups or stews.

Lifestyle

Eye Exercises. See Chapter 10 on eye exercises. Recommendations include daily practice of the following:

- Palming
- Near and far
- Hot dog
- Massaging the acupressure points around the eyes

Microcurrent stimulation (MCS), applied at home daily, helps to support healthy circulation to the retina, increases energy production (ATP) within the retinal cells, and helps the retina eliminate waste. Along with nutrients mentioned above, daily MCS helps the body get the blood and essential nutrients to the retina to help maintain healthy retinal tissue. See Chapter 10-3 for more information.

Other Modalities

Chinese Medicine

The Liver meridian supports overall healthy flow of blood and energy to the eyes and throughout the body, while the Spleen and Kidney meridians support blood production and eye nourishment. Your acupuncturist or herbalist are best able to determine which herbal formulas are most relevant for supporting your eyes regarding a weak retina, but here are some suggested eye formulas that can be helpful:

Zhu jing wan. Preserve vistas pills tonify and nourish the Liver and Kidneys, enrich the yin, and improve vision.

Ming mu di huang wan. Rehmannia pills "to brighten the eyes" address the following patterns: Liver blood deficiency, Kidney yin deficiency, Liver yin deficiency.

Gui pi tang. Restore the Spleen decoction increases qi, tonifies blood, strengthens the spleen, nourishes the heart, and helps the spleen control the blood.

On the Horizon

A nationwide clinical trial compared the use of silicone oil with long-acting intraocular gas for repairing a retinal detachment caused by proliferative vitreoretinopathy (PVR) and found that at 6 or 24 months after surgery, a higher percentage of eyes receiving silicone oil had an attached macula and a visual acuity better than 5/200 compared to control.[17]

Also See

Chapter 7, Vision Diet

Chapter 8, Nutrients

Chapter 10-4, Eye Exercises, Microcurrent Stimulation

Chapter 15-32, Vitreous Detachment

---

[1] Kang, H.K., Luff, A.J. (2008). Management of retinal detachment: a guide for non-ophthalmologists. *BMJ*, May 31;336(7655):1235-40.

[2] Mayo Clinic. Retinal Detachment. Retrieved Mar 9 2018 from https://www.mayoclinic.org/diseases-conditions/retinal-detachment/diagnosis-treatment/drc-20351348.

[3] Jia, Y.P., Sun, L., Yu, H.S., Liang, L.P., Li, W., et al. (2017). The Pharmacological Effects of Lutein and Zeaxanthin on Visual Disorders and Cognition Diseases. *Molecules*, Apr 20;22(4)

[4] Woo, T.T., Li, S.Y., Lai, W.W., Wong, D., Lo, A.C. (2013). Neuroprotective effects of lutein in a rat model of retinal detachment. *Graefes Arch Clin Exp Ophthalmol*, Jan;251(1):41-51.

[5] Calder PC. (2003). N-3 polyunsaturated fatty acids and inflammation: from molecular biology to the clinic. *Lipids*, 38(4):343–352

[6] Young, R.W. (1967). The renewal of photoreceptor cell outer segments. *J Cell Biol*, Apr; 33(1):61-72.

[7] Santos, F.F., de Turco, E.B., Gordon, W.C., Peyman, G.A., Bazan, N.G. (1996). Alterations in rabbit retina lipid metabolism induced by detachment. Decreased incorporation of [3H]DHA into phospholipids. *Int Ophthalmol*, 19(3):149-59.

[8] Thimons, J.J. (1992). Posterior vitreous detachment. *Optom Clin*, 2(3):1-24.

[9] Goto, S., Kogure, K., Abe, K., Kimata, Y., Kitahama, K., et al. (2001). Efficient radical trapping at the surface and inside the phospholipid membrane is responsible for highly potent antiperoxidative activity of the carotenoid astaxanthin. *Biochimica Biophysica Acta*, 1512:251-8.

[10] Matsunaga, N., Imai, S., Inokuchi, Y., Shimazawa, M., Yokota, S., et al. (2009). Bilberry and its main constituents have neuroprotective effects against retinal neuronal damage in vitro and in vivo. *Mol Nutr Food Res*, Jul;53(7):869-77.

[11] Yao, Y., Vieria, A. (2007). Protective activities of Vaccinium antioxidants with potential relevance to mitochondrial dysfunction and neurotoxicity. *Neurotoxicology*, 28 93–100.

[12] Zhu, Y., Xia, M., Yang, Y., Liu, F., Li, Z., et al. (2011). Purified anthocyanin supplementation improves endothelial function via NO-cGMP activation in hypercholesterolemic individuals. *Clin Chem*, Nov;57(11):1524-33.

[13] Cohen-Boulakia, F., Valensi, P.E., Boulahdour, H., Lestrade, R. Dufour-Lamarinie, J.F., et al. (2000). In vivo sequential study of skeletal muscle capillary permeability in diabetic rats: effect of anthocyanosides. *Metabolism*, Jul;49(7):880-5.

[14] Ou, H.C., Lee, W.J., Lee. I.T., Chiu, T.H., Tsai, K.L., et a;/ (2009). Ginkgo biloba extract attenuates oxLDL-induced oxidative functional damages in endothelial cells. *J Appl Physiol*, 106:1674–85.

[15] Chung, H.S., Harris, A., Kristinsson, J.K., Ciulla, T.A., Kagemann, C., et al. (1999). Ginkgo biloba extract increases ocular blood flow velocity. *J Ocul Pharmacol Ther*, 15:233–40.

[16] Mutlu, U., Ikram, M.A., Hofman, A., de Jong, P.T., Uitterlinden, A.G., et al. (2016). Vitamin D and retinal microvascular damage: The Rotterdam Study. *Medicine (Baltimore)*, Dec; 95(49): e5477

[17] Campochiaro, P. A. (1997). The Silicone Study: A Small Piece of the PVR Puzzle is Put Into Place. *Arch Ophthalmol*, Mar;115(3):407-408.

15-26. RETINAL VEIN OCCLUSION

Retinal vein occlusion (RVO) is a common vascular disorder of the retina affecting the veins. It is a leading cause of vision loss worldwide. In fact, RVO is second only to diabetic retinopathy as the most common cause of blindness.

Retinal vein occlusion is the condition in which the small veins that carry blood away from the retina become blocked. In our bodies, arteries carry blood from the heart to other parts of the body, and veins are responsible for transporting blood back to the heart. When a blockage occurs in either a retinal artery or vein, we call it an occlusion, or ocular stroke.

What is Retinal Vein Occlusion?

Retinal vein occlusion is a blockage of the small veins that carry blood away from the retina. When this occurs, it can lead to hemorrhages (bleeding) and leakage of fluid from the blocked blood vessels.

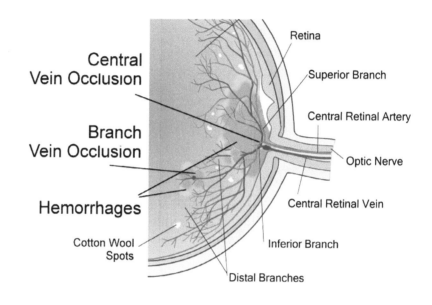

There are two types of retinal vein occlusions. One type is called **central retinal vein occlusion** (CRVO), the blockage of the main retinal vein. The second type is called **branch retinal vein occlusion** (BRVO), the blockage of one of the smaller branch veins.

Who gets Retinal Vein Occlusions?

Central retinal vein occlusion (RVO). Most patients experience the occlusion in one eye. In 6-14% of cases, RVO occurs in both eyes. An estimated 2.5 million people are affected by central retinal vein occlusion[1] with a .2% per 15-year incidence rate.[2]

Branch retinal vein occlusion is three times more common than RVO, and its incidence is higher in all ethnic populations. This type of retinal vein occlusion affects an estimated 13.9 million people[3] with a 1.8% per 15-year incidence rate.[4]

Men and women are affected equally, most are between 60 and 70 years old.

Types of Occlusion

Eye doctors also categorize retinal vein occlusions based on potential treatment strategies:

Nonischemic (also called venous stasis retinopathy) occlusions are relatively benign and account for 75-80% of all cases. The body develops alternate pathways for blood vessels that may result in macular edema but rarely in neovascularization with its accompanying problems.

Ischemic (hemorrhagic retinopathy) means that there is an inadequate blood supply, resulting in a marked decrease in vision. Hemorrhagic retinopathy results in complications such as macular edema, macular ischemia, and neovascularization that can lead to blindness in two-thirds of people diagnosed with this disorder.

Signs and Symptoms

Gradual or subtle vision loss. The severity of vision loss may depend on where the blockage or clot occurs. In some cases, this loss of vision is subtle with intermittent episodes of blurred vision.

Sudden vision loss. In other cases, vision loss may be sudden and dramatic, particularly related to those with the ischemic form of RVO. A severe blockage in an artery or vein is called an occlusion or stroke.

- Patients with CRVO generally show vision changes. It may present in sudden, painless, monocular vision loss or dense central scotoma (partial loss of vision or blind spot).
- BRVO causes a sudden and painless vision loss. If the affected area is not in the center of the eye, BRVO can go unnoticed without symptoms.

Causes and Risk Factors

The majority of causes and risk factors associated with retinal vein occlusion are lifestyle driven, meaning that they can be avoided with healthy lifestyle choices.

The exact process, known as atheroma, or atherosclerosis (hardening of the arteries), is a degenerative disorder linked to the ongoing accumulation of plaque and scar tissue (from the repair of microscopic tears due to high blood pressure) in the arterial walls and the subsequent narrowing and weakening of the walls. As these patches of deposits and scar tissue accumulate, the risk for heart attack and stroke increases, as does the risk for peripheral vascular diseases (PVD), which are marked by degeneration of the blood vessels in areas other than the heart.

Examples of PVD include stroke (brain), renal (kidney) artery disease, venous disease (problems with veins in the legs, including spider and varicose veins), and pulmonary vascular disease (lungs). So, if retinal vein occlusion occurs in a person with cardiovascular concerns, it could be considered a type of PVD.

The risk of developing retinal vein occlusion seems to increase if you have risk factors for cardiovascular disease. These include:

- **High blood pressure**. According to one study, 73% of patients with CRVO had hypertension, and 23% had diabetes.[5]
- **High cholesterol levels**. According to a study of patients with central retinal vein occlusion in people 40 years old and younger, hypercholesterolemia (identified in 65% of cases), hypertriglyceridemia (64% of cases), and hyperhomocysteinemia (42% of cases) were identified as risk factors. Three patients (14%) developed stroke, and one (5%) developed transient ischemic attacks during follow-up,[6] suggesting that the presence of CRVO may indicate serious systemic diseases.

Conditions other than cardiovascular concerns that contribute to retinal vein occlusion include:

- Diabetes
- Smoking and glaucoma (both raise pressure in the eye)
- Diseases that promote undesired or abnormal blood clotting, such as antiphospholipid antibody syndrome (APS)
- Aging (not a condition but linked to high risk, particularly if other underlying issues exist)

Related Conditions

Neovascular glaucoma. As a result of the body's natural attempt to restore blood drainage to the eye, neovascularization (new blood vessel formation) results in neovascular glaucoma.

Neovascular glaucoma begins first with the new blood vessels forming in the iris or the angle where the iris meets the cornea.

According to a 2004 study, the overall prevalence of **glaucoma** was 9.9% and the prevalence of **ocular hypertension** was 16.2% for those with central retinal vein occlusion and hemi-occlusion involving approximately half of the retina.[7]

Vitreous hemorrhage can also occur due to occlusion of retinal veins.

Retinal detachment can develop in late or severe cases of retinal occlusion.

Macula edema may develop in patients with the relatively benign non-ischemic type of occlusion.

Conventional Treatment

Unfortunately, there is no way to actually unblock retinal veins. However, your doctor may treat any health problem that seems to be related to the retinal vein occlusion. Currently, anti-VEGF drugs such as ranibizumab and bevacizumab appear to be the most frequently chosen treatment options with little potential for side effects. Steroids are another option but have more potential side effects. Some treatment strategies may use both. According to an article in *Review of Ophthalmology*, 99% of people who get anti-VEGF injections receive some improvement, at the least.[8] Injections need to be given regularly for one to two years for lasting benefits (in this review, one out of two patients show improved vision).[9] The aim of treatment is to detect and treat underlying risk factors, but also to detect and treat complications of the blocked vein, where possible. If an underlying cause such as high blood pressure, high cholesterol, or diabetes is determined, then proactive treatment for these conditions is necessary. Managing secondary effects includes the following procedures:

- Closing leaky blood vessels with laser treatment
- Administering injections of vascular endothelial growth factor (VEGF) that can temporarily resolve the neovascularization, reduce macular edema, and improve vision.
- Intravitreal injection of corticosteroid drugs to combat the inflammatory components that leads to edema (steroid implants are now also being used)
- Focal laser therapy to reduce swelling due to edema
- Pan-retinal photocoagulation therapy when patients have new blood vessel formation following the retinal vein occlusion

Also, the doctor may prescribe medications for lowering cholesterol or controlling high blood sugar that is related to diabetes, etc. Early diagnosis and treatment of retinal vein occlusion, and any complications, may make a difference to the level of visual loss in the short and long run.

Complementary Treatment

Because this disorder is largely related to lifestyle choices, preventive measures such as stopping smoking, exercising regularly, eating a healthy diet, losing weight if you are overweight, keeping blood pressure and cholesterol at healthy levels, and managing chronic stress are all exceedingly helpful in preventing or avoiding this disorder. These lifestyle choices support healthy circulation, help to keep the blood vessels unclogged, and support the free flow of essential nutrients to the retina. The goal is to maintain healthy vision as well as reduce the risk of future occurrences through proper medical and lifestyle management.

Nutrients

Certain nutrients such as zeaxanthin, lutein, ginkgo biloba, omega-3 fatty acids, bilberry, and a number of other vitamins and enzymes may help preserve vision for those who are at risk for, or those who have experienced, retinal vein occlusion. All of the following nutrients support healthy circulation, reducing free radical damage due to inflammation in the blood vessels. In the case of the enzymes, nattokinase and serrapeptase help clear clogged blood vessels.

Essential

Lutein. 6mg–20mg per day. A great deal of research has been done about the critical role lutein has in maintaining a healthy retina. In a typical study, a control group of patients with retinal deterioration who received lutein showed significant improvement in vision sharpness. With respect to atherosclerosis, researchers conclude that people given lutein, zeaxanthin, and astaxanthin, together with other nutrients, were more likely to report significant improvements.[10] Lutein may also be helpful in fighting atherosclerosis by improving circulation. Researchers found that lutein levels in the blood are tied to artery wall thickness,[11] and lutein may help reduce the accumulation of plaque by preventing oxidation of fats in the bloodstream.[12]

Zeaxanthin. 2mg–12mg per day. Numerous studies (particularly related to macular degeneration) have been done on the role of this nutrient, combined with lutein, in helping to maintain retinal health, particularly central vision. One study focused on zeaxanthin alone and found that it is more effective than lutein in protecting against oxidative stress from ultraviolet light exposure.[13]

Resveratrol. 150mg–175mg per day, (trans-resveratrol is a well absorbed form). This is a powerful antioxidant with anti-inflammatory properties, and it has the capacity to inhibit formation of extra blood vessels.[14]

Omega-3 fatty acids. 2,000 IU–3,000 IU per day. Omega-3 fatty acids have a supportive effect on the circulatory system and can reduce blood cholesterol levels.[15]

Grapeseed extract. 300mg per day. Grapeseed extract protects the central nervous system from reactive oxygen species,[16] and it helps to maintain healthy platelet function and other aspects of platelet responses.[17]

Astaxanthin. 6mg–12mg per day. This is shown to help optimize joint, immune, brain, and cardiovascular health. Astaxanthin is a fat-soluble carotenoid that is 10 times more powerful as an antioxidant than beta-carotene, lutein, or zeaxanthin, and from 60–500 times stronger than vitamin E.[18]

Ginkgo biloba. 120mg per day, *and/or* **vinpocetine**, 10mg–30mg per day. Vinpocetine enhances cerebral metabolism by helping to maintain healthy blood flow and oxygen utilization.[19] [20] [21] Controlled trials also found that ginkgo extracts support the quality of vision in patients who take them over a six-month period. This has been verified in both human and animal studies. Ginkgo appears to support the action of antioxidants.[22]

Very Important

Bilberry. 180mg–240mg per day. This fruit is a powerful antioxidant, and it helps suppress photo-oxidative processes and improve microcapillary circulation.[23] It is widely used to improve night vision and to decrease vascular permeability and capillary fragility; moreover, the berry has various other reputed health benefits, although most interest has been focused on its anthocyanin-related antioxidant effects.[24] [25] [26] [27]

Nattokinase. 150mg–300mg per day, split up before or between meals. Nattokinase helps break down debris in the blood and tissues that can contribute to blood vessel blockages and chronic inflammation that increases the risk of blood vessel blockages. It supports the circulatory system by thinning the blood and dissolving blood clots. Nattokinase was reported to have an effect on both oxidative injury-mediated arterial thrombosis[28] [29] and inflammation-induced venal thrombosis.[30]

Vitamin C (buffered and ascorbated). 2,000mg per day, split up with meals. As an antioxidant, vitamin C scavenges free radicals in the body and protects tissues from oxidative stress.[31] [32]

High-quality, whole-food, organic multivitamin. Follow dosage recommendations on the bottle.

Helpful

Taurine. 750mg–1,000mg per day. The amino acid taurine is a potent antioxidant found in the retina and is critical for nerve health, for clearing away old tissue, and regenerating old tissue. A deficiency of taurine has been shown to lead to retinal degeneration. Taurine supplementation has been used with some success to prevent, treat, and stabilize retinal changes.[33] [34] [35] [36]

Vitamin D3. 2,000 IU–5,000 IU per day. Vitamin D plays a critical role in immune support and in regulating healthy cell division and differentiation.[37]

Green tea. 500mg–750mg per day. Studies have shown that green tea has excellent scavenging ability for free radicals, such as superoxide and the hydroxyl and peroxyl radical.[38] [39] [40] [41]

Note. If you are on any blood-thinning medications such as Coumidan or Plavax, review any supplements you are interested in taking with your doctor, as some have slight blood-thinning properties.

Diet

Follow the Vision diet in Chapter 7.

Juicing. Here is a suggested list of ingredients. Choose at least 4–6 items to combine.

- Ginger root, carrot, parsley, endive, turnip, broccoli, cabbage, green leafy vegetables, celery, cucumber, tomato, radish, squash, wheatgrass, pear, and watermelon
- Do not use too many carrots or too much fruit due to their sweetness. Choose organic whenever possible.
- Try to use room temperature vegetables and fruit.
- Do not add ice or very cold liquids since cold foods and liquids will eventually extinguish the stomach's digestive fire.
- Do not juice as often during the cooler months of the year, and instead, switch to vegetable soups or stews.

Lifestyle

Eye Exercises. We recommend the regular practice of the exercises listed below for eye circulation-related conditions. See Chapter 10-4 for more information.

- Palming
- Eye massage

The health of the eyes is reflective of the health of the entire body. Therefore, your lifestyle choices, in addition to dietary choices, are important for achieving and maintaining good vision. Below are some recommendations:

Stop smoking. Eliminate smoking that produces cyanide, a retinal toxin.

Limit drug use. Limit your consumption of pharmaceutical drugs as much as possible; but be sure to work closely with your health provider on this.

Exercise daily. Engage in at least 20 minutes of aerobic exercise every day, such as walking or swimming.

Care for emotional health. Emotional health is important for maintaining physical health. Take up the practice of yoga, meditation, tai chi, outdoor walking, or prayer on a daily basis.

Microcurrent stimulation. Recommended usage is 5–10 minutes twice a day for the MCS 100ile unit. Usage may vary depending on the type of microcurrent unit, so check with your healthcare practitioner for proper instructions. If you have a history of retinal bleeding, do not use MCS, unless your eye doctor is treating you for this condition and recommends MCS. Contraindications include having a pacemaker or history of epilepsy. See Chapter 10-3 for more information.

Other Modalities

Chinese Medicine

In Chinese medicine, the Liver "opens to the eyes" and is the primary meridian for supporting overall flow of energy and circulation through the eyes. The Kidney meridian nourishes the blood to the eyes, and the Spleen meridian also nourishes the blood while helping to prevent fluids from leaking from blood vessels. Other meridians may be out of balance that can affect eye health, so an evaluation by an acupuncturist can best determine where the out-of-balances are and offer the optimal treatment strategy. The meridians involved in this condition can vary greatly, as there are a range of underlying conditions that can contribute to RVO.

Common patent formulas can include the following. Follow the directions on the bottles or ask your health care practitioner for their recommended dosage.

Ming mu di huang tang (bright eyes) is a classic formula used in Chinese medicine for eye health, helping to nourish the Kidneys and Liver. It is known to help with blurriness of vision, tearing against wind, conjunctive congestion with pain, and swelling of eye.

Qi ju di huang wan (rehmannia 6 plus chrysanthemum and lycii) nourishes Kidney and Liver blood and yin. This formula is a classic adaptation of rehmannia 6 (liu wei di huang wan) with a **special emphasis on the eyes**, in particular dry eyes, redness, and heat caused by yin (fluid) deficiency.

Zhu jing wan (preserve vistas pill) tonifies and nourishes the liver and kidneys, enriches the yin, and improves vision.

Xiao yao san is a classic Liver tonic used in Chinese medicine.

Shu gan tang + erchen tang (soothe the Liver tea + two ages tea, also known as bupleurum powder to spread the Liver) is used for many digestive issues that are aggravated by stress, especially when it effects the stomach or the intestines. This herb also stimulates movement of qi and blood and supports the Liver.

Wen dan tang (warm the gallbladder decoction) nourishes Kidney and Liver yin and brightens the eyes. This is specifically formulated for disharmony between gallbladder and stomach and the resulting phlegm heat, enabling the free flow of qi. When qi in these meridians is blocked, phlegm can develop, inhibiting proper digestion and elimination, and often resulting in frequent nausea and vomiting.

Modified xuefu zhuyu tang (move stasis in blood) invigorates the blood and dispels blood stasis. This formula supports healthy circulation, reduces cardiovascular issues, and reduces hypertension.

Yunnan baiyao. This formula helps stop bleeding, disperses blood stasis, activates blood circulation, alleviates pain, clears away toxins, and reduces swelling. It can be taken internally or applied externally (for example, in the case of cuts).

Gui pi tan (restore the Spleen decoction) increases qi, tonifies blood, strengthens the Spleen, nourishes the heart, and helps the Spleen control the blood.

Herbal formula and treatment strategies can vary significantly based on the Chinese medicine practitioners' evaluation and intake.

On the Horizon

The majority of these current treatments attempts to reduce the macular edema, but few attempts to improve the underlying retinal venous outflow, retinal perfusion, and oxygenation.

Researchers are searching for more thorough knowledge of the underlying causes to better prevent RVO and to provide more effective treatments, based on greater knowledge of the molecular and hemodynamic pathophysiology (defined as the study of the movements of the blood and the related forces that move blood).

Also See

---

[1] Rogers, S., McIntosh, R.L., Cheung, N., Lim, L., Wang, J.J. (2010). The Prevalence of Retinal Vein Occlusion: Pooled Data from Population Studies from the United States, Europe, Asia, and Australia, *Ophthalmology*. Feb;117(2):313-9.e1.

[2] Laouri, M., Chen, E., Looman, M., Gallagher, M. (2011). The burden of disease of retinal vein occlusion: review of the literature. *Eye (Lond)*, 2011 Aug;25(8): 981–988.

[3] Rogers, S., McIntosh, R.L., Cheung, N., Lim, L., Wang, J.J., et al. (2010). The prevalence of retinal vein occlusion: pooled data from population studies from the United States, Europe, Asia, and Australia. *Ophthalmology*, 2010 Feb;117(2):313-9.e1.

[4] Klein, R., Moss, S.E., Meuer, S.M., Klein, B.E. (2008). The 15-year cumulative incidence of retinal vein occlusion: the Beaver Dam Eye Study. *Arch Ophthalmol*, 126(4):513-518.

[5] National Eye Institute. Standard Care vs Corticosteroid for Retinal Vein Occlusion (SCORE) Study Results. Retrieved Jan 14 2018 from https://nei.nih.gov/score/score_background.

[6] Kuo, J.Z.C., Lai, C.C., Ong, F.S.C., Shih, C.P., Yeung, L., et al. (2010). Central Retinal Vein Occlusion in a Young Chinese Population. *Retina*, Mar;30(3):479-484.

[7] Hayreh, S.S., Zimmerman, M.B., Beri, M., Podhajsky, P. (2004). Intraocular pressure abnormalities associated with central and hemicentral retinal vein occlusion. *Ophthalmology*, Jan;111(1):133-41.

[8] Kent, C. (2012). Treating RVO: Which Options Work Best? Retrieved Jan 14 2018 from https://www.reviewofophthalmology.com/article/treating-rvo-which-options-work-best.

[9] American Academy of Ophthalmology. Boyd, K. (2017). Branch Retinal Vein Occlusion (BRVO) Treatment. Retrieved Jan 14 2018 from https://www.aao.org/eye-health/diseases/branch-retinal-vein-occlusion-treatment.

[10] Parisi, V., Tedeschi, M., Gallianaro, G., Varano, M., Saviano, S., et al. (2008). Carotenoids and antioxidants in age-related maculopathy, Ophthalmology, Feb;115(2):324-333.e2.

[11] Zou, Z., Hu, X., Huang, Y., Xiao, X., Ma, L., et al., (2011), High serum level of lutein may be protective against early atherosclerosis: the Beijing atherosclerosis study. *Atherosclerosis*, Dec;219(2):789-93.

[12] Howard, A.N., Thurnham, D.I., (2017), Lutein and atherosclerosis: Belfast versus Toulouse revisited, Med Hypotheses, Jan;98:63-68.

[13] Delcourt, C., Carriere, I., Delage, M., Berberger-Gateau, P., Schalch, W., et al, (2006), Plasma Lutein and Zeaxanthin and Other Carotenoids as Modifiable Risk factors for Age Related Maculopathy and Cataract: the POLA study. *Invest Ophthalmol Vis Sci, Jun;47(6):2329-35.*

[14] Wang, Z., Wang S., Yang, S., Yin, T., Zhang, Y., et al. (2017). Tissue Distribution of trans-Resveratrol and Its Metabolites after Oral Administration in Human Eyes, J Ophthalmol Mar 2017:4052094.

[15] Lecerf, J.M. (2009). Fatty acids and cardiovascular disease. *Nutr Rev*, May;67(5):273-83.

[16] Balu, M., Sangeetha, P., Murali, G., Panneerselvam, C. (2005). Age-related oxidative protein damages in central nervous system of rats: modulatory role of grape seed extract. *Int J Dev Neurosci*, Oct;23(6):501-7.

[17] Vitseva, O., Varghese, S., Chakrabarti, S., Folts, J.D., Fredman, J.E. (2005). Grape seed and skin extracts inhibit platelet function and release of reactive oxygen intermediates. *J Cardiovasc Pharmacol*, Oct;46(4):445-51.

[18] Maher, T.J., PhD (2000), Astaxanthin, Continuing Education Module, New Hope Institute of Healing.

[19] Horsch, S., Walther, C. (2004). Ginkgo biloba special extract EGb 761 in the treatment of peripheral arterial occlusive disease (PAOD)--a review based on randomized, controlled studies. *Int J Clin Pharmacol Ther*, Feb;42(2):63-72.

[20] Feher, G., Koltai, K., Kesmarky, G., Horvath, B., Toth, K., et al. (2009). Effect of parenteral or oral vinpocetine on the hemorheological parameters of patients with chronic cerebrovascular diseases. *Phytomedicine*, Mar;16(2-3):111-7.

[21] Bagoly, E., Feher, G., Szapary, L. (2007). The role of vinpocetine in the treatment of cerebrovascular diseases based in human studies. Orv Hetil, Jul 22;148(29):1353-8.

[22] Mashayekh, A., Pham, D.L., Yousem, D.M., Dizon, M. Barker, P.B., et al. (2011). Effects of Ginkgo biloba on cerebral blood flow assessed by quantitative MR perfusion imaging: a pilot study. *Neuroradiology*, Mar;53(3):185-191.

[23] Chu, W.K., Cheung, S.C.M., Lau, R.A.W., Benzie, I.F.F. (2011). Chapter 4 Bilberry (Vaccinium myrtillus L.). *Herbal Medicine: Biomecular and Clinical Aspects. 2nd ed.* Boca Raton, FL: CRC Press/Taylor & Francis.

[24] Camire M.E. (2000). Herbs Botanicals and Teas. *Bilberries and blueberries as functional foods and nutraceuticals*, pp. 289–319. Lancaster, PA: Technomic Publishing Company.

[25] Park, S.J., Shin, W.H., Seo, J.W., Kim, E.J. (2007). Anthocyanins inhibit airway inflammation and hyperresponsiveness in a murine asthma model. *Food Chem Toxicol,* Aug;45(8):1459-67.

[26] Mazza, G., Kay, C.D., Correll, T., Holub, B.J. (2002). Absorption of anthocyanins from blueberries and serum antioxidant status in human subjects. *J Agric Food Chem*, 50:7731–7.

[27] Zafra-Stone, S., Yasmin, T., Bagchi, M., Chatterjee, A., Vinson, J.A., et al. (2007). Berry anthocyanins as novel antioxidants in human health and disease prevention. *Mol Nutr Food Res*, Jun;51(6):675-83.

[28] Suzuki Y., Kondo K., Matsumoto Y., Zhao B.-Q., Otsuguro K., et al. (2003). Dietary supplementation of fermented soybean, natto, suppresses intimal thickening and modulates the lysis of mural thrombi after endothelial injury in rat femoral artery. *Life Sci*, 73:1289–1298.

[29] Jang J.-Y., Kim T.-S., Cai J., Kim J., Kim Y., Shin K., Kim K.-S., Park S.K., Lee S.-P., Choi E.-K., et al. Nattokinase improves blood flow by inhibiting platelet aggregation and thrombus formation. *Lab Anim Res*, 2013;29:221–225.

[30] Xu J., Du M., Yang X., Chen Q., Chen H., et al. (2014). Thrombolytic effects in vivo of nattokinase in a carrageenan-induced rat model of thrombosis. *Acta Haematol*, 132:247–253.

[31] Du, J., Cullen, J.J., Buettner, G.R. (2012). Ascorbic acid: chemistry, biology and the treatment of cancer. *Biochem Biophys Acta*, Dec;1826(2):443-57.

[32] Cangemi, R., Angelico, F., Loffredo, L., Del Ben, M., Pignatelli, P., et al. (2007). Oxidative stress-mediated arterial dysfunction in patients with metabolic syndrome: Effect of ascorbic acid. *Free Radic Biol Med*, Sep 1;43(5):853-9.

[33] Birdsall, T.C. (1998). Therapeutic applications of taurine. *Altern Med Rev*, Apr;3(2):128-36.

[34] Imaki, H., Moretz, R., Wisniewski, H., Neuringer, M., Sturman, J. (1987). Retinal degeneration in 3-month-old rhesus monkey infants fed a taurine-free human infant formula. *J Neurosci Res*, 18(4):602-14.

[35] Lombardini, J.B. (1991). Taurine: retinal function. *Brain Res Brain Res Rev*, May-Aug;16(2):151-69.

[36] Shpak, N.I., Naritsyna, N.I., Konovalova, N.V. (1989). Taufon and emoksipin in the combined treatment of sclerotic macular dystrophies. *Oftalmol Zh*, (8):463-5.

[37] Hewison, M. (2012). Vitamin D and immune function: an overview. *Proc Nutr Soc*, Feb;71(1):50-61.

[38] Chen, L., Yang, X., Jiao, H., Zhao, B. (2003). Tea catechins protect against lead-induced ROS formation, mitochondrial dysfunction, and calcium dysregulation in PC12 cells. *Chem Res Toxicol*, Sep;16(9):1155-61.

39 Kondo, K., Kurihara, M., Miyata, N., Suzuki, T., Toyoda, M. (1999) Mechanistic studies of catechins as antioxidants against radical oxidation. *Arch Biochem Biophys*, Feb 1;362(1):79-86.

40 Sinha, D., Roy, S., Roy, M. (2010). Antioxidant potential of tea reduces arsenite induced oxidative stress in Swiss albino mice. *Food Chem Toxicol*, Apr;48(4):1032-9.

41 Sun, Y., Hung, W.C., Chen, F.Y., Lee, C.C., Huang, H.W. (2009). Interaction of tea catechin (-)-epigallocatechin gallate with lipid biolayers. *Biophys J*, Feb;96(3):1026-35.

15-27. RETINITIS PIGMENTOSA

Retinitis pigmentosa comprises a group of inherited disorders, such as Leber's, in which the rods and cones that make up the photoreceptor cells in the retina are dysfunctional, due to genetic mutations. But about half of retinitis pigmentosa (RP) cases appear to be isolated with no previous family history. The condition leads to progressive vision loss and affects 1 out of 4,000 people.

What is Retinitis Pigmentosa?

Retinitis pigmentosa is a progressive degenerative disorder of the photoreceptors and/or retinal pigmented epithelium (RPE) that can cause a profound loss of vision. The vast majority of patients are over 45 years old,[1] although the symptoms of RP often appear in childhood, causing difficulty in seeing at night, and requiring longer time in adjusting from dark to light.

Retinitis pigmentosa primarily affects the side (peripheral) vision due to deterioration of the rod photoreceptors, but in later life it can affect the cones, rarely resulting in total blindness, but possibly leading to the state of "legal blindness" by age 40. Most people retain central vision with restricted side vision into their 50s. This is referred to as tunnel vision.

Genes, Photoreceptors, and Retinal Epithelium

The retinal pigment epithelium (RPE) layer lies between the Bruch's membrane and the layers of photoreceptor nerve cells, which is where light is detected and transferred to the optic nerve, and then, to the visual cortex of the brain. Not only is the RPE responsible for allowing nourishment to pass through to the photoreceptor cells, but it also protects the retina from damaging exposure and helps maintain the structural integrity of the retina.

Photoreceptors consist of rods and cones that lie behind bipolar cells that connect rods, cones, and nerve ganglions. Rods detect peripheral objects, black and white, movement, and dim light objects; they are located to the periphery of the macula. Cones, concentrated in the center of the retina, detect color, fine details, and function best in brighter light conditions.

Retinitis pigmentosa develops because the gene mutations send incorrect messages to the photoreceptor cells and RPE, causing production of the wrong types and wrong amounts of protein that would normally allow the cells to function properly.[2]

Loss of rod photoreceptors is followed by loss of cone receptors. An eye doctor can diagnose the condition by seeing dark pigment deposits on the retina.

Types of Retinitis Pigmentosa

Retinitis pigmentosa is typically genetically related. Even simple RP is highly complicated. Each genetic type is caused by mutations in several or many different genes.[3]

- **Dominant**. An abnormal gene set from one parent that can cause disease, even though the matching gene from the other parent is normal.

- **Recessive**. A copy from each parent of an abnormal gene that must be present in order for the disease or trait to develop.
- **X-linked**. The mother carries the mutated gene, and her sons have a 50% chance of being affected.
- **Rare mitochondrial and digenic forms**. Digenic inheritance (DI) is the simplest form of inheritance for genetically complex diseases.

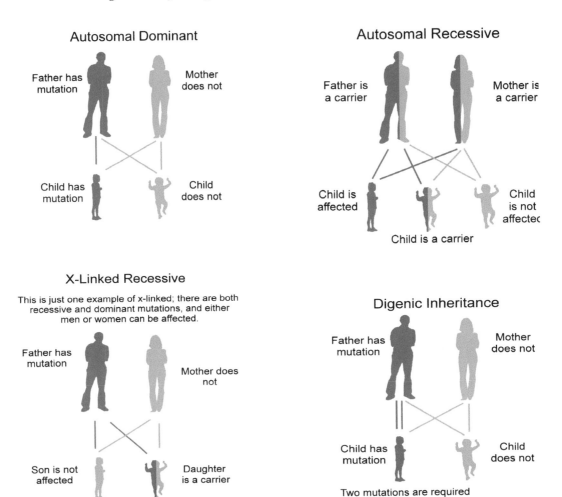

Signs and Symptoms

The typical symptoms include decreased night vision and peripheral vision. Marked loss of vision typically develops over many years. The diagnosis is made through a complete and thorough eye examination and includes a special test called an electroretinogram (ERG).

- **Night blindness loss is** the inability to see in low light conditions.
- **Peripheral vision** deteriorates giving the effect of tunnel vision.
- **Color vision** deteriorates when the patient is less able to discriminate color details.
- **Detailed vision** deterioration is also an early symptom.

Causes and Risk Factors

Gene mutations, dominant, recessive, or x-linked are carried from parent to child. Digenic inheritance, another form, requires two mutated genes. More than 100 different mutations have been identified of the gene-controlling rhodopsin, that support low light vision, and are associated with the variants of retinitis pigmentosa.

In other words, many different types of mutations of the gene controlling rhodopsin have been discovered. Rhodopsin allows our eyes to work in low-light conditions. Since the discovery of its link to retinitis pigmentosa in 1989, one hundred other mutations have been found that account for variations of retinal deterioration.

Environment. Mutations can occur during one's lifetime, often related to environmental factors that include ultraviolet radiation from the sun, exposure to toxins, or possibly additives and chemicals added to our foods. Mutations may also occur if a mistake is made when DNA copies itself during cell division.

Conventional Treatment

Avenues of research for RP treatment include gene therapy, stem-cell therapy, and drug therapy. See the "On the Horizon" section below for more information. In addition, supplemental nutrients have been shown to be helpful, although the research is mixed.

Complementary Approach

Successful approaches are not limited to the therapies you choose or to the drugs you decide to take; they can also include what drugs not to take. Case in point: do not take impotence drugs such as Viagra. Viagra obstructs an enzyme that sends light signals from the retina to the brain. Doctors have known for several years that it could cause temporary vision problems in healthy men, but a new Australian study found that its effects could be permanent. The study shows that sildenafil (Viagra) may cause permanent damage.[4]

Nutrients

Although RP is caused by genetic mutations rather than dietary deficiencies, genetic mutations may arise due to environmental conditions. In studies on both RP and other retinal disorders, it has been shown that targeted nutrient supplementation helps support the photoreceptor cells toward the goal of slowing down or stabilizing the genetic effects of RP. Researchers have noted, as reviewed below, that lower levels of antioxidants may contribute to RP progression, and therefore, increasing antioxidants may be helpful.

Essential

Vitamin A palmitate. 15,000 IU per day. Progression can be reduced by the daily intake of vitamin A palmitate.[5][6] Patients supplementing with this daily dosage of vitamin A showed a 20% slower decline in vision compared with controls. Based on this finding, researchers estimated, that an average patient in the study who began taking 15,000 IU/day of vitamin A, at age 32, would retain some useful vision until age 70; whereas a patient not on this dose, would lose useful vision at age 63.

> **Note**. Vitamin A is contra-indicated for those suffering from Stargardt disease (see Stargardt chapter for more information). Pregnant women should not take vitamin A.

DHA. 600mg, 2 times per day. Taken along with vitamin A, we recommend the following: After 2 years of DHA+vitamin A, discontinue DHA, but consume dietary sources of it (DHA). One study's findings predicted that, if someone at age 37, with typical retinitis pigmentosa starts taking 15,000 IU/day of vitamin A and eats one-or-two 3-ounce servings of omega-3-rich fish per they would not lose all central vision until the age of 78. If the average RP patient eats less than 1–2 three-ounce servings of omega-3-rich fish per week, they are predicted to lose all central vision by the age of 59.[7]

> **Note**. The research on adding vitamin E[8] or omega-3 fatty acids[9] to vitamin A intake is mixed.[10] A Harvard Medical School review determined that adding omega-3 to vitamin A is beneficial only for people not already taking vitamin A.[11] Read the cited article for more details on this protocol.

Lutein. 10mg–20mg per day. This powerful antioxidant is found both in the lens of the eye and the retina, and it helps protect the eyes from damage due to sunlight exposure by filtering out light.[12] [13] [14] [15] [16] [17] Another study showed that, daily supplementation of both lutein (12mg) and vitamin A may slow down the progression of RP.[18]

Zeaxanthin. 2mg–4mg per day. Like lutein, this antioxidant is found in the retina and lens and is important for retinal support. It may be helpful for RP patients who tend to have low zeaxanthin blood levels.[19]

Saffron. 20mg per day. Studies have shown that supplementing with saffron helps protect photoreceptor cells from damage as well as support healthy circulation in the retina.[20] [21] Although these studies were focused on macular degeneration, they may be relevant to RP. More research is needed.

Very Important

Omega-3 fatty acids. 2,000 IU–3,000 IU per day. DHA from omega-3 fatty acids accounts for approximately 50–60% of the total fatty acid content within rod outer segments of photoreceptors, and it tends to be very deficient in today's diet.[22] [23] Even though research about omega-3 significantly helping RP is not conclusive, we feel it is an important dietary addition for photoreceptor support.

Green tea. 500mg–750mg per day. The polyphenol compounds of certain green teas and their extracts are potentially neuroprotective in the photoreceptor outer segment and RPE if delivered in the proper dosages, namely about two cups of green tea per day.[24]

CoQ10. 100mg–200mg per day (ubiquinol is a more easily absorbed form). CoQ10 is found in every cell of the body, acts as a powerful antioxidant, and boosts energy production within cells. Coenzymes help enzymes work to digest food and perform other body processes, and they help protect the heart and skeletal muscles. CoQ10 also has powerful antioxidant properties, protecting important proteins and mitochondrial DNA6 from oxidative damage.[25]

Helpful

Vitamin D3. 5,000 IU per day. Lower levels of vitamin D are associated with retinal microvascular damage, suggesting inadequate nutrient delivery to the retina.[26]

Alpha-lipoic acid. 150mg–300mg per day. The alpha-R form is the most highly absorbed form with 300mg of standard alpha-lipoic acid that contains 150mg of the natural R form and 150mg of the unnatural S form. Researchers have noted that because patients with RP have signs of ocular oxidative stress without signs of systemic oxidative stress, lower levels of antioxidants may contribute to RP progression; therefore, antioxidants may be helpful.[27] Alpha-lipoic acid has been called the "universal" antioxidant, because it boosts glutathione levels in cells that are already within a normal range, and it has potent antioxidant actions.[28] [29] [30] Alpha-lipoic acid also is a cofactor for some of the key enzymes (alpha keto acid dehydrogenases) involved in generating energy from food and oxygen in mitochondria.[31] [32] [33]

Diet

Follow the recommendations in Diet, Chapter 7.

Juicing. This is a suggested list of ingredients for retinitis pigmentosa. Choose at least 4–6 items to combine.

- Ginger, leeks, garlic, parsley, cabbage, beets, carrots, celery, apples, spinach, grapes, lemon, chlorophyll, raspberries, wheatgrasses
- You can add your favorite fruits and vegetables as well, but not too much fruit or carrots due to their sugar content.
- Try to use room temperature vegetables and fruit.
- Do not add ice or very cold liquids since cold foods and liquids will eventually extinguish the stomach's digestive fire.
- Do not juice as often during the cooler months of the year, and instead, switch to vegetable soups or stews.

Lifestyle

Microcurrent stimulation (MCS). Daily sessions at home. The MCS 100ile unit is the most researched unit used for retinal health. Five research studies have been done to date showing MCS as a method to daily support retinal and photoreceptor health in the following three ways. Although most of the studies looked at macular degeneration, some of them included RP patients who had positive results as well. See Chapter 10-3 for more information.

1. Supports healthy circulation to the retina
2. Increases energy (ATP) production within the retinal cells
3. Helps the retina eliminate waste[34] [35] [36]

Eye exercises. See Chapter 10 for eye exercises and acupuncture points that are good for all eye conditions and overall eye health. The exercises we recommend to do regularly for retinitis pigmentosa include:

- Near and far
- Hot dog
- Figure eights
- Palming

Avoid microwaves. Steaming and slow cooking is the best option for retaining the maximum amount of nutrients in food. High temperature cooking and microwaving both cause greater nutritional deterioration. We feel that if you are going to use a microwave, then warming up foods in the microwave is preferable to cooking in the microwave.

Sunglasses. Wear 100% ultraviolet-blocking wrap-around sunglasses (polarized) and a hat, since ultraviolet light from the sun can cause damage to the lens of the eye and increase free radical activity and oxidative stress in the retina. Amber colored lenses are best for neutralizing blue light.

Smoking. Tobacco smoke contains many toxic, carcinogenic, and mutagenic chemicals. It also contains stable and unstable free radicals and reactive oxygen species (ROS) in the particulate and the gas phase, with the potential for biological oxidative damage.[37]

Blue-blocker glasses. Wearing blue-blocker glasses when on the computer or outdoors helps protect the retina and lens from damage. Adding a program such as "F.lux" to the computer, using blue-light blockers on iPhones and iPads, and using blue-blocking glasses when at work under fluorescent or LED lighting—all help. Replace home LED or fluorescent lighting with incandescent or low voltage halogen-lamp-operated lighting with a direct current.[38]

Exercise. Exercise regularly several times a week. Most importantly, take time away from your electronic devices! Your eyes and your body need regular breaks from computers, phones, and televisions. Electronic devices emit "hot energy" so take a break to look at green objects in the distance, such as trees. Taking rest periods for a couple of minutes, at least every hour, will do wonders for your eyes and your body. Make sure your "rest" activities are the opposite of your current preoccupation; the point is, engage your eyes and body in different ways. For example, if you've been sitting and doing close-up work, stand up and stretch while looking out a window into nature. Better yet, take a walk around the block. If, on the other hand, you've been engaged in broader visual work, a rest might include checking your emails on your phone. Doing eye exercises during your rest period is also recommended.

Meditation. Find time for meditation each day. Walking in nature, without electronic devices, can be extremely meditative; it is very relaxing to both our psyche and our physical body. Additionally, walking barefoot or with leather-soled shoes on the ground (not on man-made material such as asphalt) allows healthy negative electrons to enter into the body.[39] Free electrons have antioxidant effects and work to reduce inflammation.

Yoga. Inversion poses in yoga have been shown to aid blood flow to the heart and head that helps the body bring more oxygen and nutrients to the eyes. One of the best and safest inversion poses is lying on the floor with your legs up a wall. Beginner and advanced yoga practitioners enjoy this posture equally. See Chapter 10-7 for more information.

Other Modalities

Chinese Medicine

Although there are a number of causes of RP, as long as there are rods active in the eyes, these can be supported and nourished through acupuncture and specific herbs. In Chinese medicine, the Liver "opens to the eyes" and is the primary meridian for supporting overall flow of energy and circulation through the eyes. The Kidney and Spleen meridians nourish the blood to the eyes. Other meridians may be out of balance as well that can affect eye health, so an evaluation by an acupuncturist can best determine where the imbalances are and offer the optimal treatment strategy. Acupuncture treatments are typically done by inserting needles below the knees and elbows, then in specific points along the orbit of the eye and under the eye.

Common Chinese Medicine Patterns related to Retinitis Pigmentosa

In TCM, retinitis pigmentosa can be caused by deficient fire at the gate of life, deficient Liver and Kidney yin that causes a deficiency of essence and blood, or deficient Spleen qi, Liver yin deficiency, Liver yin deficiency with heat, Liver qi and blood stagnation with Lung qi and deficiency, Kidney yang weakness, and central (Spleen) qi weakness,

Ming mu di huang wan, "to brighten the eyes", nourishes the Liver, enriches the Kidneys and improves vision.

Herbal formula and treatment strategies can vary significantly based on the Chinese Medicine practitioner's evaluation and intake.

Acupuncture

In a small pilot study, a dozen RP patients were treated with acupuncture for two weeks. Half of them experienced "measurable, significant, visual function improvements."[40] Six of nine who were tested for dark-adapted full-field stimulus had significant improvements after one week of treatment that lasted for 10 to 12 months, well outside the variations for typical RP therapies.[41] See Chapter 9-4 for more information on Micro Acupuncture.

Other Therapies

The following therapies promote improved flow of energy and circulation throughout the body. The daily stress that we encounter due to poor diet, emotional imbalances, lack of regular exercise, and more, can cause areas within the body to tighten up. This restricts circulation, and in turn can negatively affect all retinal disorders. The eyes are the second most biologically active part of the body; only the brain is more active. So, they require a great deal of nutrition and the free flow of blood and energy to remain healthy.

The eight **acupressure points** around the orbit of the eye can be massaged periodically throughout the day to help relax the eyes and stimulate energy and circulation flow.

The **Alexander technique** is a way of learning to move mindfully through life, adjusting old habits to relieve tension in the body. By relieving tension in our daily physical habits, we affect the free flow of energy and circulation to the eyes.

Craniosacral is a method for relieving pain and tension through gentle manipulations of the skull that is regarded as harmonizing with the natural rhythm of the central nervous system.

Chiropractic is a manipulative treatment of joint misalignments, especially those of the spinal column. Misalignments are believed to cause other disorders by affecting the function of nerves, muscles, and organs.

Essential oil therapy uses plant extracts, often applied to the skin to help in many ways, including tension release, anxiety relief, sleep improvement, pain reduction, circulation enhancement, digestion improvement, and more. Some suggested oils include the following:

Carrot seed essential oil improves the eyes by protecting against macular degeneration, detoxifying blood vessels, toning the liver, relieving stress and anxiety, and providing many nourishing vitamins and minerals.

Frankincense has been around since antiquity. It is a sacred plant that can be helpful in showing us our visual blind spots. Frankincense tells us to "open up that third eye" and is our main "go to" around the eyes.

Saffron is very helpful for eye health as it helps rebalance body fluids on a cellular level, and it stimulates the "qi" in the entire body. It contains high levels of antioxidants, vitamins, and minerals.

Keep essences away from the mouth, eyes, and mucous membranes; if a few drops get in one of these sensitive areas it may be uncomfortable for 15–30 minutes, but not harmful. You can lessen discomfort by adding a pure oil like olive or coconut oil to neutralize the irritating effect. For the eye area, dab a few drops around the outside of the eye. Do not put the neutralizing oil in the eye.

Combine ¼ cup of avocado oil with ¼ cup of calendula-infused oil. Slowly add 5 drops each of the essential oils. Then close the bottle and shake well; apply 4 drops of this mixture on your clean face. Massage in gentle circular motions. Leave overnight. For more information, see Appendix 9, Essential Oils.

On the Horizon

Gene Therapy

- **Leber congenital amaurosis** due to RPE65 gene. Near-blind children with RPE65 gene dysfunction have experienced significant vision improvement through gene therapy.[42] [43]

- **Recessive RP.** Gene therapy addressing MERTK gene mutations is under trial.[44][45]
- **Dominant RP.** Gene therapy for autosomal dominant retinitis pigmentosa will go to trial soon.[46]
- **Regeneration of cone cells.** Other gene therapy research finds that non-functioning cone cells can be regenerated.[47]

Drug Therapy

- **FDA-approved drug therapy.** Valproic acid shows potential for people with dominant forms of RP.[48] One researcher notes that it may be harmful for people in non-dominant RP.[49]
- **Synthetic retinoid** is a therapeutic drug by the biopharmaceutical QLT.[50]
- **Mitochondial support** compounds are being investigated.[51]

Stem-Cell Therapy

In one stem-cell technique known as CRISPR, faulty genes are enhanced with fully functional genes by an injection into the retina of a harmless virus or "vector" to carry the specifically required gene into the retinal cells, using the patient's own stem cells.[52]

In a clinical trial completed, but not yet published, as of August, 2018, bone marrow stem cells were injected into the retina of RP patients.[53] A number of researchers have hypothesized that such a treatment might be beneficial.[54][55]

A 2012 animal study replaced photoreceptor cells where no active cells remained with transplanted stem cells (rod precursor cells) that regenerated into a distinct new layer of active photoreceptor cells (stem cells that were able to convert to rod cells).

Other Techniques

Electronic implant surgery. This provides the opportunity to restore some degree of vision with an electronic device in the subretinal space.[56]

Retinal cell transplants. Several groups around the world are investigating the use of retinal transplantation in the treatment of inherited retinal diseases, including RP and age-related macular degeneration.

Growth factors. These are substances that have specific roles in nourishing nerve cells. One of the main growth factors that have received attention is ciliary neurotrophic factor (CNTF) that has been shown to be successful in slowing retinal degeneration in animal models of retinitis pigmentosa.[57]

Also See

1 Health Research Funding. (2015). 18 Scary Retinitis Pigmentosa Statistics. Retrieved Dec 14 2017 from http://healthresearchfunding.org/18-scarey-retinitis-pigmentosa-statistics.

[2] Fighting Blindness Foundation. Retinitis Pigmentosa. Retrieved Mar 27 2018 from http://www.blindness.org/retinitis-pigmentosa.

3 Daiger, S.P., Bowne, S.J., Sullivan, L.S. (2007). Perspective on Genes and Mutations Causing Retinitis Pigmentosa. *Arch Ophthalmol*, Feb; 125(2): 151–158.

4 Nivison-Smith, L., Zhu, Y., Whatham, A., Bui, B.V., Fletcher, E.L., et al. (2014). Sildenafil alters retinal function in mouse carriers of Retinitis Pigmentosa. *Exp Eye Res*, 128: 43.

5 Sofi, F., Sodi, A., Franco, F., Murro, V., Biagini, D. (2016). Dietary profile of patients with Stargardt's disease and Retinitis Pigmentosa: is there a role for a nutritional approach? *BMC Ophthalmol.* Jan 22;16:13.

[6] Hartong, D.T., Berson, E.L., Dryja, T.P. (2006). Retinitis pigmentosa. *Lancet*, Nov 18;368(9549): 1785-809.

[7] Harvard Medical School. Massachusetts Eye and Ear. New Findings Lead to Revised Therapeutic Regimen to Slow RP. Retrieved May 5 2018 from https://www.masseyeandear.org/for-patients/patient-guide/patient-education/diseases-and-conditions/rp-and-supplements.

8 Berson, E.L., Rosner, B., Sandberg, M.A., Hayes, K.C., Nicholson, B.W. (1993). A randomized trial of vitamin A and vitamin E supplementation for retinitis pigmentosa. *Arch Ophthalmol* Jun; 111(6):761-772.

[9] Ibid. Berson. (2004).

[10] Rayapudi, S., Schwartz, S.G., Wang, X., Chavis, P. (2013). Vitamin A and fish oils for retinitis pigmentosa. *Cochrane Database Syst Rev, Dec 19;(12):CD008428.*

[11] Ibid. Harvard Medical School. New Findings Lead to Revised Therapeutic Regimen to Slow RP.

12 Bosch-Driessen, L.H., Plaisier, M.B., Stilma, J.S., Van der Lelij, A. Rothova, A. (2002). Reactivations of ocular toxoplasmosis after cataract extraction. *Ophthalmology*, 109:1780-1878.

13 Piermarocchi, S., Saviano, S., Parisi, V., Tedeschi, M., Panozzo, G., et al. (2012). Carotenoids in Age-related Maculopathy Italian Study (CARMIS): two-year results of a randomized study. *Eur J Ophthalmol*, Mar-Apr;22(2):216-25.

14 Krinsky, N.I., Landrum, J.T., Bone, R.A. (2003). Biologic mechanisms of the protective role of lutein and zeaxanthin in the eye. *Annu Rev Nutr*, 23:171-201.

[15] Moukarzel, A.A., Bejjani, R.A., Fares, F.N. (2009). Xanthophylls and eye health of infants and adults. J *Med Liban*. Oct-Dec;57(4):261-7.

[16] Semba, R.D., Dagnelie, G. (2003). Are lutein and zeaxanthin conditionally essential nutrients for eye health? *Med Hypotheses*, Oct;61(4):465-72.

17 Bahrami, H., Melia, M., Dagnelie, G. (2006). Lutein supplementation in retinitis pigmentosa: PC-based vision assessment in a randomized double-masked placebo-controlled clinical trial]. *BMC Ophthalmol*, Jun 7;6:23.

18 Berson, E.L., Rosner, B., Sandberg, M.A, Weigel-DiFranco, C., Brockhurst, R.J., (2010). Clinical Trial of Lutein in Patients With Retinitis Pigmentosa Receiving Vitamin A. *Arch Ophthalmol*, Apr;128(4):403-11.

[19] Sandberg, M.A., Johnson, E.J., Berson, E.L. (2010). The relationship of macular pigment optical density to serum lutein in retinitis pigmentosa. *Invest Ophthalmol Vis Sci*, Feb;51(2):1086-91.

20 Marangoni, D., Falsini, B., Piccardi, M., Ambrosio, L., Minnella, A.M. (2013). Functional effect of Saffron supplementation and risk genotypes in early age-related macular degeneration: a preliminary report, *J Transl Med,* Sep 25;11:228.

21 Falsini, B., Piccardi, M., Minnella, A., Savastano, C., Capoluongo, E. et al. (2010). Influence of saffron supplementation on retinal flicker sensitivity in early age-related macular degeneration, *Invest Ophthalmol Vis Sci*, Dec;51(12):6118-24.

22 Bush, R.A., Malnoe, A., Reme, C.E., Williams, T.P. (1994). Dietary deficiency of N-3 fatty acids alters rhodopsin content and function in the rat retina. *Invest Ophthalmol Vis Sci.* Jan, 35(1):91-100.

23 Stillwell, W., Wassall, S.R. (2003). Docosahexaenoic acid: membrane properties of a unique fatty acid. *Chem Phys Lipids*, Nov;126(1):1-27.

24 Jarrett, S.G., Boulton, M.E. (2012). Consequences of oxidative stress in age-related macular degeneration. *Mol Aspects Med*, Aug;33(4):399–417.

25 Littarru, G.P., Tiano, L. (2007). Bioenergetic and antioxidant properties of coenzyme Q10: recent developments. *Mol Biotechnol,* Sep;37(1):31-7.

26 Mutlu, U., Ikram, M.A., Hofman, A., de Jong, P.T., Uiterlinden, A.G., et al. (2016). Vitamin D and retinal microvascular damage: The Rotterdam Study. *Medicine (Baltimore).* 2016 Dec; 95(49): e5477.

27 Campochiaro, P.A., Strauss, R.W., Lu, L., Hafiz, G., Wolfson, Y., et al. (2015). Is There Excess Oxidative Stress and Damage in Eyes of Patients with Retinitis Pigmentosa? *Antioxid Redox Signal, Sep* 1;23(7):643-8.

28 Khanna, S., Atalay, M., Laaksonen, D.E., Gul, M., Roy, S., Sen, C.K. (1999). Alpha-lipoic acid supplementation: tissue glutathione homeostasis at rest and after exercise. *J Appl Physiol,* Apr;86(4):1191-6.

29 Hultberg, M., Hultberg, B. (2006). The effect of different antioxidants on glutathione turnover in human cell lines and their interaction with hydrogen peroxide. *Chem Biol Interact,* Nov 7;163(3):192-8.

30 Guimarães, S.B., Santos, J.M., Aragão, AA., de Sandes Kimura, O., Barbosa, P.H., et al. (2007). Protective effect of alpha-lipoic acid in experimental spermatic cord torsion. *Nutrition,* Jan;23(1):76-80.

31 Arivazhagan, P., Ramanathan. K., Panneerselvam, C. (2001). Effect of DL-alpha-lipoic acid on mitochondrial enzymes in aged rats. *Chem Biol Interact,* Nov 28;138(2):189-98.

32 Palaniappan, A.R., Dai, A. (2007). Mitochondrial ageing and the beneficial role of alpha-lipoic acid. *Neurochem Res,* 2007 Sep;32(9):1552-8.

33 Packer, L. (1998). alpha-Lipoic acid: a metabolic antioxidant which regulates NF-kappa B signal transduction and protects against oxidative injury. *Drug Metab Rev,* May;30(2):245-75.

34 Paul, E.L. (1997). The Treatment of Retinal Diseases With Micro Current Stimulation And Nutritional Supplementation.

35 Reader, A.L., Halloran, G. (1997). Bioelectrical Stimulation in an Integrated Treatment for Macular Degeneration, RP, Glaucoma, CMV, and DR. Fourth Annual Symposium on Biological Circuits, Oct. 1997, Mankato University, MN.

36 O'Clock, G.D., Jarding, J.B. (2009). Electrotherapeutic device/protocol design considerations for visual disease applications. *Conf Proc IEEE Eng Med Biol Soc,* 2133-6.

37 Valavanidis, A., Vlachogianni, T., Fiotakis, K. (2009). Tobacco Smoke: Involvement of Reactive Oxygen Species and Stable Free Radicals in Mechanisms of Oxidative Damage, Carcinogenesis and Synergistic Effects with Other Respirable Particles. *Int J Environ Res Pub Health,* Feb;6(2):445-462.

38 Facts are Facts. Energy Saving Light Bulbs can make you ill! Retrieved Apr 17 2018 from https://www.facts-are-facts.com/article/energy-saving-light-bulbs-can-make-you-ill

39 Oschman, J.L., Chevalier, G., Brown, R. (2015). The effects of grounding (earthing) on inflammation, the immune response, wound healing, and prevention and treatment of chronic inflammatory and autoimmune diseases. *J Inflamm Res,* 8:83-96.

40 Bittner, A. (2014). A pilot study of an acupuncture protocol to improve visual function in retinitis pigmentosa patients. *Clin Exp Optom,* May; 97(3): 240–247.

41 Ibid. Bittner. (2014).

42 Foundation Fighting Blindness. Retinitis Pigmentosa Research Advances. Retrieved Mar 27 2018 from http://www.blindness.org/sites/default/files/pages/pdfs/Advances-RP-June-2015.pdf.

43 Ashtari, M., Cyckowski, L.L., Monroe, J.R., Marshall, K.A., Chung, D.C. et al. (2011). The human visual cortex responds to gene therapy-mediated recovery of retinal function. *J Clin Invest,* Jun; 121(6):2160-8.

44 Ibid. Foundation Fighting Blindness. Retinitis Pigmentosa Research Advances.

45 Clemson, C.M., Tzekov, R., Krebs, M., Checchi, J.M., Bigelow, C., et al. (2011). Therapeutic potential of valproic acid for retinitis pigmentosa. *Br J Ophthalmol,* Jan;95(1):89-93.

46 Ibid. Foundation Fighting Blindness. Retinitis Pigmentosa Research Advances.

47 Ibid. Foundation Fighting Blindness. Retinitis Pigmentosa Research Advances.

48 Ibid. Foundation Fighting Blindness. Retinitis Pigmentosa Research Advances.

49 Sisk, R.A. (2012). Valproic acid treatment may be harmful in non-dominant forms of retinitis pigmentosa. *Br J Ophthalmol,* Aug;96(8):1154-5.

50 Ibid. Foundation Fighting Blindness. Retinitis Pigmentosa Research Advances.

51 Ibid. Foundation Fighting Blindness. Retinitis Pigmentosa Research Advances.

52 Bassuk, A.G., Zheng, A., Li, Y., Tsang, S.H., Mahajan, V.B. (2016). Precision Medicine: Genetic Repair of Retinitis Pigmentosa in Patient-Derived Stem Cells. *Sci Rep,* Jan 27;6:19969

53 Siquerira, R.C. (2010). Autologous Bone Marrow-Derived Stem Cells Transplantation For Retinitis Pigmentosa. Retrieved Dec 24 2017 from https://clinicaltrials.gov/ct2/show/NCT01068561

[54] Smith, L.E. (2004). Bone marrow-derived stem cells preserve cone vision in retinitis pigmentosa. *J Clin Invest*, Sep;114(6):755-7.

[55] He, Y., Zhang, Y., Liu, X., Ghazaryan, E., Li, Y., et al. (2014). Recent advances of stem cell therapy for retinitis pigmentosa. *Int J Mol Sci,* Aug 20; 15(8): 14456-74.

56 MacLaren, R.E. (2017). Electronic retinal implant surgery. *Eye* (Lond), 2017 Feb;31(2):191-195.

57 Wan, J., Zhao, X.F., Vojtek, A., Goldman, D. (2014). Retinal injury, growth factors, and cytokines converge on β-catenin and pStat3 signaling to stimulate retina regeneration. *Cell Rep*, Oct 9; 9(1): 285–297.

15-28. SJÖGREN'S SYNDROME

Sjögren's syndrome (SS), first identified in 1933 by Swedish ophthalmologist Dr. Henrik Sjögren, is an autoimmune disorder, a disease in which the body produces antibodies that attack its fluid-producing tissues and organs. After rheumatoid arthritis and lupus (which SS often accompanies), Sjögren's is the third most common rheumatic disorder.[1] According to the Sjögren's Syndrome Foundation,[2] more than 4 million Americans have been diagnosed with SS. It has been proven to affect virtually every racial and ethnic group; however, 9 out of 10 patients are women. The average age of diagnosis is late 40s, though the disorder can affect people of any age.

What is Sjögren's

In cases of Sjögren's, the body does not produce enough water, affecting all of the moist tissue of the body. The glands that produce moisture for eyes, mouth, reproductive organs, etc. can be damaged, and their outflow inhibited. The result is, for example, dry eyes due to not enough tear production by lacrimal glands, dry mouth due to not enough saliva from salivary glands, and mucous membrane dryness. The mucous membranes and the moisture-secreting glands of your eyes and mouth are usually affected first.

Pathology

Immune-system cells, usually B and T lymphocytes (small white blood cells), infiltrate the glands responsible for secreting body fluids. This infiltration causes inflammation in the glands that results in decreased water production throughout the body.

The condition is systemic. It affects the entire body. Not only may it be evidenced by dry mouth (xerostomia) and dry eyes, it can be related to keratoconjunctivitis sicca, rheumatoid arthritis, and an excess of certain proteins in the blood (hypergammaglobulinemia). The lymph nodes, lungs, kidneys, liver, bone marrow, muscle, and skin can all be involved as well.

Once symptoms appear, they tend to remain steady, or worsen, and only rarely do they go into remission. Additionally, while some people experience mild discomfort, others suffer debilitating symptoms that greatly impair their overall function. Early diagnosis and proper treatment are important, as complications can be serious, and swift action can greatly improve a patient's quality of life.

Types of Sjögren's

There are two types of Sjögren's: primary and secondary. They both tend to affect the entire body but differ in type and intensity of symptoms.

Primary Sjögren's syndrome means that the disease occurs on its own.

Secondary Sjögren's syndrome, on the other hand, occurs with another already existing autoimmune disorder involving the joints, muscles, or connective tissues such as lupus (systemic lupus erythematosus), rheumatoid arthritis, or scleroderma (hardening of the skin). Secondary SS may develop years after the onset of one of these aforementioned disorders. Other organ or gland malfunctions commonly include lung disease, kidney disease, and lymphoma.[3] Lymphomas may occur in the salivary glands, but also frequently occur in the gastrointestinal tract.[4][5]

Signs and Symptoms

The most common symptoms of Sjögren's are dry eyes and dry mouth. The symptoms include the following:

- **Generalized dryness**, including chronic dryness and possibly inflammation of the eyes and mouth. In addition to mouth dryness, inflammation of the salivary glands can lead to dental decay, mouth sores and swelling, cavities, gum disease, difficulty in swallowing (gastroesophageal reflux disease), stones, and/or infection of the parotid gland inside of the cheeks.
- **Dry skin**, including external genitalia, vaginal dryness, and dryness in the ear, nose, and throat
- **Prolonged fatigue, chronic pain, and neuropathies**
- **Decrease in gastrointestinal secretions** involving the kidneys, liver, and pancreas. This can result in poor absorption of nutrients as a lack of availability of essential enzymes to break down food in the small intestine. Patients with SS frequently have irritable bowel syndrome-like symptoms (IBS).[6] Gastrointestinal disease may occur in one quarter of the patients and include dysphagia, gastritis, motility disorders, pancreatitis, pancreatic insufficiency, pernicious anemia, autoimmune hepatitis, and symptoms consistent with IBS such as abdominal pain, diarrhea, constipation, bloating, flatulence, vomiting, and nausea.[7][8]
- **Joint pain** as well as joint swelling and stiffness
- **Persistent dry cough**
- **A sore and cracked tongue**
- **Thyroid problems** such as Hashimoto's thyroiditis, Raynaud's phenomenon, lymph node enlargement
- **Kidney, nerve, and muscle disease**
- **Vasculitis**. In rare cases, vasculitis can occur. Vasculitis is an inflammatory condition of the blood vessels that damages the tissues of the body supplied by these vessels. Complications depend on which blood vessels, organs, or other body systems are affected.
- **Other**. Sjögren's can also affect other parts of the body, including the inflammation of the lining of the breathing passages, the peripheral nervous system, and the brain. Patients with SS have a higher risk of developing lymphoma.[9]

Obtaining a diagnosis

It is estimated that Sjogren's is misdiagnosed in more than half of affected adults.[10] Data suggest that patients experience symptoms for an average of 3.9 years before a diagnosis of SS is made.[11] Such delays in diagnosis can be a source of psychological distress from unexplained symptoms.[12]

While there is no one single test for Sjögren's, doctors can generally trace the symptoms of primary SS to problems with the tear and saliva glands. When suspicious of SS, eye doctors use the Schirmer test to measure tear production and diagnostic dyes (rose bengal and lissamine green) to evaluate the corneal surface for tear production.

Medical or physical exams can also be helpful with diagnosis. Specific blood tests include:

- Analysis for antinuclear antibodies (ANA test) that are unusual antibodies directed against the nucleus of the cell. About 70% of Sjögren's patients have a positive ANA test result.
- Abnormal blood levels of inflammation biomarkers.
- Sedimentation rate, detecting whether red blood cells are tending to clump.
- C-reactive protein; concentrations increase in the presence of inflammation.
- Thyroid levels.
- Erythrocyte sedimentation rate (ESR), a marker of overall inflammation.
- Immunoglobulins (IG), a test for elevated proteins.[13]
- Other blood tests include rheumatoid factor (RF) (60–70% of Sjogren's patients test positive for RF), SS-A (or Ro) and SS-B (or La) (40% of patients are positive for SS-B, which may also be found in lupus patients).
- Other tests include urine test, chest x-ray, and saliva-gland biopsy,[14] which can be performed by a dentist to measure saliva production and flow.

People with the primary Sjögren's are more likely to have certain antibodies circulating in their blood than people with the secondary type. The Sjö test (Bausch & Lomb, Rochester, NY, USA) is a blood test for the early detection of SS. This test analysis includes a number of early biomarkers along with the classic Sjögren's biomarkers. The cumulative sensitivity of the Sjö panel has been 89.9%.[15]

Sjögren's may appear to be similar to sialadenitis, an infection of the salivary glands. Sialadenitis may include gland inflammation, but more commonly consists of inflammation that is scattered within the body and in the interstitial spaces between the body's structures, especially in front of the ear and under the chin.[16]

Causes and Risk Factors

There are more than 80 different autoimmune disorders[17] in which a person's immune system mistakenly identifies healthy tissues as an invader and creates antibodies to attack it. The exact cause or causes of Sjögren's syndrome and other autoimmune disorders is unknown.

- One theory, however, is that microorganisms (bacteria or viruses), or a toxin, such as a pharmaceutical drug or other chemical, may trigger changes in the body that confuse the immune system.[18] This may occur more often in people who carry genes that increase their risk for autoimmune disorders.[19]
- Having any autoimmune disorder is a risk for secondary Sjögren's syndrome; nearly 25% of patients with autoimmune diseases develop additional autoimmune diseases.[20]
- Helicobacter pylori infection has been implicated in onset of Sjogren Syndrome.[21]

Conventional Treatment

Currently, there is no cure for Sjögren's syndrome. The only conventional treatment is in the management of symptoms. Treatment differs patient by patient, depending on where the symptoms are being experienced. For example, for dry eyes, your eye doctor may prescribe a prescription medication such as Restasis that helps improve tear production. Additionally, thick eye ointments can be used before bedtime. Minor surgery or punctal plugs may be recommended to close the tear ducts in order to help maintain moisture in the eyes.

Other medications include pilocarpine (Salagen) and cevimeline (Evoxac) for dry mouth. These medications should be avoided by people with asthma, certain heart diseases, and possibly glaucoma. Anti-inflammatories such as prednisone and autoimmune suppressants such as azathioprine and cyclophosphamide can be helpful. Of course, antibiotics are commonly used for infections in the mouth and eye as well as for common conditions like sinusitis, bronchitis, and vaginitis.

All of these medications can pose health risks with long-term usage; so, discuss strategies with your doctor prior to beginning treatment. You will want to attempt to determine the length of time needed for treating the symptom as well as the potential risks and benefits.

Certain other medications can cause dry mouth, such as drugs used to treat allergies (antihistamines and decongestants), diarrhea, blood pressure, low body fluids, and depression. Tranquilizers and anti-psychotic drugs may also cause dry mouth.

According to one study, punctual plug placement resulted in 50% or greater improvement of symptoms, improvement in ocular-surface health, reduction in artificial tear use, and improved contact lens comfort in patients with dry eye. Serious complications from plugs were infrequent.[22]

Simple actions such as chewing gum regularly to stimulate the salivary glands, drinking water throughout the day, and using lip balm on cracked lips may help dry mouth. Medication that helps the body produce more saliva can also be helpful. Numoisyn liquid and lozenges are one example. Vitamin E oil has also been used with some success.

Saltwater (saline) nasal sprays can help dryness in the nasal passages. Vaginal lubricant should be considered for sexual intercourse if vaginal dryness is a problem.

While treatments are primarily based on symptoms, they can vary significantly. However, regardless of which type of Sjögren's, it is important to monitor for lymphoma.

Complementary Approach

There are a number of great nutrients, including antioxidants, herbs, vitamins, and minerals that help support natural tear production, internally moisten the body, reduce inflammation, and help with overall water metabolism throughout the body. These can all help reduce the symptoms of Sjögren's naturally.

Nutrients

Essential
There is evidence that anti-inflammatories can be helpful.[23]

Omega-3 fatty acids. 2,000 IU–3,000 IU per day. Fish oil contains EPA and DHA that reduce inflammation.[24] [25] It may be taken in supplement form and/or consumed as wild caught fish, such as salmon, a few times each week.

Homeopathic eyedrops for dry eyes and **over the counter eyedrops** (preservative free) are recommended.

Evening primrose or black currant oil. 500mg–1,000mg per day. Both stimulate aqueous tear secretion and reduce the production of another prostaglandin (fatty acid), PGE2 that causes inflammation that contributes to dry eyes.[26] [27] Supplementing with evening primrose oil reduces dry eye syndrome in SS patients by 68%[28] and dampens the immune response.[29] The gamma-linolenic acid (GLA) in evening primrose oil and in borage oil has been shown to improve the ocular surface of patients with tear-deficient dry eye.[30]

Vitamin D3. 5,000 IU per day. A number of studies show the relationship between vitamin D deficiencies and dry eye syndrome, including accelerated evaporation of tears and other heath symptoms such as fatigue, functional impairment, and pain.[31] [32] Vitamin D also plays an important role in keeping the immune system in balance.[33]

Digestive enzymes. Use as directed. Chronic inflammation can affect the ability to properly absorb nutrients through our digestive tract and possibly cause allergic sensitivities to a wide range of foods (see diet below). Taking digestive enzymes during meals can help make up for the lack of enzyme production that may result from chronic inflammation. Additional HCL (hydrochloric acid) in a digestive enzyme formula may help as well.

Green tea extract. 160mg per day. The polyphenols in green tea have been shown to improve meibomian gland function.[34] Green tea epicatechin's antioxidant capacity fights free radicals caused by chronic inflammation.[35] [36] [37] [38] Some research also suggests that green tea may help prevent the onset of Sjögren's.[39] In an animal model of Sjögren's, researchers found that green tea's epigallocatechin-3-gallate normalizes the level of a protein (PCNA) required for cell integrity and DNA damage repair.[40]

Vitamin A (palmitate). 5,000 IU per day. Vitamin A is necessary for mucin production in the tear film. The mucin layer allows the watery layer to spread evenly over the surface of the eye and helps the eye remain moist and lubricated. Vitamin A also serves to help nourish the cornea.[41]

> **Note**. Vitamin A is contra-indicated for those suffering from Stargardt disease (see Stargardt chapter for more information). Pregnant women should not take vitamin A without their doctor's supervision.

Very Important

Saffron. 20mg per day with food. Saffron has neuroprotective properties against oxidative damage.[42] [43] [44]

MSM capsules. 2,000mg per day, with or without food. MSM helps reduce overall inflammation in the body such as that associated with Sjögren's.[45]

Astaxanthin. 6mg–12mg per day. Astaxanthin destroys unstable free radicals and wards off their constant attack towards all parts of the body.[46]

Serrapeptase. 500mg–800mg, 1–2 times per day, taken on an empty stomach. Serrapeptase is an enzyme that helps reduce inflammation for a number of conditions.[47] [48] [49] It is believed to dissolve dead or damaged tissue without harming living tissue, thereby helping to reduce related inflammation. Excess debris in the body can stimulate an ongoing immune response. The result is chronic inflammation in the body and eyes as well as circulatory problems due to scar tissue buildup in the blood vessels.

Anti–inflammatory herbal formula. Take a high-quality formula as directed. This will help reduce higher levels of inflammation in the body. Take as directed. Common herbs used in these formulas include berberine, boswellia serrata, ginger, green tea, holy basil, hu zhang, MSM, oregano, quercetin, rosemary, rutin, skullcap, turmeric, vitamin C.

Trans-resveratrol. 175mg per day. This potent antioxidant reduces oxidative damage[50] [51] and supports a healthy inflammatory response.[52]

Sea buckthorn oil. 2,000mg a day. This special oil, from the berries of a cold weather shrub, contains helpful oils as well as a special essential fatty acid called omega-7. This little-known nutrient is extremely helpful at fortifying tears and saliva and improving lubrication throughout the body. Carotenoids and tocopherols in the oil, or eicosanoids produced from the fatty acids of the oil may have a positive effect on inflammation and differentiation of the meibomian gland cells.[53] It also can provide protection to the bowel and alleviate vaginal dryness.

Helpful

High-quality, organic, whole-food multivitamin. Take as directed.

Curcumin. 630mg daily. Various studies conclude that curcumin has anti-oxidant, anti-inflammatory, anti-angiogenic (prevents growth of new unwanted blood vessels) effects, and wound-healing benefits.[54] [55] Curcumin may help prevent corneal damage, due to ocular inflammation,[56] and it may inhibit pro inflammatory cytokines. An increase in pro inflammatory cytokines were found in the tear film of dry eye patients,[57] possibly due to chronic inflammation that contributes to dry eye syndrome and onset of conjunctivitis.[58]

Diet

Follow the Vision diet in Chapter 7 with a focus on maintaining a strong alkaline diet. Celiac sprue, a chronic, auto-immune, inflammatory condition that is primarily triggered by gluten hypersensitivity, causes symptoms such as uveitis, abdominal pain, bloating, arthritis, and various vitamin deficiencies, including vitamin D. Gluten hypersensitivity is estimated to affect 1% of the population and to be present in many patients with Sjögren's syndrome. Therefore, some SS patients should be on a gluten free diet.[59] Other food sensitivities can include wheat,[60] corn, dairy, eggs, and beef.[61] We recommend working closely with a nutritionist and allergy specialist to help determine the best diet for you.

Juicing. This is a suggested list of ingredients for Sjögren's. Choose at least 4-6 items to combine:

- Green leafy vegetables, cucumber, parsley, beets, carrots, tomatoes, persimmons, and lemon
- Use organic whenever possible. Don't use too many carrots. Add your favorite fruits and vegetables.
- Try to use room temperature vegetables and fruit.
- Do not add ice or very cold liquids since cold foods and liquids will eventually extinguish the stomach's digestive fire.
- Do not juice as often during the cooler months of the year, and instead, switch to vegetable soups or stews.

Other Dietary Tips
- Nibble on lemons or natural low-sugar candies to stimulate saliva production. Eat smaller, more frequent meals to stimulate saliva flow.
- Drink plenty of water. Frequent, small sips are more effective and comfortable than large, infrequent gulps.
- Avoid strongly flavored foods and soft drinks that may irritate an already dry mouth or interfere with digestion.

Lifestyle

Eye exercises. Recommended daily exercises include palming and massaging the acupressure points around the eyes (see Chapter 10-4).

Exercise. Regular exercise can help reduce joint pain and improve depression.[62] Daily aerobic exercise such as fast walking, swimming, yoga, and/or gym workouts are very helpful for increasing circulation and improving overall eye health. Make sure you stretch regularly as well.

Other Lifestyle Tips

- Use toothpaste without detergents (sodium lauryl sulfate or cocamidopropyl betaine) to reduce mouth irritation.
- Combat nose dryness with salt-water (saline) solutions.
- Avoid mouthwashes and rinses that contain alcohol or witch hazel. These ingredients can aggravate oral dryness and burning.
- Use a humidifier to add moisture to the air in your bedroom.
- Managing stress is crucial for managing this condition: take a walk, meditate, take a yoga class, or engage in some other stress-relieving activity on a consistent basis.
- Pay attention to drugs that harm the eyes (see Chapter 12).
- Carefully clean eyelids with warm water, or baby shampoo, or one of the commercially available eyelid cleansers.
- Apply vitamin E oil, or moisturizing gels, to dry parts or to sore parts of the mouth or tongue for long-lasting relief. You can use the liquid oil by punching a small hole in a liquid vitamin capsule.
- Always take non-steroidal anti-inflammatory drugs (NSAIDs) with food or milk to avoid stomach upset.

Other Modalities

Chinese Medicine

One of the major symptoms of "yin deficiency" is internal dryness. The Kidneys in Chinese medicine also rule over the endocrine system, which relates to, among other things, immune imbalances, and the Kidneys control water metabolism throughout the body.

Common patent formulas include:

Ming mu di huang wan. Rehmannia pills "to brighten the eyes" address Liver blood deficiency, Kidney yin deficiency, and Liver yin deficiency.

Qi ju di huang wan. Chrysanthemum, lycium fruit, and rehmannia pill tonifies Kidney yin, tonifies blood, and clears the eyes.

Zhu jing wan. "Preserve vistas" pill tonifies and nourishes the Liver and Kidneys, enriches the yin, and improves vision.

Herbal formula and treatment strategies can vary significantly based on the Chinese medicine practitioner's evaluation and intake. Therefore it is important to work with a skilled herbalist or Chinese medical practitioner.

On the Horizon

Upcoming studies look at the following possible new treatment strategies:

- A 2012 **stem cell** study showed remarkable improvement in SS patients treated with mesenchymal stem cells.[63]
- **MicroRNA expression** profiles as biomarkers of minor salivary gland inflammation in Sjögren's syndrome. MicroRNA expression patterns have shown, in our preliminary experiments, to accurately distinguish glands (from controls and SS patients) with either a low or a high degree of inflammation. [64]

Also See

[1] Tanakchi, S. (2018). Sjögren's syndrome. *Pathology Outlines,* Mar. 12.

2 Sjögren's Syndrome Foundation. About. Retrieved Dec 04 2017 from https://www.sjogrens.org/home/about-sjogrens

3 Delaleu, N., Jonsson, R., Koller, M.M. Sjogren's syndrome. (2005). Sjögren's syndrome. *Eur J Oral Sci,* 113(2):101–113.

4 Liang, Y., Yang, Z., Qin, B., Zhong, R. (2014). Primary Sjogren's syndrome and malignancy risk: a systematic review and meta-analysis. *Ann Rheum Dis,* Jun; 73(6):1151-6.

5 Mariette, X. (1999). Lymphomas in patients with Sjögren's syndrome: review of the literature and physiopathologic hypothesis. *Leuk Lymphoma,* Mar; 33(1-2):93-9.

6 Kim-Lee, C., Suresh, L., Ambrus, J.L. Jr. (2015). Gastrointestinal disease in Sjogren's syndrome: related to food hypersensitivities. *Springerplus,* 4: 766.

7 Ebert, E.C. (2012). Gastrointestinal and hepatic manifestations of Sjogren syndrome. *J Clin Gastroenterol,* Jan; 46(1):25-30.

8 Bengtsson, M., Hammar, O., Mandl, T., Ohlsson, B. (2011). Evaluation of gastrointestinal symptoms in different patient groups using the visual analogue scale for irritable bowel syndrome (VAS-IBS). *BMC Gastroenterol,* Nov 10; 11():122.

9 Cojocaru, M., Cojocaru, I.M., Silosi, I. (2010). Multiple autoimmune syndrome. *Maedica (Buchar),* Apr;5(2):132-4.

[10] Usuba, F.S., Lopes, J.B., Fuller, R., Yamamoto, J.H., Alves, M.R., et al (2014). Sjögren's syndrome: An underdiagnosed condition in mixed connective tissue disease. *Clinics (Sao Paulo),* Mar; 69(3):158-62.

[11] Sjögren's Syndrome Foundation. About Sjögren's syndrome. [Accessed May 26, 2015]. Available from: https://www.sjogrens.org/home/about-sjogrens-syndrome

[12] Segal., B, Bowman, S.J., Fox, P.C., Vivino, F.B., Murukutla, N., et al. (2009). Primary Sjögren's Syndrome: health experiences and predictors of health quality among patients in the United States. *Health Qual Life Outcomes,* May 27; 7():46.

[13] Sjögren's Syndrome Foundation. Diagnosis. Retrieved Jul 10 2018 from https://www.sjogrens.org/home/about-sjogrens/diagnosis.

[14] Ibid. Tanakchi. (2018).

[15] Beckman, K. A., Luchs, J., Milner, M.S. (2016). Making the diagnosis of Sjögren's syndrome in patients with dry eye. *Clin Ophthalmol,* 10:43-53.

[16] Ibid. Tanakchi. (2018).

17 MedlinePlus. Autoimmune disorders. Retrieved Dec 04 2017 from https://www.nlm.nih.gov/medlineplus/ency/article/000816.htm

[18] Siddiqui, H., Chen, T., Aliko, A., Mydel, P.M., Jonsson, R., et al (2016). Microbiological and bioinformatics analysis of primary Sjogren's syndrome patients with normal salivation. *J Oral Microbiol,* 8:10.3402.

19 Ibid. Tanakchi. (2018).

20 Ibid. Cojocaru. (2010).

21 Izzotti, A., Saccà, S.C., Bagnis, A., Recupero, S.M. (2009). Glaucoma and Helicobacter pylori infection: correlations and controversies. *Br J Ophthalmol,* Nov;93(11):1420-7.

22 Marcet, M.M., Shtein, R.M., Bradley, E.A., Deng, S.X., Meyer, D.R. (2015). Safety and Efficacy of Lacrimal Drainage System Plugs for Dry Eye Syndrome: A Report by the American Academy of Ophthalmology. *Ophthalmology,* Aug;122(8):1681-7.

[23] Ciutin, C., Ostas, A., Cojocaru, V.M., Walsh, S.B., Isenberg, D.A. (2015). Advances in the treatment of ocular dryness associated with Sjögren's syndrome. Semin Arthritis Rheum, Dec;45(3):321-7.

24 Laidlaw, M., Holub, B.J., et al. (2003). Effects of supplementation with fish oil-derived n-3 fatty acids and gamma-linolenic acid on circulating plasma lipids and fatty acid profiles in women. *Am J Clin Nutr,* 2003 Jan;77(1):37-42.

[25] Barham, J.B., Edens, M.B., Fonteh, A.N., Johnson, M.M., Easter, L., et al. (2000). Addition of eicosapentaenoic acid to gamma-linolenic acid supplemented diets prevents serum arachidonic acid accumulation in humans. *J Nutr,* Aug;130(8):1925-31.

26 Oxholm, P., Manthorpe, R., Prause, J.U., Horrobin, D. (1986). Patients with Sjogren's Syndrome Treated For 2 Months with Evening Primrose Oil. *Scand J Rheumatol,* 15(2):103-8.

[27] Baudouin, C. (2001). Dry eye: an unexpected inflammatory disease. *Arch Soc Esp Oftalmol,* 76: 205-206.

28 Ibid. Oxholm. (1986).

29 Wu, D., Meydani, M., Leka, L.S., Nightingale, Z., Handelman, G.J., et al. (1999). Effect of dietary supplementation with black current seed oil on the immune response of healthy elderly subjects. *Am J Clin Nutr,* Oct;70(4):536-43.

30 Barabino, S., Rolando, M., Camicione, P., Ravera, G., Zanardi, S., et al. (2003). Systemic linoleic and gamma-linolenic acid therapy in dry eye syndrome with an inflammatory component. *Cornea,* Mar;22(2):97-101.

[31] Galor, A., Gardener, H., Pouyeh, B., Feuer, W., Florez, H. (2014). Effect of a Mediterranean dietary pattern and vitamin D levels on Dry Eye syndrome. *Cornea,* May; 33(5):437-41.

[32] Kurtul, B.E., Özer, P.A., Aydinli, M.S. (2015). The association of vitamin D deficiency with tear break-up time and Schirmer testing in non-Sjögren dry eye. *Eye (Lond),* Aug 29(8):1081-4.

[33] Prietl, B., Treiber, G., Pieber, T.R., Amrein, K. (2013). Vitamin D and immune function. *Nutrients.* Jul 5; 5(7):2502-21.

34 Nejabat, M., Reza, S.A., Zadmehr, M., Yasemi, M., Sobhani, Z. (2017). Efficacy of Green Tea Extract for Treatment of Dry Eye and Meibomian Gland Dysfunction; A Double-blind Randomized Controlled Clinical Trial Study. *J Clin Diagn Res,* Feb;11(2):NC05-NC08.

35 Chen, L., Yang, X., Jiao, H., Zhao, B. (2003). Tea catechins protect against lead-induced ROS formation, mitochondrial dysfunction, and calcium dysregulation in PC12 cells. *Chem Res Toxicol,* Sep;16(9):1155-61.

[36] Skrzydlewska, E., Ostrowska, J., Stankiewicz, A., Farbiszewski, R. (2002). Green tea as a potent antioxidant in alcohol intoxication. *Addict Biol,* Jul;7(3):307-14.

[37] Kondo, K., Kurihara, M., Miyata, N., Suzuki, T., Toyoda, M. (1999). Mechanistic studies of catechins as antioxidants against radical oxidation. *Arch Biochem Biophys,* Feb 1;362(1):79-86.

[38] Caturla, N., Vera-Samper, E., Villalaín, J., Mateo, C.R., Micol, V. (2003). The relationship between the antioxidant and the antibacterial properties of galloylated catechins and the structure of phospholipid model membranes. *Free Radic Biol Med,* Mar 15;34(6):648-62.

39 Hsu, S.D., Dickinson, D.P., Qin, H., Borke, J., Ogbureke, K.U., et al. (2007). Green tea polyphenols reduce autoimmune symptoms in a murine model for human Sjogren's syndrome and protect human salivary acinar cells from TNF-alpha-induced cytotoxicity. *Autoimmunity,* Mar;40(2):138-47.

[40] Dickenson, D., Yu, H., Ohno, S., Thomas, C. Derossi, S., et al. (2014). Epigallocatechin-3-gallate prevents autoimmune-associated down- regulation of p21 in salivary gland cells through a p53-independent pathway. *Inflamm Allergy Drug Targets,* Feb;13(1):15-24.

[41] Hori, Y., Spurr-Michaud, S., Russo, C., Argüeso, P., Gipson, I.K. (2004). Differential regulation of membrane-associated mucins in the human ocular surface epithelium. *Invest Ophthalmol Vis Sci,* 45:114–122.

[42] Bisti, S., Maccarone, R., Falsini, B. (2014). Saffron and retina: neuroprotection and pharmacokinetics. Vis Neurosci, Sep;31(4-5):355-61.

[43] Marangoni, D., Falsini, B., Piccardi, M., Ambrosio, L., Minnella, A.M. (2013). Functional effect of Saffron supplementation and risk genotypes in early age-related macular degeneration: a preliminary report, J Transl Med, Sep 25;11:228.

[44] Falsini, B. (2017) Trial: Saffron Supplementation in Stargardt's Disease (STARSAF02). Retrieved May 30 from https://clinicaltrials.gov/ct2/show/study/NCT01278277.

[45] Ahn, H., Kim, J., Lee, M., Kim, Y., Cho, Y.W., et al. (2015). Methylsulfonylmethane inhibits NLRP3 inflammasome activation. *Cytokine,* Feb;71(2):223-31.

[46] Sportsnutritionist. Maher, T.J. (2000), Astaxanthin. Retrieved Dec 04 2017 from http://sportsnutritionist.info/course/wp-content/uploads/2013/04/Astaxanthin.pdf

[47] Mazzone, A., Catalani, M., Costanzo, M., Drusian, A., Mandoli, A., et al. (1990). Evaluation of Serratia peptidase in acute or chronic inflammation of otorhinolaryngology pathology: a multicentre, double-blind, randomized trial versus placebo. *J Int Med Res,* Sep-Oct;18(5):379-88.

[48] Tachibana, M., Mizukoshi, O., Harada, Y., Kawamoto, K., Nakai, Y. (1984). A muti-centre, double-blind study of serrapeptase versus placebo in post-antrotomy buccal swelling. *Pharmatherapeutica,* 3(8); 526-30.

[49] Panagariya, A., Sharma, A.K. (1999). A preliminary trial of serratiopeptidase in patients with carpal tunnel syndrome. *J Assoc Physicians India,* 47 (12); 1170-1172.

[50] Remsberg, C.M., Yáñez, J.A., Ohgami, Y., Vega-Villa, K.R., Rimando, A.M., et al. (2008). Pharmacometrics of pterostilbene: preclinical pharmacokinetics and metabolism, anticancer, anti-inflammatory, antioxidant and analgesic activity. *Phytother Res,* 2008 Feb;22(2):169-79.

[51] Perecko, T., Jancinova, V., Drabikova, K., Nosal, R., Harmatha, J. (2008) Structure-efficiency relationship in derivatives of stilbene. Comparison of resveratrol, pinosylvin and pterostilbene. *Neuro Endocrinol Lett,* Oct;29(5):802-5.

[52] Currais, A., Prior, M., Dargusch, R., Armando, A., Ehren, J., et al. (2014). Modulation of p25 and inflammatory pathways by fisetin maintains cognitive function in Alzheimer's disease transgenic mice. *Aging Cell,* 2014 Apr;13(2):379-90.

[53] Järvinen, R.L., Larmo, P.S., Setälä, N.L., Yang, B., Engblom, J.R., et al. (2011). Effects of oral sea buckthorn oil on tear film Fatty acids in individuals with dry eye. *Cornea,* 2011 Sep;30(9):1013-9.

[54] Maheshwari, R.K., Singh, A.K., Gaddipati, J., Srimal, R.C. (2006). Multiple biological activities of curcumin: a short review. *Life Sci,* Mar 27; 78(18):2081-7.

[55] Zhang, N., Li, H., Jia, J., He, M. (2015). Anti-inflammatory effect of curcumin on mast cell-mediated allergic responses in ovalbumin-induced allergic rhinitis mouse. *Cell Immunol,* Nov-Dec; 298(1-2):88-95.

[56] Kimura, K. (2010). [Molecular mechanism of the disruption of barrier function in cultured human corneal epithelial cells induced by tumor necrosis factor-alpha, a proinflammatory cytokine]. *Nippon Ganka Gakkai Zasshi.* Nov; 114(11):935-43.

[57] Solomon, A., Dursun, D., Liu, Z., Xie, Y., Macri, A., Pflugfelder, S.C. (2001). Pro- and anti-inflammatory forms of interleukin-1 in the tear fluid and conjunctiva of patients with dry-eye disease. *Invest Ophthalmol Vis Sci,* Sep; 42(10):2283-92.

[58] Chung, S.H., Choi, S.H., Choi, J.A., Chuck, R.S., Joo, C.K. (2012). Curcumin suppresses ovalbumin-induced allergic conjunctivitis. *Mol Vis,* 18():1966-72.

[59] Rashtak, S., Marietta, E.V., Murray, J.A. (2009). Celiac sprue: a unique autoimmune disorder. *Expert Rev Clin Immunol,* Sep; 5(5):593-604.

[60] Battais, F., Pineau, F., Popineau, Y., Aparicio, C., Kanny, G., et al. (2003). Food allergy to wheat: identification of immunogloglin E and immunoglobulin G-binding proteins with sequential extracts and purified proteins from wheat flour. *Clin Exp Allergy,* Jul; 33(7):962-70.

[61] Zuo, X.L., Li, Y.Q., Li, W.J., Guo, Y.T., Lu, X.F., et al. (2007). Alterations of food antigen-specific serum immunoglobulins G and E antibodies in patients with irritable bowel syndrome and functional dyspepsia. *Clin Exp Allergy,* Jun; 37(6):823-30.

62 Kawashima, M., Uchino, M., Yokoi, N, Uchino, Y., Dogru, M., et al. (2014). The Association between Dry Eye Disease and Physical Activity as well as Sedentary Behavior: Results from the Osaka Study. *J Ophthalmol,* 2014:943786.

63 Xu, J., Wang, D., Liu, D., Fan, Z., Zhang, H., et al. (2012). Allogeneic mesenchymal stem cell treatment alleviates experimental and clinical Sjögren syndrome. *Blood,* 2012 Oct 11;120(15):3142-51.

[64] Alevizos, I., Illei, G.G. (2010). MicroRNAs in Sjögren's syndrome as a prototypic autoimmune disease. *Autoimmun Rev,* Jul;9(9):618-621.

15-29. STARGARDT DISEASE

Stargardt disease (fundus flavimaculatus or Stargardt macular dystrophy) is a form of inherited macular dystrophy that affects young people. It arises from an inherited recessive gene and manifests as a very severe type of macular degeneration that begins in late childhood, resulting in legal blindness. Estimates of prevalence vary widely from 1 per 1000 people to 1 per 900,000. This very broad range could be due to poor data, variations in regional diet, behaviors, environment, etc.).[1] [2] [3]

What is Stargardt Disease?

Mutations in the gene ABCA4 (ABCR) underlie Stargardt disease and also have been implicated in cone dystrophy, cone-rod dystrophy, and retinitis pigmentosa.[4] [5] [6] [7] The ABCA4 defect, located on chromosome 1,[8] results in the eyes' inability to transport retinoids (a form of vitamin A) from the photoreceptor cells to the retinal pigment epithelial layer that is responsible for providing nourishment to retinal cells.[9] [10]

Stargardt's is similar to age-related macular degeneration but usually identified before age 20. The first symptom is decreased vision.

Early stage. Stargardt disease results in progressive central vision loss, first reported as difficulty in reading and seeing in low light situations, although vision is generally good. These problems are usually noticed between ages 6 to 12, though the symptoms may emerge as an adult.

Disease progression. With further progression, oily deposits begin to accumulate in the layer of tissue comprising the retinal pigment epithelium layer of cells (RPE) that is the layer behind the macula. The RPE is a layer lying between the retina and the choroid, providing nourishment to photoreceptor cells. These oily deposits, called lipofuscin, look like yellowish-tinted specks.

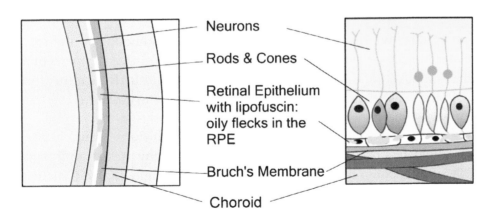

Neurons

Rods & Cones

Retinal Epithelium with lipofuscin: oily flecks in the RPE

Bruch's Membrane

Choroid

The accumulation of lipofuscin eventually causes wasting-away of the macula and the RPE.[11] [12] How fast and to what degree vision is lost, varies, especially in children. It can begin with 20/40 vision and rapidly decrease to 20/200, which is the level for legal blindness. Color vision may also be impaired in advanced Stargardt's. By age 50, about half of all patients assessed in clinical trials have visual acuities of 20/200 to 20/400.

Signs and Symptoms

The main signs and symptoms are loss of visual acuity or sharpness of vision, decreased color vision, and small blind spots.

Other symptoms may include blurriness, visual distortion, difficulty adapting to the dark after sunlight exposure, and/or light sensitivity.

In more severe stages of vision loss, patients may experience phantom vision or visual hallucinations. These episodes are not usually related to underlying psychiatric problems, but rather are normal attempts by the brain to make sense of impaired sensory information. The brain may embellish the image, making it very real, just as it does in our dreams.

Causes and Risk Factors

Stargardt disease nearly always arises from an inherited recessive gene. This means that both parents carry the gene. The child has a 25% chance of inheriting a gene from each parent. Parents themselves might not have Stargardt's since they might have only one gene and two are required.

In 1997 researchers identified the specific gene tied to Stargardt's. It is one of 19 known mutations of the ABCR gene, which produces a protein required for energy transport to, and from, photoreceptor cells in the retina. The mutations cause a non-functioning protein that is unable to perform its transport function. The dysfunctional ABCR protein allows fatty deposits to accumulate in the retina's RPE layer. The end result is that photoreceptor cells degrade with resulting vision loss.

Conventional Treatment

Currently, there is no effective treatment for Stargardt disease, although in the future, bone marrow stem-cell injections may be a therapy. Research does suggest that supplementation with beta-carotene and vitamin A should be avoided, as those with Stargardt's have difficulty breaking down this vitamin in the eyes[13] that can result in additional toxicity to the retina.

Diagnostic evaluation of Stargardt disease is based on family history, visual acuity, fundus examination, visual field testing, color testing, electroretinography (ERG), optical coherence tomography (OCT), fundus photo of the retina, and fluorescein angiography. Genetic testing is currently not performed on a routine basis.

Research shows that ongoing exposure to sunlight increases the risk of cataracts and macular degeneration,[14] and that ultraviolet-protecting sunglasses help protect the retina from damage. Researchers are investigating whether the injection of human embryonic stem cells has some benefit.[15]

Complementary Approach

Taking targeted supplements and establishing healthy lifestyle habits are still helpful at any stage of Stargardt disease, keeping in mind that the preservation of vision and the potential level of vision improvement is based on the level of vision the patient has at the time of incorporating complementary approaches. Antioxidants are essential to maintaining healthy vision, but at the same time, **vitamin A and beta-carotene should be avoided. Also, carotenoids that can be converted to vitamin A should be minimized.** However, there are certain non-vitamin-A-converting carotenoids that can be very useful in helping protect the photoreceptor cells in the retina. These include lutein, zeaxanthin, mesozeaxanthin, astaxanthin, and lycopene, all of which are not converted to vitamin A in the body.[16][17][18]

Nutrients

Essential

Lutein and zeaxanthin are two similarly structured carotenoids that make up the macular pigment in the retina. They are powerful antioxidants. Acting as a yellow filter, they help protect the light-sensitive photoreceptor cells (the cones) against damaging blue (visible) light.[19][20][21][22][23]

Lutein and zeaxanthin need fat to absorb well, so take them with food or a small amount of oil.

Lutein. 6mg–30mg per day. Lutein has also been shown to reduce eye inflammation.[24]

Zeaxanthin. 2mg–4mg per day. This essential nutrient, located more in the central part of the retina, has been found to be critical in maintaining healthy vision. Research has shown it to be a critical carotenoid for those with macular degeneration.[25]

Lycopene. 3mg per day. People with the lowest serum levels of lycopene, the most abundant carotenoid in blood, are twice as likely to develop macular degeneration when compared to those with the highest levels.[26]

Omega-3 fatty acids (not cod liver oil as it contains vitamin A). 2,000mg–3,000mg per day. Omega-3 fatty acids found in fish, are a primary component of retinal photoreceptors and of the myelin sheath that surrounds nerve fibers in the eye. DHA (a component of omega-3 fatty acid) has been found to have antioxidative, anti-inflammatory, anti-apoptotic, and anti-angiogenic (limiting growth of new blood vessels) effects.[27][28][29][30][31][32]

Astaxanthin. 6mg–12mg per day. Like other antioxidants, astaxanthin is effective in protecting against damage from light. It helps to protect the photoreceptors from oxidative damage.[33] It is 10 times more powerful than beta-carotene, lutein, or zeaxanthin; it is 550 times stronger than vitamin E; and it is 6,000 times stronger than vitamin C. For best absorption, astaxanthin should be taken with a healthy fat. Some astaxanthin supplements contain some fat in their formulation. Among other benefits, it also supports cardiovascular, brain, and mitochondria health.[34][35][36][37][38]

Mesozeaxanthin. 10mg per day. Mesozeaxanthin is a carotenoid in the lutein family that supports central vision in the retina. Studies show that supplementing with mesozeaxanthin helps protect central vision for those with macular degeneration. One 2007 study found that higher levels of all three carotenoids (lutein, zeaxanthin, and mesozeaxanthin) increased blood and macular pigment density.[39] [40]

Trans-resveratrol. 175mg per day. This potent antioxidant helps protect nerve cells from damage[41] and reduces oxidative damage.[42] [43] It also maintains the health of existing blood vessels while suppressing the growth of new ones (angiogenesis), similar to the neovascularization that can affect those with diabetic retinopathy. It reduces RPE cell degeneration that can lead to malfunctioning of the blood-retinal barrier and to loss of vision.[44] Among other functions, the RPE regulates the transport of nutrients and waste products to and from the retina and contributes to outer segment renewal by ingesting and degrading the spent tips of photoreceptor outer segments.[45]

Vitamin C (buffered and ascorbated). 2,000mg–3,000mg per day. As an antioxidant, vitamin C scavenges free radicals in the body and protects tissues from oxidative stress.[46] [47] [48]

Saffron. 20mg per day. Studies have shown that saffron helps protect photoreceptor cells from damage and supports healthy circulation in the retina.[49] [50] [51] [52] [53] [54]

Very Important

Ginkgo biloba. 120mg per day. Ginkgo helps support healthy circulation to the eyes and body, and it helps maintain the normal function and tone of blood vessels.[55] [56] [57]

Glutathione (GSH), reduced. 500mg–900mg per day. This is a potent antioxidant shown to help protect retinal cells from damage. It is best taken sublingually or intraorally, as it is not well absorbed through capsules or tablets.[58] [59] The sublingual form has 5–10 times greater absorption so the dosage will be smaller. Follow label instructions.

Taurine. 750mg–1,000mg per day. Taurine is a potent antioxidant found in the retina and essential in helping the eyes eliminate waste. Additionally, it supports the rods and cones within the retina.[60] [61] [62] One study also gave taurine a potential role in reducing the negative effects of oxidative stress for those with macular degeneration.[63]

Helpful

Green tea extract. 500mg–750mg per day. Green tea is excellent at scavenging reactive oxygen species such as superoxide and the hydroxyl and peroxyl radicals,[64] [65] and it is potentially neuroprotective in the photoreceptor outer segment and RPE, if delivered in the proper dosages (about two cups of green tea per day).[66]

CoQ10. 100mg–200mg per day. Research findings strongly suggest that a combination of acetyl-L-carnitine, n-3 fatty acids, and coenzyme Q10 can help maintain healthy vision by affecting mitochondrial lipid metabolism. It also may improve fundus alterations (the fundus includes the interior lining of the eyeball, including the retina, optic disc–the head of the nerve to the eye, and the macula) where we get our most detailed vision in patients affected by early AMD.[67]

Goji berries. A study found that daily supplementation with goji berries increased the levels of zeaxanthin in the blood and protected the retina from additional drusen formulation or loss of pigmentation.[68]

Diet

No extra vitamin A. People with Stargardt's cannot make an enzyme to get rid of the waste products from metabolized vitamin A and compounds similar to vitamin A. The build up of these waste products leads to the death of retinal cells, so supplementing with vitamin A (and beta-carotene) should be avoided.

Limit foods high in beta-cryptoxanthin that can be converted to vitamin A in the body. These carotenoids are typically found in yellow foods.[69] [70]

Limit foods highest in alpha-carotene and beta-carotene that also convert to vitamin A in the body. Beta-carotene produces as much vitamin A as alpha-carotene.

Foods high in these three categories include the following:[71] [72] [73] [74]

- Chard, Chinese cabbage, collards, corn salad, dandelion greens, lamb's quarters, raw lettuce, kale, spinach, pokeberry shoots, mustard-, beet-, and turnip-greens
- Broccoli, lettuce, peas, peppers, and tomatoes
- Pumpkin, carrot, winter squash, and sweet potato
- Basil, cilantro, chicory, parsley, and watercress
- Hot taco sauce, chili powder, cayenne, coriander, and pickles
- Moose liver, turkey liver, duck liver, and veal
- Mango, papaya, cantaloupe, and watermelon
- Apricot, Surinam-, sour-, and ground- cherry, ohelo berry, passion fruit, persimmon, plum, and peach
- Grapefruit, oranges, tangerine, loquat, and rose apple

The following foods are a little less high:

- Tomato, asparagus, broccoli, celery, and other cabbages are a little less high in beta-carotene
- Amaranth greens, and purslane are also high in vitamin A, but less so

Lifestyle

Microcurrent stimulation (MCS). Daily sessions at home. The MCS 100ile unit is the most researched unit used for retinal health related to AMD. Research studies show MCS as a method to daily support retinal and photoreceptor health in three ways:

1. Supports healthy circulation to the retina

2. Increases energy (ATP or adenosine triphosphate) production within the retinal cells through our mitochondria
3. Helps the retina eliminate waste[75] [76] [77] [78]

See Chapter 10-3 for more information.

Other Modalities

Chinese Medicine

In Chinese medicine, the Liver "opens to the eyes" and is the primary meridian for supporting overall flow of energy and circulation through the eyes. The Kidney meridian nourishes the blood to the eyes. The Spleen meridian also nourishes the blood, while helping to keep fluids from leaking from blood vessels. Other meridians may be out of balance as well that can affect eye health, so an evaluation by an acupuncturist can best determine where the out-of-balances are and offer the optimal treatment strategy. Acupuncture treatments are typically done by inserting needles below the knees and elbows, in specific points along the orbit of the eye, and under the eye (not in the eye). An evaluation by an acupuncturist is the best way to determine where the imbalances are.

Xiao yao san is a classic Liver tonic used in Chinese medicine. The Liver "opens to the eyes" and is the primary meridian (flow energy) that supports healthy circulation and the free flow of energy in the eyes, as well as throughout the body.

Ming mu di juang wan is a classic formula used in Chinese medicine for eye health, helping to nourish the Kidneys and Liver. Known to help with blurriness of vision, tearing against wind, conjunctive congestion with pain, and swelling of eye.

Herbal formula and treatment strategies can vary significantly, based on the Chinese medicine practitioner's evaluation and intake.

Essential Oil

Carrot seed essential oil improves the eyes by protecting against macular degeneration, detoxifying blood vessels, toning the liver, relieving stress and anxiety, and providing many nourishing vitamins and minerals.

Frankincense has been around since antiquity, a sacred plant that can be helpful in showing us our visual blind spots. Frankincense tells us to "open up that third eye" and is our main "go to" for application around the eyes.

Keep essences away from the mouth, eyes, and mucous membranes; if a few drops get in one of these sensitive areas it may be uncomfortable for 15–30 minutes, but not harmful. You can lessen discomfort by adding a pure oil like olive or coconut oil to neutralize the irritating effect. For the eye area, dab a few drops around the outside of the eye. Do not put the neutralizing oil in the eye.

Combine ¼ cup of avocado oil with ¼ cup of calendula-infused oil. Slowly add 5 drops each of the essential oils. Then close the bottle and shake well; apply 4 drops of this mixture on your clean face. Massage in gentle circular motions. Leave overnight.

For more information, see Essential Oils in Appendix 9.

Other Alternative Therapies

You can also consider ayurvedic medicine, craniosacral, homeopathy, and reiki that are discussed in Appendix 7.

On the Horizon

Gene therapy. Research on gene therapy is in process and offers promise for the future in regenerating lost retinal cells.

Synthetic A. Columbia University is working with a synthetic form of vitamin A, called ALK-001, that isn't readily converted into lipofuscin (currently in Phase II).[79] As part of the natural biological processes in the eye, vitamin A transforms chemically. Molecules of vitamin A sometimes bond to other vitamin A molecules and create clumps or deposits called "dimers." These dimers are found both in the elderly with AMD and in young children with Stargardt's.[80] Researchers are now working on the structure of vitamin A itself. If it is possible to reduce vitamin A's tendency to clump within the eye, scientists might be able to create a new therapy for Stargardt's.[81] [82]

Stem cell research is actively in process through a company, Ocata Therapeutics, currently in Phase I/II stages.[83]

Also See

Chapter 7, Vision Diet

Chapter 8, Nutrients

Chapter 10-4, Eye Exercises

Chapter 15-18, Macular Degeneration

Appendix 6, Amsler Test

---

[1] According to most literature (which cites Blacharski (1988) Stargardt's affects 1 in 8,000 to 10,000 people. This estimate was high because it was not epidemiological, but instead relied on the fact that Stargardt's appeared to be more common than retinoblastoma but less common than retinitis pigmentosa. See Cornish. (2017).

[2] Cornish, K.S., Ho, J., Downes, S., Scott, N.W., Bainbridge, J., Lois, N. (2017). The Epidemiology of Stargardt Disease in the United Kingdom. *Ophthalmol Ret,* Dec; 125(12): 1718-1722.

[3] Riverio-Alvarez, R., Aguirre-Lamban, J., Lopez-Martinez, M.A., Trujillo-Tiebas, M.J., Catalapiedra, D., et al. (2009). Frequency of ABCA4 mutations in 278 Spanish controls: an insight into the prevalence of autosomal recessive Stargardt disease. *Brit J Ophthalmol,* Oct; 93(10): 1369-1364.

[4] Michaelides, M., Chen, L.L., Brantley, M.A., Andorf, J.L., Isaak, E.L. et al. (2007). ABCA4 mutations and discordant ABCA4 alleles in patients and siblings with bull's-eye maculopathy. *Br J Ophthalmol,* 91: 1650–1655.

[5] Fujinami, K., Lois, N., Davidson, A.E., Mackay, D.S., Hogg, C.R., et al. (2013). A longitudinal study of Stargardt disease: clinical and electrophysiologic assessment, progression, and genotype correlations. *Am J Ophthalmol,* 155: 1075–1088.

[6] Fujinami, K., Sergouniotis, P.I., Davidson, A.E., Mackay, D.S., Tsunoda, K., et al. (2013). The clinical effect of homozygous ABCA4 alleles in 18 patients. *Ophthalmology,* 120: 2324–2331.

[7] Allikmets, R., Shroyer, N.F., Singh, N., Seddon, J.M., Lewis, R.A., et al. (1997). Mutation of the Stargardt disease gene (ABCR) in age-related macular degeneration. *Science,* 277: 1805–1807.

[8] Westerfeld, C., Mukai, S. (2008). Stargardt's disease and the ABCR gene. *Semin Ophthalmol,* Jan-Feb;23(1):59-65.

[9] Sun, H., Nathans, J. (1997). Stargardt's ABCR is localized to the disc membrane of retinal rod outer segments. *Nat Genet,* 17:15–16.

[10] Chen, Y., Okano, K., Maeda, T., Chauhan, V., Golczak, M., et al. (2012). Mechanism of all-trans-retinal toxicity with implications for Stargardt disease and age-related macular degeneration. *J Biol Chem,* 287: 5059

[11] Weng, J., Mata, N.L., Azarian, S.M., Tzekov, R.T., Birch, D.G., Travis, G.H. (1999). Insights into the function of Rim protein in photoreceptors and etiology of Stargardt's disease from the phenotype in abcr knockout mice. *Cell,* 98: 13–23.

[12] Mata, N.L., Weng, J., Travis, G.H. (2000). Biosynthesis of a major lipofuscin fluorophore in mice and humans with ABCR-mediated retinal and macular degeneration. *Proc Natl Acad Sci U S A,* 97: 7154–7159.

13 Sofi, F., Sodi, A., Franco, F., Murro, V., Biagini, D., et al. (2016). Dietary profile of patients with Stargardt's disease and Retinitis Pigmentosa: is there a role for a nutritional approach? *BMC Ophthalmol,* Jan 22;16:13.

[14] Roberts, J.E. (2011). Ultraviolet radiation as a risk factor for cataract and macular degeneration. *Eye Contact Lens,* Jul;37(4):246-9.

[15] National Eye Institute. Facts About Stargardt Disease. Retrieved Apr 16 2018 from https://nei.nih.gov/health/stargardt/star_facts.

[16] National Institutes of Health. Vitamin A. Retrieved Apr 16 2018 from https://ods.od.nih.gov/factsheets/VitaminA-HealthProfessional/.

[17] Ambati, R.R., Moi, P.S., Ravi, S., Aswathanarayana, R.G. (2014). Astaxanthin: Sources, Extraction, Stability, Biological Activities and Its Commercial Applications—A Review. *Mar Drugs,* Jan;12(1):128-152.

[18] Abdel-Aai, E.M., Akhtar, H., Zaheer, K., Ali, R. (2013). Dietary Sources of Lutein and Zeaxanthin Carotenoids and Their Role in Eye Health. *Nutrients,* Apr;5(4):1169-1185.

[19] Snellen, E.L., Verbeek, A.L., Van Den Hoogen, G.W., Cruysberg, J.R., Hoyng, C.B. (2002). Neovascular age-related macular degeneration and its relationship to antioxidant intake. *Acta Ophthalmol Scand,* Aug;80(4):368-71.

[20] Richer, S., Stiles, W., Statkute, L., Pulido, J., Frankowski, J. (2004). Double-masked, placebo-controlled, randomized trial of lutein and antioxidant supplementation in the intervention of atrophic age-related macular degeneration: the Veterans LAST study (Lutein Antioxidant Supplementation Trial). *Optometry,* Apr;75(4):216-30.

[21] Souied, E.H., Delcourt, C., Querques, G., Bassols, A., Merle, B., et al. (2013). Oral docosahexaenoic acid in the prevention of exudative age-related macular degeneration: the Nutritional AMD Treatment 2 study. *Ophthalmology,* Aug;120(8):1619-31.

[22] Landrum, J.T., Bone, R.A., Joa, H., Kilburn, M.D., Moore, L.L., et al. (1997). A one year study of the macular pigment: the effect of 140 days of a lutein supplement. *Exp Eye Res,* Jul;65(1):57-62.

[23] Bernstein, P.S., Zhao, D.Y., Wintch, S.W., Ermakov, I.V., McClane, R.W., et al. (2009). Resonance Raman measurement of macular carotenoids in normal subjects and in age-related macular degeneration patients. *Ophthalmology,* 109:1780-1878.

[24] Kijlstra, A., Tian, Y., Kelly, E.R., Berendschot, T.T. (2012). Lutein: more than just a filter for blue light. *Prog Retin Eye Res,* Jul;31(4):303-15.

[25] National Eye Institute. (2013). NIH study provides clarity on supplements for protection against blinding eye disease. Retrieved Apr 16 2018 from https://nei.nih.gov/news/pressreleases/050513.

[26] Mares-Perlman, J.A., Brady, W.E., Klein, R., Klein, B.E., Bowen, P., et al. (1995). Serum antioxidants and age-related macular degeneration in a population-based case-control study. *Arch Ophthalmol,* 1995 Dec;113(12):1518-23.

[27] Souied, E.H., Delcourt, C., Querques, G., Bassols, A., Merle, B., et al. (2013). Oral docosahexaenoic acid in the prevention of exudative age-related macular degeneration: *Ophthalmology,* Aug;120(8):1619-31.

[28] SanGiovanni, J.P., Chew, E.Y. (2005). The role of omega-3 long-chain polyunsaturated fatty acids in health and disease of the retina. *Prog Retin Eye Res,* 24(1): 87–138.

[29] Chong, E.W., Robman, L.D., Simpson, J.A., Hodge, A.M., Aung, K.Z. (2009). Fat consumption and its association with age-related macular degeneration. *Arch Ophthalmol,* May;127(5):674-80.

[30] Smith, W., Mitchell, P., Leeder, S.R. (2000). Dietary fat and fish intake and age-related maculopathy. *Arch Ophthalmol,* Mar;118(3):401-4.

[31] Cho, E., Hung, S., Willett, W.C., Spiegelman, D., Rimm, E.B., et al. (2001). Prospective study of dietary fat and the risk of age-related macular degeneration. *Am J Clin Nutr,* Feb;73(2):209-18.

[32] Delcourt, C.s, Carrière, I., Cristol, J.P., Lacroux, A., Gerber, M. (2007). Dietary fat and the risk of age-related maculopathy: the POLANUT Study. *Eur J Clin Nutr,* Nov;61(11):1341-4.

[33] Otsuka, T., Shimazawa, M., Nakanishi, T., Ohno, Y., Inoue, Y., et al. (2013). Protective effects of a dietary carotenoid, astaxanthin, against light-induced retinal damage. *J Pharmacol Sci,* 123(3):209-18.

[34] BetaForce. Astaxanthin: The Most Powerful Natural Antioxidant Ever Discovered. Retrieved Apr 2 2018 from http://www.beta-glucan-info.com/astaxanthin.htm.

[35] Chiro.org. Antioxidants: Relative Singlet Oxygen Quenching Rates. Retrieved Apr 16 2018 from http://www.chiro.org/nutrition/FULL/ Antioxidants_Relative_Singlet_Oxygen_Quenching_Rates.html.

[36] Kidd, P. (2011). Astaxanthin, cell membrane nutrient with diverse clinical benefits and anti-aging potential. *Altern Med Rev,* Dec;16(4):355-64.

[37] Song, X., Wang, B., Lin, S., Jing, L., Mao, C., et al. (2014). Astaxanthin inhibits apoptosis in alveolar epithelial cells type II in vivo and in vitro through the ROS-dependent mitochondrial signaling pathway. *J Cell Mol Med,* Nov;18(11):2198-212.

[38] Kuroki, T., Ikeda, S., Okada, T., Maoka, T., Kitamura, A., et al. (2013). Astaxanthin ameliorates heat stress-induced impairment of blastocyst development in vitro: astaxanthin colocalization with and action on mitochondria--. *J Assist Reprod Genet,* Jun;30(5):623-31.

[39] Bone, R.A., Landrum, J.T., Cao, Y., Howard, A.N., Alvarez-Calderon, F. (2007). Macular pigment response to a supplement containing meso-zeaxanthin, lutein and zeaxanthin. *Nutr Metab (Lond),* May 11;4:12.

[40] Connolly, E.E., Beatty, S., Thurnham, D.I., Loughman, J., Howard, A.N. (2010). Augmentation of macular pigment following supplementation with all three macular carotenoids: an exploratory study. *Curr Eye Res,* Apr:35(4):335-51.

[41] Anekonda, T.S., Adamus, G. (2008). Resveratrol prevents antibody-induced apoptotic death of retinal cells through upregulation of Sirt1 and Ku70. *BMC Res Notes,* Dec 1;1:122.

[4242] Remsberg, C.M., Yáñez, J.A., Ohgami, Y., Vega-Villa, K.R., Rimando, A.M., et al. (2008). Pharmacometrics of pterostilbene: preclinical pharmacokinetics and metabolism, anticancer, anti-inflammatory, antioxidant and analgesic activity. *Phytother Res,* Feb;22(2):169-79.

[43] Perecko, T., Jancinova, V., Drabikova. K., Nosal, R., Harmatha, J. (2008). Structure-efficiency relationship in derivatives of stilbene. Comparison of resveratrol, pinosylvin and pterostilbene. *Neuro Endocrinol Lett,* Oct;29(5):802-5.

[44] Antonetti, D.A., Klein, R., Gardner, T.W. (2012). Diabetic retinopathy. *N Eng J Med.* Mar, 29; 366(13):1227-39.

[45] Boulton, M. (2001). The role of the retinal pigment epithelium: Topographical variation and ageing changes. *Eye,* 15:384-389.

[46] Du, J., Cullen, J.J., Buettner, G.R. (2012). Ascorbic acid: chemistry, biology and the treatment of cancer. *Biochem Biophys Acta,* Dec;1826(2):443-57.

[47] Cangemi, R., Angelico, F., Loffredo, L., Del Ben, M., Pignatelli, P., et al. (2007). Oxidative stress-mediated arterial dysfunction in patients with metabolic syndrome: Effect of ascorbic acid. *Free Radic Biol Med,* Sep 1;43(5):853-9.

[48] Cho, E., Seddon, J.M., Rosner, B., Willett, W.C., Hankinson, S.E. (2004). Prospective study of intake of fruits, vegetables, vitamins, and carotenoids and risk of age-related maculopathy. *Arch Ophthalmol,* Jun;122(6):883-92.

[49] Falsini, B., Piccardi, M., Minnella, A., Savastano, C., Capoluongo, E., et al. (2010). Influence of saffron supplementation on retinal flicker sensitivity in early age-related macular degeneration. *Invest Ophthalmol Vis Sci,* Dec;51(12):6118-24.

[50] Marangoni, D., Falsini, B., Piccardi, M., Ambrosio, L., Minnella, A.M. (2013). Functional effect of Saffron supplementation and risk genotypes in early age-related macular degeneration: a preliminary report. *J Transl Med,* Sep 25;11:228.

[51] Alavizadeh, S.H., Hosseinzadeh, H. (2014). Bioactivity assessment and toxicity of crocin: a comprehensive review, *Food Chem Toxicol,* Feb;64:65-80.

[52] Corso, L., Cavallero, A., Baroni, D., Garbati, P., Prestipino, G., et al. (2016). Saffron reduces ATP-induced retinal cytotoxicity by targeting P2X7 receptors. *Purinergic Signal,* Mar;12(1):161-74.

[53] Broadhead, G.K., Grigg, J.R., Chang, A.A., McCluskey, P. (2015). Dietary modification and supplementation for the treatment of age-related macular degeneration, *Nutr Rev,* Jul;73(7):448-62.

[54] Broadhead, G.K., Chang, A., Grigg, J., McCluskey, P. (2016). Efficacy and Safety of Saffron Supplementation: Current Clinical Findings. *Crit Rev Food Sci Nutr,* Dec 9;56(16):2767-76.

[55] Lebuisson, D.A., Leroy, L., Rigal, G. (1986). Treatment of senile macular degeneration with Ginkgo biloba extract. A preliminary double-blind drug vs. placebo study. *Presse Med,* Sep 25;15(31):1556-8

[56] Fies, P., Dienel, A. (2002). Ginkgo extract in impaired vision--treatment with special extract EGb 761 of impaired vision due to dry senile macular degeneration. *Wien Med Wochenschr,* 152(15-16):423-6.

[57] Diamond, B.J., Shiflett, S.C., Feiwel, N., Matheis, R.J., Noskin, O., et al. (2000). Ginkgo biloba extract: mechanisms and clinical indications. *Arch Phys Med Rehabil,* May;81(5):668-78.

[58] Ayalasomayajula, S.P., Kompella, U.B. (2002). Induction of vascular endothelial growth factor by 4-hydroxynonenal and its prevention by glutathione precursors in retinal pigment epithelial cells, *Eur J Pharmacol,* Aug 9;449(3):213-20.

[59] Sternberg, P., Davidson, P.C., Jones, D.P., Hagen, T.M., Reed, R.L., et al. (1993). Protection of retinal pigment epithelium from oxidative injury by glutathione and precursors. *Invest Ophthalmol Vis Sci,* Dec;34(13):3661-8.

[60] Birdsall, T.C. Therapeutic applications of taurine. *Altern Med Rev,* 1998 Apr;3(2):128-36.

[61] Shpak, N.I., Naritsyna, N.I., Konovalova, N.V. (1989). Taufon and emoksipin in the combined treatment of sclerotic macular dystrophies]. *Oftalmol Zh,* (8):463-5.

[62] Lombardini, J.B. (1991). Taurine: retinal function. *Brain Res Brain Res Rev,* May-Aug;16(2):151-69

[63] Drobek-Słowik, M., Karczewicz, D., Safranow, K. (2007). The potential role of oxidative stress in the pathogenesis of the age-related macular degeneration (AMD). *Postepy Hig Med Dosw* (Online), 61:28-37.

[64] Chen, L., Yang, X., Jiao, H., Zhao, B. (2003). Tea catechins protect against lead-induced ROS formation, mitochondrial dysfunction, and calcium dysregulation in PC12 cells. *Chem Res Toxicol,* Sep;16(9):1155-61.

[65] Skrzydlewska, E., Ostrowska, J., Stankiewicz, A., Farbiszewski, R. (2002). Green tea as a potent antioxidant in alcohol intoxication. *Addict Biol,* Jul;7(3):307-14.

[66] Jarrett, S.G., Boulton, M.E. Consequences of oxidative stress in age-related macular degeneration. *Mol Aspects Med,* Aug;33(4):399–417.

[67] Feher, J., Kovacs, B., Kovacs, I., Schveoller, M., Papale, A., et al. (2005). Improvement of visual functions and fundus alterations in early age-related macular degeneration treated with a combination of acetyl-L-carnitine, n-3 fatty acids, and coenzyme Q10. *Ophthalmologica,* May-Jun;219(3):154-66.

[68] Bucheli, P., Vidal, K., Shen, L., Gu, Z., Zhang, C., et al. (2011). Goji berry effects on macular characteristics and plasma antioxidant levels. *Optom Vis Sci,* Feb:88(2):257-62.

[69] Burri, B.J. (2015). Beta-cryptoxanthin as a source of vitamin A. *J Sci Food Agric,* Jul;95(9):1786-94.

[70] SelfNutritionData. Foods highest in Beta Cryptoxanthin. Retrieved Dec 18 2017 from http://nutritiondata.self.com/foods-000136000000000000000.html.

[71] SelfNutritionData. Foods highest in Beta Carotene. Retrieved Apr 16 2018 from http://nutritiondata.self.com/foods-000135000000000000000.html.

[72] SelfNutritionData. Foods highest in Alpha Carotene. Retrieved Apr 16 2018 from http://nutritiondata.self.com/foods-000134000000000000000.html.

[73] SelfNutritionData. Foods highest in Vitamin A. Retrieved Apr 16 2018 from http://nutritiondata.self.com/foods-000098000000000000000.html.

[74] Ibid. SelfNutritionData. Foods highest in Vitamin A.

[75] Michael, L.D., Allen, M.I. (1993). Nutritional supplementation, electrical stimulation and age related macular degeneration. *J. Orthomol Med,* 8:168-

[76] Wallace, L. B. (1997). Treatment for Macular Degeneration Utilizing Micro-Current Stimulation. *J. Opt Photother,* Mar.

[77] O'Clock, G.D., Jarding, J. B. (2009). Electrotherapeutic device/protocol design considerations for visual disease applications. *Conf Proc IEEE Eng Med Biol Soc,* 2009

[78] Chaikin, L., Kashiwa, K., Bennet, M., Papastergiou, G., Gregory, W. (2015). Microcurrent stimulation in the treatment of dry and wet macular degeneration. *Clin Ophthalmol,* Dec 17;9:2345-53.

[79] Clinicaltrials. Phase 2 Tolerability and Effects of ALK-001 on Stargardt Disease (TEASE). Retrieved Dec 04 2017 from https://clinicaltrials.gov/ct2/show/NCT02402660.

[80] Kim, S.R., Jang, Y.P., Jockusch, S., Fishkin, N., Turro, N., et al. (2007). The all-trans-retinal dimer series of lipofuscin pigments in retinal pigment epithelial cells in a recessive Stargardt disease model. *Proc Natl Acad Sci U S A*, Dec 4;104(49):19273-19278.

[81] Ma, L., Kaufmann, Y., Zhang, J., Washington, I. (2010). C20-D3-vitamin A Slows Lipofuscin Accumulation and Electrophysiological Retinal Degeneration in a Mouse Model of Stargardt Disease. *J Biol Chem*, Mar 11;286(10) 7966-7974.

[82] Saad, L., Washington, I. (2016). Can Vitamin A be Improved to Prevent Blindness due to Age-Related Macular Degeneration, Stargardt Disease and Other Retinal Dystrophies? *Adv Exp Med Biol*, 2016;854:355-61.

[83] Blindness.org. Gene Therapy Clinical Trial Underway for Stargardt Disease. Retrieved Dec 04 2017 from http://www.blindness.org/sites/default/files/pages/pdfs/Advances-Stargardt-March-2017.pdf.

15-30. USHER SYNDROME

Usher syndrome is a group of genetic-related disorders that bring about simultaneous hearing and vision loss.

There are three types of Usher (USH), all with similar symptoms. Different genes have been identified for each type. In the U.S., types 1 and 2 are the most common; together, they account for approximately 90–95% of all cases of children who have Usher syndrome.[1]

Approximately 3–6% of all children who are deaf and another 3–6% of children who are hard-of-hearing have Usher syndrome.[2] Usher syndrome affects approximately 4 to 17 per 100,000 people[3] [4] and accounts for about 50% of all hereditary deaf-blindness cases.[5]

What is Usher Syndrome?

The eye condition of retinitis pigmentosa (RP) is responsible for the vision loss aspect of Usher syndrome. Usher is defined by the progressive degeneration of the retina, manifesting as a loss of night and peripheral vision that eventually results in "tunnel vision," or the ability to see only straight ahead. Most people with Usher also have severe balance problems.

When an eye doctor looks at the retina in a patient with Usher, the optic nerve looks very pale, the blood vessels supplying nutrients to the retina are thin, and the doctor can see that there are characteristic spots and splotches of pigment called bone spicules.[6]

Types of Usher Syndrome

Type 1 Usher. At birth, the child is severely deaf and has severe balance problems. Before the age of 10, the child may begin to develop vision problems. This type of Usher syndrome includes problems with the inner ear affecting balance that results in children being unable to sit or walk independently until later than usual.

Type 2 Usher. At birth, the child has moderate to serious deafness and normal capacity for balance. These children are assisted by hearing aids, and retinitis pigmentosa isn't noticed until they reach their teens.[7] Type 2 is thought to be the most common form of Usher syndrome, although the frequency is unknown. The vision problems of this type 2 tend to progress more slowly than those of type 1.

Type 3 Usher. These children do not have hearing problems at birth, and they have normal or almost normal balance, although some balance issues may develop with adulthood. However, hearing and vision deteriorate with time, usually by their teen years. Hearing aids are usually needed by adulthood, and blind spots appear by the late teens to early adulthood.[8]

By mid-adulthood, the person is usually legally blind. The clinical diagnosis refers to a central visual acuity of 20/200 or less in the better eye, with the best possible correction and/or a visual field of 20 degrees or less. Type 3 Usher syndrome accounts for only a small percentage of all

Usher syndrome cases in most populations. Though it is prevalent in Finland where it accounts for about 40% of all cases.[9]

Signs and Symptoms

Type 1

- Profound deafness in both ears from birth
- Decreased night vision before age 10
- Balance problems from birth

Type 2

- Moderate to severe hearing loss from birth
- Decreased night vision begins in late teens
- Balance typically remains normal

Type 3.

- At birth, children typically have normal hearing
- Near normal balance but problems can start to slowly develop over time
- Rate of decline in hearing and vision loss varies
- Vision and hearing loss often develop in adolescence
- Night blindness and the appearance of blind spots often develop in adolescence
- Legal blindness often occurs by midlife

Causes and Risk Factors

Usher syndrome is inherited as an autosomal recessive trait, which means that the mutated gene is not located on either of the chromosomes (X or Y) that determine a person's sex. This means that both males and females can have the disorder and can pass it along to a child. Because it is recessive, both parents must have the mutation; two copies of the mutated gene are required. If someone has only one mutated gene, from one parent, they have the capacity to pass the trait on to a child but do not themselves exhibit any symptoms of the condition.

Nine genes have been identified so far that can cause Ushers syndrome. These are the following:

Type 1 Usher syndrome: MY07A, USH1C, CDH23, PCDH15, SANS

Type 2 Usher syndrome: USH2A, VLGR1, WHRN

Type 3 Usher syndrome: USH3A

These genes are responsible for proper development of normal hearing, balance, vision, and function in the development and maintenance of fine hair-like cells in the inner ear that help transmit sound and motion signals to the brain. In the retina, these genes are also involved in determining the structure and function of the light-sensing cells called rods and cones.

Conventional Treatment

There is no treatment available to date for any of the three types of Usher syndrome. It is important, however, to diagnose the condition early, so that early childhood communication and development skills may be learned before too much hearing or sight is lost.

Complementary Approach

Targeted supplementation may help slow down the progression of vision loss in type 2 and type 3. Antioxidants and nutrients may "hyper-nourish" the retina by supporting the retinal cells that are lost due to retinitis pigmentosa (particularly the rod photoreceptor cells that enable us to see at night, in low light, and provide peripheral vision).[10] Certain herbs have been shown to help support hearing as well.

Nutrients

Recommended nutrients for children:

Recommended nutrients for children are lutein, zeaxanthin, bilberry, and vitamin D3. Dosages for children vary by weight and age, so parents should contact the authors at www.naturaleyecare.com to discuss.

Recommended nutrients for teens and adults:

Recommended dosages are for adults 150 pounds and over and should be adjusted by weight for teens under 15.

Essential

Lutein. 10mg–20mg per day. This powerful antioxidant, as well as zeaxanthin, is found both in the lens of the eye, and more importantly for retinitis pigmentosa, it is found in the retina. It also helps protect the eyes from damage due to sunlight exposure by filtering out light.[11] [12] [13] [14] Another study shows that supplementing with both lutein and vitamin A, may slow down the progression of retinitis pigmentosa.[15]

Zeaxanthin. 2mg–4mg per day. This is another powerful antioxidant that is essential for helping maintain the health of the retina. It also helps protect the eyes from damage due to sunlight exposure by filtering out light.[16]

Vitamin A palmitate. 15,000 IU per day. A recent study shows increased intake of vitamin A plus one to two 3-ounce servings of omega-3-rich fatty fish (salmon, sardine, mackerel, herring) supports cone health and slows down the progression of retinitis pigmentosa.[17] In another study, vitamin A was again shown to help support the photoreceptor cells.[18]

Note. Pregnant women should not supplement with vitamin A due to the increased risk of birth defects. Vitamin A is contra-indicated for those suffering from Stargardt disease (see Stargardt chapter for more information.)

Combined vitamin A and DHA. Along with vitamin A, we recommend 600mg of DHA, 2 times per day. One study's findings predicted that, if someone with typical retinitis pigmentosa starts taking 15,000 IU/day of vitamin A and eats one-or-two 3-ounce servings of omega-3-rich fish per week from age 37, they would not lose all central vision until the age of 78. If the average patient eats less than one to two 3-ounce servings of omega-3-rich fish per week, they are predicted to lose all central vision by the age of 59.[19]

Omega-3 fatty acids. 2,000 IU–3,000 IU per day. Due to the high amounts of carbohydrates eaten in today's modern diet, the amount of dietary omega-3 fatty acids that are so essential for retinal and brain health, has declined. And the amount of omega-6 fatty acids, with pro-inflammatory effects, has dramatically increased. DHA from omega-3 fatty acids accounts for approximately 50–60% of the total fatty acid content within rod outer segments of photoreceptor cells; the low levels of DHA we consume negatively impact our retinal health.[20]

Saffron. 20mg per day. Studies have shown that supplementing with saffron helps protect photoreceptor cells from damage and also supports healthy circulation in the retina.[21] [22]

Very Important

Green tea. 500mg–750mg per day. Two cups of green tea per day has been found to provide neuroprotective properties, and it is particularly relevant to helping protect photoreceptor outer segments and the retinal pigment epithelium.[23]

CoQ10. 100mg–200mg per day (ubiquinol is a more easily absorbed form). CoQ10 is found in every cell of the body. CoQ10 acts as a powerful antioxidant, boosting energy production within cells, and protecting important proteins and mitochondrial DNA from oxidative damage.[24] In vitro studies show the CoQ10 also helps reduce apoptosis (cell death) in the retina.[25]

Helpful

Vitamin D3. 5,000 IU per day. Lower levels of vitamin D are associated with retinal microvascular damage.[26] In USH, the blood vessels supplying the retina with oxygen and nutrients are thin, and vitamin D may support the integrity of those vessels.

Alpha-lipoic acid. 150mg–300mg per day. Alpha-R form is the most highly absorbed. 300mg of standard alpha-lipoic acid contains 150mg of the R form (natural) and 150mg of the S form (unnatural). Alpha-lipoic acid is a cofactor for some of the key enzymes (alpha-keto acid dehydrogenases) involved in generating energy from food and oxygen in mitochondria.[27] [28] [29]

Diet

We recommend that you follow the diet recommendations in Chapter 7 and consider food allergy testing.

Juicing. Juicing is a great way to get concentrated nutrients. Choose at least 4–6 items to combine.

- Ginger, leeks, garlic, parsley, cabbage, beets, carrots, celery, apples, spinach, grapes, lemon, chlorophyll, raspberries, wheatgrasses
- You can add your favorite fruits and vegetables as well. Do not use too many carrots or fruit due to their sweetness.
- Try to use room temperature vegetables and fruit.
- Do not add ice or very cold liquids since cold foods and liquids will eventually extinguish the stomach's digestive fire.
- Do not juice as often during the cooler months of the year, and instead, switch to vegetable soups or stews.

Lifestyle

Microcurrent stimulation (MCS). You can use daily, at home. The MCS 100ile unit is the most researched unit used for retinal health. See Chapter 10-3 for more information. Research has shown that MCS supports retinal and photoreceptor health in the following ways: [30] [31] [32] [33] [34]

1. Supports healthy circulation to the retina
2. Increases energy (ATP or adenosine triphosphate) production within the retinal cells through our mitochondria
3. Helps the retina eliminate waste

Eye exercises. We recommend these eye exercises for retinal and overall eye support (see Chapter 10 for more eye exercises):

- Daily eye massage of the 8 acupressure points around the eyes
- Palming
- Near and far

Sunglasses. Since ultraviolet light from the sun can cause damage to the retina by accelerating the rate of free radical activity, wear 100% ultraviolet-blocking wrap-around sunglasses (polarized) and a hat. Amber colored lenses are best for neutralizing blue light that can damage retinal visual cells. Sources of non-natural blue light are LED and fluorescent lighting and electronic screens such as with computers, cell phones, and televisions.

Cigarette smoking causes dramatic increases in free radical activity in the body, notwithstanding impacting good circulation and lung health. Quitting without supplementing the diet with additional vitamins and minerals doesn't seem to eliminate the increased risk of Usher for almost ten years. This is likely due to how smoking depletes antioxidant levels in the body and the eyes. Smoking reduces blood supply to the eye, enlarges the normal blind spot, reduces visual perception, and decreases macular pigment. Although research has not been done on smoking in the case of Ushers syndrome, the body is trying to maintain healthy vision despite the genetic effects. Smoking reduces the body's ability to do this.

Exercise regularly several times a week. Regular exercise helps maintain healthy circulation to the body and eyes and helps the body detox. Again, whatever you can do to help the body help itself is the best way to support healthy vision and hearing.

Other Modalities

Yoga

Inversion poses in yoga have been shown to aid blood flow to the heart and head. One of the best and safest inversion poses is lying on the floor with your legs up a wall. Beginning as well as advanced yoga practitioners enjoy this posture.

Chinese Medicine

As long as there are rods active in the eyes, these can be supported and nourished through acupuncture and specific herbs. In Chinese medicine, the Liver "opens to the eyes," and it is the primary meridian for supporting overall flow of energy and circulation through the eyes. The Liver system deals more with the function of sight. The Kidney meridian nourishes the blood to the eyes and relates to the neurological structure of the photoreceptors and optic nerve. While the Spleen meridian also nourishes the blood, it helps keep fluids from leaking out of the blood vessels that results in cases of ocular bleeding and retinal edema. Other organs may be out of balance as well that can affect eye health, so an evaluation by an acupuncturist can best determine where the imbalances are and offer the optimal treatment strategy. Acupuncture treatments are typically done by inserting needles into key points around the body to help increase blood flow to the eye and to stimulate the photoreceptors. There are both distal points away from the eyes as well as specific points around the orbit of the eye.

Common Chinese Medicine Patterns related to Retinitis Pigmentosa

You gui wan. "Restore the right Kidney" pills warm the Kidneys and tonify Kidney essence.

Ming mu di huang wan. "Brighten the eyes" formula nourishes the Liver, enriches the Kidneys, and improves vision.

Bu zhong yi qi tang. "Supplement the center and boost the qi" decoction tonifies the qi of the middle burner and raises the sunken yang.

Herbal formula and treatment strategies[35] can vary significantly based on the Chinese medicine practitioner's evaluation and intake.

Essential Oils

Essential oil therapy uses plant extracts to apply to the skin. These may help in many ways, including tension and anxiety relief, sleep improvement, pain reduction, circulation enhancement, digestion improvement, and more.

Carrot seed essential oil improves the eyes by protecting against macular degeneration, detoxifying blood vessels, toning the liver, relieving stress and anxiety, and providing many nourishing vitamins and minerals.

Frankincense has been around since antiquity, a sacred plant that can be helpful in showing us our visual blind spots. Frankincense tells us to "open up the third eye."

Saffron is very helpful for eye health as it helps rebalance body fluids on a cellular level and stimulate the "qi" in the entire body. It contains high levels of antioxidants, vitamins, and minerals.

Keep essences away from the mouth, eyes, and mucous membranes; if a few drops get in one of these sensitive areas it may be uncomfortable for 15–30 minutes, but not harmful. You can lessen discomfort by adding a pure oil like olive or coconut oil to neutralize the irritating effect. For the eye area, dab a few drops around the outside of the eye. Do not put the neutralizing oil in the eye.

Combine ¼ cup of avocado oil with ¼ cup of calendula-infused oil. Slowly add 5 drops each of the essential oils. Then close the bottle and shake well; apply 4 drops of this mixture on your clean face. Massage in gentle circular motions. Leave overnight.

For more information, see Appendix 9.

Other Therapies

The following therapies promote improved flow of energy and circulation throughout the body. The daily stresses that we encounter, such as poor diet, emotional imbalances, lack of regular exercise, and more, can cause areas within the body to tighten up and restrict circulation. This can result, eventually, in pain and disease. The eyes are the **second most biologically active part of the body**; only the brain is more active. So, they require a great deal of nutrition and the free flow of blood and energy to remain healthy.

You can periodically massage the **eight acupressure points** around the orbit of the eye, throughout the day. This will help relax the eyes and stimulate energy and circulation flow (see Chapter 10 for acupressure points).

Alexander technique is a way of learning to move mindfully through life, adjusting old habits to relieve tension in the body. By relieving tension in our daily physical habits, we affect the free flow of energy and circulation to the eyes.

Craniosacral is a method of relieving pain and tension through gentle manipulations of the skull. It is regarded as harmonizing with the natural rhythm of the central nervous system.

Chiropractic is a manipulative treatment of joint misalignments, especially those of the spinal column. Misalignments are believed to cause other disorders by affecting the function of nerves, muscles, and organs, and affecting the free flow of energy and blood to the eyes.

Shiatsu is a pressure-based therapy that works to unblock and balance the body's meridian systems. Basically, shiatsu is acupuncture with no needles. Therefore, like acupuncture, it can balance qi energy in the body.

On the Horizon

The direction of research for Ushers syndrome is to identify all of the genes that cause Usher syndrome and determine the function of those genes. The early identification of these genes offers an opportunity for better preparedness of what may come, as well as possible gene-therapy treatment for the future.

Early screening. NIDCD (National Institute on Deafness and Other Communication Disorders) researchers, along with collaborators from universities in New York and Israel, pinpointed a mutation named R245X of the **PCDH15** gene that accounts for a large percentage of type 1 Usher syndrome in today's Ashkenazi Jewish population (Jewish people who originate from Eastern Europe). This mutation provides an opportunity for early screening to identify and become prepared for Ushers with those who have the gene.

Gene therapy (CRISPR technique). Researchers are developing techniques to replace these faulty genes with fully functional genes by an injection into the retina of a harmless virus or "vector" to carry the specifically required gene into the retinal cells, using the patient's own stem cells.[36]

Stem cell research. Research using stem cells is underway for retinitis pigmentosa, for regenerating retinal cells, and for improving vision.[37]

Retinal cell transplants. Several groups around the world are investigating the use of retinal transplantation in the treatment of inherited retinal diseases, including Usher.[38]

Also See

Chapter 7, Vision Diet

Chapter 10-3, Microcurrent Stimulation

Chapter 15-27, Retinitis Pigmentosa

---

1 National Eye Institute. Usher Syndrome. Retrieved Dec 4 2017 from https://www.nidcd.nih.gov/health/usher-syndrome

2 Ibid. NIH. Usher Syndrome.

3 Boughman, J.A., et al. (1983). Usher syndrome: definition and estimate of prevalence from two high-risk populations. *J Chron Dis*, 36(8), 595–603.

4 Kimberling, W., et al. (2010). Frequency of Usher syndrome in two pediatric populations: implications for genetic screening of deaf and hard of hearing children. *Genet Med*, 12(8), 512–516.

5 National Institutes of Health. Usher syndrome. Genetics Home Reference. Retrieved Dec 4 2017 from https://ghr.nlm.nih.gov/condition/usher-syndrome

6 Ibid. National Eye Institute. Usher Syndrome.

7 Ibid. National Institutes of Health. Usher Syndrome.

[8] Ibid. National Institutes of Health. Usher Syndrome.

[9] Usher Syndrome Coalition. Frequent Questions. Retrieved Dec 4 2017 from https://www.usher-syndrome.org/what-is-usher-syndrome/frequent-questions.html.

[10] Moukarzel, A.A., Bejjani, R.A., Fares, F.N. (2009). Xanthophylls and eye health of infants and adults. *J Med Liban,* Oct-Dec;57(4):261-7.

11 Bernstein, P.S., Zhao, D.Y., Wintch, S.W., Ermakov, I.V., McClane, R.W., et al. Resonance Raman measurement of macular carotenoids in normal subjects and in age-related macular degeneration patients. *Ophthalmology,* Oct;109(10):1780-7.

12 Piermarocchi, S., Saviano, S., Parisi, V., Tedeschi, M., Panozzo, G., et al. (2012). Carotenoids in Age-related Maculopathy Italian Study (CARMIS): two-year results of a randomized study. *Eur J Ophthalmol,* Mar-Apr;22(2):216-25.

13 Krinsky, N.I., Landrum, J.T., Bone, R.A. (2003). Biologic mechanisms of the protective role of lutein and zeaxanthin in the eye. *Annu Rev Nutr,* 23:171-201.

14 Bahrami, H., Melia, M., Dagnelie, G. (2006). Lutein supplementation in retinitis pigmentosa: PC-based vision assessment in a randomized double-masked placebo-controlled clinical trial [NCT00029289]. *BMC Ophthalmol,* Jun 7;6:23.

15 Berson, E.L., Rosner, B., Sandberg, M.A., Weigel-DiFranco, C., Brockhurst, R.J., et al. (2010). Clinical Trial of Lutein in Patients With Retinitis Pigmentosa Receiving Vitamin A. *Arch Ophthalmol,* Apr;128(4):403-11.

[16] Semba, R.D., Dagnelie, G. (2003). Are lutein and zeaxanthin conditionally essential nutrients for eye health? *Med Hypotheses,* Oct;61(4):465-72.

17 Sofi, F., Sodi, A., Franco, F., Murro, V., Biagini, D., et al. (2016). Dietary profile of patients with Stargardt's disease and Retinitis Pigmentosa: is there a role for a nutritional approach? *BMC Ophthalmol,* Jan 22;16:13.

18 Berson, E.L., Rosner, B., Sandberg, M.A., Hayes, K.C., Nicholson, B.W., et al. (1993). A randomized trial of vitamin A and vitamin E supplementation for retinitis pigmentosa. *Arch Ophthalmol,* Jun;111(6):761-72.

19 Massachusetts Eye and Ear. New Findings Lead to Revised Therapeutic Regimen to Slow RP. Retrieved Dec 04 2017 from http://www.masseyeandear.org/for-patients/patient-guide/patient-education/diseases-and-conditions/rp-and-supplements

20 Stillwell, W., Wassall, S.R. (2003). Docosahexaenoic acid: membrane properties of a unique fatty acid. *Chem Phys Lipids,* Nov;126(1):1-27.

21 Marangoni, D., Falsini, B., Piccardi, M., Ambrosio, L., Minnella, A.M., et al. (2013). Functional effect of Saffron supplementation and risk genotypes in early age-related macular degeneration: a preliminary report. *J Transl Med,* Sep 25;11:228.

22 Falsini, B., Piccardi, M., Minnella, A., Savastano, C., Capoluongo, E., et al. (2010). Influence of saffron supplementation on retinal flicker sensitivity in early age-related macular degeneration. *Invest Ophthalmol Vis Sci,* Dec;51(12):6118-24.

23 Jarrett, S.G., Boulton, M.E. (2012). Consequences of oxidative stress in age-related macular degeneration. *Mol Aspects Med,* Aug;33(4):399–417.

24 Littarru, G.P., Tiano, L. (2007). Bioenergetic and antioxidant properties of coenzyme Q10: recent developments. *Mol Biotechnol,* Sep;37(1):31-7.

[25] Lulli, M., Witort, E., Papuci, L., Torre, E., Schiavone, N., et al. (2012). Coenzyme Q10 protects retinal cells from apoptosis induced by radiation in vitro and in vivo. *J Radiat Res,* Sep;53(5):695-703.

26 Mutlu, U., Ikram, M.A., Hofman, A., de Jong, P.T., Uitterlinden, A.G., et al. (2016). Vitamin D and retinal microvascular damage: The Rotterdam Study. *Medicine (Baltimore),* Dec; 95(49): e5477.

27 Arivazhagan, P., Ramanathan, K., Panneerselvam, C. (2001). Effect of DL-alpha-lipoic acid on mitochondrial enzymes in aged rats. *Chem Biol Interact,* Nov 28;138(2):189-98.

[28] Palaniappan, A.R., Dai, A. (2007). Mitochondrial ageing and the beneficial role of alpha-lipoic acid. *Neurochem Res,* Sep;32(9):1552-8.

[29] Packer, L. (1998). alpha-Lipoic acid: a metabolic antioxidant which regulates NF-kappa B signal transduction and protects against oxidative injury. *Drug Metab Rev,* May;30(2):245-75.

30 Michael, L.D., Allen, M.I. (1993). Nutritional supplementation, electrical stimulation and age related macular degeneration. *J. Orthomol Med,* 8:168-171.

31 Halloran, G. (1997). Bioelectrical Stimulation in an Integrated Treatment for Macular Degeneration, RP, Glaucoma, CMV-Retinitis, and Diabetic Retinopathy; *Fourth Annual Symposium on Biological Circuits*, Oct. Mankato University, MN.

32 Wallace, L. B. (1997). Treatment for Macular Degeneration Utilizing Micro-Current Stimulation. *J. Opt Photother,* Mar.

33 Paul, E.L. (1997). The Treatment of Retinal Diseases With Micro Current Stimulation And Nutritional Supplementation.

34 O'Clock, G.D., Jarding, J.B. (2009). Electrotherapeutic device/protocol design considerations for visual disease applications. *Conf Proc IEEE Eng Med Biol Soc*, 2009:2133-6.

35 Bittner, A.K., Rosenfarb, A., Gould, J., Dagnelie, G. (2015). Response to Re: A pilot study of an acupuncture protocol to improve visual function in retinitis pigmentosa patients. *Clin Exp Optom*, Jan;98(1):100.

36 Bassuk, A.G., Zheng, A., Li, Y., Tsang, S.H., et al. Repair of Retinitis Pigmentosa in Patient-Derived Stem Cells. Retrieved Dec 04 2017 from http://www.nature.com/articles/srep19969

37 He, Y., Zhang, Y., Liu, X., Ghazaryan, E., Li, Y., et al. (2014). Recent Advances of Stem Cell Therapy for Retinitis Pigmentosa. *Int J Mol Sci*, Aug; 15(8): 14456–14474.

38 Radtke, N.D., Aramant, R.B., Petry, H.M., Green, P.T., Pidwell, D.J., et al. (2008). Vision improvement in retinal degeneration patients by implantation of retina together with retinal pigment epithelium. *Am J Ophthalmol*, Aug;146(2):172-182.

15-31. UVEITIS

Uveitis is inflammation in the uvea, which includes the iris, the ciliary body, and the choroid in the eye. It can also affect nearby parts of the eye, like the retina, vitreous, and optic nerve. Over time, chronic inflammation due to uveitis can cause permanent vision loss, if not controlled. Chronic uveitis is often associated with other ongoing systemic inflammatory conditions. It is a contributing factor to a number of serious eye conditions, including cataracts, macular degeneration, and glaucoma. Uveitis is the third leading cause of blindness in developed nations, and the fifth leading cause of blindness in America. Without treatment, it frequently leads to vision loss.

The Uvea

The uvea consists of the following three structures:

The **iris**, the colored tissue surrounding the pupil, the **ciliary body**, located behind the iris that focuses the lens, and the **choroid**, containing blood vessels that line the back of the eye.

Inflammation occurring in any of the above structures, but not necessarily all, is termed "uveitis." Depending upon which structures are inflamed, uveitis may be further subcategorized:

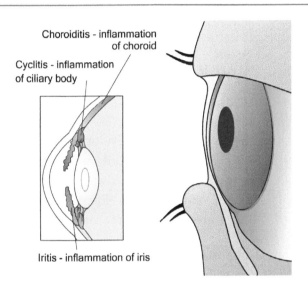

- **Iritis or anterior (front) uveitis**. Anterior uveitis can involve the iris, ciliary body, cornea, and sclera. It is the most common type of uveitis and accounts for approximately 50–60% of all uveitis cases in special care clinics.[1] Sixty-five percent of cases are related to another health condition. The remaining 35% are idiopathic (no discernible relationship to another health problem).
- **Cyclitis or intermediate uveitis**. Intermediate uveitis is the least common type of uveitis and has been found to account for 3–17% of uveitis around the world.[2]
- **Choroiditis or posterior (back) uveitis**. This category accounts for only 10–40% of uveitis cases. However, more visual loss results in these cases than from other uveitis forms. Such vision loss may be due to cystoid macular edema, retinal detachment, subretinal fibrosis, or optic nerve damage.[3] Up to 50% of patients with posterior uveitis have an associated systemic disease.[4]

Early detection and treatment are necessary to reduce the risk of permanent vision loss.

Symptoms

Depending on which part of the eye is inflamed in uveitis, a combination of the following symptoms may be present:

- Redness
- Light sensitivity
- Floaters, which may look like dark floating spots, bushy lines, or web-like structures
- Blurry vision
- Changes in vision
- Pain

These symptoms may come on suddenly, and may be experienced without any pain. The symptoms described above may not necessarily mean that you have uveitis. However, if you experience one or more of these symptoms, contact your eye doctor for a complete exam.

Causes and Risk Factors

Uveitis may arise from either infectious or non-infectious sources.

Non-infectious. Uveitis may develop following eye trauma or surgery. It is often associated with other conditions; for example, it may be linked to autoimmune diseases, such as Crohn's, ankylosing spondylitis, sarcoidosis, or rheumatoid arthritis. A cancer in the eye, such as a lymphoma, can cause uveitis. Fifty percent of cases are idiopathic (no underlying cause identified), 20% are due to trauma, and 30% are due to a systemic underlying cause.

Certain drugs can cause orbital inflammation, uveitis, and scleritis, such as bisphosphonates (including Fosamax) that for example, are prescribed to post-menopausal women to prevent calcium bone loss.[5]

Infectious. Viruses like Lyme disease, West Nile virus, herpes zoster, syphilis, tuberculosis, or toxoplasmosis may cause uveitis. Helicobacter pylori infection has also been implicated with the onset of uveitis. [6]

Conventional Treatment

Aggressive medical treatment of uveitis is needed to prevent glaucoma, scarring of the structures inside the eye, and possible blindness. If the cause is known, prescription drugs are used to control that cause and reduce inflammation.

- Eye drops are most often used for anterior uveitis, sometimes in conjunction with corticosteroid injections. But they must be postponed if the corneal surface is damaged by an ulcer, because the corticosteroids prevent healing of the ulcer or lead to a worsening of it.

- Injections and oral medication (corticosteroids) are used for posterior uveitis or panuveitis.
- Aspirin (not aspirin substitutes), Rimadyl, indomethacin, Profinal, Ocufen, Voltaren, and corticosteroids (cortisone drugs) are used to minimize inflammation.

Another possibility is the use of a capsule implanted in the eye that slowly releases corticosteroids. In 2005, the drug Retisert was approved by the FDA for this use, for severe cases of uveitis.

Complementary Approach

Taking targeted supplements and establishing healthy lifestyle habits are important over the long term to reduce inflammation and neutralize free radicals produced by ongoing inflammation. During the metabolism of cell mitochondria (the energy sources in the cell) reactive oxygen species (ROS) are generated. ROS refer to reactive molecules and free radicals that damage healthy cells. ROS play an important role in influencing inflammatory signals induced by large molecules called endotoxins that hold toxins within their cell walls (lipopolysaccharides or LPS).

A number of different antioxidants have been shown to neutralize ROS, including glutathione (best taken sublingually or intraorally).[7] Oxidative stress and inflammation associated with uveitis play critical roles in the initiation and progression of a wide range of eye diseases, including age-related macular degeneration, glaucoma, cataract, cystoid macular edema, and diabetic retinopathy that lead to progressive loss of vision and blindness if untreated.[8][9][10] There is growing evidence that supplementing with targeted nutrients that have antioxidant and anti-inflammatory properties may have a role in the prevention and treatment of these age-related eye diseases and disorders.[11]

Nutrients

Along with what your eye doctor recommends, antioxidants and herbs can help support the health of the eyes, improve circulation, reduce inflammation, and help the eyes eliminate waste naturally.

Because uveitis is often related to an overall inflammatory condition, these antioxidants can help overall body health as well.

Essential

Astaxanthin. 6mg–12mg per day. Astaxanthin is a fat-soluble carotenoid that, in its value as an antioxidant, is 10 times more powerful than beta-carotene, lutein, or zeaxanthin, and from 60 to 500 times stronger than vitamin E. Astaxanthin destroys free radicals and wards off their constant attack towards all parts of the body.[12]

Lutein. 6mg–20mg per day. This carotenoid has been proven to help support the retina and reduces eye inflammation.[13] It is well researched for retinal support and is essential for supporting the retinal pigment. One study shows that taking lutein along with zeaxanthin and astaxanthin, significantly improved visual acuity (vision sharpness).[14] Multiple animal studies on the neuroprotective effects of lutein against retinal neural damage caused by inflammation in endotoxin-induced uveitis (EIU) have shown that the lutein has a dose-dependent anti-inflammatory effect on EIU.[15] [16]

Bilberry. 180mg–240mg per day. Bilberry is neuroprotective and has been shown to improve microcirculation.[17] [18] [19] [20] [21] Keeping circulation healthy in the eyes is essential in helping the body manage inflammation, deliver essential nutrients, and detoxify the eyes.

Omega-3 fatty acids, 2,000mg–3,000mg per day *or* **DHA**, 1000mg per day. The omega-3s are essential nutrients for retinal health; they have anti-inflammatory properties.[22] [23] In the retina, DHA, one of the omega-3 fatty acids, increases mitochondrial activity as well as being anti-inflammatory, anti-oxidative, anti-apoptotic (cell death), and anti-angiogenic (growth of unwanted new eye blood vessels may leak and cause damage to the retina) effects.[24] [25] [26]

Trans-resveratrol. 175mg per day. This potent antioxidant helps protect nerve cells from damage,[27] reduces oxidative damage,[28] [29] and supports a healthy inflammatory response.[30]

Very Important

Alpha-lipoic acid. 300mg–600mg per day. This antioxidant reduces retinal oxidative stress.[31]

Ginkgo biloba. 120mg per day. Ginkgo stabilizes capillaries and makes them less fragile.[32] [33] [34] It has been found to help prevent damage in the eye due to low oxygen conditions, as well as prevent the formation of abnormal blood vessels.[35] Ginkgo improves blood circulation. Improved circulation to the eyes helps the body keep the eyes healthy and reduces the effects of uveitis by helping deliver essential antioxidants and oxygen to the retina.

Glutathione (GSH), reduced. 500mg–900mg per day. Preferably, this is taken in an intraoral or sublingual form, as glutathione is not absorbed well through the digestive system. It is synthesized in the body with 3 amino acids: L-glutamic acid, L-cysteine, and glycine. Glutathione (GSH) is one of the super antioxidants that neutralize the full range of free radicals that contribute to uveitis. The sublingual form has 5–10 times greater absorption so the dosage will be smaller. Follow label instructions.

Curcumin (as highly absorbed phospholipid blend). 630mg per day. Curcumin has potent natural anti-inflammatory and antioxidant properties.[36] [37] [38] [39] [40] [41]

Green tea extract. 500mg-750mg per day. Green teas and their extracts are potentially neuroprotective in the photoreceptor outer segment and retinal pigment epithelium (RPE).[42]

MSM. 2,000mg per day, split up with meals or with water. MSM helps nourish and strengthen body tissues and has natural anti-inflammatory properties.[43]

Taurine. 750mg–1,000mg per day. Taurine is found naturally in high concentrations in the heart and retina; smaller amounts are found in the brain, kidneys, intestine, and skeletal muscle.

Taurine deficiency may lead to retinal degeneration. Supplementation has been used with some success to prevent, treat, and stabilize retinal changes.[44] [45] [46] [47]

Superoxide dimutase. 250mg per day, is helpful in treating uveitis; it has a greater antioxidant effect compared to the drug dexamethasone. Adding it to therapy with the corticsteroid dexamethasone results in lower inflammation intensity and enhanced dexamethasone effect.[48]

Helpful

Serrapeptase. 500mg–800mg, 1–2 times per day on an empty stomach. Serrapeptase can help reduce inflammation for a number of conditions.[49] [50] [51] It is believed to dissolve fibrin and other dead or damaged tissue without harming living tissue, thereby helping to reduce related inflammation. Excess debris in the body can stimulate an ongoing immune response. The result is chronic inflammation in the body and eyes as well as circulatory problems due to scar tissue buildup in the blood vessels. Circulatory issues are directly linked to inflammation and cell damage.

Lycopene. 3mg per day. Lycopene's strong lipid antioxidant properties make it very effective in protecting against free radicals and maintaining healthy LDL cholesterol. LDL oxidation can lead to circulatory problems over time that can affect eye and overall health.[52] [53] [54] [55]

Diet

Maintain a healthy diet with plenty of vegetables, fruits, and grains. We recommend the Mediterranean diet,[56] or any diet that is an alkaline and anti-inflammatory (see Chapter 7 for more information).

Juice daily. Our recipe to help support overall eye health and reduce inflammation naturally is a combination of the following (try using at least 4–6 of the nutrients recommended).

- Green leafy vegetables, celery, cucumber, carrot, parsley, beets, all types of berries, apple, lemon, ginseng, garlic, green tea

Add your favorite fruits and vegetables. Avoid using too many carrots or beets or too much fruit because of their high natural sugar content. Choose organic, if possible.

Supplement your diet. Supplement with a good daily multivitamin and/or a good organic green drink. We recommend the green drink daily (typically 1 scoop in an 8oz glass of water, fruit juice, rice milk, or almond milk).

Go organic. Organic products are more nutritious than conventional produce, and do not carry the high levels of added synthetic hormones, pesticides, herbicides, antibiotics, and other toxins that conventional produce maintains.

Limit refined products. Lessen sugar intake (particularly white or refined sugar), and refined carbohydrates. Sugar has a number of negative side effects, including inflammation, reducing the immune system, and potentially affecting healthy circulation. Try stevia as a sweetener rather than sugar. Stevia is an herb and does not affect blood sugar levels; it is far more concentrated, so you only need a small amount.

Avoid aspartame and other artificial sweeteners (and foods labeled "diet"). Aspartame is known to cause a wide range of symptoms including headaches (also migraines), heart palpitation, memory loss, insomnia, anxiety attacks, skin problems, loss of hearing and taste, seizures, diabetes, and vision problems.

Avoid certain fats. These include corn oil, safflower oil, hydrogenated vegetable oils, canola oil, and most margarines that contain trans fats. Also avoid any foods made with shortening or partially hydrogenated vegetable oils, such as doughnuts, biscuits, pies, cookies, crackers, muffins, and cakes. Consumption of trans fats has shown to increase the risk of coronary heart disease that ultimately affects circulation to the eyes and can result in inflammation.[57]

Limit alcohol consumption to one glass of red wine daily. Alcohol reduces protective glutathione levels, and it interferes with liver functioning. The liver stores fat and filters our blood, so it is critical for eye and overall health.

Cut down on caffeine, coffee, and soft drinks. Watch your intake of soft drinks (three tablespoons of sugar per can!) and processed foods that contain sugar. Sugary sodas are linked to a 23% greater risk of heart failure. Again, poor circulation can cause eye disease and contribute to inflammation.

Avoid monosodium glutamate (MSG). This flavor enhancer has potential retinal toxins.[58]

Avoid fat blockers like olestra. These impair the absorption of carotenoids.

Eliminate or significantly reduce fast foods and fried foods.

Read the labels. When you buy processed foods, avoid artificial flavorings and colorings. As noted above, avoid foods that contain hydrogenated fats and trans-fatty acids that disrupt the digestive process.

Lifestyle

Wear wrap-around sunglasses with 100% UVA and UVB protection whenever out in the sun. The best lens color is amber, which neutralizes blue light. Brown is the next best color. Cheaper glasses may have a coating to block out UV light that can rub off over time. Many people think it is the tint that helps protect one's eyes, but it is actually the UV filter on, or in, the lens. So, if the filter coating wears off, a dark lens actually increases pupil dilation, allowing more light to enter the eyes.

Eliminate smoking. Smoking produces cyanide, a retinal toxin. A 2005 review of 17 research studies determined that the risk of macular degeneration in smokers is 2–3 times higher than in non-smokers. A 2015 study looked at this issue again, this time investigating specific damage to the macula as a result of smoking, and finding significant damage to many tissue layers of the macula. By smoking you are significantly increasing the level of free radicals in the body that can cause or contribute to chronic inflammation and disease.

Limit the amount of medications. Talk to your doctor or get a second opinion to make sure that you are not taking more medication (both prescription and non-prescription) than you really need and that your medications do not conflict.

Exercise every day. Get 20 minutes of aerobic exercise per day by walking, swimming, or other sports or activities that you enjoy.

Manage your mental health. Emotional well-being is very important to good physical health. Fear, anger, stress, etc. are important factors in many diseases. You can help balance your emotions through meditation, prayer, exercise, martial arts, etc.

Do yoga. Research has suggested that daily yoga results in not only reduced stress, but also reduced inflammation, which is an issue in inflammatory conditions like uveitis.

Eye exercises. Specifically, we recommend the following exercises for uveitis:

- Palming
- Eye massage
- Acupressure points massaged daily

Other Modalities

Chinese Medicine

In Traditional Chinese Medicine, uveitis can be related to a number of different meridians, depending on the underlying cause and imbalance. These meridians that are related include the Liver (opening the eyes for healthy circulation of blood and energy), the Spleen (breakdown of essential nutrients and dispersion of these nutrients throughout the body), and the Kidney (oversees the endocrine system and includes maintaining the balance of our immune system). In Chinese medicine, inflammation is also considered related to "blocked energy," which if unblocked through acupuncture and/or herbs, helps the body heal.

Chinese herbs for uveitis

Common patent formulas your acupuncturist may consider for uveitis include:

Xiao yao san. Classic Liver tonic used in Chinese medicine. The Liver "opens to the eyes" and is the primary meridian (flow energy) that supports healthy circulation and the free flow of energy in the eyes, as well as throughout the body.

Tien ma gou teng yin. Nourishes yin, clears inflammation (Liver wind).

Shi hu ye guang wan. Nourishes yin, clears inflammation (Liver wind).

Herbal formula and treatment strategies can vary significantly, based on the Chinese medicine practitioner's evaluation and intake.

Also See

1 Albert, D.M., Jakobiec, F.A., editors. (2000). *Principles and Practice of Ophthalmology.* 2nd ed. Philadelphia, PA: WB Saunders Co.

2 Ibid. Albert. (2000).

3 Jabs, D.A., Akpek, E.K. (2005). Immunosuppression for posterior uveitis. Retina, Jan; 25(1):1-18.

4 Ibid. Albert. (2000).

5 Michelle Stephenson. (2011). Systemic Drugs with Ocular Side Effects. Retrieved Dec 04 2017 from https://www.reviewofophthalmology.com/article/systemic-drugs-with-ocular-side-effects

6 Izzotti, A., Saccà, S.C., Bagnis, A., Recupero, S.M. (2009). Glaucoma and Helicobacter pylori infection: correlations and controversies. *Br J Ophthalmol,* Nov;93(11):1420-7.

7 Ray, P.D., Huang, B.W., Tsuji, Y. (2012). Reactive oxygen species (ROS) homeostasis and redox regulation in cellular signaling. *Cell Signal,* May;24(5):981-990.

8 Levkovitch-Verbin, H. (2015). Retinal ganglion cell apoptotic pathway in glaucoma: Initiating and downstream mechanisms. *Prog. Brain Res,* 220:37–57.

9 Kowluru, R.A., Mishra, M. (2015). Oxidative stress, mitochondrial damage and diabetic retinopathy. *Biochem. Biophys. Acta.* 1852:2474–2483.

10 Dib, B., Lin, H., Maidana, D.E., Tian, B., Miller, J.B., et al. (2015). Mitochondrial DNA has a pro-inflammatory role in AMD. *Biochem. Biophys. Acta,* 1853:2897–2906.

11 Rhone, M., Basu, A. (2008). Phytochemicals and age-related eye diseases. *Nutr. Rev,* 66:465–472.

12 Sportsnutritionist. Maher, T.J. (2000). Astaxanthin. Retrieved Dec 04 2017 from http://sportsnutritionist.info/course/wp-content/uploads/2013/04/Astaxanthin.pdf

13 Kim, J.E., Clark, R.M., Park, Y., Lee, J., Fernandez, M.L. (2012). Lutein decreases oxidative stress and inflammation in liver and eyes of guinea pigs fed a hypercholesterolemic diet. *Nutr Res Pract,* Apr;6(2):113-119.

14 Parisi, V., Tedeschi, M., Gallianaro, G., Varano, M., Saviano, S., et al. (2008). Carotenoids and antioxidants in age-related maculopathy, *Ophthalmology,* Feb;115(2):324-333.e2.

15 Sasaki, M., Ozawa, Y., Kurihara, T., Noda, K., Imamura, Y. (2009). Neuroprotective effect of an antioxidant, lutein, during retinal inflammation. *Invest Ophthalmol Vis Sci,* Mar; 50(3):1433-9.

16 Jin, X.H., Ohgami, K., Shiratori, K., Suzuki, Y., Hirano, T., et al. (2006). Inhibitory effects of lutein on endotoxin-induced uveitis in Lewis rats. *Invest Ophthalmol Vis Sci,* Jun; 47(6):2562-8.

17 Matsunaga, N., Imai, S., Inokuchi, Y., Shimazawa, M., Yokota, S. (2009). Bilberry and its main constituents have neuroprotective effects against retinal neuronal damage in vitro and in vivo. *Mol Nutr Food Res,* Jul;53(7):869-77.

18 Yao, Y., Vieira, A. (2007). Protective activities of Vaccinium antioxidants with potential relevance to mitochondrial dysfunction and neurotoxicity. *Neurotoxicology,* Jan;28(1):93-100.

19 Zhu, Y., Xia, M., Yang, Y., Liu, F., Li, Z. (2011). Purified anthocyanin supplementation improves endothelial function via NO-cGMP activation in hypercholesterolemic individuals. *Clin Chem,* Nov;57(11):1524-33.

20 Cohen-Boulakia, F., Valensi, P.E., Boulahdour, H., Lestrade, R., Dufour-Lamartinie, J.F. (2000). In vivo sequential study of skeletal muscle capillary permeability in diabetic rats: effect of anthocyanosides. *Metabolism,* Jul;49(7):880-5.

21 Ibid. Zhu. (2011).

22 Udell, I.J., Abelson, M.B. (1983). Chemical mediators of inflammation. *Int Ophthalmol Clin*, 23:1:15-26.

23 Abelson, M.B., Butrus, S.I., Kliman, G.H., Larson, D.L., Corey, E.J., et al. (1987). Topical arachidonic acid: A model for screening anti-inflammatory agents. *J Ocul Pharmacol*, 3:63-75.

24 SanGiovanni, J.P., Chew, E.Y. (2005). The role of omega-3 long-chain polyunsaturated fatty acids in health and disease of the retina. *Prog Retin Eye Res*, 24(1): 87–138.

25 Bazan, N.G. (2006). Cell survival matters: docosahexaenoic acid signaling, neuroprotection and photoreceptors. *Trends Neurosci*, May;29(5):263-71.

26 Mukherjee, P.K., Marcheselli, V.L., Serhan, C.N., Bazan, N.G. (2004). Neuroprotectin D1: a docosahexaenoic acid-derived docosatriene protects human retinal pigment epithelial cells from oxidative stress. *Proc Natl Acad Sci USA*, Jun 1;101(22):8491-6.

27 Anekonda, T.S., Adamus, G. (2008). Resveratrol prevents antibody-induced apoptotic death of retinal cells through upregulation of Sirt1 and Ku70. *BMC Res Notes*, Dec 1;1:122.

28 Remsberg, C.M., Yáñez, J.A., Ohgami, Y., Vega-Villa, K.R., Rimando, A.M., et al. (2008). Pharmacometrics of pterostilbene: preclinical pharmacokinetics and metabolism, anticancer, anti-inflammatory, antioxidant and analgesic activity. *Phytother Res*, Feb;22(2):169-79.

29 Perecko, T., Jancinova, V., Drabikova, K., Nosal, R., Harmatha, J. (2008). Structure-efficiency relationship in derivatives of stilbene. Comparison of resveratrol, pinosylvin and pterostilbene. *Neuro Endocrinol Lett*, Oct;29(5):802-5.

30 Currais, A., Prior, M., Dargusch, R., Armando, A., Ehren, J, et al. (2014). Modulation of p25 and inflammatory pathways by fisetin maintains cognitive function in Alzheimer's disease transgenic mice. *Aging Cell*. 2014 Apr;13(2):379-90.

31 Kowluru, R.A., Odenbach, S. (2004). Effect of long-term administration of alpha-lipoic acid on retinal capillary cell death and the development of retinopathy in diabetic rats. *Diabetes*, Dec;53(12):3233-8.

32 Welt, K., Weiss, J., Martin, R., Hermsdorf, T., Drews, S., et al. (2007). Ginkgo biloba extract protects rat kidney from diabetic and hypoxic damage. *Phytomedicine*, Feb;14(2-3):196-203.

33 Qiu, Y., Rui, Y.C., Li, T.J., Zhangj, L., Yao, P.Y. (2004). Inhibitory effect of extracts of Ginkgo biloba leaves on VEGF-induced hyperpermeability of bovine coronary endothelial cells in vitro. *Acta Pharmacol Sin*, Oct;25(10):1306-11.

34 Huang, S.Y., Jeng, C., Kao, S.C., Yu, J.J., Liu, D.Z. (2004). Improved haemorrheological properties by Ginkgo biloba extract (Egb 761) in type 2 diabetes mellitus complicated with retinopathy. *Clin Nutr*, Aug;23(4):615-21.

35 Oh, J.H., Oh, J., Togloom, A., Kim, S.W., Huh, K. (2013). Effects of Ginkgo biloba Extract on Cultured Human Retinal Pigment Epithelial Cells under Chemical Hypoxia. *Curr Eye Res*, 38(10): 1072–1082.

36 Kurup, V.P., Barrios, C.S. (2008). Immunomodulatory effects of curcumin in allergy. *Mol Nutr Food Res*, Sep;52(9):1031-9.

37 Karaman, M., Arikan, A.Z., Firinci, F., Kiray, M., Bagriyanik, A., et al. (2011). Effects of curcumin on lung histopathology and fungal burden in a mouse model of chronic asthma and oropharyngeal candidiasis. *Arch Med Res*, Feb;42(2):79-87.

38 Oh, S.W., Cha, J.Y., Jung, J.E., Chang, B.C., Kwon, H.J., et al. (2011). Curcumin attenuates allergic airway inflammation and hyper-responsiveness in mice through NF-κB inhibition. *J Ethnopharmacol*, Jul 14;136(4):414-21.

39 Nugroho, A.E., Ikawati, Z., Sardjiman, Maeyama, K. (2009). Effects of benzylidenecyclopentanone analogues of curcumin on histamine release from mast cells. *Biol Pharm Bull*, May;32(5):842-9.

40 Meghana, K., Sanjeev, G., Ramesh, B. (2007). Curcumin prevents streptozotocin-induced islet damage by scavenging free radicals: a prophylactic and protective role. *Eur J Pharmacol*, Dec 22;577(1-3):183-91.

41 Calabrese, V., Bates, T.E., Mancuso, C., Cornelius, C., Ventimiglia, B., et al. (2008). Curcumin and the cellular stress response in free radical-related diseases. *Mol Nutr Food Res*, Sep;52(9):1062-73.

42 Jarrett, S.G., Boulton, M.E. (2012). Consequences of oxidative stress in age-related macular degeneration. *Mol Aspects Med*, Aug;33(4):399–417.

43 Batawan, M., Benjamin, R.L., Bloomer, R.J. (2017). Methylsulfonylmethane: Applications and Safety of a Novel Dietary Supplement. *Nutrients*, Mar;9(3):290.

44 Birdsall, T.C. (1998). Therapeutic applications of taurine. *Altern Med Rev*, Apr;3(2):128-36.

45 Shpak, N.I., Naritsyna, N.I., Konovalova, N.V. (1989). Taufon and emoksipin in the combined treatment of sclerotic macular dystrophies. *Oftalmol Zh*, (8):463-5.

46 Lombardini, J.B. (1991). Taurine: retinal function. *Brain Res Brain Res Rev*, May-Aug;16(2):151-69.

47 Imaki, H., Moretz, R., Wisniewski, H., Neuringer, M., Sturman, J. (1987). Retinal degeneration in 3-month-old rhesus monkey infants fed a taurine-free human infant formula. *J Neurosci Res*, 18(4):602-14.

[48] Chesnokova, N.B., Neroev, V.V., Beznos, O.V., Beyshenova, G.A., Panova, I.G., et al. (2015). Effects of dexamethasone and superoxide dismutase instillations on clinical course of uveitis and local biochemical processes (experimental study). *Vestn Oftalmol*, May-Jun;131(3):71.75.

49 Mazzone, A., Catalani, M., Costanzo, M., Drusian, A., Mandoli, A., et al. (1990). Evaluation of Serratia peptidase in acute or chronic inflammation of otorhinolaryngology pathology: a multicentre, double-blind, randomized trial versus placebo. *J Int Med Res*, Sep-Oct;18(5):379-88.

50 Tachibana, M., Mizukoshi, O., Harada, Y., Kawamoto, K., Nakai, Y. (1984). A multi-centre, double-blind study of serrapeptase versus placebo in post-antrotomy buccal swelling. *Pharmatherapeutica*, 3(8); 526-30.

51 Panagariya, A., Sharma, A.K. (1999). A preliminary trial of serratiopeptidase in patients with carpal tunnel syndrome. *J Assoc Physicians India*, Dec;47(12):1170-2.

52 Balestrieri, M.L., De Prisco, R., Nicolaus, B., Pari, P., Moriello, V.S., et al. (2004). Lycopene in association with alpha-tocopherol or tomato lipophilic extracts enhances acyl-platelet-activating factor biosynthesis in endothelial cells during oxidative stress. *Free Radic Biol Med*, Apr 15;36(8):1058-67.

53 Erdman, J.W., Ford, N.A., Lindshield, B.L. (2009). Are the health attributes of lycopene related to its antioxidant function? *Arch Biochem Biophys*, Mar 15;483(2):229-35.

54 Xu, X., Zhu, M., Hu, M. (2011). Effects of lycopene on blood cells and fibrinolytic activity in hyperlipidemic rats. *Wei Sheng Yan Jiu*, Sep;40(5):620-3.

55 Hsiao, G., Wang, Y., Tzu, N.H., Fong, T.H., Shen, M.Y. (2005). Inhibitory effects of lycopene on in vitro platelet activation and in vivo prevention of thrombus formation. *J Lab Clin Med*, Oct;146(4):216-26.

56 National Eye Institute. NIH study provides clarity on supplements for protection against blinding eye disease. Retrieved Dec 04 2017 from https://nei.nih.gov/news/pressreleases/050513.

57 Lopez-Candalaes, A., Burgos, P.M.H., Hernandez-Suarez, D.F., Harris, D. (2017). Linking Chronic Inflammation with Cardiovascular Disease: From Normal Aging to the Metabolic Syndrome. *J Nat Sci*, Apr;3(4):e341.

58 Vorwerk, C.K., Lipton, S.A., Zurakowski, D., Hyman, B.T., Sabel, B.A., et al. (1996). Chronic low-dose glutamate is toxic to retinal ganglion cells. Toxicity blocked by memantine. *Invest Ophthalmol Vis Sci*, Jul;37(8):1618-24.

15-32. VITREOUS DETACHMENT

Posterior vitreous detachment (PVD) affects 75% of people over the age of 65, though it may be helped with dietary and nutritional changes. The prevalence of a spontaneous PVD has been reported to be as high as 24% among patients aged 50–59 years and 87% among patients aged 80–89 years.[1][2] After occurring in one eye, PVD usually occurs in the other eye within 6 months to 2 years.[3]

In patients with symptoms of a PVD, there is an incidence of retinal tears of 14.5% and hemorrhages of 22.7%.[4][5] One study shows floaters in 42%, flashes in 18%, and both floaters and flashes in 20% of patients with PVD and secondary retinal pathology.[6]

Only about 10% of patients with PVD develop a retinal tear; around 40% of patients with an acute retinal tear, if left untreated, will develop a retinal detachment.[7] So, it is crucial to get an immediate evaluation at any first signs of symptoms.

A vitreous detachment is not sight threatening and requires no medical treatment.

In some cases with a partial vitreous tear, the remaining fibers can continue to pull on the retina, resulting in a macula hole, or potentially, a tear in the retina or retinal blood vessel. Again, this needs to be monitored by your eye doctor.

What is the Vitreous?

The jelly-like vitreous gel (vitreous humor) is 99% water and takes up the space between the retina and the inner lens of the eye. As we get older, the vitreous becomes more liquid, and it causes a strain on the connective tissue and fibers between the vitreous humor and the retina, often resulting in a tear or detachment from the retina. The vitreous is composed of collagen fibers (about 0.5%), hyaluronic acid (about 0.5%), a small amount of ascorbic acid, and water (about 99%).[8][9]

Structure

The vitreous humor fills the center of the eyeball, filling the space through which light passes between the lens of the eye and the retina at the back of the eye. Millions of fine fibers contained in the vitreous attach to the retina surface. There are no blood vessels in the vitreous. If a substance enters the vitreous humor, it will typically remain suspended in the gel. These substances can include blood, pieces of connective tissue, or clumps of cells, which are collectively referred to as "floaters." Although 99% water, the vitreous does contain hyaluronic acid, hyalocytes that reprocess the hyaluronic acid, ascorbic acid, salts, sugars, vitrosin (a type of collagen), a network of collagen type II fibers, and a wide array of proteins in micronutrients. It also contains cells called "phagocytes" that remove waste cellular material over time.

A thin membrane of collagen called the vitreous membrane or hyaloid membrane encloses the vitreous. It is clear, transparent, gelatinous (2–4 times the viscosity of water), and thins with age. Relatively speaking, the few cells that it contains are mostly phagocytes, whose function is to remove debris. The hyaloid membrane, surrounding the vitreous, is attached only at the optic disc, where nerves pass from the photoreceptor system to the optic nerve, at the ora serrata, and on the top side of the lens, which is the junction of photo-sensitive and non-photosensitive areas of the retina. Vitrosin fibers floating within the vitreous are kept apart by electrical charges.

The most obvious purpose of the vitreous humor is to maintain a constant pressure, holding the shape of the eyeball in place.

Types of Vitreous Detachment

The pathology of PVD is always the same; however, its effects are different. There is no telling where the separation or tears will occur. It can occur:

At the **ora serrata** (the junction of the retina and the ciliary body) and the vitreous humor straddles it,

At the **optic disc**, where the membrane is attached to the retina,

Or at a random place along the side of the **hyaloid membrane** (a thin transparent membrane enveloping the vitreous humor of the eye), leaving a space between the vitreous membrane and retina into which fluid can accumulate.

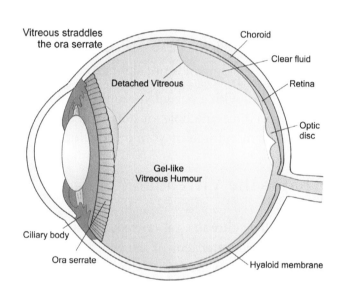

Signs and Symptoms

It is suggested that as much as up to 20% of PVDs are without symptoms.[10] While they do not usually cause any permanent vision loss, they can be annoying, particularly related to an influx of vitreous floaters. Here are some symptoms to be on the lookout for:

- Sudden detachment of the vitreous from the retina, often causing flashes that look like lightning or electric sparks
- Sudden change in the type, and/or increase in number, of floaters
- Sudden ring of floaters to the temporal side of vision (toward the ears)

These symptoms may last days to weeks; however, it is critical to see your eye doctor immediately, at the first sign of any of these symptoms, to rule out the possibility of a retinal tear or detachment that is considered a medical emergency and a severe threat to vision. Your eye doctor will perform an immediate dilated retinal examination to determine whether you are dealing with a vitreous or retinal tear or detachment, or another condition altogether.

It is important to note that the risk of retinal detachment is greatest in the first six weeks following a vitreous detachment, but can occur over three months after the event. Between 8% and 26% of patients with acute PVD symptoms have a retinal tear at the time of the initial examination.[11]

Causes and Risk Factors

Aging. As the vitreous thins with age, the risk is greater.[12]

Myopia. People who are highly myopic (more than 6 diopters) are at greater risk of vitreous and retinal tears and detachments.[13] Patients with myopia experience PVD approximately 10 years earlier than those who are farsighted (hyperopia).[14] [15]

Cataract surgery. This increases the risk for PVD. In one study, 75% of people with cataract surgery developed PVD.[16] This includes cataract surgery by phacoemulsification, ultrasound to break up the lens that is then removed manually and replaced with an artificial lens.[17]

Trauma. Blows to the head, other trauma, and even vigorous nose blowing can cause vitreous detachments.

Computer use. Excessive computer use may contribute to vitreous detachment, as it restricts the free flow of blood and energy to the eyes.

Menopause. Menopause lowers levels of estrogen and hyaluronic acid that may lead to changes in the vitreous. In premenopausal women, high levels of vitamin B6 may be connected to more frequent PVD due to their estrogen-dampening effect.[18]

Drugs. Injection of various intravitreal drugs that are typically used for retinal bleeding in such disorders as wet macular degeneration, increase the risk of a PVD. [19]

Conventional Treatment

There is no specific treatment for posterior vitreous detachment, unless there is a retinal tear that needs to be surgically repaired. In more severe cases requiring a vitrectomy, there are several serious vision-threatening concerns that include bleeding into the vitreous humor, corneal edema, infection, elevated IOP, retinal detachment, and cataract formation.

Complementary Approach

Targeted supplementation, a healthy diet, and regular exercise can help maintain a healthy retina and vitreous. For those that may be prone to vitreous tears/detachments, such as seniors, particularly if they are very nearsighted, targeted supplements can help keep the retina strong and healthy. We highly recommend regular checkups with your eye doctor to monitor your progress.

Nutrients

Essential

Lutein. 6mg–20mg per day. This carotenoid is well researched for retinal support and is essential for supporting the retinal pigment.[20] Another study shows that taking lutein, zeaxanthin, and astaxanthin, significantly improves visual acuity (vision sharpness).[21]

Zeaxanthin. 2mg–12mg per day. Taken with lutein, zeaxanthin is a potent antioxidant found in the retina that helps maintain the health of the retina.[22]

Omega-3 fatty acids. 2,000mg–3,000mg per day. Fifty percent of the retina is comprised of essential fatty acids. Research shows it has anti-inflammatory properties.[23] [24]

Hyaluronic acid. 100mg–200mg per day. This helps strengthen connective tissue. It is found in the vitreous along with ascorbic acid (believed to help support the integrity of the vitreous and related connective tissue to the retina).[25]

Vitamin C (buffered and ascorbated). 2,000mg–3,000mg per day, split up with meals. Vitamin C helps support the vitreous and connective tissue in the eye, and has been postulated to react with oxygen in the ocular fluids.[26] [27] Depletion of ascorbate in the eyes reduces the ability of the vitreous to consume needed oxygen.[28]

Very Important

Silica. 40mg per day. This helps support connective tissue (as well as bone health).[29]

Helpful

Bilberry. 120mg–180mg per day. Along with supporting night vision, bilberry is neuroprotective and has been shown to improve microcirculation.[30] [31] [32]

Ginkgo biloba. 120mg per day. Ginkgo contains many different flavonoids, including polyphenolic flavonoids that have been proven to exert antioxidative properties.[33] Numerous studies have shown that ginkgo biloba improves overall circulation[34] that helps the body deliver essential nutrients and oxygen to the retina and eyes.

Vitamin D3. 2,000 IU–5,000 IU per day. Lower levels of vitamin D are associated with retinal microvascular damage.[35]

A good whole-food, organic multivitamin. Follow directions on the bottle.

Proteolytic enzymes. 60,000 IU split up between meals in 8oz of water. When taken between meals, proteolytic enzymes such as serrapeptase, can travel through the bloodstream and enter the vitreous to help dissolve floaters. Another proteolytic enzyme that works similarly is nattokinase; the recommended dosage is 150–200mg per day, taken between meals (larger dosages can be taken with your healthcare practitioner's guidance).

Diet

Healthy eating programs like the Mediterranean diet goes a long way in preserving healthy vision and overall eye health. With this diet, it is important to avoid refined foods, that is, foods containing white flour, added sugars, fried food, and so forth. This includes fast or processed foods. Keep overall sugar consumption low, and include healthy oils such as first cold-pressed extra-virgin olive oil. Also consume plenty of fresh fruits and vegetables, and when possible, use organic products.

Juicing. Use some combination of the following:

- Ginger, leeks, garlic, parsley, cabbage, beets, carrots, green-leafy vegetables (such as spinach, kale, and Swiss chard), apples, celery, grapes, lemon, raspberries, wheatgrasses, and chlorophyll
- You can add your favorite fruits and vegetables but not too much fruit, due to their high natural-sugar content (berries are lower in sugar).
- It is best to use room-temperature vegetables and fruit and not add ice (or drink very cold liquids), since cold foods and liquids eventually extinguish the stomach's digestive fires, reducing its ability to break down food effectively.
- Do not consume juices as often during the cooler months of the year; instead, switch to vegetable soups or stews.

Lifestyle

Eye exercises. See eye exercises in Chapter 10 for different daily exercises. Include the following into your daily routine:

- Palming
- Hot dog
- Near and far
- Figure eights

Other Modalities

Chinese Medicine

In Chinese medicine, the Liver (meridian) "opens to the eyes," and is responsible for supporting overall eye health and the free flow of energy and blood to the eyes. So, for any eye issue, always consider Liver support through both herbs and acupuncture.

The Spleen and Kidney meridians also help nourish the eyes and support production of blood. From a Chinese medical perspective, a common pattern to look for with PVD is "excess Liver-Gallbladder yang rising." Also, since PVDs often occur as we age, and they are related to reduced circulation and availability of essential nutrients, the formulas below help nourish and support these specific aspects.

Zhu jing wan. Preserve vistas pill tonifies and nourishes the Liver and Kidneys, enriches the yin, and improves vision.

Ming mu di huang wan. Rehmannia pills to "brighten the eyes" is related to the following patterns: Liver blood deficiency, Kidney yin deficiency, and Liver yin deficiency.

Gui pi tang. Restore the Spleen decoction increases qi, tonifies blood, strengthens the Spleen, nourishes the heart, and helps the Spleen control the blood.

Herbal formula and treatment strategies can vary significantly, based on the Chinese medicine practitioner's evaluation and intake.

Cell Salts

Cell salts may help posterior vitreous detachment. To make a cell salt solution, put up to 10 tablets of each cell salt in a 16- to 24-ounce bottle; fill with water and swirl to dissolve tablets. Sip throughout the day. Cell salts are prepared in a homeopathic manner, and they typically contain 12 minerals that include forms of calcium, potassium, magnesium, sodium, iron, and silica. This formula can be purchased online from different companies.

Homeopathy

Homeopathic remedies are non-toxic, natural medicines that are safe for everyone, including infants and pregnant or nursing women. You may use 6X, 10X, 30X, 6C, or 30C potencies.

#1 Calc fluor 6X for tissue integrity

#2 Calc phos 6X for calcium strength

#12 Silicea 6X to support connective tissue health

Also See

---

[1] Hollands, H., Johnson, D., Brox, A.C., Almeida, D., Simel, D.L., et al. (2009). Acute-onset floaters and flashes: is this patient at risk for retinal detachment? *JAMA*, Nov 25; 302(20):2243-9.

[2] Rahman, R., Ikramm K., Rosen, P.H., Cortina-Borja, M., Taylor, M.E. (2002). Ocular and systemic posaconazole(SCH-56592) treatment of invasive Fusarium solani keratitis and endophthalmitis. *Br J Ophthalmol*, Jul; 86(7):829.

[3] Hikichi, T. (2007). Time course of posterior vitreous detachment in the second eye. *Curr Opin Ophthalmol*, May; 18(3):224-7.

[4] Ibid. Coffee. (2007).

[5] Dayan, M.R., Jayamanne, D.G., Andrews, R.M., Griffiths, P.G. (1996). Flashes and floaters as predictors of vitreoretinal pathology: is follow-up necessary for posterior vitreous detachment? *Eye (Lond)*,10 (Pt 4)():456-8.

[6] Ibid. Dayan. (1996).

[7] RNIB. Understanding posterior vitreous detachment. Retrieved Jan 14 2018 from http://www.rnib.org.uk/eye-health/your-guide-posterior-vitreous-detachment-pvd/posterior-vitreous-detachment-PVD.

[8] Thimons, J.J. (1992). Posterior vitreous detachment. *Optom Clin*. 1992; 2(3):1-24.

[9] Stolyszewski, I., Niemcunowicz-Janica, A., Pepinski, W., Spolnicka, M., Zbiec, R., et al. (2007). Vitreous humour as a potential DNA source for postmortem human identification, *Fola Histochem Cytobiol*, 45(2):135-6.

[10] Richardson, P.S., Benson, M.T., Kirkby, G.R. (1999). The posterior vitreous detachment clinic: do new retinal breaks develop in the six weeks following an isolated symptomatic posterior vitreous detachment? *Eye (Lond)*, Apr; 13 (Pt 2)():237-40.

[11] Coffee, R.E., Westfall, A.C., Davis, G.H., et al. (2007). Symptomatic posterior vitreous detachment and the incidence of delayed retinal breaks: case series and meta-analysis. Am J Ophthalmol, 2007;144:409-13

[12] Foos, R.Y. (1972). Posterior vitreous detachment. *Trans Am Acad Ophthalmol Otolaryngol*, 76:480-497.

[13] Gelia, L., Raman, R., Pal, S.S., Ganesan, S., Sharma, T. (2017). Incidence, Progression, and Associated Risk Factors of Posterior Vitreous Detachment in Type 2 Diabetes Mellitus: *Semin Ophthalmol*, 32(2):191-197.

[14] Akiba, J. (1993). Prevalence of posterior vitreous detachment in high myopia. *Ophthalmology*, 1993 Sep;100(9):1384-8.

[15] Wagle, A.M., Lim, W.Y., Yap, T.P., Neelam, K., Au Eong, K.G. (2011). Utility values associated with vitreous floaters. *Am J Ophthalmol*, Jul; 152(1):60-65.e1.

[16] Ibid. Gelia. (2017).

[17] Hilford, D., Hilford, M., Mathew, A., Polkinghome, P.J. (2009). Posterior vitreous detachment following cataract surgery. *Eye (Lond)*, Jun;23(6):1388-92.

[18] . Chuo, J.Y., Lee, T.Y.Y., Hollands, H., Morris, A.H., Reyes, R.C., et al. (2006). Risk Factors for Posterior Vitreous Detachment: A Case-Control Study. *Am J Ophthalmol*, 142(6):931-937.

[19] Geck, J., Pustolla, N., Baraki, H., Atili, A., Feltgen, N., et al. (2013). Posterior vitreous detachment following intravitreal drug injection. *Graefes Arch Clin Exp Ophthalmol*, Jul; 251(7): 1691–1695.

[20] Landrum, J.T., Bone, R.A., Joa, H., Kilburn, M.D., Moore, L.L., et al. (1997). A one year study of the macular pigment: the effect of 140 days of a lutein supplement. *Exp Eye Res*, Jul;65(1):57-62.

[21] Piermarocchi, S., Saviano, S., Parisi, V., Tedeschi, M., Panozzo, G., et al. (2012). Carotenoids in Age-related Maculopathy Italian Study (CARMIS): two-year results of a randomized study. *Eur J Ophthalmol*, Mar-Apr;22(2):216-25.

[22] NIH. (2013). NIH Study provides clarity on supplements for protection against blinding eye disease. Retrieved Nov 10 2017 from https://nei.nih.gov/news/pressreleases/050513.

[23] Udell, I.J., Abelson, M.B. (1983). Chemical mediators of inflammation. *Int Ophthalmol Clin*, 23:1:15-26.

[24] Abelson, M.B., Butrus, S.I., Kliman, G.H., Larson, D.L., Corey, E.J., et al. (1987). Topical arachidonic acid: A model for screening anti-inflammatory agents. *J Ocul Pharmacol*, 3:63-75.

[25] Ibid. Thimons. (1992).

[26] Takano, S., Ishiwata, S., Nakazawa, M., Mizugaki, M., Tamai, M. (1997). Determination of ascorbic acid in human vitreous humor by high-performance liquid chromatography with UV detection. *Curr Eye Res*, 16(6):589–594.

[27] Eaton, J.W. (1991). Is the lens canned? *Free Radic Biol Med*. 11(2):207–213.

[28] Shui, Y.B., Holekamp, N.M., Kramer, B.C., Crowley, J.R., Wilkins, M.A., et al. (2009). The Gel State of the Vitreous and Ascorbate-Dependent Oxygen Consumption. *Arch Ophthalmol*, Apr;127(4):475-482.

[29] Jugdaohsingh, R. (2009). Silicon and Bone Health. *J Nutr Health Aging*, Mar-Apr;11(2):99-110.

[30] Matsunaga, N., Imai, S., Inokuchi, Y., Shimazawa, M., Yokota, S., et al. (2009). Bilberry and its main constituents have neuroprotective effects against retinal neuronal damage in vitro and in vivo. *Mol Nutr Food Res*, Jul;53(7):869-77.

31 Cohen-Boulakia, F., Valensi, P.E., Boulahdour, H., Lestrade, R. Dufour-Lamarinie, J.F., et al. (2000). In vivo sequential study of skeletal muscle capillary permeability in diabetic rats: effect of anthocyanosides. Metabolism, Jul;49(7):880-5. *NeuroToxicology*, 28 (2007) 93–100.

32 Zhu, Y., Xia, M., Yang, Y., Liu, F., Li, Z., et al. (2011). Purified anthocyanin supplementation improves endothelial function via NO-cGMP activation in hypercholesterolemic individuals. *Clin Chem*, Nov;57(11):1524-33.

33 Ou, H.C., Lee, W.J., Lee, I.T., Chiu, T.H., Tsai, K.L., et al. (2009). Ginkgo biloba extract attenuates oxLDL-induced oxidative functional damages in endothelial cells. *J Appl Physiol*, 2009;106:1674–85.

34 Chung, H.S., Harris, A., Kristinsson, J.K., Ciulla, T.A., Kagemann, C., Ritch, R. (1999). Ginkgo biloba extract increases ocular blood flow velocity. *J Ocul Pharmacol Ther*, 15:233–40.

35 Mutlu, U., Ikram, M.A., Hofman, A., de Jong, P.T., Uitterlinden, A.G., et al. (2016). Vitamin D and retinal microvascular damage: The Rotterdam Study. *Medicine (Baltimore)*, Dec; 95(49): e5477.

16-1. BAGS AND RINGS UNDER THE EYES

Many times, we are very self-conscious of baggy eyes or dark rings under our eyes. They are a natural part of aging or genetics, caused by factors we can modify to some extent.

Signs and Symptoms

Bags under the eyes are seen as mild swelling in the skin below the eyes. How chronically the eye puffiness continues, really depends on the cause(s), and if these causes become resolved. Bagginess under the eyes may also be due to genetics, and in these cases, are difficult to resolve and may be more permanent. They may appear almost overnight, may develop over time, and may stay for as long as the underlying cause is unresolved.

Dark rings/circles under the eyes can be brownish or blueish, depending on whether skin pigmentation (associated with genetics) or thin skin is involved. Thin skin reveals fine veins and is associated with skin transparency.

What are Baggy Eyes?

It helps to decipher baggy eyes if we see the area around and below the eyes as hills and valleys.

There are three valleys below the eye: the **tear trough** (orbital rim hollow), the **eyelid crease hollow**, and the **zygomatic hollow**.

The hills are called the **orbicularis roll**, the orbital **fat bag, the fluid bag,** and the **malar mound**.[1] As fat and musculature change and shift with aging, their placement on these hills and valleys change the surface appearance.

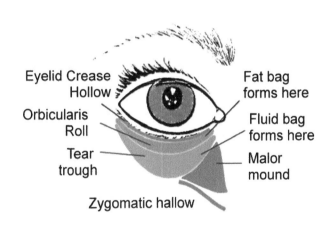

The **triangular malar mound**'s appearance varies, depending on whether genetics, thyroid disorder, allergies, or aging affect it.[2] The changeability of the different hills or bags varies. For example, the changes in the fat bag increase slowly over time, while changes in the fluid bag vary from day to day.[3]

What are Dark Rings/Circles?

We think of dark rings under our eyes as being due to fatigue, and while fatigue may worsen appearance, the rings have an underlying cause.

Blueish rings/circles. The skin under the eyes is normally thick enough to conceal blood underneath the skin. But some people's skin is very transparent; it also thins as we age. In addition, as we age, collagen and fat beneath the skin decrease. In these cases, a blueish tint appears due to oxygenated blood pooled beneath the under-eye skin. This is known as a vascular type of dark ring and accounts for about 35% of all dark ring cases.[4]

Brown rings/circles arise from the skin pigmentation, usually due to genetics. Eye rubbing or sun exposure can make the circles worse. Circles from skin pigmentation especially affect people of Asian and African-American heritage. This is known as a pigmented type of dark ring/circle. About 54% of dark-circle cases are a combination of pigmented and vascular types.[5]

Causes and Risk Factors

Bags Under Eyes

Changes due to the **fat bag** tend to develop gradually over time, though not always.

- **Aging**. As we age, the muscles supporting the eyelids sag, fat in the lower eyelid moves downward, and gravity generally shifts everything downward over the hills and valleys below the eye.
- **Genetics**. Inherited causes tend to be long-term and difficult to resolve, and they are often a permanent problem without a natural solution.

Changes due to the **fluid bag** tend to be of a shorter duration and/or a more rapid onset.

- **Fluid retention**. Nutrition, poor diet, and especially foods that increase fluid retention such as salty foods.
- **Allergies**. Seasonal and other allergies, including food allergies.
- **Sensitivities**. Other environmental sensitivities.
- **Lack of sleep**.
- **Stress**

Other causes include the following:

Medications such as stimulants that affect sleep patterns, long-term use of pain killers that cause adrenal fatigue, and long-term use of antibiotics that affect proper digestion. Medications that may cause swelling under the eyes include ACE inhibitors, such as benazepril (Lotensin), captopril, enalapril (Vasotec), fosinopril, lisinopril (Prinivil, Zestril), moexipril, perindopril (Aceon), quinapril (Accupril), ramipril (Altace), and trandolapril (Mavik).

Thyroid and/or kidney problems and disorders may occasionally, not often, cause baggy eyes.

Adrenal deficiency may be a cause, such as excessive stress, poor diet, lack of exercise, and lack of sleep, or medications.

Dark Rings/Circles Under Eyes

Blueish colored rings under the eyes are due to very thin skin; oxygenated pooled blood can show through. This is more noticeable in the morning. The thin layer of fat under the skin normally shields this coloring, but as one ages, the fat layer also thins and/or sags, revealing the blue color.

Rings that are more brown colored result from hyperpigmentation, triggered by chronic eye rubbing, sun exposure, or genetics.

Conventional Treatment

Bags under eyes are usually a cosmetic concern and don't require specific treatment, though they may indicate underlying health concerns.

Conventional treatments include:

- **Rest** and relaxation.
- **Allergy medications** for hay fever and other sensitivities.
- **Surgical interventions** such as laser resurfacing, chemical peels, and fillers that may improve skin tone and tighten the skin.
- **Eyelid surgery** (blepharoplasty) is an option to remove bags under eyes, which is usually an outpatient procedure. The risks of eyelid surgery include eye infection, and dry eyes (resulting in problems with vision, tear ducts, and eyelid repositioning).

Rings/Circles Under Eyes

Blue rings/circles are sometimes reduced with topical creams that have stimulating ingredients like caffeine that can constrict blood vessels and temporarily boost circulation.[6] Potent hydrators, such as hyaluronic acid may plump the area, pushing the skin up and away from the pooled blood. Retinoic acid creams may be able to thicken the outer layer of the skin to conceal shadows.

Brown rings/circles might be reduced by over-the-counter creams that contain soy or citrus and which claim to lighten circles over a period of four to six weeks.

Note. Avoid hydroquinone, a go-to lightener for sunspots and scars. It reduces melanin production in the skin that lightens the skin, but it can impact allergies, liver or kidney disease, and use of antibiotics. It can cause burning, stinging, itching, or redness. It can make you sunburn more easily and make your skin more sensitive to cold and wind.[7]

Complementary Approach

Natural approaches have the best chance of working when the bagginess under the eyes is due to lifestyle considerations rather than genetics. This is because sometimes they are a symptom caused by poor diet, lack of sleep, chronic stress, and more. If the bagginess is due to these causes or other health issues such as allergies, hypothyroidism, and chronic fatigue syndrome, etc., natural approaches (along with your doctors' suggestions) will help support energy and overall health. Supplements by themselves may help reduce the bagginess as well as support overall health, but lifestyle changes may also be needed to make the natural approach more effective and enduring.

Sufficient sleep, good stress management, and a healthy diet are the simplest home remedies. As part of natural eye care, the healing aspects of flowers and plants are frequently used to treat minor problems, such as puffiness under the eyes.

These remedies are not really effective if the dark rings/circles are related to genetics.

Nutrients

Essential (depending on the underlying cause)

Kidney qi tonic (adrenal boosting formula). Consult with your local acupuncturist or herbalist who can provide this for you.

Kidney yin tonic or a similar Kidney qi tonic offered by your local acupuncturist.

Natural cream for under the eyes to move and increase circulation in that area and to help repair the skin cells. Creams and lotions that contain some combination of the following nutrients can be helpful: hyaluronic acid, vitamin A, vitamin E, rose hips, cucumber, and green tea.

Helpful

Eye creams containing coffee and hyaluronic acid and/or retinol.

Diet

Minimize sugar, salt, and **refined carbohydrates** in your diet. Follow our Vision diet in Chapter 7.

Drink plenty of water and keep your alcohol consumption to a minimum.

Juicing. We recommend some combination of the following along with your favorite fruits and vegetables:

- Ginger, leeks, garlic, parsley, cabbage, beets, carrots, leafy-green vegetables, apples, celery, lemon, raspberries, tomato, watermelon, cucumber, wheatgrasses, and chlorophyll
- Not too much fruit due to its natural sugar content.
- Try to use room temperature vegetables and fruit.
- Do not add ice or very cold liquids since cold foods and liquids will eventually extinguish the stomach's digestive fire.
- Do not juice as often during the cooler months of the year, and instead, switch to vegetable soups or stews.

Lifestyle

Don't rub your eyes. Massage around your eyes if you want to help move circulation and energy. Constant rubbing of your eyes can end up breaking small blood vessels around the eyes, possibly resulting in a tired look. Rubbing may also damage the cornea and increase the risk of infection.

Stop smoking. Besides causing circulatory problems, smoking can cause a thinning of skin due to interference with blood flow to the skin. The smoke rising from the cigarette can also aggravate the eyes. Smoking also depletes the body of essential nutrients such as vitamin C that is essential in repairing skin. Smokers are also four times more likely than non-smokers to feel tired after a night's sleep.[8]

Change your sleeping position. If you sleep on your side or stomach, try sleeping on your back, and even add an extra pillow under your head.

Curb allergies. If you have hay fever or allergies, Neti Pot may help reduce excess fluid buildup.

Remove makeup. Makeup contains substances that can irritate eye tissue; always remove makeup when you can, and definitely before you go to bed. Use only natural, organic makeup.

Use cold compresses. Close your eyes and gently cover them with a cold washcloth for about five minutes, several times a day. This can improve circulation and slightly reduce the puffiness that some people experience.

Moisturize. You can plump up your skin slightly by using a good moisturizer that contains vitamin C, licorice, fennel, and stabilized oxygen. Vitamin C is an antioxidant that protects skin cells from damage and supports collagen production. Licorice and fennel remove inflammation, and stabilized oxygen is a form of hydrogen peroxide that promotes circulation.

Use sunscreen daily. Use a natural sunscreen, especially made for the face, with a sun protection factor (SPF) of at least 15, but preferably 20. Use all day and every day to protect the skin under your eyes.

A Few Old-School Remedies

Tea

Black tea. First, steep in warm water, then squeeze out the excess water and apply under the eyes. There are tannins in the black tea that reduce blood vessel dilation.

Rosemary tea. Try applying a cold compress of rosemary tea to increase circulation that helps reduce swelling around the eyes. Bring a half-cup of fresh rosemary and a quart of water to a boil. Steep for 20 minutes, then strain, and chill. Soak a washcloth in the tea, ring out extra liquid, and place over eyes for 15 to 20 minutes—once a day, or as needed.

Vegetable slices

Cucumber slices. Take thinly sliced cucumber and cool the slices by placing them in the refrigerator. These slices can be placed over closed eyes and left for 15 minutes every day. This is an excellent way to keep wrinkles and dry skin away.

Raw potato slices. Close your eyes and cover eyelids with slices of raw potato for 15–20 minutes. Then rinse with warm water and apply a hydrating herbal cream, or an eye- or facial-moisturizer.

Compresses

Cucumber juice. Grate a cucumber, remove the juice by squeezing the pulp, and refrigerate. Make a mixture of lemon juice, lanolin cream, and cucumber juice, and apply around the eye for 10–15 minutes.

Combination of potato and cucumber juices. Dip some cotton cloth or cotton pads in a 1:1 mixture of potato and cucumber juices. Put the cotton on your eyelids and rest for 20 minutes. Rinse your eyelids with cold water afterward.

Hot and cold. To increase circulation, alternately apply hot (but comfortable) and cold water under your eyes with a washcloth, for 30 seconds each time, for 10 minutes.

Other Self-Help Ideas

Parsley contains vitamin K that can help increase circulation under the eyes and reduce puffiness. There are a couple of ways you can apply this herb:

- Mix a handful of fresh parsley with one tablespoon of plain yogurt in a food processor until a paste is formed. To apply, rub the paste under your eyes and let it stay for 20 minutes, then rinse with lukewarm water. For this to work most efficiently, repeat once a week.
- Freeze parsley into ice cubes, wrap the ice cubes in a soft small towel then apply under the eyes. The parsley ice cube will soothe the eyes, and at the same time, work on diminishing the dark circles. Parsley is also packed with chlorophyll that helps fade darkness. The ice cubes reduce the swelling.

Egg whites are astringent and can tighten pores, and can reduce puffy bagginess. Egg whites also have lots of the B-vitamins that promote good circulation and reduce inflammation.

- If you are concerned that an egg is old, a home test that is pretty reliable is to pour room temperature water into a glass, then drop the eggs into the water. If they float, they are NOT good. If they sink, they should be fine.
- Dab half a teaspoon of one raw egg white on the clean, dry skin around your eyes only. Important: don't get it in your eyes. Leave it on for about 15 minutes until it dries, then, rinse well with warm water. Finally, wash your hands with soap and water.

Homemade rose water contains both vitamins A and C and has strong astringent and anti-inflammatory properties. Simmer rose petals in just enough distilled water to cover them. When the petals have lost their color, strain the liquid and let it cool. Dip a cotton ball into the rosewater and dab under eyes to reduce dark circles and refresh the skin. You can save the rosewater in a jar for future use.

Lemon and tomato combinations can also be helpful for dark circles. Apply a mixture of lemon and tomato juice (equal parts) two times a day. Make a paste out of the following:

- 1 tsp. tomato juice
- 1/2 tsp. lemon juice
- a pinch of turmeric powder
- 1 tsp. of flour

Apply around eyes. Leave on for 10 minutes before rinsing.

Turmeric-pineapple paste (paste of turmeric with pineapple juice) on the skin under your eyes may help.

Mint crushed may be applied around the eyes.

Almond oil massaged under and around eyes at bedtime, daily for two weeks helps remove dark circles and is an excellent "skin food."

Other Modalities

Massage and acupressure are helpful because they aid in increased circulation that can eliminate the fluid build-up associated with bags.

Massage

Types of massage include Swedish massage, aromatherapy massage, hot stone massage, deep tissue, shiatsu, Thai massage, and reflexology.

Acupressure

Here is a great circulation-boosting exercise that is easy, which you can do yourself.

- Close your eyes and gently press your ring finger underneath one eye on the bone, moving from the inside corner to the outside corner along the eye orbit (on the bone structure around the eyes).
- Do this exercise 10 to 15 times.
- Then repeat under the other eye.

You might also refer to our eye exercises and eye acupressure points in Chapter 10 to help relax the muscles around your eyes.

Chinese Medicine

From a Chinese medicine perspective, the causes and risk factors are the same as above, particularly lack of sleep, poor diet, and chronic stress conditions that can cause the Kidney energy to become depleted. In Chinese medicine, the Kidneys "rule" over the endocrine system that includes the adrenals (controlled by the pituitary gland, another part of the endocrine system). One of the resulting symptoms of depleted Kidney energy is bags under the eyes and possibly general fatigue.

The common pattern imbalances are Kidney yin or Kidney qi deficiencies. Your acupuncturist is able to determine this during the initial intake and create an appropriate treatment strategy.

Chinese Patent Formulas

Qi ju di huang wan. Rehmania 6 plus chrysanthemum and lycii nourishes Kidney and Liver blood and yin.

Zhu jing wan. Preserve vistas pill tonifies and nourishes the Liver and Kidneys, enriches the yin, and improves vision.

On the Horizon

A pilot study indicates that the daily use of epidermal growth-factor (EGF) serum reduced the appearance of eye bagginess.[9]

See Also

Chapter 7, Vision Diet

---

[1] Naik, M.N. (2016). Hills and Valleys: Understanding the Under-Eye. *J Cutan Asethet Surg*, Apr-Jun;9(2);61-4.

[2] Ibid. Naik. (2016).

[3] Ibid. Naik. (2016).

[4] Park, S.R., Kim, H.J., Park, H.K., Kim, J.Y., Kim, N.S., et al. (2016). Classification by causes of dark circles and appropriate evaluation method of dark circles. *Skin Res Technol*, Aug;22(3):276-83.

[5] Ibid. Park. (2016).

[6] McNight, C. (2017). Does Caffeine Constrict Blood Vessels? Retrieved Sep 8 2018 from https://www.livestrong.com/article/395736-does-caffeine-constrict-blood-vessels/.

[7] Everyday Health. What is Hydroquinone Topical? Retrieved Jun 10 2018 from https://www.everydayhealth.com/drugs/hydroquinone-topical.

[8] Philips, B.A., Danner, F.J. (1995). Cigarette smoking and sleep disturbance. *Arch Intern Med*, Apr 10;155(7):734-7.

[9] Seidel, R., Moy, R.L. (2015). Reduced appearance of under-eye bags with twice-daily application of epidermal growth factor (EGF) serum: a pilot study. *J Drugs Dermatol*, Apr;14(4):405-10.

16-2. BLEPHARITIS

When the eyelids are inflamed and sore, the condition is often called blepharitis. The inflammation may develop due to irritations, allergies, infections, and insect bites. It may be due to mild conditions such as allergies or dry eyes. It is often a chronic condition that is difficult to treat, though it is not contagious. Blepharitis can be uncomfortable and may be unsightly, but it usually doesn't cause permanent damage to your eyesight.

Blepharitis is very common. Ophthalmologists report that 37% of their patients experience it, and optometrists report 47% of their patients do as well. But according to one telephone survey, it seems to be more common than clinical reports. Younger people appear to have the condition more often than older people.[1] It is found across all age groups and all ethnic groups.

What is Blepharitis?

Behind the eyelids and eyelashes are several glands. The Meibomian glands secrete a fatty substance called meibum that spreads (via blinking) over the surface of the eye and slows the evaporation of tears. Tear-secreting glands also lie behind the eyelids.

Blepharitis is identified by the presence of "greasy scales" between the eyelashes and by redness on the lid around the eyelashes caused by the body's immune response (increased blood flow). Sometimes tiny veins expand and are noticeable (telangiectasia); the eyelid can become swollen.

Types of Blepharitis

There are two types of blepharitis: anterior and posterior.

Anterior blepharitis is found on the front and outside of the eyelid along the line of eyelashes. Bacteria and scalp dandruff are the most common causes of the inflammation there. Increased Meibomian gland activity may also occur.[2]

Posterior blepharitis is found on the innermost part of the eyelid that touches the eyeball. It occurs when the Meibomian glands are not functioning properly. Two skin disorders can also cause posterior blepharitis: scalp dandruff and acne rosacea.[3]

Blepharitis may occur as acute (often sudden onset) or chronic (ongoing).

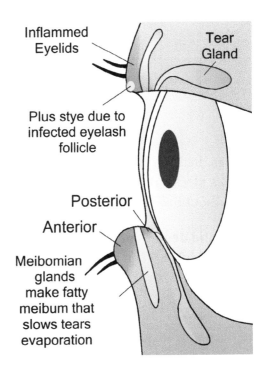

Inflammed Eyelids

Tear Gland

Plus stye due to infected eyelash follicle

Posterior

Anterior

Meibomian glands make fatty meibum that slows tears evaporation

Symptoms

Blepharitis manifests in a wide variety of symptoms. Common symptoms are redness and/or swelling of the eyelids, itching, scaling, swelling, or crusting around the eyelashes (especially on waking up). There can also be vision blurriness, dry eyes, or sensitivity to light, as well as a burning sensation or sense of a foreign body in the eye.

Blepharitis may be accompanied by styes and chalazia and is also linked to acne rosacea and dry eyes. Symptoms worsen in dry, windy weather, especially when it is also hot.

Signs & Symptoms				
	Posterior	Anterior Staph	Anterior Seborrehic	Anterior Demodex
Red eyes and thickened edges	✓ ✓	✓ ✓	✓	✓
Itching	✓	✓ ✓	✓ ✓	✓ ✓
Dryness and burning	✓ ✓	✓	✓	✓
Grit in eye	✓	✓ ✓	✓ ✓	
Oily eyelashes			✓ ✓	
Crusty scales at eyelid base		✓ ✓	✓ ✓	✓ ✓
Watering eyes	✓ ✓	✓	✓	✓
Erosion of eyelid edge	✓ ✓			
Light sensitivity, blurry vision	✓ ✓	✓		
Ropey, white mucous	✓ ✓			

Risks

Dry eyes. Patients with blepharitis are at increased risk of dry eyes. When scaling around the eyelashes blocks glands, the oils they produce are unable to get out of the glands onto the tear film. Without this protective oily layer, the water layer quickly evaporates, leading to dry eyes.

Anxiety and depression. Patients with blepharitis are at elevated risk of anxiety and depression. The risk is higher when the condition is first diagnosed; it declines with time.[4]

Causes

Bacteria, dandruff, and fungi are commonly thought to be causes of blepharitis. But what may be more important is that the presence of these toxins that change the healthy environment of the eyelid and produce pro-inflammatory cytokines, toxins, and free radicals.[5]

Anterior Blepharitis

Bacteria may cause this type of blepharitis, including several types of staphylococcus and propionibacterium acne.[6]

Scalp dandruff (seborrheic dermatitis) or a mix of bacteria and dandruff is also very common. This form of blepharitis allows increased growth of malassezia yeasts that live in the sebum oil of the skin. This type of blepharitis is not as severe as a staph infection, but the eyelids will look greasy and scaly. The patient may also have dandruff, acne, or eczema.

Fungi have also been found to be present with blepharitis and may be a cause. These include penicillium, candida, and trichophyton.[7] Researchers have also identified pityrosporum yeasts.[8]

Demodex mites have also been found in blepharitis eyelids.[9] The presence of mites or microbes on the eyelids does not prove that they caused the condition. Rather all that can be said is that, they found the changed eyelid habitat more hospitable than that of a healthy eyelid. In fact, in such cases, treatment with antibiotics or steroids may change the microbial life of the healthy eyelid in favor of specific antibiotic-resistant strains.[10]

Irritation from insect bites, scratches, or infections.

Allergies from pollen or environmental pollutants.

Posterior Blepharitis

Meibomian gland dysfunction is the most common cause of posterior blepharitis; although it may also contribute to anterior blepharitis.

Skin conditions such as rosacea and scalp dandruff can also cause posterior blepharitis.

Conventional Treatment

Conventional treatment depends on the specific type and severity of blepharitis. Mild symptoms may only require warm soaking and daily lid hygiene. Diluted baby shampoo may be recommended for cleansing of the lids. Other varieties may require antibiotics and/or cortisone cream, or even oral antibiotics, any of which should only be used under medical supervision.

Complementary Approach

There are a number of natural ways to help manage mild cases of blepharitis, reduce symptoms, and help keep the eyelids clean and the eyes moist.

Essential

Preservative free eyedrops. These will help keep the eyes moist. Homeopathic eyedrops are available that can help with natural tear production and with dry eyes.

Blepharitis treatment protocol.

1. Add a dropper full[1] of **EyeEase** herbal formula to eight ounces of water and boil for three minutes.
2. When the heated herbal water cools just enough for you to be able to touch it, then put a clean compress into the herbal heated water, wring out the excess, and place on your closed eye lids.
3. When the compress starts to lose its heat, put the warm **Bruder** eye mask (which has been heated in the microwave for 20 seconds) on your eyes for ten minutes.
4. After removing the eye mask, put 1 **MSM** drop into each eye.

Do this two to three times a day.

Daily warm compresses. These will sooth the eyes. Herbs can be included in the infusion, such as burdock, calendula, chamomile, chrysanthemum flower, eyebright, echinacea angustifolia, forsythia, golden seal, honeysuckle, marigold, and red raspberry leaf.

Important

Immune boosting formula. This may contain herbs such as red clover flowers, echinacea root, astragalus, reishi mushroom (medicinal), milk thistle, thymus extract, and cat's claw.

Self help

Tea tree shampoo. This may be effective for blepharitis caused by mites,[11] and combined with geranium oil, effective against staphylococcus.[12] A combination of grapefruit seed extract (citricidal) and geranium oil was found effective against untypable staph strains.[13]

Self help for general symptom relief

Eye rubbing. Avoid rubbing your eyes.

Compress. Apply a warm, wet washcloth as a compress to the affected area, and hold it in place until cool. Repeat this application 3–4 times a day. This is effective because it warms the glands on the eyelid, allowing the oils to become more fluid.

Dry warmth. You can also use commercial eyelid heating pads or a warm hard-boiled egg wrapped in a cloth.

Massage. After warming the glands, gentle finger pressure at the base of the eyelids may help remove accumulated oils. An eye doctor can also help to remove accumulated material.

Lid scrub. Use a commercial lid "scrub" or baby shampoo on a cotton swab to wash your lids.

---

[1] A dropper full is about ½ the dropper, the amount that can be pulled into the dropper with one squeeze. It is approximately 30 drops.

Castor oil (fresh and from the health food store). Place a small bit on a Q-tip and apply to the inner lower-lid margin.

Honey. Use the same application method as with castor oil. Mix with sterile spring water to reduce stinging. This can be done while doing the "sunning" eye exercise (see eye exercises in Chapter 10), because it really brings on tearing. Honey has antibiotic, antifungal, and antiviral properties.

Salt and baking soda. Mix 1/4 teaspoon of salt *plus* 1/4 teaspoon baking soda *in* 1/2 cup of warm water that has been boiled. Dip finger in the mixture and rub on eyelid margins with eyes closed, once in the morning and once at night before bed.

Massage protocol. One study reports beneficial results with the following specific massage protocol for blelpharitis[1]:

- Under a comfortably warm shower, close the affected eyelid(s); using the thumb(s) and index finger(s), gently massage the upper lid downward with your index finger(s) and the lower lid upward with your thumb(s) for 30 seconds.

- After showering, use a warm water-moistened Q-tip to gently but firmly scrub all eyelid edges from where the lashes grow (not the red inside of the eyelid), being careful to not touch the sensitive cornea.

  o For the lower lid, hold the Q-tip in your hand and near enough to the tip for stability, perhaps an inch or two from the end. Use the index finger of the other hand to gently pull down the skin below your eye, to turn out the eyelid, so that it is further from the sensitive cornea. Scrub in small sections (1/5 of the eyelid length) across the edge, for 3 seconds each.

  o For the upper lid, hold and turn out the upper eyelid by reaching your hand over your head from above, so that again, the eyelid is turned away from the sensitive surface of the cornea. It may work best to use two fingers to pull up the eyelid.

Chinese Medicine

Repeated blepharitis can be due to chronic dry eyes. Our tears contain natural antibiotics that help us neutralize normal bacteria around our eyes. With less tears, come fewer natural antibiotics. In Chinese medicine, chronic dry eyes can often be due to Kidney yin deficiency. Below are some formulas that may help.

Preserve vistas pill (zhu jing wan). Tonifies and nourishes the Liver and Kidneys, enriches the yin, and improves vision.

Ming mu di huang wan (rehmannia pills "to brighten the eyes"). Related to the following patterns: Liver blood deficiency, Kidney yin deficiency, and Liver yin deficiency

Your acupuncturist may modify these formulas or recommend other formulas based on his/her intake evaluation.

Herbal Tea

Chrysanthemum and goji berry tea. Chrysanthemum flowers have heat-clearing properties that are important to help cool off red and dry eyes. Goji berries are beneficial for the kidneys, the lungs, the liver, and to build yin fluids such as tears. Brew the chrysanthemum flowers like you would any loose tea, and then put a small handful of goji berries into the made tea. After drinking the tea, you can eat the berries.

Anti-inflammatory and hydrating tea. Combine 10g dried chrysanthemum flowers, 10g goji berries, 5g jin yin hua (honeysuckle), and 5g glycyrrhiza uralensis fisch (licorice root). Soak these for 30 minutes in spring water, bring to a boil, reduce heat, cover, and simmer for 10 minutes. Strain them, and set the tea aside. Add more spring water to the herbs, boil, and simmer again. Combine both batches in a jar, and drink 2 cups a day. This will keep in your refrigerator for five days.

Essential Oils

Carrot seed properties include antiseptic, disinfectant, detoxifier, and antioxidant.

Frankincense helps relieve chronic stress and anxiety, reduces pain and inflammation, and boosts immunity.

Keep essences away from the mouth, eyes, and mucous membranes; if a few drops get in one of these sensitive areas it may be uncomfortable for 15–30 minutes, but not harmful. You can lessen discomfort by adding a pure oil like olive or coconut oil to neutralize the irritating effect. For the eye area, dab a few drops around the outside of the eye. Do not put the neutralizing oil in the eye.

Combine ¼ cup of avocado oil with ¼ cup of calendula-infused oil. Slowly add 5 drops each of the essential oils. Then close the bottle and shake well; apply 4 drops of this mixture on your clean face. Massage in gentle circular motions. Leave overnight.

For more information, see Appendix 9.

Also See

Chapter 7, Vision Diet

Chapter 8, Nutrients

Appendix 5, Recommended Products (for homeopathic eyedrops)

---

1 Lemp, M.A., Nichols, K.K. (2009). Blepharitis in the United States 2009: a survey-based perspective on prevalence and treatment. *Ocul Surf*, Apr;7(2 Suppl):S1-S14.

2 National Eye Institute. Facts About Blepharitis. Retrieved Feb 10 2018 from https://nei.nih.gov/health/blepharitis/blepharitis.

[3] Ibid. National Eye Institute. Facts About Blepharitis.

4 Chiang, C.C., Lin, C.L., Tsai, Y.Y., Peng, C.L., Liao, Y.T., et al. (2013). Patients with Blepharitis Are at Elevated Risk of Anxiety and Depression. *Plos One*, 8(12):e83335.

[5] Dadaci, Z., Kilinc, F., Ozer, T.T., Sahin, G.O., Acir, N.O., et al. (2015). Periodic acid-Schiff staining demonstrates fungi in chronic anterior blepharitis. *Eye (Lond)*, Dec;29(12):1522-7.

[6] Ibid. Dadaci. (2015).

[7] Ibid. Dadaci. (2015).

[8] Nelson, M.E., Midgley, G., Blatchford, N.R. (1990)). Ketoconazole in the treatment of blepharitis. *Eye (Lond)*, 4(PI1:151-9.

[9] Ibid. Dadaci, (2015).

[10] Ibid. Dadaci. (2015).

[11] Ibid. Dadaci. (2015).

[12] Edwards-Jones, V., Buck, R., Shawcross, S.G., Dawson, M.M., Dunn, K. (2004). The effect of essential oils on methicillin-resistant Staphylococcus aureus using a dressing model. *Burns,* Dec;30(8):772-7.

[13] Ibid. Edwards-Jones. (2004).

16-3. CONJUNCTIVITIS

Conjunctivitis, commonly known as pink eye, affects three to six million Americans annually.[1] It has been one of the most treatable of any eye conditions. It is, however, becoming increasingly prevalent due to resilient bacterial strain infections, changing climate, increased pollen loads, pollution, and the resulting heightened immunological response to environmental changes.

Pink eye infection generally starts in one eye and easily spreads to the other, causing red and irritated eyes that usually resolve from three to seven days. If the symptoms last longer than a week, then you should see your eye doctor. This is important because, if the infection enters the cornea (the transparent surface of the eyeball), scars can form, causing cloudy areas that may harm your vision. In addition, if you experience sensitivity to light, pain, vision loss, or signs of herpes, you should consult your healthcare provider.

About the Conjunctiva

The conjunctiva is the membrane forming the moist lining of the eyelids and covering the surface of the cornea. If the conjunctiva becomes infected, conjunctivitis is the result. This protective layer is more exposed to the exterior environment than any other part of the body, and it is therefore open to more microorganisms than any other membrane.

The conjunctiva is made up of flattened and columnar epithelium cells and goblet cells that secrete mucin. It also secretes tears, but than the tear glands. It contains both nerve cells and microcapillaries that deliver nutrients and remove waste.[2] It is connected to the sclera (the white of the eye) by a thin vascular membrane called the episclera. The types of conjunctiva are:[3]

- **Tarsal** (palpebral) conjunctiva lines the eyelids.
- **Fornix** conjunctiva forms the junction between tarsal and ocular conjunctiva. This type of conjunctiva is very flexible and permits eyelids and eyeballs to move freely.
- **Ocular** (bulbar) conjunctiva covers the white part of the eye and is tightly bound to the underlying layer of sclera. This type of conjunctiva moves as the eyeball moves.

Types of Conjunctivitis

Eye doctors refer to conjunctivitis types as follows:

Allergic conjunctivitis, inflammation due to allergies, is caused by the immune system's release of histamine and other biochemicals.

Viral conjunctivitis, which can occur along with colds or flu and is contagious. Most often, rubbing the eyes with contaminated hands causes it to spread.

Bacterial conjunctivitis that generally requires antibiotics for treatment.

- Various organisms can cause conjunctivitis including: contagious herpes keratitis, gonococcal, and chlamydia (not common). The incidence has increased in recent years and may be due, in part, to increased antibiotic-resistant strains.[4]
- Neonatal conjunctivitis (ophthalmia neonatorum) is found in newborn children, passed from the mother's birth canal.[5]

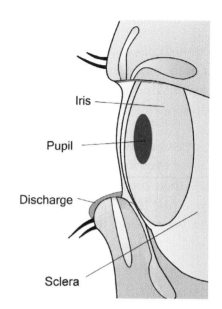

Chemical origins may be due to an acidic or alkaline material getting in the eye.[6]

Related disorders include episcleritis and scleritis.[7]

Symptoms

Symptoms of conjunctivitis include:

- Red and irritated eyes
- Morning "glued" eyelids, from night discharges
- Sensitivity to light
- Feeling of itchiness
- Feeling of griminess

Repeated conjunctivitis can be due to chronic dry eyes. Our tears contain natural antibiotics that help neutralize normal bacteria around our eyes. With less tears, come fewer natural antibiotics.

Causes

Infections

Infections, including infected insect bites and scratches, are a common cause of conjunctivitis.

- **Bacteria.** Bacteria, such as pneumococcus, staphylococcus, or streptococcus, are the cause of some cases. Bacterial conjunctivitis is more common in children.[8]
- **Virus.** Pink eye can also be caused by an adenovirus that spreads by many means, including swimming pools, wet towels, or touching your eyes with dirty hands. Viral conjunctivitis is more common in adults.[9]

Irritants

Insect bites, debris, and rubbing the eyes can contribute to pink eye. Chronic dry eyes may contribute to the cause. The tear film provides protective, lubricating, nutritional, and antimicrobial functions, and plays an important role in visual acuity. A lack of natural tears, therefore, reduces our ability to fight bacterial infection.[10]

Drugs that can cause dry, irritated eyes include antihistamines, acne medicine, antidepressants, Parkinson's medications, sleeping pills, birth control pills, blood pressure medications, pain relievers such as NSAIDS (for example, ibuprofen), and nasal decongestants.[11]

Allergies

Allergies and sensitivities that manifest in the eyes often cause pink eye. This includes environmental pollution, pollen, and other allergens.

- **Vernal keratoconjunctivitis.** This condition typically occurs only seasonally, and it is thought to be an allergic disorder. Patients experiencing conjunctivitis only during allergy seasons, often have other family members with allergy-related conditions, such as asthma or hay fever. It is more common in boys than girls, and more common under 20 years old. It occurs most often in hot-climate summers.
- **Allergic conjunctivitis.** Some people are susceptible to allergic conjunctivitis brought on by the use of drugs. See the information on drugs that harm the eyes in Chapter 12.

Conventional Treatment

After other potential problems have been ruled out, conventional medicine usually prescribes sulfa-based eyedrops. These usually work within three days. If not, broad-spectrum antibiotic eyedrops or ointment is prescribed; these only work with bacterial infections. Use preservative-free allergy or antihistamine eyedrops to help keep the eyes lubricated and reduce itching. Antihistamines or steroids may be prescribed by an eye doctor and should only be used under the doctor's direction. Whenever taking antibiotics, make sure you take probiotics as well.

Patients who wear contacts and those who have a sexually-transmitted disease must be treated.[12]

Complementary Approach

There are natural ways to improve pink eye and reduce the symptoms and risk of future onsets.

Nutrients

Essential

Vitamin A (palmitate). 2,500 IU–5,000 IU per day. Vitamin A is especially important in promoting health in all skin and membrane tissues, including epithelial and corneal healing.

> **Note.** Vitamin A is contra-indicated for those suffering from Stargardt disease (see Stargardt chapter for more information.) Do not supplement with Vitamin A if pregnant.[13]

Riboflavin. Conjunctivitis may be triggered by a vitamin B2 deficiency. Supplementing with the entire B complex can increase the availability of vitamin B2 without inducing deficiencies of the other B vitamins. Riboflavin plays an essential role in maintaining the structure and function of the ocular surface. Riboflavin deficiency induces ocular surface damage.[14]

Preservative-free eyedrops. To keep the eyes moist, homeopathic eyedrops are available. They can help with natural tear production and for those with dry eyes (see Appendix 5).

Use warm compresses daily. Herbs can be included in an infusion, such as burdock, chamomile, chrysanthemum flower, eyebright, echinacea, goldenseal, marigold and red raspberry leaf.

Important

Immune boosting formula. This may contain herbs such as red clover flowers, echinacea root, astragalus, reishi mushroom (medicinal), milk thistle, thymus extract, and cat's claw.

Curcumin. 635mg per day. Curcumin reduces conjunctiva inflammation from allergies in an experimental model.[15] An herbal complex (Norflo) with curcumin and phospholipids reduced inflammatory symptoms in almost 80% of the patients after several weeks.[16]

Diet

Eat yogurt or kefir. Kefir typically contains about three times as much beneficial bacteria as yogurt.[17] The acidophilus in yogurt/kefir combats bacterial infection. Likewise, we also suggest acidophilus supplements. Eat 1/2 cup of yogurt with live cultures, 3 times per day, or take an acidophilus supplement (with about six billion live or probiotic organisms), 3 times per day.

Lifestyle

Avoid rubbing your eyes.

Compress. Apply a warm, wet washcloth as a compress to the affected area, and hold it in place until cool; cold compresses are used for allergic-related conjunctivitis. Repeat this application 5–10 minutes, 3–4 times per day. Yogurt can also be used in a soothing compress to the eyes. You don't need to put the yogurt directly in your eyes, but instead, use it in a compress.

Lid scrub. Use a commercial lid scrub or baby shampoo on a cotton swab to wash your lids.

Castor oil or honey Place a small bit of fresh, natural castor oil on a Q-tip, and apply to the inner lower lid margin. Mix honey with sterile spring water to reduce stinging. Honey has antibiotic, antifungal, and antiviral properties.

Calendula. This herb is soothing and reduces swelling, itching, and inflammation. It is helpful in infections like conjunctivitis, irritation due to pollution, allergies, and minor injuries. It is antiseptic. Apply as a compress, or use as an eyewash or eyedrop.

Salt and baking soda. Mix 1/4 teaspoon of salt plus 1/4 teaspoon baking soda in 1/2 cup of warm water that has been boiled. Dip your finger in the mixture and rub on eyelid margins with eyes closed, once in the morning and once at night before bed.

Colloidal silver eyedrops. When used as eyedrops, 1–2 drops, 3–4 times per day, this has the potential to resolve conjunctivitis. It should not be used for longer than one week at a time.

Massage protocol. One study reports beneficial results with the following specific massage protocol for eyelid irritations:

- Under a comfortably warm shower, close the affected eyelid(s), and using the thumb(s) and index finger(s), gently massage the upper lid downward with your index finger(s) and the lower lid upward with your thumb(s) for 30 seconds.
- After showering, use a warm water-moistened Q-tip to gently but firmly scrub all eyelid edges from where the lashes grow (not the red inside of the eyelid), being careful to not touch the sensitive cornea.
- For the lower lid, hold the Q-tip in your hand and near enough to the tip for stability, perhaps an inch or two from the end. Use the index finger of the other hand to gently pull down the skin below your eye, to turn out the eyelid, so that it is further from the sensitive cornea. Scrub in small sections (1/5 of the eyelid length) across the edge, 3 seconds each.
- For the upper lid, hold and turn out the upper eyelid by reaching your hand over your head from above, so that again, the eyelid is turned away from the sensitive surface of the cornea. It may work best two use two fingers to pull up the eyelid.

Chinese Medicine

In Chinese medicine, chronic dry eyes are often due to Kidney yin deficiency. Below are some formulas that may help.

Preserve vistas pill (zhu jing wan). Tonifies and nourishes the Liver and Kidneys, enriches the yin, and improves vision.

Ming mu di huang wan (rehmannia pills "to brighten the eyes"). Related to the following patterns: Liver blood deficiency, Kidney yin deficiency, and Liver yin deficiency

Your acupuncturist may modify these formulas or recommend other formulas based on his/her intake evaluation.

Herbal Tea

Chrysanthemum and goji berry tea. Chrysanthemum flowers have heat-clearing properties that are important to help cool off red and dry eyes. Goji berries are beneficial for the kidneys, the lungs, the liver, and to build yin fluids such as tears. Brew the chrysanthemum flowers like you would any loose tea, and then put a small handful of goji berries into the made tea. After drinking the tea, you can eat the berries

Essential Oils

Carrot seed properties include antiseptic, disinfectant, detoxifier, and antioxidant.

Frankincense helps relieve chronic stress and anxiety, reduces pain and inflammation, and boosts immunity.

Keep essences away from the mouth, eyes, and mucous membranes; if a few drops get in one of these sensitive areas it may be uncomfortable for 15–30 minutes, but not harmful. You can lessen

discomfort by adding a pure oil like olive or coconut oil to neutralize the irritating effect. For the eye area, dab a few drops around the outside of the eye. Do not put the neutralizing oil in the eye.

Combine ¼ cup of avocado oil with ¼ cup of calendula-infused oil. Slowly add 5 drops each of the essential oils. Then close the bottle and shake well; apply 4 drops of this mixture on your clean face. Massage in gentle circular motions. Leave overnight.

For more information, see Appendix 9.

Also See

Chapter 7, Vision Diet

Chapter 8, Nutrients

Chapter 12, Drugs that Harm the Eyes

Appendix 5, Recommended Products

[1] Wikipedia. Conjunctivitis. Retrieved Apr 25 2018 from https://en.wikipedia.org/wiki/Conjunctivitis.

[2] Wikipedia. Conjunctiva. Retrieved Apr 24 2018 from https://en.wikipedia.org/wiki/Conjunctiva.

[3] Roat, M.I. (2016). Overview of Conjunctival and Scleral Disorders. Retrieved Apr 24 2018 from https://www.merckmanuals.com/professional/eye-disorders/conjunctival-and-scleral-disorders/overview-of-conjunctival-and-scleral-disorders.

[4] McAnena, L., Knowles, S.J., Curry, A., Cassidy, L. (2015). Prevalence of gonococcal conjunctivitis in adults and neonates. *Eye (Lond)*, Jul:29(7):875-880.

[5] Wikipedia. Neonatal conjunctivitis. Retrieved Apr 25 2018 from https://en.wikipedia.org/wiki/Neonatal_conjunctivitis.

[6] Ibid. Wikipedia. Conjunctivitis.

[7] Ibid. Roat. (2016).

[8] Ibid. Wikipedia. Conjunctivitis.

[9] Ibid. Wikipedia. Conjunctivitis.

10 Bron, A.J., Tiffany, J.M., Gouveia, S.M., Yokoi, N., Voon, L.W. (2004). Functional aspects of the tear film lipid layer. *Exp Eye Res,* Mar; 78(3):347-60.

[11] WebMD. Is Your Medication Causing Dry Eye? Retrieved May 1 2018 from https://www.webmd.com/eye-health/medication-cause-dry-eye#1.

12 Ibid. Wikipedia. Conjunctivitis.

[13] Kruse, F.E., Tseng, S.C., (1994). Retinoic acid regulates clonal growth and differentiation of cultured limbal and peripheral corneal epithelium. *Invest Ophthalmol Vis Sci,* Apr;35(5):2405-20.

[14] Takami, Y., Gong, H., Amemiya, T. (2004). Riboflavin deficiency induces ocular surface damage. *Ophthalmic Res,* May-Jun;36(3):156-65.

15 Chung, S.H., Choi, S.H., Choi, J.A., Chuck, R.S., Joo, C.K. (2012). Curcumin suppresses ovalbumin-induced allergic conjunctivitis. *Mol Vis,* 18:1966-72.

16 Allegri, P., Mastromarino, A., Neri, P. (2010). Management of chronic anterior uveitis relapses: efficacy of oral phospholipidic curcumin treatment. Long-term follow-up. *Clin Ophthalmol,* Oct 21; 4():1201-6.

17 The Globe and Mail. What's the difference between yogurt and kefir? Retrieved Feb 10 2018 from https://www.theglobeandmail.com/life/health-and-fitness/ask-a-health-expert/whats-the-difference-between-yogurt-and-kefir/article7904569/

16-4. OCULAR HERPES

When one of the herpes viruses, herpes simplex 1 or herpes zoster, manifests in the eyes, it is called ocular herpes or herpetic eye disease. Ocular herpes may cause scarring, chronic inflammation, lesions, and ulcers that damage different layers of the cornea. It is the most common infectious cause of corneal blindness in the U.S.[1]

Many people become infected with one of these viruses during childhood; they can be passed from one person to the other because the virus is contained in the moist skin that lines the mouth. In many people, the primary infection does not cause any symptoms. The most common time for a first active infection is between the ages of 30 and 40, and it may be more common in people who wear contacts. Because it affects the nerves directly, herpetic eye disease can be very painful.

Both viruses never leave the body after an initial infection; this can result in periodic flare-ups through one's life, causing potential pain, including in the face and eyes. It is not known why the virus can suddenly flare-up, but it may be due to stress, low immunity, and/or trauma.

Most flare-ups will resolve within a few weeks in non-immunocompromised people, and in some, flare-ups can recur through one's lifetime, possibly posing sight threatening eye problems.

Two Types of Herpes Viruses

Two types of viruses are found: herpes simplex 1 (cold sores, herpes) and varicella zoster (chicken pox, shingles), causing herpes simplex keratitis and herpes zoster ophthalmicus, respectively.

Herpes simplex 1 virus is common; 50–80% of Americans carry the antibodies, depending on the socioeconomic group, and ocular infection from this virus affects about .008% to .03% of the population.[2]

Varicella zoster virus was once very common; in the pre-inoculation era, 95% of children had the varicella antibodies before age 20.[3] It is still carried by about 20% of the population.[4] About 1% of these people develop herpes zoster ophthalmicus.[5]

What is Ocular Herpes

Herpes Simplex Keratitis

Herpes simplex keratitis occurs when the herpes simplex 1 virus (HSV) infects the cornea or the white part of the eye. The term keratitis means an inflammation of the cornea. The virus first attacks the corneal epithelium,[6] the thin outer layer of the cornea. This layer plays an important role in protecting the eye. It blocks intrusion from foreign materials and provides a smooth surface to absorb oxygen and cellular nutrients that are delivered through the tear film that lies on top of it. The epithelium also contains many nerve endings; it's very sensitive.

When a virus attacks the cornea, this outer epithelium layer becomes red, irritated, and painful, because the nerve endings serving the cornea also become infected. The extent of damage can vary widely, sometimes healing by itself within a week to ten days. If the virus recurs at a latter time, however, the results can be more serious, including ulcers and lesions that extend to the stroma layer of the cornea. The stroma layer is a thick layer comprised of water, layers of protein fibers, and cells delivering nourishment.

There are two major types of this virus. Type I is the most common and is not sexually transmitted, while Type II typically infects the genitals. Of the two types, Type I more commonly affects the eye, often resulting in symptoms such as eye infections, cold sores, or blisters.

Herpes Zoster Ophthalmicus

This condition, with initial symptoms that may be similar to herpes simplex keratitis, occurs when the varicella zoster virus, dormant in most people, attacks the ophthalmic nerve. It spreads to the epithelial layer of the cornea, then to the stroma layer. In 40–50% of cases, anterior uveitis also develops. Skin rashes around the eyes are another characteristic result.[7]

Types of Ocular Herpes

Herpes Simplex Keratitis

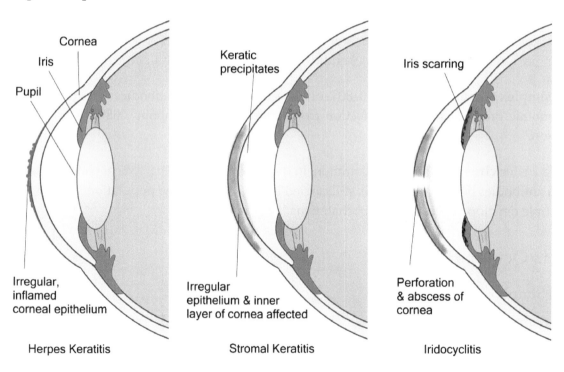

Herpes Keratitis   Stromal Keratitis   Iridocyclitis

Primary HSV. Once a person is infected, this virus may manifest as herpes simplex 1 or become dormant. If dormant, it remains dormant until some stress triggers an outbreak. This initial outbreak is rarely noticed and rarely affects the cornea. Sometimes a patient will have an episode of conjunctivitis or blepharitis that resolves itself.[8]

Recurrent HSV. If HSV recurs, it most often affects the cornea, resulting in herpes simplex keratitis. Although it usually affects the cornea, it can cause retinitis, trabeculitis (inflammation of the trabecular meshwork), anterior uveitis, and optic neuritis.[9]

Epithelial keratitis. This is the most common and mildest form. It affects only the top epithelial layer of the cornea. Inflammation of the epithelial layer of the cornea takes the form of several types of sores or ulcers. They are identified according to their shape and location, including dendritic, geographical, marginal, and metaherpetic. This form of ocular herpes affects about 1 in 700 people in the U.S.[10]

Stromal keratitis. Inflammation of a deeper layer of the cornea, the stroma, is more often associated with immune system issues; it can be quite serious, resulting in permanently blurred vision and blindness. It can manifest as a wide range of interrelated conditions. Some of these include interstitial keratitis (affecting spaces between cells), necrotizing keratitis, disciform keratitis (disc-shaped corneal swellings), and keratouveitis (uveitis predominates). Stromal keratitis develops in about 25% of those people who have epithelial keratitis.[11]

Recurrence. Recurrence of epithelial or stromal keratitis is 10% after 1 year, 23% after 2 years, and 50% after 10 years.[12]

Herpes Zoster Ophthalmicus

Like the herpes simplex 1 virus, the herpes zoster virus can cause an initial outbreak, or it can remain dormant in the body. If there is a recurrence, often triggered by emotional or environmental stress, not only the skin (shingles) but the cornea can be impacted. And, like the herpes keratitis, the epithelial or stroma layer can be affected.

Epithelial punctate. Epithelial erosions manifest with ulcers or lesions on the surface of the cornea.

Nummular keratitis. If the stroma layer is involved, it is called nummular keratitis, which occurs with granular deposits in the stroma layer, or **necrotising interstitial keratitis**, which occurs with leaking into the stroma, corneal thinning, and sometimes perforated cornea.[13]

Disciform keratitis. This form displays corneal edema, and it folds in the Descemet's membrane.[14]

Neurotropic. This form involves damage to the nerves in the cornea, causing corneal damage, thinning, and sometimes perforation.[15]

Iridocyclitis or anterior uveitis. These can develop from the zoster virus. Not only is the cornea affected, but also the deeper tissues of the iris is affected that causes severe light sensitivity, blurred vision, pain, and redness.

Signs and Symptoms

Many of the symptoms of ocular herpes are common to both types. These symptoms include:

- Pain in and around only one eye
- Redness and irritation
- Corneal swelling and cloudiness
- Small white itchy lesions or swellings on the cornea
- Recurring eye infections
- Conjunctivitis

There are a few other symptoms that help differentiate between the two forms.

Herpes Simplex Keratitis[16]

- A feeling of grit or dirt in the eye
- Tearing and discharge
- Pain, especially when looking at bright light
- Conjunctiva infection that heals without scarring

Herpes Zoster Ophthalmicus[17]

- Headache and fever
- Rash or sores on forehead, eyelids, around the eyes, and sometimes the tip of the nose
- Blurry vision

Causes and Risk Factors

Ocular herpes is caused by infection from others or self-infection from a cold sore. Because the virus can lie dormant for years, it may be inactive and then become active during times of stress, or when catalyzed by an event such as sunburn, exposure to toxins, general trauma to the eyes, and other situations. The elderly (and others who are immunocompromised) are prone to recurrence of a breakout and more serious effects, due to reduced ability to fight infection.

Here are some other possible risk factors:

- An imbalance in the ratio of the amino acids arginine and lysine in the body make people more vulnerable. People who have had ocular herpes should avoid arginine supplementation.[18] Lysine in the body helps fight the herpes infection, reducing both the recurring incidence rate and healing time.[19]
- Stress causes the immune system to be less effective and can cause an increase in the risk of outbreaks.[20] Certain lower immune factors can lead to a higher incidence of outbreaks.[21]
- Excess sugar increases the risk and severity of outbreaks, as it reduces our ability to fight infection.[22]

- In some cases, Bell's facial nerve palsy has been shown to have herpes simplex or herpes zoster as causative factors.[23] [24]
- Certain medications have been linked to ocular HSV reactivation, including beta-blockers, immunosuppressing drugs, particularly those with topical ocular corticosteroids, epinephrine, and prostaglandins. There is also a possible link to excimer laser treatment.[25]

Conventional Treatment

Treatment depends on the form of the condition. Initial treatment is with either topical eyedrops or oral antiviral medication, such as Viroptic (trifluridine, GlaxoSmithKline), which is the cornerstone of topical treatment for herpes simplex keratitis. Treatments typically last 1–2 weeks, depending on healing time. Eyedrops called corticosteroids can help control the disease, but they can also raise the pressure in the eyes for some people, in which case additional eyedrops may be prescribed along with the corticosteroids to keep the pupil dilated that helps prevent the eye pressure from increasing due to corticosteroids.

In certain less-common cases, intravenous medication may be necessary, using antiviral drugs such as Acyclovir, and more recently Valacyclovir, to suppress the reproduction of the virus. Multiple treatments with steroids may be required if the middle layer of the cornea (herpetic stromal keratitis), back layer of the cornea (herpetic endotheliitis), and/or the iris (herpetic iritis) are affected.

Herpetic iritis is also treated with aggressive steroid use, including hourly prednisolone acetate and cycloplegia as cornerstone therapies.

Complementary Approach

Consider the following recommendations in addition to your eye doctor's recommendations. These are particularly helpful in milder versions of an outbreak and help reduce the risk of additional outbreaks. Taking targeted antioxidants are important to help neutralize free radicals that result from inflammation, and certain natural eyedrops can help reduce the symptoms.

Nutrients

Essential

L-lysine (the L form is best absorbed). 1000mg–3000mg per day. L-lysine appears to be an effective agent for reduction of the occurrence, severity, and healing time for recurrent HSV infection.[26] Talk to your doctor about your proper dosage. It is considered safe, but high dosages might cause gallstones and renal dysfunction.[27] People with kidney or liver disease and pregnant women should consult their doctor before supplementing with lysine.

Curcumin (as highly absorbed phospholipid blend). 630mg daily. Curcumin may prevent corneal epithelial barrier-function disruption related to ocular inflammation.[28] It also inhibits proinflammatory cytokines (an increase in proinflammatory cytokines have been found in the tear film of dry eye patients)[29] that may possibly be due to chronic inflammation that contributes to dry eye syndrome and the onset of conjunctivitis.[30]

Licorice root. 450mg–900mg per day. Licorice has been shown to have antiviral properties.[31] [32] Licorice extract in liquid form is said to break the DNA chain of herpes, so that it cannot multiply.[33] If you have high blood pressure, consult your doctor before taking licorice.

A high-quality, natural immune-boosting formula. See Appendix 5 for product recommendations.

Very Important

Glutathione (GSH), reduced. 500mg–900mg per day. This is taken preferably in an intraoral or sublingual form, as glutathione is not absorbed well through the digestive system. Glutathione is one of the super antioxidants that neutralizes the full range of free radicals in the body. GSH levels decline in human eyes with age.[34] It is normally present in high levels in the ocular lens, cornea, aqueous humor, and retina, where it performs multiple roles, including maintaining normal tissue hydration and lens transparency and protecting against oxidative damage. Inflammation causes onset of free radicals. The sublingual form has 5–10 times greater absorption so the dosage will be smaller. Follow label instructions.

Lutein. 6mg–20mg per day. Lutein is identified by researchers as having therapeutic potential in managing uveitis, inflammatory eye conditions, and dry eye.[35] [36] Multiple animal studies on the neuroprotective effects of lutein against retinal neural damage that is caused by inflammation in endotoxin-induced uveitis (EIU) have shown that lutein has a dose-dependent anti-inflammatory effect on EIU.[37] [38]

Trans-resveratrol. 175mg per day. This potent antioxidant helps protect nerve cells from damage,[39] reduces oxidative damage,[40] and supports a healthy inflammatory response.[41]

MSM capsules. 2,000mg per day, split up with meals or with water. MSM helps nourish and strengthen body tissues and has natural anti-inflammatory properties.[42]

Helpful

Bilberry. 180mg–240mg per day. Bilberry is neuroprotective and has been shown to improve microcirculation.[43] [44] [45] [46]

Omega-3 fatty acids. 2,000mg–3,000mg per day. These essential nutrients for retinal health have anti-inflammatory properties,[47] or take **DHA** (one of the omega-3 fatty acids, 1000mg daily).

Homeopathic eyedrops. Choose those that have anti-inflammatory properties, including those that contain the following homeopathic elements:

- Nat mur
- Rhus tox
- Graphitis
- Sulph or hepar sulph

Antivirals. These include wild oregano oil (150mg–300mg per day, based on your healthcare practitioner's recommendations), monolaurin capsules (300mg–600mg per day, also as advised by your medical provider), coconut oil (1–4 tablespoons per day, use in cooking, frying, baking, or in smoothies), and camu powder (1 tablespoon per day, mixed with juice, smoothies, or yogurt).

Anti-inflammatory/anti-scar tissue supplements. These include bromelain or proteolytic enzymes like Zygest.

Toxin absorption supplements. King chlorella absorbs the toxins released by dying herpes virus.

Diet

Diet can be an important way to help manage ocular herpes and reduce the intensity of the outbreak. Overconsumption of sugar and refined carbohydrates that have been shown to lower one's immune system, tend to favor viruses. Chronic stress also reduces one's ability to fight infections. Identify and avoid foods and/or chemicals to which you may be allergic.

Follow the Vision diet in Chapter 7.

A potential risk factor for ocular herpes outbreaks is an imbalance in the ratio between the essential amino acids L-lysine and arginine. Arginine, only essential under certain conditions, is necessary for the herpes virus (HSV) to grow. Reducing one's consumption of foods high in l-Arginine, such as cashews, chocolate, peanuts, and almonds can be helpful. Lysine has been shown to block the activity leading to HSV development. Supplementing with lysine, or consuming foods with higher ratios of lysine to arginine, such as organic yogurts and cheeses, may prove helpful for combating outbreaks.

For those who do not eat animal products, higher ratios of lysine to arginine can be found in papaya, beets, mango, apricot, pears, figs, and avocado.

Juicing. We recommend juicing with some combination of the following foods, along with your favorite fruits and vegetables:

- Celery, cabbage, carrot, leafy-green vegetables, blueberries, cherries, other berries, garlic, parsley, dandelion greens, lemons, pomegranate, ground flaxseeds, and raw honey.
- Try to use room temperature vegetables and fruit.
- Do not add ice or very cold liquids since cold foods and liquids will eventually extinguish the stomach's digestive fire.
- Do not juice as often during the cooler months of the year, and instead, switch to vegetable soups or stews.

Lifestyle

Try to maintain a low stress life. Daily meditation, prayer, daily walks in the park, regular low-stress exercise—all can help reduce the reoccurrence rate.

Other Modalities

Chinese Medicine

From a Chinese medical perspective, blistering and erosion of genital tissue, plus burning and itching are the key symptoms of the pattern of "damp heat." Overconsumption of candy and sugar that promote the formation of active damp heat, precipitates outbreaks. Poor dietary habits, including the eating of hot and spicy foods, heavy and greasy foods, and alcohol, all lead to recurrent outbreaks.

The leading Chinese herbal formula to treat this pattern is *damp heat clearing* (long dan xie gan wan).

See Also

Chapter 7, Vision Diet

Chapter 8, Nutrients

Chapter 15-31, Uveitis

1 Clinicaltrials.gov. Herpetic Eye Disease Study (HEDS) I. Retrieved Feb 10 2018 from https://clinicaltrials.gov/ct2/show/NCT00000138.

[2] White, M.E., Chodosh, J. (2014). Herpes Simplex Virus Keratitis: A Treatment Guideline - 2014. *American Academy of Ophthalmology*, Jun. Retrieved Apr 27 2018 from https://www.aao.org/clinical-statement/herpes-simplex-virus-keratitis-treatment-guideline.

[3] Kelley, P.W., Petruccelli, B.P., Stehr-Green, P., Erickson, R.L., Mason, C.J. (1991). The susceptibility of young adult Americans to vaccine-preventable infections. A national serosurvey of US Army recruits. *JAMA*, 226(19):2724.

4 Opstelten, W., Zaal, M.J. (2005). Managing ophthalmic herpes zoster in primary care. *BMJ*, Jul 16; 331(7509): 147–151.

[5] Tran, K.D., Falcone, M.M., Choi, D.S., Goldhardt, R., Karp, C.L., et al. (2016). Epidemiology of Herpes Zoster Ophthalmicus: Recurrence and Chronicity. *Ophthalmology*, Jul;123(7):1469-1476.

[6] Wikipedia. Herpes simplex keratitis. Retrieved Apr 27 2018 from https://en.wikipedia.org/wiki/Herpes_simplex_keratitis.

[7] Wikipedia. Herpes zoster ophthalicus. Retrieved Apr 27 2018 from https://en.wikipedia.org/wiki/Herpes_zoster_ophthalmicus.

[8] Ibid. White. (2014).

[9] Ibid. White. (2014).

10 Right Diagnosis. Statistics about Ocular Herpes. Retrieved Feb 10 2018 from http://www.rightdiagnosis.com/o/ocular_herpes/stats.htm

11 Ibid. Right Diagnosis. Statistics about Ocular Herpes.

12 Barker, N.H. (2008). Ocular herpes simplex. *BMJ Clin Evid*, 23;2008. pii: 0707.

[13] Ibid. Wikipedia. Herpes zoster ophthalmicus.

[14] Ibid. Wikipedia. Herpes zoster ophthalmicus.

[15] Ibid. Wikipedia. Herpes zoster ophthalmicus.

[16] WebMD. Introduction to Herpes and the Eye. Retrieved Apr 27 2018 from https://www.webmd.com/genital-herpes/guide/eye-herpes#1.

[17] Ibid. WebMD. Introduction to Herpes and the Eye.

[18] Moore, S. (2017). Cold Sores from L-Arginine. Retrieved Mar 30 2018 from https://www.livestrong.com/article/197872-cold-sores-from-l-arginine/.

[19] Griffith, R.S., Walsh, D.E., Myrmel, K.H., Thompson, R.W., Behforooz, A. (1987). Success of L-lysine therapy in frequently recurrent herpes simplex infection. Treatment and prophylaxis. *Dermatologica,* 175(4):183-90.

[20] WebMD. (1999). Long-Term Stress May Trigger Herpes Outbreaks. Retrieved Mar 30 2018 from https://www.webmd.com/balance/stress-management/news/19991111/long-term-stress-trigger-herpes-outbreaks#1

[21] Seppanen, M., Meri, S., Notkola, I.L., Seppala, I.J.T., Hiltunen-Back, E., et al. (2006). Subtly Impaired Humoral Immunity Predisposes to Frequently Recurring Genital Herpes Simplex Virus Type 2 Infection and Herpetic Neuralgia. *J Infect Dis,* Sep;194(5):571-78.

[22] WebMD. Six Immune System Busters & Boosters. Retrieved Mar 30 2018 from https://www.webmd.com/cold-and-flu/cold-guide/10-immune-system-busters-boosters#1.

[23] Murakami, S., Mizobuchi, M., Nakashiro, Y., et al. (1996). Bell palsy and herpes simplex virus: identification of viral DNA in endoneurial fluid and muscle. *Ann Intern Med,* Jan 1;124(1 Pt 1):27-30.

[24] Furuta, Y., Ohtani, F., Chida, E., et al. (2001). Herpes simplex virus type 1 reactivation and antiviral therapy in patients with acute peripheral facial palsy. *Auris Nasus Larynx,* May;28 Suppl:S13-7.

[25] [No authors listed] Herpetic Eye Disease Study Group. Predictors of recurrent herpes simplex virus keratitis. *Cornea,* Mar;20(2):123-8.

[26] Griffith, R.S., Walsh, D.E., Myrmel, K.H., Thompson, R.W., Behforooz, A. (1987). Success of L-lysine therapy in frequently recurrent herpes simplex infection. Treatment and prophylaxis. *Dermatologica,* 175(4):183-90.

[27] Verzola, D., Fama, A., Villaggio, B., Di Rocco, M., Simonato, A., et al. (2012). Lysine triggers apoptosis through a NADPH oxidase-dependent mechanism in human renal tubular cells. *J Inherit Metab Dis,* Nov;35(6):1011-9.

[28] Kimura, K. (2010). Molecular mechanism of the disruption of barrier function in cultured human corneal epithelial cells induced by tumor necrosis factor-alpha, a proinflammatory cytokine. *Nippon Ganka Gakkai Zasshi,* Nov; 114(11):935-43.

[29] Solomon, A., Dursun, D., Liu, Z., Xie, Y., Macri, A., et al. (2001). Pro- and anti-inflammatory forms of interleukin-1 in the tear fluid and conjunctiva of patients with dry-eye disease. *Invest Ophthalmol Vis Sci,* Sep; 42(10):2283-92.

[30] Chung, S.H., Choi, S.H., Choi, J.A., Chuck, R.S., Joo, C.K. (2012). Curcumin suppresses ovalbumin-induced allergic conjunctivitis. *Mol Vis,* 18:1966-72.

[31] Fiore, C., Eisenhut, M., Krausse, R., Ragazzi, E., Pellati, D., et al. (2008). Antiviral effects of Glycyrrhiza species. *Phytother Res,* Feb; 22(2):141-8.

[32] Ghannad, M.S., Mohammadi, A., Safiallahy, S., Faradmal, J., Azizi, M., et al. (2014). The Effect of Aqueous Extract of Glycyrrhiza glabra on Herpes Simplex Virus 1. *Junidshapur J Microbiol,* Jul;7(7):e11616.

[33] Ibid. Ghannad. (2014).

[34] Harding, J.J. (1970). Free and protein-bound glutathione in normal and cataractous human lenses. *Biochem J,* May; 117(5):957-60.

[35] Chao, S.C., Vagaggini, T., Nien, C.W., Huang, S.C., Lin, H.Y. (2015). Effects of Lutein and Zeaxanthin on LPS-induced Secretion of IL-8 by Uveal Melanocytes and Relevant Signal Pathways. J Ophthalmol. 2015:152854.

[36] Chao, S.C., Nien, C.W., Iacob, C., Hu, D.N., Huang, S.C., et al. (2016). Effects of Lutein on Hyperosmoticity-Induced Upregulation of IL-6 in Cultured Corneal Epithelial Cells and Its Relevant Signal Pathways. J Ophthalmol. 2016:8341439.

[37] Sasaki, M., Ozawa, Y., Kurihara, T., Noda, K., Imamura, Y., et al. (2009). Neuroprotective effect of an antioxidant, lutein, during retinal inflammation. *Invest Ophthalmol Vis Sci.* Mar; 50(3):1433-9.

[38] Jin, X.H., Ohgami, K., Shiratori, K., Suzuki, Y., Hirano, T., et al. (2006). Inhibitory effects of lutein on endotoxin-induced uveitis in Lewis rats. *Invest Ophthalmol Vis Sci,* Jun; 47(6):2562-8.

[39] Anekonda, T.S., Adamus, G. (2008). Resveratrol prevents antibody-induced apoptotic death of retinal cells through upregulation of Sirt1 and Ku70. *BMC Res Notes,* Dec 1;1:122.

[40] Perecko, T., Jancinova, V., Drabikova, K., Nosal, R., Harmatha, J. (2008). Structure-efficiency relationship in derivatives of stilbene. Comparison of resveratrol, pinosylvin and pterostilbene. *Neuro Endocrinol Lett,* Oct;29(5):802-5.

[41] Ghadiri, S. E., Arbabi-Aval, M., Rezaei, K.M., Ahmadieh, H. (2015). Anti-inflammatory properties of resveratrol in the retinas of type 2 diabetic rats. *Clin Exp Pharmacol Physiol,* Jan;42(1):63-8.

[42] Butawan, M., Benjamin, R.L., Bloomer, R.J. (2017). Methylsulfonylmethane: Applications and Safety of a Novel Dietary Supplement. *Nutrients,* Mar; 9(3): 290.

43 Matsunaga, N., Imai, S., Inokuchi, Y., Shimazawa, M., Yokota, S., et al. (2009). Bilberry and its main constituents have neuroprotective effects against retinal neuronal damage in vitro and in vivo. *Mol Nutr Food Res,* Jul;53(7):869-77.

44 Zhu, Y., Xia, M., Yang, Y., Liu, F., Li, Z., et al. (2011). Purified anthocyanin supplementation improves endothelial function via NO-cGMP activation in hypercholesterolemic individuals. *Clin Chem,* Nov;57(11):1524-33.

45 Yao, Y., Vieira, A. (2007). Protective activities of Vaccinium antioxidants with potential relevance to mitochondrial dysfunction and neurotoxicity. *Neurotoxicology,* Jan;28(1):93-100.

46 Cohen-Boulakia, F., Valensi, P.E., Boulahdour, H., Lestrade, R. Dufour-Lamarinie, J.F., et al. (2000). In vivo sequential study of skeletal muscle capillary permeability in diabetic rats: effect of anthocyanosides. *Metabolism,* Jul;49(7):880-5.

47 Udell, I.J., Abelson, M.B. (1983). Chemical mediators of inflammation. *Int Ophthalmol Clin,* 23:1:15-26.

16-5. OCULAR ROSACEA

Ocular rosacea is an inflammation of the white of the eye caused by immune system weakness. It can also affect the cornea and usually develops only in the eyes. It appears in combination with the skin version of rosacea in 20% of facial rosacea patients.

Rosacea is fairly common and is experienced by as many of 10% of adults, especially people with fair skin and light-colored hair and eyes. More than half of these patients also have ocular rosacea and/or related problems, such as blepharitis and conjunctivitis.[1] Ocular rosacea primarily affects people between ages 30 and 60. Women who are going through menopause are also vulnerable to ocular rosacea, as is anyone with a tendency toward flushing or blushing. Consequently, women tend to experience ocular rosacea twice as often as men.

What is Ocular Rosacea?

The cornea is the lens in front of the eyes that does most of the refracting of light to the retina, and it is separated by a thin opaque layer called the sclera (also referred to as the white of the eyes). The sclera contains connective tissue and is continuous with the stroma layer of the cornea. Ocular redness caused by ocular rosacea is due to inflammation of the sclera that can extend to, and damage, the cornea.

This condition is caused by inherent defects in the body's immune system and vasoregulatory processes (related to vessels in the body that carry blood and lymph fluid, particularly arteries and veins). Usually the condition develops only in the eyes, but sometimes it is experienced in combination with the skin version of rosacea. Ocular rosacea can also affect the cornea of your eye, especially if you have dry eyes. It affects roughly 20% of facial rosacea patients.

Pathology

Researchers suspect that ocular rosacea derives from a mix of immune system and vascular irregularities and weaknesses.[2] Increased eyelid bacteria produce several fatty or waxy substances[3] that, in turn, cause increased levels of toxic biochemicals that irritate the cornea and surfaces adjacent to the cornea.[4]

In the healthy eye, oily meibum covers the surface of the cornea, helping to slow evaporation of tears. But increased toxic and irritating biochemicals (proinflammatory cytokine and matrix metalloproteinase) cause the meibum to thicken that in turn reduces its ability to protect the tear film.[5] In this way, the process toward chronic inflammation reinforces itself.[6] Chronic inflammation in turn, suppresses meibomian gland function that further reinforces development of ocular rosacea,[7] not to mention dry eye syndrome.

Microscopic demodex mite infection also develops. Demodex brevis lives in the meibomian glands. Demodex folliculorum specializes in the area around the eyelids and eyelashes where it feeds on skin cells and increases the number of skin cells on the surface of the eyelash.[8] To further the self-reinforcing cycle of dysfunction, these mites carry bacteria that stimulate enzymes that degrade cellular proteins.[9]

Forty percent of ocular rosacea patients also develop damage to the outer protective epithelium layer of the cornea. Damage takes the form of pinpoint indentations called punctate epithelial erosions that by themselves cause redness, irritation, and light sensitivity.[10] Other corollary corneal conditions include corneal ulcers, edema, keratitis, scarring, corneal thinning, neovascularization, stem cell deficiencies, and cell death.[11]

Sign and Symptoms

The following ocular rosacea symptoms are most related to, and include, the symptoms of blepharitis, conjunctivitis, and dry eye syndrome.[12]

- Eye redness of conjunctiva, sclera, and/or eyelids
- Dry eyes
- Itching, burning, irritation of eyelids and surface of the eye
- Blurred vision
- Sensitivity to light
- Tearing
- Recurring instances of blepharitis, conjunctivitis, or dry eye syndrome

Signs that your eye doctor will identify include:

- Clogged meibomian glands
- Growth of new blood vessels in the cornea[13]
- Capillary leakage, resulting in corneal scarring and loss of transparency[14]
- There are a number of other conditions that can occur along with ocular rosacea, sometimes as an apparent cause or result of the ocular inflammation. These can include a number of other conditions, such as:
  - Styes or chalazia
  - Eye infections such as iritis and episcleritis
  - Corneal or scleral ulcers and perforations
  - Conjunctivitis

Causes and Risk Factors

- Blocked meibomian glands that lie along the base of the eyelashes
- Demodex mites along the base of the eyelashes
- Bacterial involvement
- Environmental irritants

- Heredity
- Hot baths and saunas
- Strenuous exercise
- Hot spicy foods
- Exposure to sunlight and hot weather
- Medications such as cortisone creams and drugs

Conventional Treatment

Conventional medicine offers no "cure" for ocular rosacea. Doctors may prescribe:
- Oral antibiotics for severe cases, such as tetracycline, doxycycline, cyclosporine, erythromycin, and minocycline
- Retinoids, vitamin A derivatives that suppress sebum production
- Immunomodulators that decrease the immune response
- Temporary use of oral corticosteroids that reduce inflammation
- Artificial tears to reduce associated dry eye symptoms
- A lid hygiene protocol, such as a diluted solution of tea tree oil, used once or twice daily along the eyelid margins and where there is facial rosacea

Complementary Approach

As ocular rosacea may be aggravated or caused by an overactive immune response, we suggest addressing the chronic inflammation of ocular rosacea through targeted supplementation, an alkaline diet, overall corneal health, healthy eye lubrication, and paying attention to eyelid health through warm compresses and lid scrubs.

Nutrients

Essential

Black currant seed oil. 500mg per day with a meal. In one study, black currant seed supports increased prostaglandin (a fatty compound with hormone-like effects). PGE1 is a prostaglandin that both stimulates aqueous tear secretion and reduces the production of another prostaglandin, PGE2 that causes inflammation that contributes to dry eyes.[15]

Turmeric (curcumin). 500mg–800mg per day with a meal. Curcumin is generally effective as an anti-inflammatory nutrient. In animal models, curcumin has been found in the sclera, and it has been shown to help reduce inflammation.[16] It also has been found to reduce matrix metalloproteinases, one of the irritant biochemicals produced in excess by bacteria on the eyelid that causes the meibum to thicken.[17]

MSM capsules. 2,000mg per day, split up with meals or with water. MSM helps nourish and strengthen body tissues and has natural anti-inflammatory properties.[18] Combined with silymarin, it has been found to be helpful in treating skin rosacea[19] and may be beneficial for ocular rosacea.

Omega-3 fatty acids. 2,000mg–3,000mg per day. Omega-3s have anti-inflammatory properties.[20] One of the omega-3s, **DHA** (1000mg daily), can be substituted. Generally, DHA increases mitochondrial activity and has antioxidative, anti-inflammatory, anti-apoptotic, and anti-angiogenic effects.[21] It has been found to be helpful in protecting the corneal epithelium after surgery.[22] In rosacea patients who also had dry eye symptoms, omega-3s in the diet for three to six months improved the condition significantly.[23]

Glutathione (GSH), reduced. 500mg–900mg per day. This is taken preferably in an intraoral or sublingual form, as glutathione is not absorbed well through the digestive system. The sublingual form has 5–10 times greater absorption so the dosage will be smaller. Follow label instructions. Glutathione is a key component of the antioxidant system of the cornea, ciliary body, sclera, and iris of the eye,[24] where it is normally present in high levels.[25] GSH levels are noted to be low in lab animals with corneal epithelium wound issues.[26] It may be important in preventing more serious corneal damage in ocular rosacea cases.[27] In an animal model, eyedrops containing glutathione were effective in treating corneal neovascularization.[28]

Very Important

Calendula. This is good for healing the cornea and can be taken as a tea or tincture (follow directions on the bottle).

Helpful

Ginger. 1,000mg–2,000mg per day. Ginger is a member of a plant family that includes cardamom and turmeric. Ginger has strong antioxidant properties,[29] reduces oxidative stress,[30] and decreases inflammation and swelling.[31]

Bilberry. 180mg–240mg per day. Bilberry is neuroprotective and has been shown to improve microcirculation.[32] [33] [34]

Diet

Drink plenty of water throughout the day.

Food choices play a key role in controlling all forms of rosacea. The following foods can trigger a rosacea flare-up, and therefore, possibly contribute to ocular rosacea.[35]

- Spicy foods
- Very hot soups or beverages
- Broad-leaf beans and pods, including lima, navy, or pea
- Dairy products like yogurt or sour cream
- Chocolate
- Some citrus fruits
- Foods high in histamine such as cheese (except cottage cheese), eggplant, spinach, vinegar, and soy sauce

Juicing. Juicing is a good way to deliver nutrients to your body. Here are suggested foods for people with rosacea. You can select from any combination of these, plus add your favorite fruits and vegetables.

- Celery, carrot, leafy-green vegetables, blueberries, cherries, other berries, parsley, watermelon, lemons, bananas, ginger, avocado, coconut, and lemon
- Try to use room temperature vegetables and fruit.
- Do not add ice or very cold liquids since cold foods and liquids will eventually extinguish the stomach's digestive fire.
- Do not juice as often during the cooler months of the year, and instead, switch to vegetable soups or stews.

Lifestyle

- Keep your eyelids clean by gently washing them daily.
- Try commercially prepared lid wipes and/or, incorporate a very dilute solution of tea tree oil, once or twice daily along the eyelid.
- Temporarily suspend wearing contact lenses while you have the condition.
- Avoid rubbing your eyes.
- Use a warm, wet washcloth as a compress, holding it in place until it cools. Repeat this several times a day.
- While at your computer, take frequent breaks, and don't forget to blink.
- Use a humidifier at home. Dry eye syndrome is a common problem for those with ocular rosacea. Keeping the air moist at home, along with regular use of preservative free eyedrops, can help reduce dry eye symptoms, and possibly avoid further complications due to chronic dry eyes.
- Make sure your eye makeup is non-toxic and non-irritating, preferably organic, and remove all makeup at night.
- Wear 100% UVA/UVB protecting sunglasses (preferably wrap-around sunglasses with either amber or brown lenses) when outdoors.

Other Modalities

Chinese Medicine

In Chinese medicine, the Kidneys control the endocrine system that includes immune response. Overactive chronic immune response, such as shown in autoimmune diseases, can be attributed to excess yang (heat) in the body. Supporting the yin (anti-inflammatory benefits) helps balance the excess yang and helps reduce overall inflammation.

Common Patent Formulas

Ming mu di huang wan. Rehmannia pills "to brighten the eyes" address the following patterns: Liver blood deficiency, Kidney yin deficiency, and Liver yin deficiency.

Preserve vistas pill. Zhu jing wan tonifies and nourishes the Liver and Kidneys, enriches the yin, and improves vision.

Your acupuncturist/herbalist can best determine which formulas are best for you.

Exercises

Yoga and qi gong are excellent exercise modalities for supporting the free flow of energy in the body. They can also help reduce chronic inflammation.

Also See

Chapter 8, Nutrients

[1] Weidmayer, S. (2015). Seeing Red: How Ocular Rosacea Impacts the Cornea. Retrieved Apr 30 2018 from https://www.reviewofoptometry.com/article/seeing-red-how-ocular-rosacea-impacts-the-cornea.

[2] Donaldson, K.E., Karp, C.L., Dunbar, M.T. (2007). Evaluation and treatment of children with ocular rosacea. *Cornea*, 26(1):42-6.

[3] Ta, C.N., Shine, W.E., McCulley, J.P., et al. (2003). Effects of minocycline on the ocular flora of patients with acne rosacea or seborrheic blepharitis. *Cornea*, 22(6):545-8.

[4] Dougherty, J.M., McCulley, J.P. (1986). Bacterial Lipases and Chronic Blepharitis. *Invest Ophthalmol Vis Sci*, 27(4):486-91.

[5] Mastrota K. (2009). Ocular surface disease. Optometric Management. Retrieved Nov 14 2017 from www.optometricmanagement.com/printarticle.aspx?articleID=102974.

[6] Onaran, Z., Karabulut, A.A., Usta, G., Örnek, K. (2012). Central corneal thickness in patients with mild to moderate rosacea. *Can J Ophthalmol*, 47(6):504-8.

[7] Kharod-Dholakia, B. (2017). Ocular Rosacea. *Medscape*, Apr 7.

[8] Leonard, J. (2017). What is Demodox brevis? *Med News Today*. Retrieved Apr 30 2018 from https://www.medicalnewstoday.com/articles/320159.php.

[9] Wikipedia. Matrix metalloproteinase. Retrieved Apr 30 2018 from https://en.wikipedia.org/wiki/Matrix_metalloproteinase.

[10] Wikipedia. Punctate opithelial erosions. Retrieved Apr 30 2018 from https://en.wikipedia.org/wiki/Punctate_epithelial_erosions.

[11] Ibid. Weidmayer. (2015).

12 Quarterman, M.J., Johnson, D.W., Abele, D.C., Lesher, J.L., Hull, D.S., et al. (1997). Ocular rosacea. Signs, symptoms, and tear studies before and after treatment with doxycycline. *Arch Dermatol*, Jan;133(1):49-54.

[13] Ghanem VC, Mehra N, Wong S, Mannis M. (2003). The prevalence of ocular signs in acne rosacea. Cornea. 22(3):230-3.

[14] Ibid. Weidmayer. (2015).

15 Baudouin C. (2001). Dry eye: an unexpected inflammatory disease. *Arch Soc Esp Oftalmol*, Apr;76(4):205-6.

[16] Zhang, J., Zhou, N., Zhang, B., Ma, J. (2018). Effect of Biodegradable Scleral Plugs Containing Curcumin on Proliferative Vitreoretinopathy. *Ophthalmic Res*, 59(1):30-36.

[17] Zhang, Y., Gu, Y., Lee, H.M., Hambardjieva, E., Vrankova, K., et al. (2012). Design, synthesis and biological activity of new polyenolic inhibitors of matrix metalloproteinases: a focus on chemically-modified curcumins. *Curr Med Chem*, 19(25):4348-58.

18 Butawan, M., Benjamin, R.L., Bloomer, R.J. (2017). Methylsulfonylmethane: Applications and Safety of a Novel Dietary Supplement. *Nutrients*, Mar;9(3): 290.

[19] Berardesca, E., Cameli, N., Cavollotti, C, Levy, J.L., Pierard, G.E., et al. (2008). Combined effects of silymarin and methylsulfonylmethane in the management of rosacea: clinical and instrumental evaluation. *J Cosmet Dermatol*, Mar;7(1):8-14.

20 Udell, I.J., Abelson, M.B. (1983). Chemical mediators of inflammation. *Int Ophthalmol Clin*, 23:1:15-26.

21 SanGiovanni, J.P., Chew, E.Y. (2005). The role of omega-3 long-chain polyunsaturated fatty acids in health and disease of the retina. *Prog Retin Eye Res*, 24(1): 87-138.

22 Kenchegowda, S., He, J., Bazan, H.E. (2013). Involvement of pigment epithelium-derived factor, docosahexaenoic acid and neuroprotectin D1 in corneal inflammation and nerve integrity after refractive surgery. *Prostaglandins Leukot Essent Fatty Acids*, Jan;88)1):27-31.

23 Bhargava, R., Chandra, M., Bansal, U., Singh, D., Ranjan, S., et al. (2016). A Randomized Controlled Trial of Omega 3 Fatty Acids in Rosacea Patients with Dry Eye Symptoms. *Curr Eye Res*, Oct;41(10):1274-1280.

24 Bogdanova, I.A., Gerasimov, A.M., Komarov, O.S. (1987). Glutathione: dehydroascorbate oxidoreductase activity in rabbit eye tissues. *Vopr Med Khim*, May-Jun;33(3):104-7.

25 Kolin, C., Reichi, S. (2016). Expression of glutathione transferases in corneal cell lines, corneal tissues and a human cornea construct. Int J Pharm, Jun 15;506(1-2):371-81.

26 Zhang, Z., Hu, X., Qi, X., Di, G., Zhang, Y., et al. (2018). Resolvin D1 promotes corneal epithelial wound healing and restoration of mechanical sensation in diabetic mice. *Mol Vis*, Apr 1;24:274-285.

27 Yogananarajah, V., Li, B., Umapathy, A., Donaldson, P.J., Lim, J.C. (2017). Regional differences in glutathione accumulation pathways in the rat cornea: Mapping of amino acid transporters involved in glutathione synthesis. *Exp Eye Res*, Aug;161:89-100.

28 Oquido, A.P.M.T., Hohmann, M.S.N., Pinho-Ribeiro, F.A., Crespigio, J., Domiciano, T.P., et al. (2017). Naringenin Eye Drops Inhibit Corneal Neovascularization by Anti-Inflammatory and Antioxidant Mechanisms. *Invest Ophthalmol Vis Sci*, Nov 1;58(13):5764-5776.

29 Ahmad, N., Katiyar, S.K., Mukhtar, H. (2001). Antioxidants in chemoprevention of skin cancer. *Curr Probl Dermatol*, 29:128–39.

30 Topic, B., Tani, E., Tsiakitzis, K., Kourounakis, P.N., Dere, E., et al. (2002). Enhanced maze performance and reduced oxidative stress by combined extracts of zingiber officinale and ginkgo biloba in the aged rat. *Neurobiol Aging*, 23(1):135–43.

31 Young, H.Y., Luo, Y.L., Cheng, H.Y., Hsieh, W.C., Liao, J.C., et al. (2005). Analgesic and anti-inflammatory activities of [6]-gingerol. *J Ethnopharmacol*, 96(1-2):207–10.

32 Matsunaga, N., Imai, S., Inokuchi, Y., Shimazawa, M., Yokota, S., et al. (2009). Bilberry and its main constituents have neuroprotective effects against retinal neuronal damage in vitro and in vivo. *Mol Nutr Food Res*, Jul;53(7):869-77.

33 Yao, Y., Vieira, A. (2007). Protective activities of Vaccinium antioxidants with potential relevance to mitochondrial dysfunction and neurotoxicity. *Neurotoxicology*, 28 93-100.

34 Zhu, Y., Xia, M., Yang, Y., Liu, F., Li, Z., et al. (2011). Purified anthocyanin supplementation improves endothelial function via NO-cGMP activation in hypercholesterolemic individuals. *Clin Chem*, Nov;57(11):1524-33.

35 Everyday Health. Are Diet and Alternative Treatments Effective for Rosacea? Retrieved Apr 30 2018 from https://www.everydayhealth.com/rosacea/experts-are-diet-and-alternative-treatments-effective.aspx.

16-6. PTOSIS

Ptosis (also called blepharoptosis) occurs when eyes are open and the eyelid droops below normal level. It may affect one or both lids and may be constant or intermittent. Often referred to as droopy eyelid, it may affect daily living, due to the interference of the eyelid over the eyes. One study in England shows that 11.5% of people over 50 years of age have some signs of ptosis.[1]

How Ptosis Affects You

This condition causes people to raise their eyebrows or tilt their head back in order to see properly. This results in a sore forehead or sore neck muscles.[2] Since the eyelids do not close properly, ptosis may result in dry eye, because the process of blinking coats the surface of one's eye with nourishing tear film. You should frequently use preservative-free natural eyedrops throughout the day, and if necessary, use a thick ointment in your eye at night, to prevent severe dryness that could lead to corneal scarring.

About the Eyelid

The levator muscle, along with the superior rectus muscle, controls movement of the eyelid. The levator palpebrae superioris (elevating muscle of the upper eyelid) arises on the bone behind the eyebrow and continues forward to the eyelid. It is comprised of smooth muscle layers (called the levator aponeurosis) at the thinner end of the eyelid.[3] When the levator muscle contracts, it raises and retracts the eyelid,[4] and the layers of the levator aponeurosis pull on eyelid fat pads and skin.

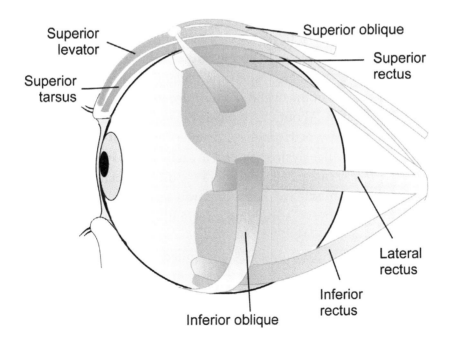

Damage to the levator muscle or inadequate messaging from the nervous system causes the muscle to be unable to function properly. Damage to or loss of nervous-system connection to other muscles near the levator muscle can also affect vision. These include the superior rectus muscle and the superior tarsal muscle.

The tarsal muscle (also known as the Mueller's muscle) adjoins the levator muscle and helps raise the upper eyelid; it accounts for 1–2mm of eyelid rise.[5] The rectus muscle turns the eye up and down.

Types and Causes of Ptosis

Congenital ptosis. In children, ptosis is usually the result of developmental failure of the levator muscle of the eyelid. It may occur in association with dysfunction of the superior rectus muscle, and it accounts for about 10% of all ptosis cases. Almost 15% of children with amblyopia have ptosis.[6] Some children with amblyopia and ptosis may need surgery.[7] Twenty percent of children with strabismus also have ptosis.[8] A DNA variant has been found in several children with congenital ptosis.[9]

Acquired ptosis develops later in life due to aging or associated conditions.

- **Age-related**. Sixty percent of all cases of ptosis are associated with stretching or dehiscence (wound damage from a surgical procedure) of the levator aponeurosis.[10] Another cause that may arise due to aging is enophthalmos, which is the change in eyeball socket (orbit) bone loss. This affects placement of the eyeball within the orbit. In one long-term study conducted over 6 to 24 years, researchers found that most patients with ptosis also had enophthalmos.[11]
- **Trauma-related**. About 11% of ptosis cases arise due to physical damage to the eyelid from injury. Most cases of ptosis in young adults are trauma-related.[12]
- **Mechanical**. Physical changes, such as swelling and increased weight due to inflammation or tumors of the eyelid, account for 9% of ptosis instances.
- **Nervous system-related**. About 6% of ptosis cases are due to nervous system conditions, such as third-nerve palsy or Horner syndrome.[13] Ptosis of one or both eyes is often the first symptom of muscular dystrophy and myasthenia gravis; ptosis eventually becomes evident in 95% of these cases. Bell's palsy is a condition that affects the nerves of your face, and this may result in muscle weakness or paralysis of eyelid muscles. Any condition that affects the third cranial nerve, supplying information to the eyelid muscles, will be linked to ptosis.
- **Muscle-related**. Four percent of cases are linked to weak muscles or deterioration of muscle tissue. Muscle paralysis due to stroke can cause ptosis.
- **Contact lens**. One study, evaluating 286 sets of identical twins, found that people wearing soft (1.41mm droop) or hard (1.84mm droop) contact lenses were more likely to develop ptosis.[14] [15] Another study of 98 patients found that hard contact-lens wear was a contributing factor, and that duration of wear increased the severity of ptosis.[16] And a third study found that one-third of young adults with ptosis wore soft contact lenses.[17]

- **Medication**. Prostaglandin analogues used to treat glaucoma or used cosmetically to increase eyelash length, such as Latisse (bimatoprost 0.03%), affect the metabolism of fat cells and cause them to shrink. The result is mild enophthalmus and ptosis.[18]

Pseudoptosis is a related condition in which the droopiness is caused by excess eyelid skin and/or fat, rather than any weakness of eyelid muscles.

Conventional Treatment

If recommended by your eye doctor, ptosis surgery to repair eyelid muscles that have stretched due to aging is accomplished through tightening the muscle and sometimes removing excess fat. If the muscle is weak, then tightening it won't help, and a procedure called a frontalis suspension is often used in which silicon strands are added and tightened to raise the eyelid by raising and lowering the eyebrows.[19] [20]

This surgery is not an exact science, and the final position of the eyelid depends upon how the tissue heals; sometimes, additional surgery is needed for adjustment. Ptosis surgery can decrease the amount and quality of tears supplying the essential tear film, resulting in dry eyes.[21] Ptosis surgery can also impact the topography of the cornea that contributes to the quality of vision and requires corrective action.[22]

Complementary Approach

A complementary approach that supports overall health and muscle integrity may be helpful.

Nutrients

Helpful

Adrenal supporting formula helps the adrenals and "raises energy to the eyes" (see VisionBoost Formula in Appendix 5).

Vitamin A (palmitate), 5,000 IU–15,000 IU per day is recommended, but not for pregnant women or women trying to become pregnant, as safe levels have not been properly determined.

> **Note**. Vitamin A is contra-indicated for those suffering from Stargardt disease (see Stargardt's chapter for more information.)

Whole-food, organic multivitamins.

Vitamin B12 with vitamin **B6** and **zinc.** These help restore proper function related to Bell's palsy. Dosages can vary, based on the severity of the symptoms.

Vitamin B1 and **B6** were used in a case study. It reported a child with leukemia that had ptosis in both eyes (caused by the cancer drugs). Treatment with 5mg thiamine (B1) and 10mg pyridoxine (B6) resulted in complete recovery from the ptosis after four weeks.[23]

Lids by Design is a new inexpensive home procedure that can be quickly effective in helping with Ptosis (see Appendix Chapter 5 for more information).

Diet

In Traditional Chinese Medicine, the upper eyelids relate to the Spleen organ. If the eyelids are drooping, it indicates that the Spleen energy is not strong enough to keep "things in place." Therefore, strengthen the Spleen energy by minimizing cold food and drinks, raw foods, sweet foods and drinks (including fruits), and over-working/thinking.

Juicing. This is a suggested list of ingredients for juicing. Choose at least 4–6 items to combine.

- Aloe, parsnip, pumpkin, strawberry, carrots, cherry, sweet potato
- Do not use too many carrots due to their sugar content.
- Add your favorite fruits and vegetables.
- Try to use room temperature vegetables and fruit.
- Do not add ice or very cold liquids since cold foods and liquids will eventually extinguish the stomach's digestive fire.
- Do not juice as often during the cooler months of the year, and instead, switch to vegetable soups or stews.

Follow the Vision diet described in Chapter 7.

Lifestyle

Eye exercises. We recommend daily eye massage of acupressure points around the eyes.

See Chapter 10 for eye exercises and acupuncture points that are good for all eye conditions and overall eye health.

Other Modalities

Essential Oils

Coriander seed is a blood sugar equalizer, intestinal cleaner, and overall body purifier that tonifies the digestive system, improves appetite, and strengthens the Spleen-Pancreas meridian. The Spleen meridian in Chinese medicine helps hold organs and eyelids up, and when weak, it can cause drooping.

Frankincense helps relieve chronic stress and anxiety, reduces pain and inflammation, and boosts immunity.

Keep essences away from the mouth, eyes, and mucous membranes; if a few drops get in one of these sensitive areas it may be uncomfortable for 15–30 minutes, but not harmful. You can lessen discomfort by adding a pure oil like olive or coconut oil to neutralize the irritating effect. For the eye area, dab a few drops around the outside of the eye. Do not put the neutralizing oil in the eye.

Combine ¼ cup of avocado oil with ¼ cup of calendula-infused oil. Slowly add 5 drops each of the essential oils. Then close the bottle and shake well; apply 4 drops of this mixture on your clean face. Massage in gentle circular motions. Leave overnight. For more information, see Appendix 9.

Chinese Medicine

Spleen (and Stomach) deficiency is often associated with drooping eyedrops as one of the functions of the Spleen (meridian). In Chinese medicine, a healthy Spleen (meridian) holds body parts up, such as preventing prolapse of the organs. It also keeps blood within the vessels (preventing leakage).

Acupuncture

In addition to acupuncture treatment, massaging LU10 is useful when the eyelids feel like they are drooping.

Recommended Patent Formula

Bu zhong yi qi tang. Central qi tea is a popular formula used for coordinating Spleen and Stomach that supports healthy digestion and the distribution of nutrients through the body when onset of ptosis is gradual.

Your acupuncturist may adjust the formula above or recommend a different one, depending on his/her intake and evaluation.

Also See

Chapter 7, Vision Diet

Chapter 8, Nutrients

Chapter 10-4, Eye Exercises

1 Wesley, K., Vislisel, J.M., Allen, R.C. (2015). A Primer on Ptosis. Retrieved Feb 10 2018 from http://webeye.ophth.uiowa.edu/eyeforum/tutorials/ptosis/index.htm

2 McInnes, C.W., Lee-Wing, M. (2015). Eyelid Ptosis. *CMAJ*, Oct 6;187(14):1074.

3 Wikipedia. Levator Palpebrae Superioris Muscle. Retrieved May 1 2018 from https://en.wikipedia.org/wiki/Levator_palpebrae_superioris_muscle.

3 Ibid. McInnes. (2015).

4 Ibid. Wikipedia. Levator Palpebrae Superioris Muscle.

5 Klejch, W., Vislisel, J.M., Allen, R.C. (2015). A Primer on Ptosis. *U Iowa Opthalmol Vis Sci*, Apr.

6 Griepentrog, G.J., Diehl, N., Mohney, B.G. (2013). Amblyopia in childhood eyelid ptosis. *Am J Ophthalmol*, Jun;155(6):1125-1128.

7 SooHoo, J.R., Davies, B.W., Allard, F.D., Durairaj, V.D. (2014). Congenital ptosis. *Surv Ophthalmol*, Sept-oct;59(5):483-92.

8 Griepentrog, G.J., Mohney, B.G. (2014). Strabismus in childhood eyelid ptosis. *Am J Ophthalmol*, Jul;158(1):208-210.

9 Phowthonkum, P., Sun, A. (2017). Novel truncating variant in DNA2-related congenital onset myopathy and ptosis suggests genotype-phenotype correlation. *Neuromuscul Discord*, Jul;27(7):616-618.

[10] Ibid. McInnes. (2015).

[11] Guyuron, B., Harvey, D. (2016). Periorbital and Orbital Aging: Senile Enophthalmos as a Cause of Upper Eyelid Ptosis. *Plast Reconstr Surg,* Jul;138(1):31e-7e.

[12] Rasiah, S., Hardy, T.G., Elder, J.E., Ng, C.Y., Lenake, M., et al. (2018). Aetiology of acquired blepharoptosis in young adults. *Orbit,* Feb;37(1):59-64.

[13] Ibid. McInnes. (2015).

[14] Satariano, N., Brown, M.S., Zwiebel, S., Guyuron, B. (2015). Environmental factors that contribute to upper eyelid ptosis: a study of identical twins. *Aesthet Surg J,* Mar;35(3):235-41.

[15] This study (Satariano, 2015) also found that ptosis was not linked to body mass index, smoking, sun exposure, alcohol use, work stress, or sleep.

[16] Watanabe, A., Imai, K., Kinoshita, S. (2013). Impact of high myopia and duration of hard contact lens wear on the progression of ptosis. *Jpn J Ophthalmol,* Mar;57(2):206-10.

[17] Ibid. Rasiah. (2018).

[18] Berke, S.J. (2012). PAP: New Concerns for Prostaglandin Use. *Rev Opthomol.* Retrieved May 2 2018 from https://www.reviewofophthalmology.com/article/pap-new-concerns-for-prostaglandin-use.

[19] Sthapit, P.R., Saiju, R., Limbu, B. (2014). Frontalis Sling Operation using Silicone Rod Compared with Autogenous Fascia Lata for Simple Congenital Ptosis. *JNMA J Nepal Med Assoc,* Jul-Sep;52(195):897-901.

[20] Bansal, R.K., Sharma, S. (2015). Results and complications of silicone frontalis sling surgery for ptosis. *J Pediatr Ophthalmol Strabismus,* Mar-Apr; 52(2):93-7.

[21] Bagheri, A., Najmi, H., Salim, R.E., Yazdani, S. (2015). Tear condition following unilateral ptosis surgery. *Orbit,* Apr;34(2):66-71.

[22] Savino, G., Battendieri, R., Riso, M., Traina, S., Poscia, A., et al. (2016). Corneal Topographic Changes After Eyelid Ptosis Surgery. *Cornea,* Apr;25(4):501-5.

[23] Hatzipantelis, E., Kyriakidis, I., Pavlou, E., Pavlidou, E. (2015). Bilateral Eyelid Ptosis, Attributed to Vincristine, Treated Successfully with Pyridoxine and Thiamine in a Child with Acute Lymphoblastic Leukemia. *Toxicol Int,* Jan-Apr;22(1):162-4.

16-7. PTERYGIUM AND PINGUECULAE

A pterygium (also referred to as "surfer's eye") is a raised, cream-colored growth, usually on the white of the eye, near the nose. It sometimes gets yellowish or reddish. Before the growth extends onto the cornea, it is called a pinguecula; after it extends onto the cornea, it is called a pterygium.

Although they can be removed surgically, the rate of recurrence is as high as 40%, and they tend to come back bigger and faster.

These growths more frequently develop in people who live in dry, hot, windy environments, and are found often on people that spend a lot of time outdoors. A pterygium is not dangerous, and it is not cancerous, but can become uncomfortable. The main problem is that it can eventually distort vision, due to the fact that it can grow onto the cornea, and eventually, even onto the central part of the eye, blocking light from entering.

The prevalence of having pterygium in the general population is 10.2%, slightly higher among men (14.5%) than women (13.6%).[1] In sunny, warm climates, the prevalence is much higher. In a study done on Barbados, the pterygium rate in the population was 23.4%.[2]

Pathology of Pterygium

Pterygium is a benign but uncontrolled growth of conjunctive cell tissue. The conjunctiva is a thin layer that lies on the sclera, the white of the eye. Researchers have found that pterygium is linked to less dense corneal endothelial cell tissue, as well as an increase in astigmatism.[3] Researchers are beginning to understand what brings about these changes, possibly due to factors that include genetic modification and virus infection.

Although pterygium is traditionally considered to be degenerative in nature, certain gene characteristics (WWOX) suggest that it is actually "premalignant" tissue, and that the WWOX gene may play a role in the growth and recurrence of pterygiums.[4]

Symptoms

A **raised, cream-colored growth** occurs, usually on the nasal side of the white of the eye.

Other symptoms include an itchy or gritty feeling in the eye, redness, and possibly a sense of burning. As it becomes more advanced, it can become inflamed, causing redness and irritation as well as affecting vision if it starts to cover the cornea.

Causes and Risk Factors

Overexposure to sunlight. This is the biggest risk factor; UV radiation is a factor in sunlight overexposure. Researchers can measure the amount of time spent out of doors via a biomarker known as conjunctival ultraviolet autofluorescence (CUA). Cell tissues emit light when they have absorbed light, and this can be measured.[5] In Australia, a large cross-sectional population-based study of more than 1,300 participants was assessed using CUA to determine the amount of sunlight exposure. The participants with the highest CUA levels also had the highest incidence of pterygium.[6] Similarly, this method has been used to determine that patients with pinguecula also have high levels of CUA.[7]

Oxidative stress and diminished antioxidant levels may also play a role on the onset of pterygium.[8]

Chronic dry eyes.

Environmental irritants, such as dust and wind.

Genetic changes. Researchers have also discovered that genes are associated with pterygium. These include tumor suppressor gene p53, and WWOX, and other genes that are linked to the maintenance of DNA, cell growth, cell movement, and cell death.[9] [10]

Virus. Human papillomavirus infection is also a risk factor in some parts of the world.[11] This virus is associated with pterygium, and it has been implicated in stomach cancer.[12]

Renal failure. Although renal failure results in conjunctival lesions that may appear to be pinguecula, there is one study that found that patients with renal failure had a higher rate of pinguecula than healthy-eyed patients.[13]

Conventional Treatment

In the early stage, your eye doctor may just recommend lubricating eyedrops, and possibly prescription steroid eyedrops to ease redness, itching, swelling, and pain.

If the pterygium is interfering with your vision, then typically it is surgically removed. In one study, the rate of recurrence after 1 year was 18.8%,[14] and they tend to come back bigger and faster.

The main complication of pterygium surgery is recurrence after removal. Some studies have reported pterygium returning at rates of 15–25% when a graft is used to replace the removed tissue (tissue underneath the pterygium is also removed and replaced with eyelid skin); the pterygium return rate is up to 76% when no graft is used. Even after the pterygium is removed a second time, it can keep coming back.[15]

A grafting technique called conjunctival-limbal autograft, using corneal epithelial stem cells (limbal cells), appears to have a lower recurrence rate.[16]

Surgical complications may also include corneal scarring and perforation of the white part of the eye. In some cases, surgical removal of pterygium can cause astigmatism.

It is recommended to wear 100% UVA/UVB wrap-around protecting sunglasses whenever outside (preferably with polarized lenses), along with a hat with a brim. Amber colored lenses are the best for neutralizing blue light from sunlight and electronic devices.

Complementary Approach

Certain natural eyedrops may be helpful in managing the pterygium and possibly improving them. Certain formulas can also help support healthy circulation in the outside of the eyes and throughout the eyes overall.

Nutrients

Very Important

Homeopathic eyedrops that help with circulation in the eyes and reduce inflammation (see Appendix 5 for eyedrops). Eyedrops can include, among other herbs, cineraria maritima, silica, euphrasia, sepia, and calcarea fluroica. Best to take at least an hour or more apart from other eyedrops.

MSM eyedrops. 1 drop in each affected eye, 2 times per day or as needed. These drops help soften tissue (to allow better transport for nutrients in the outside of the eyes), reduce inflammation, and have natural antibacterial properties. MSM in general has been found to have antioxidant properties.[17] Numerous studies have shown it to have anti-inflammatory and immune modulating properties.[18]

Castor oil eyedrops. 1 drop in each affected eye before bedtime. These help reduce inflammation and detoxify, and they also include natural healing properties.

Eyedrops that contain antioxidants, including glutathione and vitamin C.

Helpful

Whole-food eye formula to support overall eye health.

Activated charcoal. This is highly alkaline, so it realigns the body's alkalinity level. Taken orally, it helps absorb most organic toxins floating around in the body and can reduce chronic inflammation and reduce the appearance of pterygium. This would go along with an alkaline diet (see Chapter 7 for more information)

Diet

Pure water. Drink plenty of water daily.

Juicing. Choose at least 4–6 items to combine in juice.

- Ginger, parsley, beets, cabbage, carrots, endive, leafy-green vegetables, chlorophyll, wheatgrasses, and berries, (preferably all organic)
- Do not use too many carrots due to their sweetness.

- Add your favorite fruits and vegetables.
- Try to use room temperature vegetables and fruit.
- Do not add ice or very cold liquids since cold foods and liquids will eventually extinguish the stomach's digestive fire.
- Do not juice as often during the cooler months of the year, and instead, switch to vegetable soups or stews.

Lifestyle

Sunglasses. Wear 100% UVA/UVB protecting wrap-around sunglasses whenever outside. Amber colored lenses are the best for neutralizing blue light.

UV protection. Have a clear UV film placed on the side windows of your car since you get a lot of UV exposure when driving. Left-sided skin cancer on the face and left-sided cataracts are more common because of drivers' UV exposure in the car.

Apple cider vinegar. This is highly acidic. When diluted with water and applied to the affected eye, the acid in the vinegar balances the pH of the eye and naturally minimizes the growth.

Turmeric. This is an anti-inflammatory agent that helps reduce symptoms such as redness, itching, and burning sensations. Add a tablespoon of turmeric in a bowl of water. Use this mixture to rinse your eyes at least 2 times per day.

Eye exercises. We recommend palming and eye massage of acupressure points around the eyes, daily. See Chapter 10 for eye exercises and acupuncture points that are good for all eye conditions and overall eye health.

Other Modalities

Chinese Medicine

In Chinese medicine, a pterygium may occur when the initial heat in the conjunctiva is not properly addressed, or as a result of poor diet and lifestyle choices that cause damp heat in the spleen and stomach. This inhibits free flow of qi and causes stagnation in the sclera. Lung yin deficiency, inadequate fluids, liver and kidney deficiency, or yin and blood deficiency (also causing decreased fluids and tears) can cause the sclera to become malnourished.

Xiao yan san, or Chinese Liver tonic (see ReVision Formula in appendix), helps support the Liver and energy movement in the eyes. A "deficient" Liver can result in fat build-up in the tissues of the body.

Sang bai pi tang, or mulberry bark decoction, is for lingering evil heat.

San ren tang, or three kernels decoction, is for Lung yin deficiency.

Qi ju di huang wan (lycium berry, chrysanthemum, and rehmannia pill) is for Liver and Kidney yin deficiency.[19]

On the Horizon

Injection with bevacizumab, a drug used for certain cancers, including eye cancer, has been found to improve ptyergium; however repeated application is necessary.[20] Treatment with cyclosporine A is also being investigated, as it appears to down-regulate cell behavior that produces pterygium.[21]

One of the earliest signs that UV damage has caused pinguecula and pterygium is the presence of Fuchs' flecks that accumulate at the leading edge of pterygium. These are epithelial stem-like cells, and they may be used to predict the future severity of the condition or more serious conditions.[22]

Also See

Chapter 8, Nutrients

Chapter 10, Self Help

1 Liu, L., Wu, J., Geng, J., Yuan, Z., Huang, D. (2013). Geographical prevalence and risk factors for pterygium: a systematic review and meta-analysis. Retrieved Feb 10 2018 from http://bmjopen.bmj.com/content/3/11/e003787

2 Luthra, R., Nemesure, B.B., Wu, S.Y., Xie, S.H., Leske, M.C. (2001). Frequency and risk factors for pterygium in the Barbados Eye Study. *Arch Ophthalmol*, Dec;119(12):1827-32.

3 Hsu, M.Y., Lee, H.N., Liang, C.Y., Wei, L.C., Wang, C.Y., et al. (2014). Pterygium is related to a decrease in corneal endothelial cell density. *Cornea*, Jul;33(7):712-5.

4 Huang, Y.H., Chang, N.S., Tseng, S.H. (2015). Expression of WW domain-containing oxidoreductase WWOX in pterygium. *Mol Vis*, Jun 25;21:711-7.

5 Wikipedia. Conjunctival ultraviolet autofluorescence. Retrieved May 1 2018 from https://en.wikipedia.org/wiki/Autofluorescence.

6 McKnight, C.M., Sherwin, J.C., Yazar, S., Forward, H., Tan, A.X., et al. (2015). Pterygium and conjunctival ultraviolet autofluorescence in young Australian adults: the Raine study. *Clin Exp Ophthalmol*, May-Jun;43(4):300-7.

7 Kim, T.H., Chun, Y.S., Kim, J.C. (2013). The pathologic characteristics of pingueculae on autofluorescence images. *Korean J Ophthalmol*, Dec;27(6):416-20.

8 Kormanovski, A., Parra, F., Jarillo-Luna, A., Lara-Padilla, E., Pacheco-Ypez, J., et al. (2014). Oxidant/antioxidant state in tissue of primary and recurrent pterygium. *BMC Ophthalmol*, Nov 27;14:149.

9 Liu, T., Liu, Y., Xie, L., He, X., Bai, J. (2013). Progress in the pathogenesis of pterygium. *Curr Eye Res*, Dec;38(12):1191-7.

10 Ibid. Huang. (2015).

11 Ibid. Liu. (2013).

12 Di Girolamo, N. (2012). Association of human papilloma virus with pterygia and ocular-surface squamous neoplasia. *Eye (Lond)*, Feb;26(2):202-11.

13 Cohen, S.L., Gorchein, A., Hayward, J.A. (1974). Pingueculae - An Association with Renal Failure. *QJM*, Apr;43(2):281-291.

14 Han, S.B., Jeon, H.S., Kim, M., Lee, S.J., Yang, H.K., et al. (2016). Risk Factors for Recurrence After Pterygium Surgery: An Image Analysis Study. *Cornea*, Aug;35(8):1097-103.

15 American Academy of Opthalmology. After my surgery for pterygium, is it conceivable that it will grow back for the third time? Retrieved Feb 18 2018 from https://www.aao.org/eye-health/ask-ophthalmologist-q/how-many-times-can-pterygium-grow-back

[16] Masters, J.S., Harris, D.J. (2015). Low Recurrence Rate of Pterygium After Excision With Conjunctival Limbal Autograft: A Retrospective Study With Long-Term Follow-Up. *Cornea,* Dec;34(12):1569-72.

[17] Dan Dunn, J., Alvarez, L.A., Zhang, X., Soldati, T. (2015). Reactive oxygen species and mitochondria: A nexus of cellular homeostasis. *Redox Biol,* Dec; 6():472-85.

[18] Butawan, M., Benjamin, R.L., Bloomer, R.J. (2017). Methylsulfonylmethane: Applications and Safety of a Novel Dietary Supplement. *Nutrients,* Mar 16;9(3).

19 Qinghua, P., Frank, C.O., Barnblatt, P. (2014). Chapter 10, Chronic Conjunctivitis. (pp. 73-79), TCM Case Studies: Eye, Ear, Nose and Throat Disorders] Beijing, China. People's Medical Publishing House.

[20] Sarac, O., Demirel, S., Ottulu, R. (2014). Efficacy of intralesional bevacizumab administration in primary pterygium: a quantitative analysis. *Eye Contact Lens,* Jan;40(1):46-50.

[21] Kim, Y.H., Jung, J.C., Jung, S.Y., Kim, Y.I., Lee, K.W., et al. (2015). Cyclosporine A Downregulates MMP-3 and MMP-13 Expression in Cultured Pterygium Fibroblasts. *Cornea,* Sep;34(9):1137-43.

[22] Ip, M.H., Chui, J.J., Tat, L., Coroneo, M.T. (2015). Significance of Fuchs Flecks in Patients With Pterygium/Pinguecula: Earliest Indicator of Ultraviolet Light Damage. *Cornea,* Dec;34(12):1560-3.

16-8. STYE AND CHALAZION

A **stye, or hordeolum**, is a bump in the upper or lower eyelid due to one of the oil glands that is blocked and inflamed, causing redness in the surrounding area. It is caused by a bacterial infection and is quite common.

The exact number of people who get styes is not known; however, they are very common, and more common than chalazia. In the U.S., over a five-year period, 3.8% of emergency room visitors had styes.[1] Styes are quite common in teenagers; most people experience at least one or two at some point in their life.

A **chalazion, or meibomian cyst**, is a similar bump that occurs due to a blocked and inflamed meibomian or Zeis gland on the eyelid. Chalazia are more common in adults than children and most frequently occur in people aged 30-50,[2] presumably because of hormone changes.[3]

Similar, But Not the Same

While chalazia (plural) and styes can look similar, they have different causes and characteristics.

Styes

Styes are the result of a bacterial infection of the meibomian glands, or the glands of Zeis and Moll (glands supplying oil to the eyelashes). Staph infections are usually the cause. This means that styes almost always involve redness, soreness, and localized swelling in the eye, which is not typically the case with chalazia. Styes are tender and painful to the touch. Ordinarily, they swell for about three days, and then they break open and drain, with healing usually occurring within a week.[4]

Chalazia

Chalazia are not caused by infection. Rather they are caused by foreign body cell reactions with the oily sebum secreted by the meibomian glands. Chalazia usually, but not always, do not involve redness, soreness, and swelling. Twenty-five percent of chalazia show no symptoms other than the visible bump, and they usually disappear without treatment. But they can grow to a bothersome size and even blur vision, because they distort the shape of the eye. Chalazia tend to take longer than styes to resolve, sometimes up to several months.[5]

Some chalazia, however, do act more like styes, becoming red, swollen, and tender. In these cases, they are more easily mistaken for styes. Other characteristics distinguish the two:

- Chalazia tend to develop farther from the edge of the eyelid than styes.[6]
- Chalazia grow more slowly than styes and are typically larger.
- Styes are smaller and more superficial than chalazia.
- Styes almost always look like a pimple.
- Styes have a small white dot in their center, signaling an infection.[7]

Eyelid and Gland Anatomy

The upper and lower eyelids contain several kinds of glands that can become inflamed.

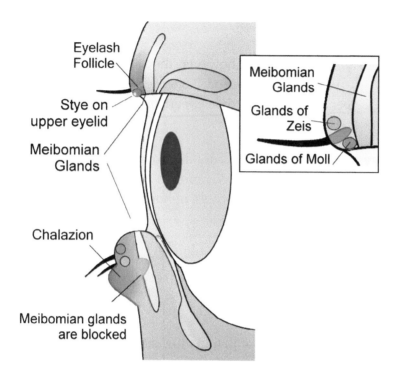

Meibomian glands, also known as tarsal glands, are located along the edge of the eyelids. They are an essential part of the eye, keeping it healthy and lubricated. They secrete fatty and oily meibum, and with every blink (with help from a tiny muscle called the Riolan's muscle), they spread a thin film over the tear film to slow the tear film's evaporation.[8] Meibum also protects tears from spilling down to the cheek by trapping tears between the edge of the eyelid and the eyeball. It also makes the eyelid airtight when closed. Meibomian glands are located on both the upper (about 50 glands) and lower (about 25 glands) eyelids.[9]

Glands of Zeis are also sebaceous (oil) glands that protect the surface of the eyelid, adding a protective layer to the top of the tear film.[10] These glands secrete sebum to the middle section of the eyelash follicle, keeping it lubricated, and keeping the eyelashes from becoming brittle.[11]

Glands of Moll are located at the base of the eyelashes. They are modified sweat glands, secreting sebum. However, unlike Zeis glands, these secretions contain immune system ingredients: the enzyme lysozyme, mucin 1, and immunoglobulin A, which suggest that they are part of the localized eyelid immune system. Their function is not precisely known, but they may be protecting against pathogens on the surface of the eye.[12] Further research supports this hypothesis with the discovery of additional immune-system components.[13]

Tear glands are not located on the eyelid, but the presence and irritation caused by styes can stimulate extra tear production.

Categories

Styes

There are two types of styes:[14]

- **External.** This type of stye emerges along the edge of the eyelid at the base of an eyelash. It can become yellow, filled with pus, and painful when touched.
- **Internal.** With internal styes, swelling develops inside of the eyelid. Generally, this type of stye is much more painful.

It is also possible for the eyelid itself to become infected. This is known as cellulitis, and it can result from the stye on the surface of the eyelid, or from the sinus cavity adjacent to the eyelid.

Chalazia

Chalazia can be categorized as either superficial or deep, depending on the glands that are blocked.

- Inflammation of a meibomian gland leads to a deep chalazion.
- Inflammation of a Zeis gland leads to a superficial chalazion.

As mentioned above, chalazia often disappear, on their own. If recurring, or if the chalazia does not resolve, see an eye doctor, as in rare cases the chalazia may be cancerous. The eye doctor will drain the contents and review the test results, if needed.

Signs and Symptoms

Styes

- Have a red bump with white center that looks like a pimple, typically on the edge of the eyelid, and closer to the eyelid surface than a chalazion.
- Almost always have localized swelling, redness, and pain, due to bacterial infection. Sometimes the entire eyelid can become swollen.
- Styes rapidly mature in size (over about three days) prior to bursting and receding.
- The skin around the eye is tender to the touch.
- Have increased eye watering due to irritation.
- Are possibly sensitive to light.

Note. Styes are contagious, so washing hands regularly is important.

Chalazia

- Are a hard, typically painless nodule or swelling in the eyelid, generally located away from the edge of the eyelid, and sometimes on the underneath side of the eyelid.
- Cause a red and swollen eyelid in some cases, but often, there is no inflammation.
- The skin outside of the chalazion usually isn't tender.
- If swelling that is due to a chalazion on the upper lid is enough to press on the cornea, blurry vision can result.

Other Eyelid Bumps

There are a few other bumps found on eyelids that are fairly common:

Milia. These are tiny white cysts (look like whiteheads) in the eyelid's outer-skin layer, near the nose, due to accumulated dead skin. They are filled with keratin, a fibrous type of protein. They are trapped at the base of sweat glands or eyelash follicles. They are common in babies, but in adults, milia may need a doctor's attention.[15]

Xanthelasma. This is a skin condition with typical distinct yellowish bumps under the skin, on or near the eyelid, generally toward the nose. They are caused by fat (cholesterol) buildup under the skin. They are not accompanied by symptoms and can be removed surgically.[16]

Causes and Risk Factors

Styes

Styes are caused by staph bacteria, and they are highly contagious. Therefore, any activity that exposes your eyelids to bacteria, such as the staphylococcus bacteria found on the skin and mucous membranes in humans, can cause styes.

Here are some examples.

- Touching your eyes without washing your hands can spread staph if you've rubbed your nose, inserted contact lenses without washing your hands, or not disinfecting your lens.
- Chronic dry eye is often associated with the onset of styes. This is because a lack of sufficient tears results in a reduction in the natural antibiotics in our tears to protect us from bacterial infection.
- Styes sometime accompany blepharitis, an inflammation along the edge of the eyelid.
- Leaving on eye makeup overnight can be a source of infection, especially if it is old makeup, or makeup you share with others, including tester makeup samples.
- Having rosacea, a skin condition characterized by facial redness, is a risk factor.

Note. Most staphylococcus bacteria are harmless; however, it is best not to touch your eyes without washing your hands first; this will cut down on the risk of infection.

Chalazia

Chalazia occur when an oil gland becomes blocked; they arise from a variety of causes, such as:

- Blepharitis or eyelid inflammation
- Meibomian gland dysfunction
- Changes in hormones during pregnancy
- Adult-onset (type 2) diabetes, possibly due to chronic inflammation linked to diabetes[17]
- Prior history of chalazia
- Touching eyes with unwashed hands

- Stye infection; the infection heals, but the white blood cells and fatty cell secretions remain, forming a hard bump.
- Skin conditions such as acne, rosacea, or seborrhea dermatitis
- Contaminated or old cosmetics
- Other conditions or habits such as smoking, gastritis, IBS, or anxiety[18]

Conventional Treatment

Styes

While styes generally resolve within a few days, there are measures that can be taken to potentially help the situation.

- Apply warm, wet compresses at the first sign of a lump for 5–10 minutes, 2–4 times a day, and for a couple of days after the lump subsides. This usually helps the area heal faster. It may also help open a blocked pore so that it can drain and start to heal.
- In the case of pain, medicine such as acetaminophen may be helpful.
- An eye doctor may prescribe topical antibiotics in the form of eyedrops or an ointment.
- Occasionally, oral antibiotics are given when the stye does not resolve, when there are multiple styes, or if there are additional complications such as blepharitis or rosacea.
- People who have rosacea, along with a stye, may require treatment of their cheeks with an antibiotic cream, an oral antibiotic, or both.
- Oral or IV antibiotics are usually given if the infection has spread to other parts of the eye or to a larger area of the eyelid.
- An eye doctor may drain a large or painful stye by making a small incision on the inside of the lid. **Do not incise the stye yourself**.

Chalazia

Even though a lump in the eyelid is unappealing cosmetically, it is benign, and with simple self-care as noted in the section below, will often resolve within several weeks.

If the chalazion does not resolve, becomes infected, inflamed, large enough to press on the cornea, or if it becomes a persistent problem, see your eye doctor. An ophthalmologist may drain the contents by making a small incision on the inside of the eyelid. The lesion can also be injected with a corticosteroid to help reduce the swelling.

If chalazia recur in the same location, the doctor may take a sample to test for tumorous growth. Sebaceous carcinoma, an uncommon but aggressive malignant tumor of the skin, may arise from the glands within the eyelids, the red prominence at the inner corner of the eye called the caruncle, or the eyebrow. They are more commonly found on the upper eyelid and in middle-aged patients. Sebaceous carcinomas are a very rare form of eye cancer; however, they can look like a chalazion or stye. So, it is important for eye care specialists to take a look at the possibility of this tumor in any patient with persistent conjunctivitis, blepharoconjunctivitis, or chronic/recurrent chalazion. As a general rule, any conjunctivitis or chalazion that is not getting better after three months of observation should be biopsied.

Complementary Approach

Diet

Juicing. Daily juicing will supply needed nutrients. As chalazia may be related to a lowered immune system, juicing daily helps keep the immune system strong. Choose from the following foods:

- Celery, cabbage, carrot, leafy-green vegetables, garlic, ginger, blueberries, other berries, parsley, dandelion greens, and lemon
- Add your favorite fruits and vegetables.
- Not too much fruit with high sugar content or carrots, as sugar lowers our ability to fight infection.
- Try to use room temperature vegetables and fruit.
- Do not add ice or very cold liquids since cold foods and liquids will eventually extinguish the stomach's digestive fire.
- Do not juice as often during the cooler months of the year, and instead, switch to vegetable soups or stews.

General Recommendations

- Eliminate cold drinks and foods, including raw foods straight from the refrigerator that extinguish the stomach's fire and reduce digestive ability.
- Eliminate sugar and refined grains. High consumption of sweet flavors negatively effects the Spleen meridian and reduce the ability to fight infection.[19]
- Eliminate late night eating or overeating.
- Eliminate milk, yogurt, and ice cream from cows as they produce dampness and mucus.
- Eliminate fried and processed foods.
- Consume kefir (from goat or cow milk, or coconut water) to boost beneficial bacteria.
- Eat plenty of fresh fruit, vegetables, and whole grains.
- Add fresh garlic to your meals; garlic is a powerful natural antibiotic and immune system booster.

Follow the Vision diet in Chapter 7.

Traditional Chinese Medicine Diet Recommendations

TCM diet recommendations look to foods that support the Spleen and Stomach meridian system that are essential for processing food and distributing nutrients throughout the body. Good nutrient distribution is required to maintain eye and overall health.

For Spleen. Include mildly sweet foods, or golden and round foods, such as beets, tomatoes, sweet peppers, and sweet potatoes.

- Other helpful Spleen foods include organic miso, natto and tempeh, oats, spelt, garbanzo beans, cabbage, rutabaga, peas, carrots, millet, corn, amaranth, sweet rice, apricots, cantaloupe, squash, potato, sweet potato, and fennel.

For Stomach/Pancreas include carbohydrate rich vegetables such as turnips, winter squash, parsnips, garbanzo beans, black beans, carrots, yams, and pumpkin. Include pungent vegetables and spices, such as ginger, cinnamon, garlic, onions, leeks, nutmeg, and black pepper. We do not recommend soybeans because most are GMO, and also contain aflatoxin and phytic acid, which in large amounts can suppress the thyroid.

Lifestyle

Complementary approaches for both chalazia and styes are the same, with few minor exceptions. They fall under two basic approaches as follows:

- Preventative treatment to reduce symptoms
- Strengthening of the immune system and improvement of meibomian gland circulation

Essential

Daily compress. The recommended first treatment for a chalazion is always very warm, wet compresses. At the first sign of a lump:

- Place a warm, clean washcloth for 5–10 minutes over the eyelid, 2–4 times a day.
- In many cases, the chalazion will subside within about five days.
- The warm washcloths increase circulation and may also open a blocked pore, so that it can drain and start to heal.
- Herbs that can help as part of the compress include burdock, chamomile, chrysanthemum flower, eyebright, echinacea angustifolia, forsythia, golden seal, honeysuckle, marigold, and red raspberry leaf.

Lid cleanser. Apply a lid cleanser each day to keep the eyelids clean. Using baby shampoo is one option.

Castor oil. Using a clean cotton swab, apply castor oil along the lid of the eye. This helps reduce inflammation and supports healing.

Eyedrops. Apply daily to keep the eye moist, preferably use only preservative-free eyedrops.

Helpful

Hydrating mask. This helps with moisturizing the eyes and unblocking the meibomian gland. Also see Appendix 5, Bruder Eye Hydrating Mask and Stye Compress.

Herbal formula. This boosts your immune system. Also see Appendix 5, Jason's ImmunoBalance Formula.

Eyelid Washes

- Alum works well as a wash for a stye. Add a couple of alum granules to one cup of water, and use the solution to wash the affected eye. This can be purchased online.

- Coriander seeds are believed to be one of the most beneficial home remedies for a stye. Add one teaspoon of coriander seeds to a cup of water and bring to a boil. Use the solution to cleanse the eyes, 3 times per day.
- Add some salt to warm water, allow it to cool slightly, and then soak a cotton ball in it. Dab the wetted cotton ball over the affected eye; use a fresh cotton ball each time. Salt has analgesic, antiseptic, and anti-inflammatory properties. In Traditional Chinese Medicine (TCM), salt reduces and breaks up lumps.
- Dandelion tea serves as an effective anti-bacterial eyelid wash. Steep the tea or bags for 5–6 minutes, and allow it to cool to a warm, or room temperature.

Vegetable Slices

- Cucumber is a soothing home remedy for styes. Place slices of chilled cucumber over the infected eyelid to reduce swelling and soreness.

You can also apply tomato slices to the affected area. Make sure to use the dense or fleshy part of a tomato, and remove the seeds. Tomato has a cooling effect.

Eye Drops

- Apply colloidal silver solution. Put two drops of colloidal silver, 2 times per day, in each affected eye, for up to 3 days if needed.
- Turmeric is a popular antiseptic home remedy. Add a teaspoon of turmeric powder to two cups of water, and bring to a boil. Continue to boil until the solution reduces to half; strain it until the water runs clear (rinse strainer between each use). Apply as eye drops, 2–3 times per day.

Compresses

- Brewed black tea bags. Brew yourself a cup of plain black tea, preferably organic, then squeeze and place the wet bag over the closed eyelid for about ten minutes. Tea contains tannins that will help provide relief from a stye. Black tea contains the most tannin of any type of tea; however, green tea can be used, if you don't have black tea.
- Prepare a paste of raw, grated potato with a little water, add to a clean cloth, and place the cloth over the affected eyes. This helps alleviate pain and swelling.
- Add a handful of acacia leaves (can be purchased online) to two cups of boiled water. Let cool, then dip a clean washcloth in the solution, and use it as a compress on the affected eye. This helps alleviate pain.
- Add some cleaned, fresh parsley leaves to a bowl, and pour boiling water over it. Steep it for a few minutes, allowing the solution to cool down a bit; then dip a clean cloth into the solution, ring out excess water, and place the cloth over your closed eyelid. Repeat this treatment before going to bed at night. This will help reduce swelling and tenderness.

Other

Aloe vera gel is a popular treatment for styes. Extract the pulpy gel from a cleaned aloe leaf by slitting it lengthwise. Remove the gel from the leaf or rub the moist pulpy side of the leaf over the infected eyelid. Aloe is an antioxidant, is antibacterial, and supports skin health.

Note 1. If a stye is not getting better with home treatment, talk to your doctor. If the infection has spread to the eyelid or eye, you may need a prescription for an antibiotic eye ointment, eyedrops, or antibiotic pills.

Note 2. In case you have blepharitis, make sure that you take the appropriate treatment. For more information, see Blepharitis, Chapter 16-2.

Other Modalities

Chinese Medicine

In Chinese medicine, diseases of the eyelid are generally a result of the relationship between poor diet and poor digestion. Problems on the upper eyelid often correspond to the Spleen meridian, while lower-lid problems correspond to the Stomach meridian. The Spleen (also related to the pancreas) and Stomach are responsible for proper digestion and the distribution of food and nutrients throughout the body. When these meridians are not flowing properly, your ability to fight colds and infections is greatly reduced.

If there is an imbalance in Spleen/Pancreas energy, symptoms can include chronic tiredness, weak digestion, abdominal bloating, loose stools, mental and physical fatigue, nausea, and poor appetite. Weak spleen function can result in "dampness" in the body, resulting in mucus, edema, joint pain, tumors or lumps (such as styes or chalazia), foggy thinking or heaviness in the head, excess yeast, and infections (bacterial, parasitic, or viral).

Chinese Patent Formulas

Er chen tang drains mucus and dampness; opens clear yang passages to the eyes.

Gui pi tang (Restore the Middle Way) is an excellent Spleen formula that controls the raising of the qi, helps contain blood within blood vessels, and transforms and transports foods and fluids.

Also See

Chapter 7, Vision Diet

Chapter 8, Nutrients

Chapter 10-4, Eye Exercises

Chapter 15-7, Dry Eye

Chapter 16-2, Blepharitis

Chapter 16-3. Conjunctivitis

[1] Channa, R., Zafar, S.N., Canner, J.K., Haring, R.S., Schneider, E.B., et al. (2016). Epidemiology of Eye-Related Emergency Department Visits. *JAMA Ophthalmol,* Mar;134(3):312-9.

2 American Optometric Association. Chalazion. Retrieved Feb 10 2018 from http://www.aoa.org/patients-and-public/eye-and-vision-problems/glossary-of-eye-and-vision-conditions/chalazion?sso=y

3 Medscape. Chalazion. Retrieved Feb 10 2018 from http://emedicine.medscape.com/article/1212709-overview#a5

4 WebMD. What Is a Stye? Retrieved Feb 20 2018 from http://www.webmd.com/eye-health/tc/styes-and-chalazia-topic-overview.

5 Ibid. WebMD. What Is a Stye?

6 Quigley Eye Specialists. Chalazion. Retrieved Feb 10 2018 from http://www.eyehealthcenteroflorida.com/eye-conditions/chalazion/.

7 Segre, L. (2018). Eye Stye (Sty) Facts: Symptoms, Causes And Treatment. Retrieved Feb 10 2018 from http://www.allaboutvision.com/conditions/styes.htm.

[8] Abelson, M.B., Ousler, G., Shapiro, A., Rimmer, D. (2016). The Form and Function of Meibomian Glands. *Rev Ophthalmol,* May 16.

[9] Wikipedia. Meibomian Gland. Retrieved May 5 2018 from https://en.wikipedia.org/wiki/Meibomian_gland.

[10] Ibid. Abelson. (2016).

[11] Quizlet. Anatomy and Physiology of The Eye. Retrieved May 5 2018 from https://quizlet.com/28127043/anatomy-and-physiology-of-the-eye-flash-cards/.

[12] Stoeckelhuber, M., Messmer, E.M., Schubert, C., Stoeckelhuber, B.M., Koehler, C., et al. (2008). Immunolocalization of defensins and cathelicidin in human glands of Moll. *Ann Anat,* 190(3):230-7.

[13] Stoeckelhuber, M., Stoeckelhuber, B.M., Welsch, U. (2003). Human glands of Moll: histochemical and ultrastructural characterization of the glands of Moll in the human eyelid. *J Invest Dermatol,* Jul;121(1):28-36.

14 Nordqvist, C. (2018). Everything you need to know about stye. Retrieved Feb 10 2018 from http://www.medicalnewstoday.com/articles/220551.php.

15 Wikipedia. Milium. Retrieved May 2 2018 from https://en.wikipedia.org/wiki/Milium_(dermatology).

16 Wikipedia. Xanthelasma. Retrieved May 2 2018 from https://en.wikipedia.org/wiki/Xanthelasma.

17 Adeoti, C., Isawumi, M., Ashaye, A., Olomola, B. (2012). The anterior segment of the eye in diabetes. *Clin Ophthalmol,* 2012; 6: 667–671.

18 Ibid. Chalazion. http://emedicine.medscape.com/article/1212709-overview.

[19] Sanchez, A., Reeser, J.L., Lau, H.S., Yahiku, P.Y., Willard, R.E., et al. (1973). Role of sugars in human neutrophilic phagocytosis. Am J Clin Nutr, Nov;26(11):1180-4.

16-9. SUBCONJUNCTIVAL HEMORRHAGE

Subconjunctival hemorrhages have an alarming appearance but are rarely serious. They are seen when a tiny capillary in the sclera (white part of the eye) leaks (hyposphagma) under the conjunctiva, causing what would look like blood on the outside of the eye, or bloodshot eyes.

The condition is frequently seen in older people, and if recurring, may indicate another condition, such as high blood pressure[1] or a disorder in which blood does not coagulate properly.[2]

When the Conjunctiva Bleeds

The blood vessels in the conjunctiva are so tiny as to usually be barely visible, but they can enlarge or break under duress. The condition looks serious, appearing as a bright red or dark red patch on the eye, but usually it is not consequential and tends to resolve itself within a few days. It can occur as the result of trauma (68%) or spontaneously (32%),[3] and typically it does not need to be treated. The patch of red may initially enlarge for the first 24 hours, and then gradually get smaller. As the affected area dissipates, it spreads in the eye, and it may seem green or yellow (like a bruise clearing up), but typically the condition is gone within a week or two. If not cleared up within two weeks, see your eye doctor.

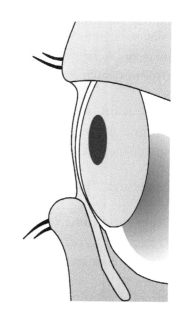

We experience similar trauma to other parts of the body as bluish bruises, due to the pooled blood seen through skin. The reason this type of trauma appears bright or dark red is that the conjunctiva is transparent and does not hide the discoloration.[4]

If the condition recurs frequently, then your doctor will recommend checking for severe hypertension, bleeding disorders, malignancies (both ocular or systemic, as in leukemia),[5] and side effects of medication.[6]

Symptoms

You will see a bright or dark red blood area in the white of the eye that may even cover the entire white of the eye.[7] It is typically painless and not noticed until seen in the mirror, or until someone else comments on it. It may, but rarely, feel itchy or scratchy. There may be some discomfort, but it is not typically associated with pain. At first occurrence, a sense of fullness or pressure might be noticed.[8]

Causes and Risk Factors

Aging. As we age, blood vessels tend to become increasingly fragile, and minor trauma can cause a hemorrhage, or it may occur spontaneously.[9] In older people, hypertension is the most common cause.[10] [11] Arteriosclerosis is a common risk factor. [12]

Trauma. Examples include putting in contact lenses,[13] diving underwater,[14] heavy lifting, strenuous activity, or head injury. These are major risk factors for younger people.[15] Trauma-linked subconjunctival bleeding is most closely linked to injury or trauma to the side of the head, the temporal area (40.5%)[16] more than other areas.

Non-accidental trauma. If subconjunctival bleeding is seen in infants and children, it could be a red flag for child abuse[17] or a sign of scurvy.[18]

Surgery. A hemorrhage can occur after eye or eyelid surgery, including LASIK[19] and other surgeries, such as bronchoscopy,[20] ear surgery,[21] and facial plastic surgery.

Medication. Any medication that promotes bleeding or inhibits clotting,[22] such as Plavix, and warfarin (Coumadin, Jantoven), as well as high doses of vitamin E, or Ranibizumb injections (sometimes prescribed for advanced macular degeneration) can cause subconjunctival bleeding.[23]

Life issues. These include excess stress or anxiety, lack of sleep, or excessive drinking.

Other conditions. Other diseases and health conditions can cause subconjunctival bleeding, such as extreme hypertension, Ebola, leptospirosis, or bone fracture around the face. Sometimes an infection like conjunctivitis can weaken the vessels, allowing them to bleed.[24]

Forceful actions. This may include actions such as sneezing, coughing, wheezing, vomiting, or blowing the nose while pinched shut (Valsava maneuver).[25] [26]

Genetics. Some people have a genetic tendency towards bruising easily.

Conventional Treatment

Usually no treatment is required. Avoid use of aspirin or other medications that inhibit clotting, if possible. If the subconjunctival hemorrhage is due to an infection, antibiotics may be prescribed. If related to trauma, the eye doctor may want to examine the eye to make sure there are no other complications associated with the trauma.

Complementary Approach

Herbs and vitamins can help strengthen blood vessels, support healthy circulation, and often speed up healing.

Helpful

Vitamin C (buffered and ascorbated). 2,000mg per day split up with meals. Take to promote healing.[27]

Arnica homeopathic remedy. To support healing, topically apply around the eyes or take pellets internally.[28]

Hypertension. If hypertension is involved, then there are nutrients (along with what your eye doctor prescribes) that can help lower blood pressure naturally, such as:

- **Coleus forskohlii.** Take 125mg-180mg per meal two to three times per day in root form.[29] Contraindicated for those with low blood pressure or hyperthyroid issues.
- **Taurine.** 750mg–1,000mg per day.[30] This also supports healthy heart and retinal health.
- **Omega-3 essential fatty acids.** 2,000mg–3,000mg per day.[31] This is also good for heart, retinal, and brain health.
- **Trans-resveratrol.** 175mg per day. Trans-resveratrol helps to reduce hypertension[32] and promotes a healthy inflammatory response.[33]

Other herbs and nutrients that may help lower blood pressure include garlic, celery, guan mu tong, breadfruit, black tea, green oats, Chinese hawthorne, flaxseed, tomato extract, pycnogenol, pomegranate, chocolate (dark), cat's claw herb, and ginger.[34]

Home Remedies

Washes and Compresses

- **Raspberry leaf tea.** This tea can help reduce the redness and bloodshot eyes. Make a tea infusion, let cool, then dip a clear washcloth or sterile cotton pad into the infusion. Apply to closed eyes for 10 minutes or more, 2 times per day.
- **Rose water.** Take 2 cotton balls and soak them in chilled rose water. Place over closed affected eye for 5–10 minutes. Repeat this 1–2 times per day for 2–3 days. You can also drop 1–2 drops of rose water in the eye as well.
- **Milk remedy.** This can provide instant relief from discomfort and help speed up the resolution. Dip a cotton ball into chilled milk, and squeeze out the excess. Leave on the closed affected eye for 10–15 minutes, and then discard. Repeat 2–3 times per day.
- **Water and clean washcloth.** Dip a clean washcloth in cold water, then place over the closed affected eye for 1–2 minutes. Repeat this 4–5 times per 8–10 minutes daily. You can also use an ice cube in a washcloth.
- **Witch hazel remedy.** Saturate a cotton ball with witch hazel. Place on closed affected eye for 10–15 minutes, then discard cotton pad. Repeat this 2–3 times per day for 2–3 days.
- **Chamomile tea.** This remedy can help resolve the blood, and it has natural anti-inflammatory properties. Boil a cup of water, place 1 tablespoon of chamomile tea into the water, steep for 5 minutes, then let cool. Strain out the chamomile. You can warm the tea

afterward. Apply to closed affected eye for 10–15 minutes and repeat 2–3 times per day for 2–3 days.

Vegetable Slices

- **Cucumber** has astringent properties. Refrigerate slices of cucumber in the refrigerator for half an hour. Place the cucumber slices on your closed eye for 10–15 minutes, 2–3 times per day. Repeat daily.
- **Raw potato** can help resolve blood pressure quickly. Take a medium sized potato and slice into thin slices. You can also grate the potato and pack it together. Place on closed affected eye for 10–15 minutes, and then discard. If needed, splash cold water on the closed eyelid to remove leftover potato. Repeat 1–2 times per day.

Other Modalities

Chinese Medicine

There are a number of patterns that can be related to contributing to a subconjunctival hemorrhage. Common patterns include Spleen qi deficiency. One of the functions of the Spleen (meridian) in Chinese medicine is to hold blood and fluids in blood vessels; heat excess patterns such as Liver heat or Heart heat rising can cause stress on the blood vessels.

Your acupuncturist can best determine treatment strategy and herbal formulas, based on the intake and evaluation.

Essential Oils

When essential oils are applied to the skin, their healing components are absorbed into the bloodstream through the pores and hair follicles. Once inside the bloodstream, they disperse to the specific organs and systems in which they work.

You can sample with a mixture or combination of oils, together with a carrier oil. You can use these oils every night.

Keep essences away from the mouth, eyes, and mucous membranes; if a few drops get in one of these sensitive areas it may be uncomfortable for 15–30 minutes, but not harmful. You can lessen discomfort by adding a pure oil like olive or coconut oil to neutralize the irritating effect. For the eye area, dab a few drops around the outside of the eye. Do not put the neutralizing oil in the eye.

Combine ¼ cup of avocado oil with ¼ cup of calendula-infused oil. Slowly add 5 drops each of the essential oils. Then close the bottle and shake well; apply 4 drops of this mixture on your clean face. Massage in gentle circular motions. Leave overnight.[35]

Cypress oil is known for its antiseptic, antispasmodic, antibacterial, stimulating, and antirheumatic properties.

Parsley seed oil has antimicrobial, antiseptic, circulatory, detoxifying, and hypotensive qualities.

Lemon oil has the ability to cleanse toxins from the body, stimulate lymphatic drainage, and fight bacteria and fungi.

Rosemary oil is highly anti-bacterial, has strong antioxidant qualities, and boosts the immune system.

Geranium oil can reduce inflammation and improve hormonal balance.

Also See

[1] Sahinoglu-Keskek, N., Cevher, S., Ergin, A. (2013). Analysis of subconjunctival hemorrhage. *Pak J Med Sci,* Jan;29(1):132-4.

[2] Brodie, S.E. (2010). Conjunctiva. In Fillit, H.M., Rockwood, K., Woodhouse, K. (Eds.). *Brocklehurst's Textbook of Geriatric Medicine and Gerontology.* Toronto, Canada: Elsevier, Ltd.

[3] Ibid. Sahinoglu-Keskek. (2013).

[4] Wikipedia. Subconjunctival Hemorrhage. Retrieved Jun 11 2018 from https://en.wikipedia.org/wiki/Subconjunctival_hemorrhage.

[5] Taamallah-Malek, I., Chebbi, A., Bouladi, M., Nacef, L., Bouguila, H., et al. (2013). Massive bilateral subconjunctival hemorrhage revealing acute lymphoblastic leukemia. *J Fr Ophtalmol,* Mar;36(3):e45-8.

[6] Tarlan, B., Kiratli, H. (2013). Subconjunctival hemorrhage: risk factors and potential indicators. *Clin Ophthalmol,* 2013;7:1163-70.

[7] Ibid. Dahl. Medicinenet.

[8] Ibid. Dahl. Medicinenet.

[9] Dahl, A.A. Subconjunctival Hemorrhage. Retrieved Jun 11 2018 from https://www.medicinenet.com/subconjunctival_hemorrhage/article.htm#subconjunctival_hemorrhage_facts.

[10] Ibid. Sahinoglu-Keskek. (2013).

[11] Ibid. Tarlan. (2013).

[12] Ibid. Tarlan. (2013).

[13] Ibid. Dahl. Medicinenet.

[14] Ibid. Dahl. Medicinenet.

[15] Ibid. Tarlan. (2013).

[16] Ibid. Sahinoglu-Keskek. (2013).

[17] DeRidder, C.A., Berkowitz, C.D., Hicks, R.A., Laskey, A.L. (2013). Subconjunctival hemorrhages in infants and children: a sign of nonaccidental trauma. *Pediatr Emerg Care,* Feb;29(2):222-6.

[18] Ibid. Wikipedia. Subconjunctival Hemorrhage.

[19] Ibid. Dahl. Medicinenet.

[20] Lim, H.Y., Puah, S.H., Ang, L.J., Teo, E.Q., Lau, S.Y. (2015). Subconjunctival haemorrhage from bronchoscopy: A case report. *Respir Med Case Rep,* Sep 3;16:97-100.

[21] Rajati, M., Bakhshaee, M., Khazaeni, K. (2013). Periorbital Ecchymosis and Subconjunctival Hemorrhage following Ear Surgery. *ISRN Otolaryngol,* Sep 30;2013:791068.

[22] Ibid. Dahl. Medicinenet.

[23] Yun, C., Oh, J., Hwang, S.Y., Kim, S.W., Huh, K. (2015). Subconjunctival hemorrhage after intravitreal injection of anti-vascular endothelial growth factor. *Graefes Arch Clin Exp Ophthalmol*, Sep;254(9):1465-70.

[24] Ibid. Wikipedia. Subconjunctival hemorrhage.

[25] Ibid. Dahl. Medicinenet.

[26] Wikipedia. Valsava Maneuver. Retrieved Jun 11 2018 from https://en.wikipedia.org/wiki/Valsalva_maneuver.

[27] Ringsdorf, W.M, Cheraskin, E. (1982). Vitamin C and human wound healing. *Oral Surg Oral Med Oral Pathol*, Mar;53(3):231-6.

[28] Paradox, P. (2017). How Does Arnica Work? Retrieved Jun 8 2018 from https://www.livestrong.com/article/171432-how-does-arnica-work/.

[29] Jagtap, M., Chandola, H.M., Ravishaankar, B. (2011). Clinical efficacy of *Coleus forskohlii (Willd.) Briq. (Makandi)* in hypertension of geriatric population. *Ayu*, Jan-Mar; 32(1): 59-65.

[30] Sun, Q., Wang, B., Li, Y., Sun, F., Li, P., et al. (2016). Taurine Supplementation Lowers Blood Pressure and Improves Vascular Function in Prehypertension. *Hypertension*, Mar;67(3):541-9.

[31] Morris, M.C., Sacks, F., Rosner, B. (1993). Does fish oil lower blood pressure? A meta-analysis of controlled trials. *Circulation*, Aug;88(2):523-33.

[32] Javkhedkar, A.A., Quiroz, Y., Rodriguez-Itrube, B., Vaziri, N.D., Lokhandwala, M.F., et al. (2015). Resveratrol restored Nrf2 function, reduced renal inflammation and mitigated hypertension in spontaneously hypertensive rats. *Am J Physiol Regul Integr Comp Physiol*, May 15;308(10):R840-6.

33 Abu-Amero, K.K., Kondkar, A.A., Chalam, K.V. (2016). Resveratrol and Ophthalmic Diseases. *Nutrients*, Apr; 8(4): 200.

[34] Tabassum, N., Ahmad, F. (2011). Role of natural herbs in the treatment of hypertension. *Pharmacogn Rev*, Jan-Jun;5(9):30-40.

[35] 7 Essential Oils for Broken Capillaries on the Face. Retrieved Jun 8 2018 from https://www.themiracleofessentialoils.com/essential-oils-for-broken-capillaries-on-the-face/.

Appendix

A-1. JUICING RECIPES FOR VISION

Here are general recommendations for different juicing recipes. You can select some combination of the recommended produce, as well as add your favorites.

Keep It Alkaline

- Include vegetables.
- Don't include too much fruit, beets, or carrots because of their high natural sugar content.

Protect the Digestive Fires

- Try to use room temperature vegetables and fruit.
- Do not add ice or very cold liquids since cold foods and liquids will eventually extinguish the stomach's digestive fire.
- Do not juice as often during the cooler months of the year, and instead, switch to vegetable soups or stews.

Go Organic

Try to use only organically grown produce. At a minimum, stay away from non-organic produce known as the "dirty dozen," (strawberries, spinach, nectarines, apples, grapes, peaches, cherries, pears, tomatoes, celery, potatoes, and sweet bell peppers). Learn more about the dirty dozen in Appendix 15, and see the full list of pesticides found in produce at www.ewg.org/foodnews/full-list.php.

Macula Support

Macular degeneration. Broccoli, basil, green and red bell pepper, raspberries, apples, leafy greens, grapes, and flaxseed or chia seeds.

Here's an example of how you might use the macular support juicing recipe.

- 2 kale leaves
- 5 small or 2 large basil leaves
- 1 tomato or 1 yellow bell pepper
- 1 carrot
- 10 grapes or 1/4 cup blueberries or 1 apple
- 1 tablespoon flaxseed

- 1 teaspoon flaxseed or hemp seed oil
- 1 teaspoon lemon juice or 1 slice ginger to brighten the flavor.

This combination provides lutein, zeaxanthin, omega-3, resveratrol, beta-carotene, lycopene, vitamin C, and other nutrients.

Lens Support

Cataracts. Carrot, celery, spinach, endive, blueberry, parsley, apple, watermelon, and radish.

Cornea and General Eye Support

Dry eyes. Carrot, celery, spinach, kale, apple, walnuts, pumpkin seeds, and yogurt.

Eye fatigue. Carrot, celery, spinach, ginger, ginseng, blueberry, parsley, and apple.

Conjunctivitis. Carrot, celery, spinach, endive, blueberry, parsley, and apple.

Ocular herpes. Celery, cabbage, carrot, green-leafy vegetables, blueberry, cherry, other berries, parsley, dandelion greens, garlic, lemons, pomegranate, ground flaxseeds, and raw honey.

Sugar Balance Support

Diabetic retinopathy. Ginger, asparagus, garlic, leeks, Jerusalem artichokes, spinach, parsley, beets, pumpkin, flaxseed or chia seed, celery, carrots, cabbage, raspberries, and chlorophyll.

Optic Nerve Support

Glaucoma. Celery, cucumber, carrots, radish, parsley, turnip, beets, raspberries, cabbage, flax seed or chia seed, apple, and plums.

Optic neuritis, optic nerve atrophy, Leber's. Ginger, beets, parsley, cabbage, endive, carrots, wheatgrasses, chlorophyll, and berries.

Retinal Support

Lattice degeneration. Ginger, leeks, garlic, parsley, cabbage, beets, carrots, spinach, apples, celery, grapes, lemon, raspberries, tomatoes and/or watermelon, wheatgrasses, and chlorophyll.

Best's disease. Ginger, leeks, garlic, beets, parsley, carrot, cabbage, celery, apple, spinach, tomatoes and/or watermelon, raspberries, grapes, lemon, wheatgrasses, and chlorophyll.

Central serous retinopathy (choroidopathy), choroidal neovascularization. Broccoli, green and red bell pepper, raspberries, apple, and leafy greens.

Photoreceptor Related Conditions

Retinitis Pigmentosa and **rod cone dystrophy.** Ginger, flaxseed or chia seed, leeks, garlic, parsley, cabbage, beets, carrots, celery, apples, spinach, grapes, lemon, chlorophyll, raspberries, and wheatgrasses.

Vitreous Support

Floaters. Garlic, beets, parsley, carrots, apple, parsnip, celery, and raspberries.

Stargardt Disease

Stargardt's is similar to macular degeneration. But because vitamin A and beta-carotene should be avoided, it is probably better to avoid juicing; the carotenoids in food may be converted to vitamin A in the body. Additionally, juicing intensifies the possible vitamin A precursor concentration.

Recommended Reading

Fresh Vegetable and Fruit Juices: What's Missing in Your Body? N.W. Walker, D.Sc.

Healing with Whole Foods, Paul Pitchford, N.D.

The Complete Book of Juicing, Michael T. Murray, N.D.

A-2. SUPPLEMENT ABSORPTION

The following is a chart that compares the absorption rates of different delivery systems.

Delivery Systems and Absorption Rates[1]

Delivery System	Rate of Absorption
Pills or tablets	10-20%
Capsules	20%
Transdermal patch	45%
Sublingual (droppers)	85-90%
Intramuscular	90%
Intraoral spray (under the tongue)	95%
Intravenous	100%

Health professionals often know how much nutrients patients should take therapeutically, but what is not known is how much will be absorbed into the patients' bloodstream through their digestive tracts. It is necessary to consider not only nutrients needed, but the likelihood of adequate digestion of those nutrients based on the patient's age (for example).

We need to consider:

1. The quality of the nutrients
2. Whether they are buffered and time-released
3. How the nutrients are combined with other nutrients

More nutrients in a pill or capsule is not necessarily better. What is important is how accurately we can insure the intake of "therapeutic dosages" recommended.

Improving Absorption

Why Sublingual Works

One solution is to take the most important nutrients orally (under the tongue) if available. Again, it's not how much you take, but how much your body tissues absorb that is important. Intraoral and sublingual absorption have become viable solutions with the introduction of liposomes. Liposomes are little fat containers that can hold nutrients and provide an efficient transport system that allows maximum absorption by the body. These fat containers bypass the stomach and take a quicker route by slipping through the sub-mucosal membrane under the tongue and directly into the bloodstream. With a greater concentration of nutrients in the blood, more nutrients reach their intended destination, thereby requiring a lower dosage intake.

The intraoral spray or sublingual method of delivery is also very helpful for individuals who have difficulty swallowing pills or capsules, and it is also cost effective since a lower dosage of nutrients is needed. It is particularly relevant for persons with poor digestion, medical issues such as diabetes, Lyme disease, or chronic inflammatory conditions, as well as the aging population in which enzyme production is reduced.

What Inhibits Absorption

Poor digestion. Enzymes are needed to metabolize food to extract nutrients. Inflammatory conditions[2] and diabetes can affect digestion. Diabetes can impact the vagus nerve, causing food to stay in the stomach longer. This is known as gastroparesis,[3] and it often affects good digestion, thereby reducing nutrients taken into the body and therefore the eyes. Lowering the acid environment of the stomach allows pathogens to survive when they otherwise might not, and this may reduce the availability of vitamin B12 and certain minerals, resulting in bone loss. Studies also indicate it may increase risk of dementia, including Alzheimer's disease.[4]

Medications. Taking medications that reduce stomach acid will reduce one's ability to absorb nutrients through the digestive tract; particular drugs and over the counter pills such as Nexium, Prevacid and Prilosec. Heartburn drugs can increase the risk of premature death. [5]

Aging. As we get older, our nutrient absorption rate through the intestinal tract is reduced, sometimes significantly.[6] Some researchers feel that the problem is not due solely to aging, but is closely linked to disease,[7] particularly when it is combined with serious health conditions or particular digestive disorders, such as ulcers, diverticulitis, gastric problems, and acid reflux.

Antibiotics. People that have been on long term antibiotics may also have reduced absorption as good bacteria in the gut, needed to breakdown food, die off as a side effect.[8] In these cases, we recommend supplementing with probiotics to replenish the good bacteria.

Stress. This restricts the flow of blood in the body by tightening muscles and restricting the free flow of fluids. Meditation, yoga, or even daily walks in nature can all help reduce stress significantly.

Eat slowly. We should be eating our food slowly and thoughtfully. Try never to eat on the run, and don't eat while conversing, writing, surfing the internet, or working. Make eating a special time for yourself.

Exercise. Daily exercise helps the body rid itself of harmful toxins that build-up. Many studies have shown that even a brisk walk of 20 minutes per day can have a major impact on reducing development of disease such as heart disease, and it has even been shown to reduce high eye pressures in cases of glaucoma.

Positive thinking. In Chinese medicine, excessive thoughts of anger, worry, resentment, grief, and fear all have effects on the free flow of energy in our body. Excess anger and/or stress often bring imbalance to the Liver, affecting the Stomach and Spleen meridians, and impacting both the ability to absorb nutrients and the ability to distribute the nutrients throughout the body.

Eating healthy food. Our bodies crave fresh food, particularly fruits, vegetables, and grains that provide not only vitamins and minerals but natural enzymes. Excessive intake of fast or highly processed foods requires our body to use its own enzymes and energy to digest food in an attempt to extract whatever limited nutrients may be available. Eat fruits and vegetables raw (juiced) or slightly steamed for best absorption. Stews and soups are good as well. Cooked carrots and tomatoes provide more antioxidants than when eaten raw.

Symptoms of Poor Absorption

Certain sugars may cause bloating, gas, or explosive diarrhea.

Protein may cause dry hair, hair loss, fluid retention, or possible edema due to fluid retention.

Fats may cause stools that are soft and bulky, light-colored, or foul-smelling. Stools may also be difficult to flush, may float, or may stick to the sides of the toilet bowl.

How to Take Nutrients

With Food

Generally, take vitamins with food. Digestive enzymes are stimulated when eating and aid in nutrient absorption. Taking some supplements with food reduces the chance of diarrhea or upset stomach. However, some supplements and herbs are better taken away from meals. Always follow the label instructions unless your health provider has advised otherwise.

Antibiotics

If taking antibiotics, add acidophilus supplements between dosages. This will help build up the good bacteria in the digestive tract that were destroyed by the antibiotics. It is important for elderly patients to take acidophilus or a probiotic formula on a regular basis.

Meals

- **Limit fluids, cold drinks.** During meals, limit fluid to improve digestion. Especially avoid cold or iced drinks when eating.
- **Stimulate digestion**. A small amount of apple cider vinegar taken just prior to a meal will stimulate production of digestive juices. Likewise, a slice of ginger with a few drops of lemon juice and a tiny pinch of salt on it will stimulate digestion before a meal.

- **Timing**. Ayurveda recommends having the largest meal mid-day, between 12:00 and 2:00 when the digestive fire is the greatest. Dinner can be a smaller meal, eaten before 8:00pm so that digestion is mostly complete by bedtime.

Nutrient Delivery

- **Liquid/sublingual**. This is the preferred, most easily absorbed and assimilated delivery method for taking vitamins and supplements.
- **Organic or wild crafted nutrients** are preferred when possible.
- **Capsules** are the next best choice. If vitamin capsules cannot be swallowed, open up the capsule and mix the contents with juice or yogurt.

Nutrients

- **Take vitamin A and lutein separately**. Otherwise, they compete for absorption. N-acetyl-carnosine also competes with vitamin A.
- **Vitamins A, D, E, K** are all fat soluble; they are best taken with a little fat such as with fish oil or in a meal with fat.[9]
- **C and iron**. Vitamin C enhances the absorption of iron found in plant foods (eating iron-rich foods with tea or milk has the opposite effect).
- **Vitamin C** is best absorbed when in ascorbated form (attached to a mineral, typically calcium, magnesium, and/or sodium) and with some combination of bioflavonoids and/or additional minerals.
- **Vitamin D3.** D is important for calcium absorption. D3 is a more readily absorbed form.

Enzymes

Although some enzymes are taken with food, others such as serrapeptase and nattokinase, are taken on an empty stomach to help break down debris and reduce overall chronic inflammation.

---

[1] Physician Desk Reference NPPDR #18

[2] Peuhkuri, K., Vapaatalo, H., Korpela, R. (2010). Even low-grade inflammation impacts on small intestine function. *World J Gastroenterol*, Mar 7; 16(9):PMC2835780.

[3] WebMD. When Diabetes Causes Stomach Problems. Retrieved Jun 18 2018 from https://www.webmd.com/diabetes/type-1-diabetes-guide/diabetes-and-gastroparesis#1.

[4] Weintraub, K. (2017). Studies Link Some Stomach Drugs to Possible Alzheimer's Disease and Kidney Problems. Retrieved Jun 18 2018 from https://www.scientificamerican.com/article/studies-link-some-stomach-drugs-to-possible-alzheimer-rsquo-s-disease-and-kidney-problems/.

[5] Xie, Y., Bowe, B., Li, T., Xian, H., Yan, Y., et al. (2017). Risk of death among users of Proton Pump Inhibitors: a longitudinal observational cohort study of United States veterans. *BMJ Open*, Jul; 7(6).

[6] Providing Healthy and Safe Foods As We Age: Workshop Summary. Retrieved Jun 18 2018 from https://www.ncbi.nlm.nih.gov/books/NBK51837/.

[7] Russell, R.M. (2001). Factors in Aging that Effect the Bioavailability of Nutrients. *J Nutr*, Apr;131(4):1359S-1361S.

[8] Langdon, A., Crook, N., Dantas, G. (2018). The effects of antibiotics on the microbiome throughout development and alternative approaches for therapeutic modulation. *Genome Med*, Apr 13;8:39.

[9] Ibid. ConsumerLab. 2018.

A-3. EFFECTS OF MOBILE DEVICES ON VISION

Smart mobile devices are used daily throughout our society and as part of daily life. Even with the latest in display technology, a wide range of eye complaints are increasing due to eyestrain from extended electronic device use. Complaints include eye fatigue, dry eyes, neck and shoulder tightness, poor concentration, irritated and watery eyes.[1] With the widespread use of smart mobile devices, smart device addiction is now a serious health problem worldwide.[2][3]

Computer eye syndrome affects 64%-90% of computer and mobile device users.[4][5][6][7]

Dry eye syndrome is associated with electronic device use in excess of four hours a day.[8] In addition, significant damage to the retina and cornea is caused by the blue light emitted from mobile devices, which results in phototoxicity and oxidative stress.[9][10][11]

Blue light. The damage to the retina caused by blue light is compounded by nighttime use of mobile devices. Children, teens, and adults often use their mobile devices in a dark place such is in the car at night or in their bedroom. When the environment is dark, the pupils are dilated, and more blue light reaches the back of the eye.

Insomnia. Not only does the increased exposure to blue light damage the retina, but blue light suppresses the secretion of melatonin which influences the circadian rhythm and our ability to fall asleep and get a good night's sleep. In one study, researchers compared exposure to 6.5 hours of blue light to 6.5 hours of green light. The results? Melatonin secretion from blue light exposure was half that of green light, and the circadian rhythm was delayed by 3 hours compared to 1.5 hours for green light exposure.[12]

Transient smartphone blindness. This temporary "blindness" in one eye can be alarming. It occurs after looking at a mobile device while lying on one's side and seeing the device mostly with one eye. One eye adapts to the bright device light and the other does not. It takes several to fifteen minutes for the 'blind' eye to adapt to the darkness again.[13]

Recommendations

Lifestyle

Limit cell phone use to under two hours per day. Prolonged daily exposure to smart mobile devices is a significant risk factor for inducing multiple types of ocular discomfort.[14] Wear blue blocking glasses when on the computer or mobile devices to filter out blue light.

Take regular breaks from mobile device or computer use to relax the eyes and do eye exercises such as *palming, near and far* and *hot dog*. See Chapter 10 for more information.

Take "sun breaks" during the day. Get outside and exercise such as walking, jogging, hiking, and as much as possible try to "ground" or touch the earth with bare feet.

Wear 100% UVA/UVB sunglasses (preferably polarized) when outside. Best color lenses are amber which neutralizes blue light. Best lighting is natural light or incandescent lighting. Do not use devices in the dark. Make sure you have plenty of ambient light around you.

Install a blue blocking program onto your computer or cell phone which will automatically adjust the brightness and blue light according to the time of day.

Nutrients

Certain nutrients help filter out light entering the eyes and act as powerful antioxidants to help protect them from damage due to UV and blue light exposure (from ongoing use of mobile devices and computers). The fact that many different antioxidants can reduce this type of damage suggests that the damage is associated with oxidative processes.

Essential

Lutein. 6mg–20mg per day. Lutein and zeaxanthin are two similarly structured carotenoids that make up the macular pigment in the retina. They are powerful antioxidants and help protect against damaging blue and UV light. These carotenoids are also used in the eye lens, acting as a sort of internal pair of sun-glasses that protect the eyes from damage against sunlight.[15][16][17][18][19]

Zeaxanthin. 2mg–12 mg per day. Like lutein, zeaxanthin protects against photo-oxidative damage to retinal epithelial cells and against oxidative damage to inflammation-related genes.[20]

Vitamin C with bioflavonoids (buffered and ascorbated). 2,000mg–3,000mg per day. As an antioxidant, vitamin C scavenges free radicals in the body and protects tissues from oxidative stress.[21][22][23]

Astaxanthin. 6mg–12mg per day. Astaxanthin has been shown to be effective in protecting against damage from light, due to its antioxidant effect.[24][25]

Diet

Eat a healthy diet including lots of green, leafy vegetables. Avoid excess sugar, refined carbohydrates, trans-fatty acids (such as in many chips and margarine), and fried food. We recommend the Vision diet (see Chapter 7).

Juicing. We recommend some combination of the following fruits and vegetables to support skin health and to help protect against the effects of UV light exposure.

- Green, leafy vegetables including kale and turnip greens, grapes, cranberries, orange, kiwi, strawberries, pineapple, apples, figs, carrots, broccoli, cabbage, peppers (green, red and yellow), and walnuts

Additional helpful herbs, vitamins, and oils that have potent antioxidant properties, protect against sun damage, and potentially protect against skin cancer include curcumin, resveratrol, vitamin E, quercetin, milk thistle, green and black teas, walnuts, borage oil, evening primrose oil, and avocado oil.[26]

---

[1] Kim, D.J., Lim, Chi, Y., Gu, N., Park, C.Y. (2017). Visual Fatigue Induced by Viewing a Tablet Computer with a High-resolution Display. *Korean J Ophthalmol,* Oct;31(5):388-393.

[2] Davey, S., Davey, A. (2014). Assessment of Smartphone Addiction in Indian Adolescents: A Mixed Method Study by Systematic-review and Meta-analysis Approach. *Int J Prev Med,* Dec; 5(12):1500-11.

[3] Nathan, N., Zeitzer, J. (2013). A survey study of the association between mobile phone use and daytime sleepiness in California high school students. *BMC Public Health,* Sep 12; 13():840.

[4] Ibid. Gowrisankaran. (2015).

[5] Rosenfield, M. (2011). Computer vision syndrome: a review of ocular causes and potential treatments. *Ophthalmic Physiol Opt,* Sep; 31(5):502-15.

[6] Blehm, C., Vishnu, S., Khattak, A., Mitra, S., Yee, R.W. (2005). Computer vision syndrome: A review. Surv Ophthalmol, May-Jun; 50(3):253-62.

[7] Klamm, J., Tarnow, K.G. (2015). Computer Vision Syndrome: A Review of Literature. *Medsurg Nurs,* Mar-Apr; 24(2):89-93.

[8] Portello, J.K., Rosenfield, M., Chu, C.A. (2013). Blink rate, incomplete blinks and computer vision syndrome. *Optom Vis Sci,* May;90(5):482-7.

[9] Niwano, Y., Kanno, T., Iwasawa, A., Ayaki, M., Tsubota, K. (2014). Blue light injures corneal epithelial cells in the mitotic phase in vitro. *Br J Ophthalmol,* Jul; 98(7):990-2.

[10] Lee, J.B., Kim, S.H., Lee, S.C., Kim, H.G., Ahn, H.G., et al. (2014). Blue light-induced oxidative stress in human corneal epithelial cells: protective effects of ethanol extracts of various medicinal plant mixtures. *Invest Ophthalmol Vis Sci,* Jun 12; 55(7):4119-27

[11] Jaadane, I., Boulenguez, P., Chahory, S., Carré, S., Savoldelli, M., et al. (2015). Retinal damage induced by commercial light emitting diodes (LEDs). *Free Radic Biol Med,* Jul; 84():373-384.

[12] Harvard Health Letter. (2018). Blue light has a dark side. Retrieved Sep 12 2018 from https://www.health.harvard.edu/staying-healthy/blue-light-has-a-dark-side.

[13] Alim-Marvasti, Al., Bi, W., Mahroo, O.A., Barbur, J.L., Plant, G.T. (2016). Transient Smartphone "Blindness" {Letter to Editor]. *N Eng J Med,* Jun 23;374:2502-2504.

[14] Kim, J., Hwang, Y., Kang, S., Kim, M., Kim, T.S., et al. (2016). Association between Exposure to Smartphones and Ocular Health in Adolescents. *Ophthalmic Epidemiol,* Aug; 23(4):269-76.

[15] Snellen, E.L., Verbeek, A.L., Van Den Hoogen, G.W., Crysberg, J.R., Hoyng, C.B. (2002). Neovascular age-related macular degeneration and its relationship to antioxidant intake. *Acta Ophthalmol Scand,* Aug;80(4):368-71

[16] Richer, S., Stiles, W., Statkute, L., Pulido, J., Frankowski, J., et al. (2004). Double-masked, placebo-controlled, randomized trial of lutein and antioxidant supplementation in the intervention of atrophic age-related macular degeneration: the Veterans LAST study (Lutein Antioxidant Supplementation Trial). *Optometry,* Apr;75(4):216-30

[17] Souied, E.H., Delcourt, C., Querques, G., Bassols, A., Merle, B., et al. (2013). Oral docosahexaenoic acid in the prevention of exudative age-related macular degeneration: The Nutritional AMD Treatment 2 Study. *Ophthalmology,* Aug;120(8):1619-31.

[18] Landrum, J.T., Bone, R.A., Joa, H., Kilburn, M.D., Moore, L.L., et al. (1997). A one year study of the macular pigment: the effect of 140 days of a lutein supplement. *Exp Eye Res,* Jul;65(1):57-62

[19] Bernstein, P.S., Zhao, D.Y., Wintch, S.W., Ermakov, I.V., McClane, R.W., et al. (2002). Resonance Raman measurement of macular carotenoids in normal subjects and in age-related macular degeneration patients. *Ophthalmology,* Oct;109(10):1780-7.

[20] Bian, Q., Gao, S., Zhou, J., Qin, J., Taylor, A., et al. (2012). Lutein and zeaxanthin supplementation reduce photooxidative damage and modulates the expression of inflammation-related genes in retinal pigment epithelial cells. *Free Radic Biol Med,* Sep 15;53(6):1298-307.

[21] Chew, E.Y., Clemons, T.E., Agron, E., Sperduto, R.E., Sangiovanni, J.P., et al. (2013). Long-term effects of vitamins C and E, β-carotene, and zinc on age-related macular degeneration: AREDS report no. 35. *Opthalmology,* Aug;120(8):1604-11.

[22] Du, J., Cullen, J.J., Buettner, G.R. (2012). Ascorbic acid: chemistry, biology and the treatment of cancer. *Biochem Biophys Acta*, Dec;1826(2):443-57.

[23] Cangemi, R., Angelico, F., Loffredo, L., Del Ben, M., Pignatelli, P., et al. (2007). Oxidative stress-mediated arterial dysfunction in patients with metabolic syndrome: Effect of ascorbic acid. *Free Radic Biol Med*, Sep 1;43(5):853-9.

[24] Piermarocchi, S., Saviano, S., Parisi, V., Tedeschi, M., Panozzo, G., et al. (2012). *Carotenoids in Age-related Maculopathy Italian Study (CARMIS): two-year results of a randomized study.* Eur J Ophthalmol. Mar-Apr;22(2):216-25.

[25] Otsuka, T., Shimazawa, M., Nakanishi, T., Ohno, Y., Inoue, Y., et al. (2013). *Protective effects of a dietary carotenoid, astaxanthin, against light-induced retinal damage.* J Pharmacol Sci. 123(3):209-18.

[26] Korac, R.R., Khambholja, K.M. (2011). Potential of herbs in skin protection from ultraviolet radiation. *Pharmacogn Rev,* Jul-Dec;5(10):164-173.

A-4. PROTECTION FROM SUN DAMAGE

Exposure to light of specific wavelengths or intensity may induce severe damage to the retina.[1]

Ongoing exposure to the sun without the protection of 100% UVA/UVB sunglasses can cause or contribute to a range of eye conditions, including macular degeneration,[2] cataracts,[3][4][5][6] corneal erosion,[7][8] and the onset of pterygium or pinguecula.[9] Proper protection from UV light can significantly reduce the risk of macular degeneration and cataracts.[10]

Sunlight exposure accelerates cellular activity in the eyes, resulting in an increase of free radicals. Again, exposure to sunlight or ultraviolet radiation increases the risk for ocular damage.[11]

UV radiation is divided into three distinct bands in order of decreasing wavelength and increasing energy: UVA (320-400 nm), UVB (290-320 nm), and UVC (200-290 nm). Different wavelengths and energy associated with UV subdivisions correspond to distinctly different effects on living tissue.[12] UV radiation is strongest between 10 am and 4 pm.[13]

Compared to UVB, UVA can penetrate deeper through the skin[14][15] and is not filtered by window glass. It has been estimated that about 50% of exposure to UVA occurs in the shade.[16][17]

Blue light is part of the sunlight spectrum, and in some ways it is even more dangerous due to our extensive additional exposure from mobile devices, computers, tablets, and large LCD screens. Blue light prevails in red, green, blue (RGB), and SSL illumination systems that did not exist a decade ago.

Conventional Approach

Wear 100% UVA/UVB sunglasses (preferably polarized) when outside. The best lens color is amber which neutralizes blue light. Yellow, copper, brown, and orange are better than green, grey, or blue.

People who drive frequently find that brown and copper tinted lenses improve visual acuity and enhance recognition of red warning lights. When it is overcast or when hazy blue light is scattered, it decreases depth perception and visual acuity and contributes to eye fatigue. Yellow and amber lenses help neutralize the blue light and protect our eyes. Using yellow tinted glasses when working on the computer, or setting your computer display to a warm color, helps protect against computer screen blue light.

There are a number of companies that are marketing sunscreen pills. According to the NIH, these do not actually provide protection against sun exposure (they may offer some protection against cell damage and inflammation); Using sunscreen (SPF 30 or higher) when outside still offers the best protection. The FDA stated that the marketing campaigns for these pills is "putting people's health at risk by giving consumers a false sense of security that a dietary supplement could prevent sunburn, reduce early skin aging caused by the sun, or protect from the risks of skin cancer."[18]

Complementary Approach

Follow recommendations above. Certain nutrients act as powerful antioxidants in the eyes and help filter out UV and blue light that cause oxidative damage.

Lutein. 6mg–20mg per day. Lutein, a powerful antioxidant, makes up the macular pigment in the retina and helps protect against damaging blue light.[19] [20] [21] [22]

Zeaxanthin. 2mg–12 mg per day. Like lutein, zeaxanthin protects the eye from blue light that causes damage from oxidative stress. [23]

Vitamin C (buffered and ascorbated). 2,000mg–3,000mg per day. As an antioxidant, vitamin C scavenges free radicals in the body and protects tissues from oxidative stress.[24] [25] [26] [27]

Astaxanthin. 6mg–12mg per day. Astaxanthin protects against damage from light due to its antioxidant effect.[28] [29]

Additional herbs, vitamins and oils that have potent antioxidant properties, protect against sun damage, and potentially protect against skin cancer include curcumin, resveratrol, vitamin E, quercetin, milk thistle, green and black teas, walnuts, borage and evening primrose oils, and avocado oil.[30]

For sunburns, tea tree oil applied to the skin can relieve sunburn by increasing blood flow in capillaries, bringing nutrients to damaging skin.[31] [32]

Juicing Recipe

We recommend some combination of the following fruits and vegetables to support skin health and help protect against the effects of UV light exposure:

- Green-leafy vegetables (including kale and turnip greens), grapes, cranberries, orange, kiwi, strawberries, pineapple, apples, figs, carrots, broccoli, cabbage, peppers (green, red and yellow), and walnuts

---

[1] Wenzel, A., Grimm, C., Samardzija, M., Remé, C.E. (2005). Molecular mechanisms of light-induced photoreceptor apoptosis and neuroprotection for retinal degeneration. *Prog Retin Eye Res*, Mar; 24(2):275-306.

[2] Chalam, K.V., Khetpal, V., Rusovici, R., Balaiya, S. (2011). A review: role of ultraviolet radiation in age-related macular degeneration. *Eye Contact Lens*, Jul;37(4):225-32.

[3] Hockwin, O., Kojima, M., Sakamoto, Y., Wegener, A., Shui, Y.B., et al. (1999). UV damage to the eye lens: further results from animal model studies: a review. *J Epidemiol Japan Epidemiol Assoc*, 1999;9(6):S39–S47.

[4] Varma, S.D., Kovtun, S., Hegde, K.R. (2011). Role of ultraviolet irradiation and oxidative stress in cataract formation-medical prevention by nutritional antioxidants and metabolic agonists. *Eye Contact Lens*, Jul; 37(4):233-45.

[5] Neale, R.E., Purdie, J.L., Hirst, L.W., Green, A.C. (2003). Sun exposure as a risk factor for nuclear cataract. *Epidemiology*, 2003;14(6):707–712.

[6] Linetsky, M., Raghavan, C.T., Johar, K., Fan, X., Monnier, V.M., et al. (2014). UVA light-excited kynurenines oxidize ascorbate and modify lens proteins through the formation of advanced glycation end products: implications for human lens aging and cataract formation. *J Biol Chem*, Jun 13;289(24):17111-23.

[7] El Chehab, H., Blein, J.P., Herry, J.P., Chave, N., Ract-Madoux, G., et al. (2012). Ocular phototoxicity and altitude among mountain guides. *J Fr Ophtalmol*, Dec; 35(10):809-15.

[8] Black, A.T., Gordon, M.K., Heck, D.E., Gallo, M.A., Laskin, D.L., et al. (2011). UVB light regulates expression of antioxidants and inflammatory mediators in human corneal epithelial cells. *Biochem Pharmacol*, Apr 1; 81(7):873-80.

[9] Ibid. El Chehab. (2012).

[10] Roberts, J.E. (2011). Ultraviolet radiation as a risk factor for cataract and macular degeneration. *Eye Contact Lens*, Jul;37(4):246-9.

[11] Remé, C., Reinboth, J., Clausen, M., Hafezi, F. (1996). Light damage revisited: converging evidence, diverging views? *Arch Clin Exp Ophthalmol*, Jan; 234(1):2-11.

[12] Tuchinda, C., Srivannaboon, S., Lim, H.W. (2006). Photoprotection by window glass, automobile glass, and sunglasses. *J Am Acad Dermatol*, May; 54(5):845-54.

[13] Kullavanijaya, P., Lim, H.W. (2005). Photoprotection. *J Am Acad Dermatol*, Jun; 52(6):937-58; quiz 959-62.

[14] Ibid. Tuchinda. (2006).

[15] Ibid. Kullavanijaya. (2005).

[16] Ibid. Kullavanijaya. (2005).

[17] Schaefer, H., Moyal, D., Fourtanier, A. (1998). Recent advances in sun protection. *Semin Cutan Med Surg*, Dec; 17(4):266-75.

[18] FDA Statement. (2018). Statement from FDA Commissioner Scott Gottlieb, M.D., on new FDA actions to keep consumers safe from the harmful effects of sun exposure, and ensure the long-term safety and benefits of sunscreens. *U.S. Food Drug Admin,* May 18.

[19] Snellen, E.L., Verbeek, A.L., Van Den Hoogen, G.W., Crysberg, J.R., Hoyng, C.B. (2002). Neovascular age-related macular degeneration and its relationship to antioxidant intake. *Acta Ophthalmol Scand*, Aug;80(4):368-71.

[20] Richer, S., Stiles, W., Statkute, L., Pulido, J., Frankowski, J., et al. (2004). Double-masked, placebo-controlled, randomized trial of lutein and antioxidant supplementation in the intervention of atrophic age-related macular degeneration: the Veterans LAST study (Lutein Antioxidant Supplementation Trial). *Optometry*, Apr;75(4):216-30.

[21] Landrum, J.T., Bone, R.A., Joa, H., Kilburn, M.D., Moore, L.L., et al. (1997). A one year study of the macular pigment: the effect of 140 days of a lutein supplement. *Exp Eye Res*, Jul;65(1):57-62.

[22] Bernstein, P.S., Zhao, D.Y., Wintch, S.W., Ermakov, I.V., McClane, R.W., et al. (2002). Resonance Raman measurement of macular carotenoids in normal subjects and in age-related macular degeneration patients. *Ophthalmology*, Oct;109(10):1780-7.

[23] Delcourt, C., Carriere, I., Delage, M., Barberger-Gateau, P., Schalch, W. (2006). Plasma Lutein and Zeaxanthin and Other Carotenoids as Modifiable Risk Factors for Age-Related Maculopathy and Cataract: The POLA Study. *Inves Ophthal Vis Sci*, Jun:47:2329-35.

[24] Chew, E.Y., Clemons, T.E., Agron, E., Sperduto, R.E., Sangiovanni, J.P., et al. (2013). Long-term effects of vitamins C and E, β-carotene, and zinc on age-related macular degeneration: AREDS report no. 35. *Opthalmology*, Aug;120(8):1604-11.

[25] Du, J., Cullen, J.J., Buettner, G.R. (2012). Ascorbic acid: chemistry, biology and the treatment of cancer. *Biochem Biophys Acta*, Dec;1826(2):443-57.

[26] Cangemi, R., Angelico, F., Loffredo, L., Del Ben, M., Pignatelli, P., et al. (2007). Oxidative stress-mediated arterial dysfunction in patients with metabolic syndrome: Effect of ascorbic acid. *Free Radic Biol Med,* Sep 1;43(5):853-9.

[27] Ibid. Cho. (2004).

[28] Piermarocchi, S., Saviano, S., Parisi, V., Tedeschi, M., Panozzo, G., et al. (2012). Carotenoids in Age-related Maculopathy Italian Study (CARMIS): two-year results of a randomized study. *Eur J Ophthalmol*, Mar-Apr;22(2):216-25.

[29] Otsuka, T., Shimazawa, M., Nakanishi, T., Ohno, Y., Inoue, Y., et al. (2013). Protective effects of a dietary carotenoid, astaxanthin, against light-induced retinal damage. *J Pharmacol Sci*, 123(3):209-18.

[30] Korac, R.R., Khambholja, K.M. (2011). Potential of herbs in skin protection. *Pharmacog Rev,* Jul 1;5(10):164-173.

[31] Mufti J. (2003). UV Protection. *House Pers Prod Ind*, Jun.

[32] Burgess CM. (2009). Cosmetic products. In: Kelly, A.P., Taylor, S.C., (Eds.). Dermatology for Skin of Color. New York: McGraw-Hill Medical.

A-5. RECOMMENDED PRODUCTS

Go to www.naturaleyecare.com for more details or call us at 845-255-8222. See individual eye condition chapters for more details of nutrients related to that condition.

Allergies

Allergy Desensitization Homeopathic Eyedrops

Jason's AllergEase Formula

Quercitin Bromelain Complex

Vitamin D3

Anti-Inflammation Formulas

Advanced Eye and Vision Support (whole food, organic) Formula

Astaxanthin

Carlsons Fish Oil or Nordic Natural Fish Oil

CBD (Pure) Oil

Enz-Flame Formula

Retinal Support (wild-crafted) Formula 2oz

Serrapeptase or Nattokinase Enzymes

Turmeric

Zyflamend Whole Body

Brain Support

Astaxanthin

Brain Cell Support 60 caps

Cognitive Factors 120 Vcaps

CoQ10

Connective Tissue Support

Advanced Eye and Vision Support (whole food, organic) Formula

Dr. Grossman's Bilberry/Gingko (wild-crafted) Formula

Hyaluronic Acid

Krill Oil

Retinal Support (wild crafted) Eye Formula

Corneal Support

Castor Oil Eyedrops

Ortho K Thin Homeopathic Eyedrops

Ortho K Thick Homeopathic Eyedrops

Dry Eyes

Bruder Eye Hydrating Mask and Stye Compress

Carlsons Fish Oil or Nordic Natural Fish Oil

Castor Oil Eyedrops

Green Tea Extract

HydroEye Gelcaps

Oasis Plus Eyedrops

Tear Stimulation Forte Homeopathic Eyedrops

Women's Tear Stimulation Homeopathic Eyedrops

Tranquileyes Basic Kit

VisionTone Formula

Vitamin D3

Eye Inflammation (external and mild)

Dr. Grossman's EyeEase Formula

LidHydgenix

MSM Drops

Eyestrain

Astaxanthin

Black Currant Seed Oil

Dr. Grossman's Vision Boost Formula

Eye Fatigue Homeopathic Pellets

Tear Stimulation Forte Homeopathic Eyedrops

General Eye Health

Advanced Eye and Vision Support (whole food, organic) Formula

Astaxanthin

Carlsons Fish Oil or Nordic Natural Fish Oil

Dr. Grossman's Maxivision Formula

Vitamin D3

Viteyes Complete

General Immune Support

Advanced Eye and Vision Support (whole food, organic) Formula

Astaxanthin

Carlsons Fish Oil or Nordic Natural Fish Oil

BioMax III (whole food, organic) Multivitamin

Jason's ImmunoBalance Formula

Jason's Famous Cold and Flu Formula

Vitamin D3

General Anti-Inflammation Support

Advanced Eye and Vision Support (whole food, organic) Formula

Astaxanthin

CBD Oil

Green Tea

Pro Omega Lemon

Vitamin D3

Zyflamend Whole Body

Lens Support

ACG Glutathione Spray (oral)

Brite Eyes III Eyedrops

Can-C Eyedrops

Castor Oil Eyedrops

Cataract Homeopathic Pellets

Cineraria Homeopathic Eyedrops

Oclumed Eyedrops

VisionTone (wild-crafted) Formula

Macula Support

Advanced Eye and Vision Support Formula

Biomax Food Multi III

Dr. Grossman's Bilberry/Ginkgo Formula

Dr. Grossman's Blood Vessel Formula

Krill Oil

Maxivision Meso

Resveratrol with Quercitin

Vitamin D3

Mitochondria Support

Acetyl-L-Carnitine

ACG Glutathione Spray (oral)

Advanced Eye and Vision Support (whole food, organic) Formula

BioMax III (whole food, organic) Multivitamin

D-Ribose

L-Carnosine

PQQ (Pyrroloquinoline quinone)

Super DHA

Taurine (liquid)

Vitamin C

Optic Nerve Support

ACG Glutathione Spray

Advanced Eye and Vision Support (whole food, organic) Formula

AminoPro (aminoguarnadine)

CBD Oil

Dr. Grossman's Coleus Ultra Formula

Eye Pressure Support with Mirtogenol

Glaucoma Homeopathic Pellets

Germanium

Krill Oil

Pure Focus (sublingual) Formula

ReVision (wild-crafted) Herbal Formula

Viteyes Complete Formula OR

Viteyes Optic Nerve Support Formula

Night Vision

Astaxanthin

Black Currant Seed Oil

Dr. Grossman's Advanced Eye and Vision Support (whole food) Organic eye formula

Dr. Grossman's Bilberry/Gingko (wild-crafted) Formula

Retinal Support

Astaxanthin

Biomax Food Multi III

Dr. Grossman's Advanced Eye and Vision Support (whole food) Organic eye formula

Dr. Grossman's Bilberry/Gingko (wild-crafted) Formula

Dr. Grossman's Blood Vessel Support Formula

Dr. Grossman's Maxivision Formula

Carlsons Fish Oil or Nordic Natural

Krill Oil

Maxivision Meso

Retinal Support (wild crafted) Eye Formula

Resveratrol with Quercitin

ReVision (wild crafted) Eye Formula

Saffron

Taurine

Vitamin D3

Sugar Balance and Blood Vessel Support

Viteyes Optic Nerve Support

Dr. Grossman's Blood Vessel Formula

Glycoease (sublingual)

Resveratrol with Quercitin

Advanced Eye and Vision Support Formula

Krill Oil

Vitreous Support

Advanced Eye and Vision Support (whole food, organic) Formula

Floater Homeopathic Pellets

Hyaluronic Acid

ReVision (wild crafted) Eye Formula

Vitamin C

Sources:

NaturalEyeCare.com

NordicNaturals.com

FiveElementHealing.net

GaiaHerbs.com

Physiologics.com

Natoph.com

InnateResponse.com

A-6. AMSLER TEST

Take this test to monitor changes in your vision. Test with adequate lighting. If you wear glasses for near work, put them on to view the grid. Sit with your eyes about 16″ from the grid.

1. Cover one eye, but do not close it or press on it.
2. Stare directly at the spot in the center of the grid, and do not look away from this spot.
3. Notice the horizontal and vertical lines in your periphery. Ask yourself as you check each eye separately: Are any of the lines wavy, missing, blurry, or discolored?

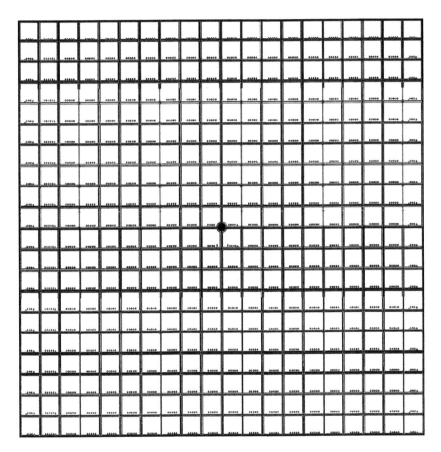

If you have not noticed problems with your vision, yet you detect broken, curved, or distorted lines (metamorphopsia) while viewing the Amsler grid, it could be that you have an early stage of macular degeneration. Try doing the same test later today or tomorrow. If the results are repeated, you should make an appointment to have your eyes examined by an optometrist, an optometric physician, or an ophthalmologist. In any case, continue using the Amsler grid test 2–3 times a week to monitor any changes.

A-7. ADDITIONAL THERAPIES

Acupressure

Acupressure is the art of stimulating targeted acupuncture points with your finger(s) and without the use of needles. Acupressure is often combined with "trigger-point" therapy to alleviate pain and muscle spasms. Acupressure and massage are most often the treatment of choice for pediatric cases.

Benefit for vision. Using acupressure points relaxes the eyes, relieves stress, and has the potential to reduce pain. See also Chapter 10-4.

Acupuncture

Acupuncture is a medical model that started in China over 3,000 years ago to help with healing the body and reducing pain. It can be used to help with eye conditions toward healthier vision. Acupuncture uses tiny, sterilized needles to stimulate points on the body for healing and health.

Benefit for vision. Acupuncture helps bring balance to the entire body, relieves stress, reduces pain, enlivens dormant nerve cells, and increases energy circulation, which in turn supports vision health. See also Chapter 9-4.

Alexander Technique

The Alexander technique is a way of learning to move mindfully through life and to adjust old habits that relieve tension in the body. The technique has been found to help reduce back and neck pain and may be helpful in improving posture, respiratory function, and general pain.[1] By relieving tension in our daily physical habits, we affect the free flow of energy and circulation to the eyes.

Benefit for vision. This technique enhances awareness of our own body, including our capacity for better vision.

Ayurvedic Medicine

Ayurvedic medicine is one of the oldest systems of medicine in the world, originating in India thousands of years ago. This practice is based on balancing the body's constitution (prakriti) and life forces (dosha) through specific lifestyle recommendations, including diet, exercise, herbal supplements, rest, and detoxification programs. The term "Ayurveda" combines the Sanskrit words ayur (life) and veda (science or knowledge).

Benefit for vision. According to Ayurvedic medicine, most vision problems arise from a pitta dosha imbalance. The aim of Ayurveda is to restore fundamental balance.

Chinese Medicine

Chinese medicine goes back over 3,000 years and primarily uses a combination of herbs, acupuncture, movement techniques such as qigong, and diet. There are 20 primary meridians (flows of energy) in the body that are evaluated by practitioners in order to determine the imbalances that cause or contribute to pain and disease. The goal is to get these meridians back into balance to support the body's natural healing process. Acupuncture is often known for reducing pain, though it has many other applications for health, including eye disease.

Benefit for vision. Traditional Chinese Medicine provides a variety of complementary approaches to treat and improve the underlying causes of vision conditions. See also Chapter 9.

Chiropractic

Chiropractic is a manipulative treatment of joint misalignments, especially those of the spinal column. Misalignments are believed to cause other disorders by affecting the function of nerves, muscles, and organs. One branch of chiropractic is Atlas Adjustment that specializes in adjusting the top vertebrae of the spine in a non-manipulative manner.

The connection between chiropractic care and visual health may be summed up in one word: tone. Traditionally, the public associates chiropractic with spinal health and perhaps proper muscle tone. Some people understand that chiropractic care addresses altered and asymmetrical patterns of nerve tension. Still fewer relate tone to optimal brain-body coordination. We can connect all those dots to the developmental, behavioral, and social dynamics that intertwine vision with posture. All of these factors, and more, contribute to our vitality and go way beyond the biomechanical perception of chiropractic contribution to our visual and overall well-being.[2]

Benefit for vision. Misalignments in the top five cervical vertebrae may impact blood flow to the eyes, pinch nerves, and cause tension and stress, all of which can contribute to vision problems.

Color Therapy

Color therapy (chromotherapy, syntonics, light therapy) has the potential to help manage eye disease.

Glaucoma. In one study of 19 patients, medication used to lower eye pressure (IOP) was withheld and green spectrum glasses were worn by the patients for 2 days straight. One group was also given adrenalin (1:1,000), thought to increase the eyes' sensitivity to green light. Results of this study showed there was a pronounced tendency for the IOP to decrease in patients wearing the green glasses, particularly when combined with very small dosages of pilocarpine (0.5 percent). The pressures decreased by 6.0mm Hg in 8 cases, 10mm Hg in 9 cases, and 10mm Hg and more in 3 cases. The results were more striking when combined with small dosages of adrenalin.[3]

Macular degeneration. Though research is limited on this, the green blue color therapy for about 20 minutes daily may be helpful.

Retinitis pigmentosa. Again, research is very limited, but red light exposure may be helpful.

In general, vision therapy using color may be helpful for accommodation, binocular conditions, visual information processing, and a constricted function visual field (the ability to make use of what we see around us.) This is means being able to use our peripheral vision, rather than relating to peripheral vision itself.[4]

Craniosacral

Craniosacral therapy is a method of relieving pain and tension through gentle manipulations of the skull that are regarded as harmonizing with the natural rhythm of the central nervous system, and they are designed to balance the flow of cerebrospinal fluid. The research has been limited. That being said, craniosacral may have some benefit.

Benefit for vision. Craniosacral may have benefits as indicated in the following. High (or low)[5] estimated cerebrospinal fluid pressure has been linked to a number of eye conditions,[6] including diabetic retinopathy[7] and glaucoma[8] [9] (including normal-tension glaucoma)[10].

Emotional Freedom Technique

Emotional Freedom Technique (EFT) is a therapeutic approach based on the premise that emotions are key to identity, and that unpleasant and unresolved emotions can cause harm. It is commonly referred to as "tapping," and has been called "acupuncture without the needles" because it consists of gently tapping with the fingers on the face and upper body, on some of the same points where an acupuncturist would insert needles. We stimulate these energy meridian points with EFT tapping, while bringing up an issue we feel stuck about, to help us move the energy through our system and clear the issue.[11]

Benefit for vision. Our vision may be directly connected to how we feel, therefore EFT helps relax the mind and our body, so we can see more clearly and with less strain. Stating the problem such as "I'm worried my vision is getting worse" engages the mind, while tapping on the acupuncture meridian points at the same time engages the body. This mind/body combination seems to give better results than healing modalities, which focus on only the mind, or only the body.

Essential Oil Therapy

Essential oil therapy uses plant extracts, usually applied to the skin, to help in many ways, including relief of tension and anxiety, improvement of sleep, reduction of pain, enhancement of circulation, improvement of digestion, and more. See Appendix 9, Essential Oils.

Benefits for vision. Essential oils can help promote healthy vision by reducing inflammation related to specific eye conditions, fighting unfriendly bacteria, aiding in digestion, boosting the immune system, supporting respiratory health, improving mood, and reducing depression.

Feldenkrais Method

Feldenkrais teaches efficient methods of movement to reduce stress of the body. The theory is that movements can repair impaired connections between the motor cortex and the body, thereby benefiting the quality of body movement and improving overall well-being.[12] When working with a practitioner, sessions include slow repetition of new movements to change habitual patterns that can also be practiced at home.

Benefit for vision. One study found these methods to be effective in treating patients with vision impairment and neck pain[13] (perhaps resulting from computer eye strain).

Grounding (Earthing)

Yoga, tai chi, meditative walks in the woods, and meditation are all great examples of ways to become grounded, to get back into the here and now, away from anxiety and worry that may cause chronic stress.

With respect to electricity, earthing means connecting directly to the ground. Grounding does not mean connecting directly, but having zero electrical potential. As a therapy, earthing is an inexpensive and easy way to reduce inflammation in the eyes and body.[14] Simply walking barefoot on the earth/grass or sand helps us absorb negative electrons from the earth. Additionally, grounding can be achieved by purchasing and using grounding bed sheets (to be used during sleep) and mats (to be used while on the computer or watching television).

Benefit for vision. Grounding the body and picking up electrons from the earth helps keep the body in balance, allowing for movement of energy, blood, and nutrients throughout.

Herbal Medicine

Herbal medicine goes back many thousands of years and has been an integral part of using nature to heal and maintain health. Some research indicates that plants were used as far back as the Neanderthal period for health and healing.

Benefit for vision. Thousands of studies verify the use of plants for health and healing, including many of those recommended in this guide.

Homeopathic

Homeopathic medicine goes back to the late 1800's and was started by a German physician, Samuel Hahnemann (1755-1843). It is the principle of "like treats like," which means that when certain substances in nature are ingested in large amounts, they can cause or mimic disease, but when reduced to extremely small amounts, leaving only the energy signature of the substances, they have the opposite effect of helping the body heal.

Benefit for vision. There are many homeopathic preparations that can help a wide range of eye conditions, including macular degeneration, glaucoma, cataracts, eye floaters, and dry eyes.

Massage

There are many types of massage, but overall the goal is to relieve both emotional stress and muscle tension. Getting a weekly or bi-weekly massage can go a long way in helping maintain health and balance.

Benefit for vision. The eye relies on the body's good blood circulation, good digestion, and good energy flow. Massage can relieve body tensions that may inhibit the free flow of energy, blood, and nutrients to the eyes, particularly due to tension in the neck and shoulder areas.

Naturopathy

Where traditional medical training includes coursework in prescription medication to treat health problems, naturopathic doctors, with similar medical training, study the use of herbs in combination with other holistic modalities that may include homeopathy, acupuncture, diet, and nutrition.

Benefit for vision. Naturopathic doctors look at the individual and the whole person in relation to their health condition, offering a holistic approach to support natural healing ability.

Reflexology

Reflexologists use pressure, primarily in points in the feet that relate to different organs and parts of the body. This process promotes tension relief, circulation improvement, and normal functioning support in any affected area of the body.

Benefit for vision. Reflexology focuses on improving circulation and energy flow to parts of the body that need healing. There are points on the feet that are related to the eyes.

Reiki

The word reiki comes from the Japanese word "rei," which means "universal life" and "ki" which means "energy." It is administered by the "laying on of hands" to stimulate and improve an individual's life force energy.

Benefit for vision. Similar to other energy methods, it helps reduce stress and focuses on the body's natural healing potential.

Rolfing

Rolfing is a system of soft tissue manipulation that releases tension and lengthens fascia (connective tissue) in order to ease strain patterns and reduce related pain. It has a physical impact on the peripheral nervous system and on upper-back pain (myofascial pain).[15] Rolfing may reduce chronic stress, reduce spinal curvature in subjects with lordosis (sway back), and enhance neurological functioning.

Benefit for vision. Rolfing relieves chronic stress and pain and enhances neurological functioning.

---

[1] Wodman, J.P., Moore, N.R. (2012). Evidence for the effectiveness of Alexander Technique lessons in medical and health-related conditions: a systematic review. *Int J Clin Pract,* Jan;66(1):98-112).

[2] Filippi, M., Chiropractic and Vision

[3] Zaretskaya, R.B. (1948). Some experiments with green spectacles prescribed to glaucomatous patients. *Am J Ophthalmol,* Aug;31(8):985-989.

[4] Mischio, G. (2013). Syntonic Phototherapy Yields Eye-Opening Results. Retrieved Sep 17 2018 from http://www.thevisiontherapycenter.com/discovering-vision-therapy/bid/83035/Syntonic-Phototherapy-Yielding-Eye-Opening-Results.

[5] Wang, N., Yang, D., Jonas, J.B. (2013). Low cerebrospinal fluid pressure in the pathogenesis of primary open-angle glaucoma: epiphenomenon or causal relationship? The Beijing Intracranial and Intraocular Pressure (iCOP) study. *J Glaucoma,* Jun-Jul;22 Suppl 5:S11-2.

[6] Morgan, W.H., Balaratnasingam, C., Lind, C.R., Colley, S., Kang, M.H., et al. (2016). Cerebrospinal fluid pressure and the eye. *Br J Ophthalmol,* Jan;100(1):71-7.

[7] Jonas, J.B., Xu, L., Xu, J., Wei, W.B., Wang, Y.X. (2015). Prevalence of Diabetic Retinopathy and Vision Loss in the Beijing Eye Study: the Potential Role of the Cerebrospinal Fluid Pressure. *Curr Diab Rep,* Oct;15(10):71.

[8] Jonas, J.B., Ritch, R., Panda-Jonas, S. (2015). Cerebrospinal fluid pressure in the pathogenesis of glaucoma. *Prog Brain Res,* 221:33-47.

[9] Fleischman, D., Berdahl, J., Stinnett, S.S., Fautsch, M.P., Allingham, R.R. (2015). Cerebrospinal fluid pressure trends in diseases associated with primary open-angle glaucoma. *Acta Ophthalmol,* May;93(3):3234-6.

[10] Wostyn, P., De Groot, V., Van Dam, D., Audenaert, K., De Deyn, P.P. (2013). Senescent changes in cerebrospinal fluid circulatory physiology and their role in the pathogenesis of normal-tension glaucoma. *Am J Ophthalmol,* Jul;156(1):5-14.

[11] Neff, N.L., NancyLNeff.com.

[12] Stalker, D., Glymour, C., eds. (1989). *Examining Holistic Medicine.* p. 373. Prometheus Books. Buffalo, NY.

[13] Lundqvist, L.O., Zetterlund, C., Richter, H.O. (2014). Effects of Feldenkrais method on chronic neck/scapular pain in people with visual impairment: a randomized controlled trial with one-year follow-up. *Arch Phys Med Rehabil,* Sep;95(9):1656-61.

[14] Oschman, J.L., Chevalier, G., Brown, R. (2015). The effects of grounding (earthing) on inflammation, the immune response, wound healing, and prevention and treatment of chronic inflammatory and autoimmune diseases. *J Inflamm Res,* Mar 24;8:83-96.

[15] Jones, T.A. (2004). Rolfing. *Phys Med Rehabil Clin N Am,* Nov;15(4):799-809.

A-8. MAGIC EYE 3D IMAGES

Magic Eye books ignited the worldwide 3D explosion of the 1990's, breaking bestselling list records worldwide. Today, popular uses for Magic Eye images still include retail products, other uses, and vision therapy uses. Viewing Magic Eye images help make one's vision more flexible (like yoga for the eyes), helping keep the eye muscles more adaptable and relaxed.

Magic Eye images are an advanced form of autostereogram. Its predecessor, the single image black and white random dot stereogram, was used to study depth perception.

Autostereograms allow you to see a three-dimensional image imbedded in a 2D picture without the need for special glasses. The surface level of some Magic Eye images sometimes appear to be random splashes of color and always at first appear to be 2D. In all the Magic Eye images, there is a deeper level with a hidden image or a 3D dimension to the image.

When you are viewing a Magic Eye image you are using your ability to use your two eyes together as a focused team. This information is then sent to your brain, and if processed successfully, the intended 3D illusion will be seen (binocular depth perception).

For many of us, our eyes feel the negative effects of working at our computers all day. But it wasn't always this way. The human eye is a remarkable tool that evolved to help our hunter-gatherer ancestors perform such tasks as spotting game, or danger, from a distance. However, the vision skills that served our ancestors so well are used very differently in today's society, particularly when we use our computers and mobile devices. Because we spend so much time at our computers, they have become the top cause of eyestrain in the United States, and many of us suffer from computer eye fatigue. Symptoms of computer eye fatigue include eyestrain, headaches, blurry vision, poor concentration, dry irritated eyes, and shoulder and neck pain.

Benefits of doing Magic Eye exercises can include the following:

- Makes the eyes more flexible regarding focusing (convergence) and seeing distance and peripherally (divergence).
- Reduces strain related to high volume computer use which can lead to blurriness of vision, poor concentration, headaches, blurred vision and body fatigue. Seeing the 3D images requires the eye muscles to work in the opposite direction of how we focus on the computer, allowing them relax and rebalance.
- Increases one's ability to recall printed information
- Improve your depth perception for sports and daily activities
- Helps relieve overall stress similar to the benefits received from meditation
- Helps integrate the physical, mental and spiritual energies together creating an enhanced sense of health and well-being as well as enhancing overall intuition

For more information, go to www.magiceye.com – much of the material above is from the book *Magic Eye Beyond 3D: Improve Your Vision*.

A-9. ESSENTIAL OILS

By Sam Berne, O.D.

When I discovered medicinal essential oils, I often applied them before my meditation or spiritual practice, and after a few months I started receiving intuitive information about how to solve different challenges in my life. My left brain discounted these messages, but after a while I realized that the plants did have an ability to help me at deeper levels, beyond symptoms. When I began using the oils on patients for their vision and health problems, many reported the same experiences. Not only did their symptoms go away, but they also found that they became more connected to themselves.

Plants communicate in ways that are outside of our normal hearing and vision. They may release chemicals via aroma, or cause a temperature change when they touch your skin, or affect you via color, as with blue tansy or lavender. As we open to this kind of subtle awareness, our spirituality grows and we connect to ourselves and others in ways beyond the material plane.

Our bodies are extremely clever when it comes to healing, and high-quality plant medicines offer us a way to connect with our biological intelligence. Many different forms of plant medicines are available. In my practice, I have had great success with the use of therapeutic grade medicinal essential oils, also known as aromatherapy oils.

When used in conjunction with other healing modalities, the improvements in physical, emotional, and energetic health are greater than when the other modality is used alone. Because of their complexity and their antibacterial, antiviral, and fungicidal properties, medicinal essential oils can improve our lymph and immune systems. Biophysicists who study the energy field to find and measure health conditions have learned that essential oils have the ability to protect, repair, and clean the energy field.

Most mainstream medicine promotes the use of synthetic pharmaceuticals for our ailments. But pharmaceuticals are problematic. They may help control symptoms, but because they don't address the factors that cause illness, they can actually cause our immune systems to switch off. Designed to work by "killing" a specific "bug," these drugs take us further away from our biological intelligence.

Medicinal essences work differently. They help us connect more deeply to our healing capabilities, and because of their complexity, help create a balance that sets limits on the bugs' behavior. They work with the body to stimulate our immune systems, helping us to heal not just the symptoms, but the causes behind our diseases and disorders. Because plants contain such a rich and complex blend of naturally occurring minerals, vitamins, and more, they can adapt to the ever-changing organisms that affect our health, keeping them in balance and improving our ability to connect to our own biology.

Plant essences do not, themselves, contain nutrients. However, they support the bioavailability of food nutrients.

Essential Oil Eye Protocol for Vision

In my years of studying and treating eye problems, I have found that in most cases, a large part of the problem is that the eye tissue is starved for nutrients. Our eyes need a great deal of oxygenation, as well as high amounts of glutathione, vitamin C, beta carotene, B complex, and other vitamins and minerals. Many people with vision problems also suffer from toxicities. The liver is always involved when someone is dealing with toxicity, and we know from Chinese medicine that the liver rules the eyes. I have found that the medicinal essences offer many properties for both improving nutrient accessibility and detoxification.

Here are some of my "go to essences" for the eyes:

Carrot seed improves the eyes by protecting against macular degeneration, detoxifying blood vessels, toning the liver, and relieving stress and anxiety.

Frankincense has been around since antiquity, a sacred plant that can be helpful in showing us our visual blind spots. Frankincense tells us to "open up that third eye" and is my main "go to" around the eyes.

Saffron is very helpful for eye health as it helps rebalance body fluids on a cellular level and stimulates the Chi in the entire body.

Sweet fennel, with its spicy sweet scent similar to black licorice, is a detoxifier, blood purifier, and diuretic, reduces swelling, headaches, and dizziness, and restores and stimulates the overall digestive system.

Yarrow reduces pain, severe rashes, respiratory difficulties, and inflammation, especially with vision conditions like optic neuritis and conjunctivitis.

To use the following protocols for some common eye problems, I recommend layering each essence below the eyes and about 2–3 inches above the eyes at the temples. Do this 2–3 times per day. If you get an essence in your eyes, dab a little coconut oil near the edge of the eye to neutralize the burning (never in the eye). Don't use water or saline as it will spread the oil in the eyes.

Medicinal essences are both harmonizing and healing, and the more deeply we connect to nature and our bodies, the more effectively the essences will do their job. They are a versatile powerhouse and offer us many gifts, without the side effects that often come with pharmaceuticals and surgery. Use them with care. If used correctly they can help assist better vision and wellness.

How to Apply Medical Essential Oils

Please be gentle when first starting to use medicinal essences. I like to start by breathing in their aroma and then take as much time as necessary to feel what my body does with the energy. The more we slow down, the more we can connect to our own rhythms, and this practice helps us nourish and reconnect to our depleted selves.

Topical use

While some practitioners state that essences must always be blended in a carrier oil and should never be put directly on the skin, I have found that the greatest medicinal power is achieved by using the essences undiluted. The most powerful and medically effective way to apply medicinal essences is topically: directly on the skin, undiluted, or neat.

The first rule of aromatherapy is to apply the essence(s) on the area of concern or as close to it as possible (e.g., for a headache at the temples, apply the essence(s) to the temple area; for an eye, apply around the outside of the eye socket – NEVER IN THE EYES). When using more than one essence, they should be layered, one at a time, on the skin. Massage each gently into the skin before applying the next essence.

When using essences on the skin, sometimes it can be important to apply or layer them in a certain order. Oils that have a yang or hot quality like oregano or clove bud tend to be skin irritants and should be used with great care on the skin. Using a "cold-hot-cold" format allows you to safely apply such essences almost anywhere on the body. I recommend beginning and ending with an essence that has a yin, or cool quality. Apply the sensitive or hot essence(s) in between, using slightly fewer drops to assure that the area they cover is within the "boundaries" of the area covered by the initial yin essence.

While for the most part essences do not have side effects, they may cause skin irritation, either because of a reaction to the essence itself or because the essence triggers a detoxification reaction (which is a good thing!). Always do a test patch when using a new essence, and consider skin type (fair skinned people are more sensitive than most) when selecting and applying essences. Tip for those with sensitive skin: the soles of the feet are full of receptors and can usually take any essence.

However careful we are, almost everyone will have a skin reaction one time or another when using essential oils. This is because the skin is a major dumping ground for hidden toxicities that are stored in the tissues, and the essences are great detoxifiers. If the skin reaction is extreme, either use some essences to help neutralize the skin reaction or reduce the dosage until the skin reaction clears.

Please try to keep the essences away from the mouth, eyes and mucous membranes. But do not be alarmed if a few drops do get in one of these sensitive areas; while it might be quite uncomfortable for 15–30 minutes, it will not do any damage. To alleviate the discomfort, you can apply a pure oil like olive oil or coconut oil to the area to neutralize the irritating effect of the essence. For the eye area, dab a few drops around the outside of the eye. Do not put the neutralizing oil in the eye.

If you have questions or are concerned for any reason—the person being treated is larger or smaller than average, in poor health, pregnant, or very young or old—it is best to work with an experienced medicinal aromatherapist until you have developed depth of knowledge in this area.

For digestive issues, I usually apply four drops twice a day on the area of concern around the stomach and digestive tract. I usually use two essences at a time, and will utilize this pair for about two weeks before moving to the next pair.

Anise seed. Aside from being great for clearing out intestinal parasites, anise seed is also a wonderful heart tonic and helps improve circulatory and nervous system imbalances.

Basil (sweet) works with digestion on many levels, including the gall bladder and liver detoxification, also offering anti-inflammatory action. If my stomach is upset, I put a few drops in a glass of water and sip after a meal.

Black pepper provides support for the intestines, liver, and pancreas, helps us become more yin (cooling), and is also helpful with irritable bowel syndrome, parasites, and constipation.

Carrot seed's properties include being an antiseptic, disinfectant, detoxifier, and antioxidant.

Clary sage helps balance the endocrine system

Coriander seed is a blood sugar equalizer, intestinal cleaner, and overall body purifier, tonifies the digestive system, improves appetite, strengthens the spleen-pancreas meridian, and is also a great analgesic and wonderful aphrodisiac. On an emotional level, coriander seed helps reduce worry and over-thinking.

Cypress oil is known for its antiseptic, antispasmodic, antibacterial, stimulating, and antirheumatic properties.

Fennel (sweet) helps balance the blood sugar, is a strong diuretic, and also helps reduce flatulence. Fennel is also one of my favorites for my eye protocol and is a powerful anti-bacterial agent.

Frankincense helps relieve chronic stress and anxiety, reduces pain and inflammation, and boosts immunity.

Geranium reduces inflammation, alleviates anxiety, and balances hormones.

Ginger, known as the queen of digestion and stomach disorders, helps to reduce nausea, sea sickness, and heartburn; it also helps to increase bowel movements and clean out the intestinal tract. It supports the kidneys and brings an overall yang (warming) energy to the digestive system. It can also help with chronic fatigue, provide a storehouse of extra energy, and increase mental clarity. On a spiritual level, sweet and spicy ginger is a fantastic catalyst for enhancing one's ability to follow through in life, promoting courage, purification, vibrancy, and success on all levels.

Green cardamom seed strengthens the spleen, improves digestive fire, reduces intestinal parasites, nausea, flatulence, diarrhea, and stimulates the movement of digestion. It is a gentle tonic for the brain, heart, and nervous system and helps to improve circulation and reduce mental activity and anxiety.

Hyssop officianalis supports the liver and strengthens the spleen and pancreas. It also protects against viruses, is an adrenal stimulant, offers immune and lung support, and can be used as an expectorant. On an emotional level, hyssop can help heal unresolved grief, stimulate forgiveness, and strengthen our sense of boundaries.

Laurel leaf supports the lymph system, lessens muscle pain, promotes perspiration, is a disinfectant, and is good for low self-esteem.

Lavender essential oil benefits include its ability to eliminate nervous tension, relieve pain, disinfect the scalp and skin, enhance blood circulation, and treat respiratory problems.

Lavender (spike) helps reduce stress, pain, helps with headaches, and has anti-inflammatory properties.

Lemon oil cleans toxins from the body and stimulates lymphatic drainage, rejuvenates energy, purifies skin, and fights bacteria and fungi.

Marjoram (sweet) has the amazing qualities of being able to strengthen and relax in the same moment. It is restorative, reduces anxiety, and quiets the mind. Sweet marjoram has both analgesic and anti-spasmodic characteristics and is warming, relaxing, and nurturing.

Parsley has antimicrobial, antiseptic, circulatory, detoxifying, and hypotensive qualities.

Patchouli can improve the spleen and pancreas, help reduce hemorrhoids, and decrease loose stools. It also improves immune system function and works as a heavy metal detoxifier. Its strong anti-inflammatory properties offer help with skin disorders such as eczema. Patchouli also offers anti-bacterial and anti-viral properties, is grounding and earthy, and helps reduce mental activity and anxiety.

Peppermint is supportive for the digestive system. It relieves dyspepsia, nausea, distension, and flatulence, and is also effective at reducing inflammation, especially in the digestive tract and colon. It offers ultimate cooling and refreshment. Energetically dry and cool, peppermint can stimulate the nerves and brain and reduce fevers and flu symptoms. On a spiritual level, it helps connect us to the healing awareness of sacred geometry.

Purple sage has anti-parasitic, anti-worm, and anti-fungal properties and stimulates overall digestion, as well as liver and gallbladder function. It is also a fantastic aura cleaner.

Rosemary cineole is highly anti-bacterial. It helps improve sluggish digestion, and can reduce candida, chronic fatigue, and cardiac fatigue. Rosemary helps improve poor concentration and muscle health and is a good expectorant for coughs and bronchitis.

Saffron's is antibacterial and is a blood purifier, antioxidant, decongestant, and memory enhancer.

Spearmint is a liver cleaner, a nervine (calms the nerves), a mouth freshener, and helps in overall detoxification. It is very yin, or cooling.

Spikenard is an overall body regulator and can reduce heartburn and help with hemorrhoids. It is highly sedative, with anti-fungal and analgesic qualities, and can open the heart, calm the mind, settle the emotions, lower anxiety, improve our sleep, and soothe the skin. On a spiritual level, spikenard can consecrate and offer a surrender through serenity and humility. I use spikenard to help with life transitions, release fears, and assist in personal evolution.

Tagetes (marigold) helps relax the stomach's digestive process, reduces parasites and worms in the stomach, and helps with candida caused by fungus. It also offers mental clarity and works as a decongestant, anti-inflammatory agent, and anti-fungal agent.

Tangerine helps support bile production and aids in draining the gallbladder. It is very relaxing and uplifting and is helpful for reducing insomnia.

Tansy (blue) has great anti-inflammatory properties. It improves both digestion and the immune system and is a good sedative.

Tarragon helps reduce loose stools and helps with many other colon and digestive imbalances, including Crohn's disease. It also helps support the kidneys when our fears rise to the surface.

Tea tree lemon reduces candida and is also calming and uplifting, with strong anti-bacterial and anti-viral properties. It supports healthy skin and reduces toe fungus.

Turmeric, a yang (warming) medicinal essence, is a great liver detoxifier and aids in clearing gallstones and colitis. It is uplifting, has anti-inflammatory and antiseptic qualities, and is good for insomnia. Turmeric offers anti-cancer support and is said to reduce tumors and cancers both internally and externally.

Verbena (lemon) aids digestion while reducing diarrhea and rectal inflammation. It reduces deficiencies in the pancreas, liver, and gallbladder. It improves depression and reproductive health in both men and women.

Yarrow is a stimulant that supports a healthy liver. It can also reduce indigestion, intestinal colic, irritable bowel, insufficient bile production, and flatulence. Yarrow reduces pain, severe rashes, respiratory difficulties, and inflammation, and is helpful with vision conditions like optic neuritis and conjunctivitis. This essence has anti-viral properties and helps support the heart and kidneys.

Zanthoxylum, a highly sedative essence, supports digestion and helps decrease anxiety, toothaches, and gum disease.

For both children and adults, medicinal essences used properly offer a non-intrusive, 100% natural treatment option for a wide range of health and wellness issues. Each essence has unique properties, and in combination, the potential for healing is vast, especially when they are used in conjunction with other modalities.

These essences have a complexity that connects us to a higher vibration and frequency, and when we use them we reunite our own diverse energies to a more united consciousness. Medicinal essences can help awaken us to a deeper connection to Mother Earth and to spiritual as well as physical and emotional healing.

Auricular Use

Application behind the ears is great for head congestion, headaches, sinus problems, general malaise, and cold and flu symptoms. This is a very powerful treatment option. Use about five drops each of 5–7 essences. Apply them on the area about midway behind the ear down to the bottom of the neck, layering over the eustachian tubes. Put the first essence behind one ear, then the other ear, and continue going back and forth until you have used all your selected essences. Use respiratory essences, antihistamine essences, and antibacterial essences.

Oral Use

Oral use of essences should be approached with care and only done under the supervision of an experienced aromatherapist. The digestive process breaks down the essences, so oral usage is generally not as powerful as topical use, but this method can be used in conjunction with topical application for an additive effect. The average absorption rate with oral usage is 20–25%.

Sublingual Use

Sublingual use (under the tongue) is more effective than swallowing the essence due to the higher level of receptors in this area. The average absorption rate there is 30–35%. Do this only under the supervision of an experienced aromatherapist.

Inhalation

Using this protocol is a great application for sinus problems, respiratory congestion, lung infections, etc. Boil a cup or mug of water (preferably on the stove, not in a microwave), then add your essences. Some essences that are commonly used in this approach are eucalyptuses, pines, spruces, peppermints, laurel leaf, himalayan soti, and tea tree. If you are using three or four essences, put about 5–7 drops of each in the hot water and hold a towel over your head, making a tent over the cup, capturing the steam. Breathe deeply, inhaling the essences carried by the steam. When the water cools, drink it. I have seen that people who use this protocol for bacterial infections may completely avoid the need for antibiotics.

How Much to Use

Determining how many drops of essence to use is an art, not a science. "One size does not fit all." Every situation is different and must be considered individually. Also, the application method influences how much of the essence will be absorbed by the body. Here are some factors to consider.

How serious is the condition? For someone in a crisis situation you might use more than for "routine maintenance." A person's height and weight are important. The larger the person, the more drops one uses. A good place to start is 8–10 drops each of up to four or five essences if the person is of average height and weight. For a large or overweight person, the amount should be increased accordingly. For a small or underweight person, the amount should be decreased.

Other factors make a difference too. Consider the person's eating habits, exercise level, and emotional state. People with unhealthy lifestyles need larger amounts of the essences than people with healthy lifestyles. Age makes a difference. For elders, children, and infants, the amount used should be reduced. Since working with babies and children requires much judgment and discretion, it is best to consult an experienced medicinal aromatherapist until you have developed depth of knowledge in this area.

Medicinal essences bring the body's systems into balance. Essences that work with blood pressure bring it into balance. Essences that work with thyroid functioning bring it into balance. Essences that are anti-bacterial kill only harmful bacteria, bringing the body back into balance, all while supporting the immune system.

A-10. VISION AND ALZHEIMER'S

It may be possible to detect very early stages of Alzheimer's disease—15 to 20 years before clinical diagnosis. Cedars-Sinai Medical Center has developed an optical imaging technique[1] that may enable doctors to detect very early amyloid plaque buildup. A large clinical study of volunteers from Australia and the U.S. is investigating the possibilities for early detection. Two other universities, the University of San Diego and Emory in Atlanta, are testing whether the equipment recognizes plaque buildup in existing Alzheimer's patients.

The problem is to figure out whether plaque observed in a retinal scan is correlated to plaque detected in a positron emission tomography (PET) scan. PET scans are invasive, use radioactive tracers, and are very expensive, so this new technique is very promising.

Early results indicate that the non-invasive test can detect Alzheimer's with 100% sensitivity and 80.6% specificity. Sensitivity of 100% means that the test doesn't overlook any actual positives by mis-identifying them; 80.6% specificity means that the test rarely identifies something else as amyloid plaque. Sensitivity avoids false-negatives; specificity avoids false-positives.[2] In other words, it errs on the side of caution.

Even more exciting is that current tests can't identify Alzheimer's until the disease is well progressed, but this new technique will allow diagnosis 15–20 years before symptoms appear. This makes it possible to address the problem by other means early on.

---

[1] Cedars-Sinai. (2018). Cedars-Sinai Device May Provide Early Detection of Alzheimer's Disease. Retrieved Aug 24 2018 from https://www.cedars-sinai.edu/Research/Research-Areas/Neurosciences/Featured-Stories/Cedars-Sinai-Device-May-Provide-Early-Detection-of-Alzheimers-Disease.aspx.

[2] Wikipedia. Sensitivity and specificity. Retrieved Aug 24 2018 from https://en.wikipedia.org/wiki/Sensitivity_and_specificity

Make These Foods 80% of Your Diet

Veggies & Salad
Asparagus
Beets
Celery
Cabbage family (collards, kale broccoli, brussels sprouts)
Chard, spinach
Chili, capsicum
Cucumber
Dandelion
Eggplant
Endive
Green beans, peas
Lettuce
Onion, garlic, leeks
Peppers, sweet
Scallions
Radishe
Rutabaga
Seaweeds
Sprouts
Squash, pumpkin
Sweet potato
Swiss chard
Tomatoes
Watercress
Zucchini

Fruit
Avocado
Coconut
Citrus (grapefruit, lemon, lime, orange)
Persimmon
Pineapple
Pomegranate
Rhubarb

Grains, Seeds, Beans
Amaranth
Beans (lima, mung, pinto, red, white)
Buckwheat
Chickpeas (garbanzos)
Lentils, dhal
Kamut
Millet
Quinoa
Pumpkin seed butter
Spouted seeds
Sprouted breads

Oil
Olive oil, extra virgin
Avocado, coconut, flaxseed

Fresh Herbs
Basil
Chives
Cilantro
Coriander
Fennel, anise
Ginger
Mint/spearmint
Oregano
Parsley
Rosemary
Tarragon
Thyme

Herbs/Spice
Cardamom
Coriander
Cumin
Garam masala
Oregano
Nutmeg
Pepper
Paprika
Sea salt

Limit These to 20% of Your Diet

Meat & Seafood
Pork, beef, lamb,
 turkey, chicken,
 venison, rabbit,
 seafood

Dairy
Eggs
Milk products (cheeses,
 creams, yogurt, whey)
Soy cheese

Sweet Fruit
Most are mildly acidic,
 one per day is fine
Apples, pears, etc.
Dates
Melons
Stone fruit (plums, etc.)
Cherries (sweet)

Vegetables
Vegetables that have been
 stored or frozen
Horseradish
Parsnips
Turnips

Flavorings
Lemon, orange,
 coconut, maple,
 lemon, orange,
 peppermint

Oils
All other cooking oils
Margarines

Sweeteners
Artificial sweeteners
Sugar, honey, syrups

Drinks
Alcohol
Cocoa
Coffee
Milk
Soft or sports drinks
Tap water
Tea (black, green)

Other
Candy
Chocolate
Miso
Mushrooms
Pizza
Snack foods
White breads, pastas
White rice, noodles

A-12. SOAKING AND SPOUTING GUIDE

For the average healthy person with a nutrient rich diet, here is a simple way to reduce phytates from your diet.

- Soak all nuts, seeds, legumes, and grains in warm un-chlorinated water. You can add about a tablespoon of something acidic to each cup to be soaked.[1]
- For grains, soak 7–8 hours or overnight.
  - ○ Grains, such as oats and corn, require longer soaking. It can help to add (1 Tbsp) freshly ground rye flour, sourdough rye culture, or some other acidic ingredient to the warm water, such as of yogurt, raw apple cider vinegar, lemon juice, whey, or kefir.
  - ○ Rinse in the morning before cooking.
- Soft nuts, such as walnuts, pecans, and cashews only need about 4 hours of soaking.
  - ○ You can add unrefined salt to the water when you soak nuts to activate enzymes that neutralize enzyme inhibitors.
  - ○ Rinse after soaking.
  - ○ Nuts that will be eaten later can be dehydrated on the lowest heat possible in the oven until completely dried. It is best to stir them occasionally and make sure they do not get burnt.

Soaking and Sprouting Times

Nuts

- Almond: 8–12 hours soaking, 12 hours sprouting.
- Cashew: 2–6 hours soaking, does not sprout.
- Pecan: 4–7 hours soaking, does not sprout.
- Walnut: 4-7 hours soaking, does not sprout.
- Brazil, pistachio, pine nut: Do not soak, do not sprout.

Seeds

- Alfalfa: 8 hours soaking, 2–5 days sprouting.
- Flax: 8 hours soaking, does not sprout.
- Pumpkin: 8 hours soaking, 1–2 days sprouting.
- Sesame: 8 hours soaking, 1–2 days sprouting.
- Sunflower: 2 hours soaking, 12-18 hours sprouting.

Grains

- Buckwheat: 15 minutes soaking, 1–2 days sprouting.
- Barley: 6 hours soaking, 2 days sprouting.
- Corn: 12 hours soaking, add lemon, etc., 2–3 days sprouting.
- Millet: 8 hours soaking, 2–3 days sprouting.

- Oats: 6 hours soaking, 2–3 days sprouting.
- Quinoa: 2 hours soaking, 1–2 days sprouting.
- Rice: 9 hours soaking, 3–5 days sprouting.
- Spelt/Rye: 8 hours soaking, 2–3 days sprouting.
- Wheat/Kamut: 7 hours soaking, 2–3 days sprouting.

Legumes

- Adzuki: 8 hours soaking, 3–5 days sprouting.
- Chickpea: 12 hours soaking, 12 hours sprouting.
- Lentil: 8 hours soaking, 12 hours sprouting.
- Mung: 1-day soaking, 2–5 days sprouting.
- Other beans and dried peas: overnight soaking, 2–3 days sprouting.

Note. Times can vary, depending on water, room temperature, and freshness. Try not to use too much water, and don't soak too long as they can spoil (especially if kept warm). If they spoil, you can usually tell by the rancid odor.

---

[1] Chaudhary, N. Soak Your Nuts Grains & Legumes. Retrieved Apr 18 2018 from http://myindianroots.blogspot.com/2015/03/soak-your-nuts-seeds-grains-legumes.html.

A-13. VISION RELATED ORGANIZATIONS

Vision Organizations

AMD Alliance International - amdalliance.org – 212-821 9200

American Foundation for the Blind (AFB) - afb.org – 214-352-7222

American Macular Degeneration Foundation - macular.org - 888-622-8527

American Optometric Association - aoa.org – 800-365-2219

BrightFocus Foundation - brightfocus.org - 800-437-2423

Cambridge Institute for Better Vision as well - bettervision.com – 978-768-3937

The Coalition for Usher Syndrome Research - usher-syndrome.org - 855-998-7437

College of Optometrists in Vision Development (COVD) - covd.org -330-995-0718

The Foundation Fighting Blindness - blindness.org - 800-683-5555

Glaucoma Research Foundation - glaucoma.org - 800-826-6693

Glaucoma Service Foundation to Prevent Blindness - willsglaucoma.org - 215-928-3190

Jack McGovern Coats Disease Foundation- coatsdiseasefoundation.org - 888-314-8853

Lighthouse International - lighthouseguild.org- 800-284-4422

MD Support - mdsupport.org - 888-866-6148

National Eye Institute - nei.nih.gov - 301-496-5248

National Keratoconus Foundation - nkcf.org - 800-521-2524

Natural Vision Improvement – visioneducators.com - 207-439-9821

Prevent Blindness - preventblindness.org - 800-331-2020

Humanitarian Eye Care Organizations

American Academy of Optometry Foundation - aaopt.org - 844-323-3937

The mission of the American Academy of Optometry Foundation (AAOF) is to develop and provide financial support for optometric research and education in vision and eye health to improve patient clinical care. The AAOF's record of achievement is a strong history of dedication to the improved visual welfare of the public.

Blindskills - blindskills.com - 800-860-4224

Blindskills is a unique self-help organization through which people who are blind or visually impaired offer support to each other as they seek to overcome this serious sensory challenge and live their own lives without unnecessary dependence on others.

Essilor Vision Foundation - essilorvisionfoundation.org - 866-385-0447

Essilor Vision Foundation is a 501(c)(3) public charity, founded in 2007 by Essilor of America, with the mission to eliminate poor vision and its lifelong consequences.

Eye Care 4 Kids - eyecare4kids.org - 801-285-5443

Eye Care 4 Kids (EC4K) is a 501(C)(3) charitable organization founded in Salt Lake City, Utah, in 2001 by Joseph Carbone. The organization has served almost 200,000 children and their families, including thousands of refugees. It has provided the equivalent of more than $50 million in vision services to indigent people. EC4K has eight clinics in Arizona, New Jersey, Nevada, and Utah.

SEE International - seeintl.org – 877-937-3133

SEE International is a leading sight-restoring nonprofit humanitarian organization. SEE works to create a world where everyone has access to high-quality vision care, regardless of their ability to pay. Each year, SEE organizes 175+ sight-restoring programs, and runs a free vision care program in its hometown of Santa Barbara, CA. These programs provide free vision screenings and surgery to people who do not have access to affordable eye care. SEE also trains medical professionals to provide comprehensive eye care worldwide. Since 1974, SEE has screened more than 3.68 million individuals and restored the sight of nearly half a million people.

Seva Foundation – seva.org – 510-845-7382

Seva works with local communities around the world to develop self-sustaining programs that preserve and restore sight.

RestoringVision - restoringvision.org – 209-980-7323

RestoringVision provides new reading and sunglasses at low cost to organizations who send glasses to developing countries. Since 2003, we have supplied more than 1.7 million glasses to more than 600 different organizations. Both reading and sunglasses are easy to dispense and make a dramatic difference in people's lives

Volunteer Optometric Services to Humanity - vosh.org - 209-980-7323

Established in 1971, Volunteer Optometric Services to Humanity (VOSH) provides vision care services to those below poverty level and without access to eye care. VOSH programs supply eyeglasses, treat eye disease, and refer or perform vision surgery to more than 100,000 people around the world each year.

World Blind Union - worldblindunion.org – 416-486-9698

The World Blind Union (WBU) is the global organization representing an estimated 285 million people worldwide who are blind or partially sighted. Members are organizations of, and for, the blind in 180 countries, as well as international organizations working in the field of vision impairment.

A-14. DENTAL CARE AND VISION

Although typically safe, local anesthesia is often used in dental care for fillings, root canals, and removing teeth. Nerves are anesthetized to reduce or eliminate pain during a procedure, particularly the maxillary (upper jaw) and mandibular (lower jaw) divisions of the trigeminal nerve (the 5th cranial nerve).[1] The trigeminal nerve is the largest cranial nerve, and it is responsible for feeling sensations in the face and motor functions such as chewing.

However, there are other nerves in the same area that if inadvertently injected, can result in eye problems, including oculomotor paralysis that manifests as the eye drooping outward and downward, and vision loss. Ptosis, (drooping eyelid), or mydriasis (pupil dilation) can also result.

In one case, anesthesia backflowed into the middle meningeal artery causing instantaneous blindness in that eye that lasted for 25–30 minutes. The condition mimics a far more serious condition, carotid artery embolus, that fortunately, is quite rare. More serious complications like permanent amaurosis, orbital cellulitis, orbital abscess, and endophthalmitis, have been reported in the literature.[2][3]

Other case studies indicate unusual but possible side effects on the eyes including diplopia (double vision), strabismus, ptosis, amaurosis fugax (painless loss of vision), and retinal thickening.

If you have any symptoms like these, contact your eye doctor immediately.

---

[1] Boynes, S.G., Echeverria, Z., Adlwahab, M. (2010). Ocular complications associated with local anesthesia administration in dentistry. *Dent Clin North Am*, 2010 Oct;54(4):677-86.

[2] Wilkie, G.J. (2000). Temporary uniocular blindness and ophthalmoplegia associated with a mandibular block injection. A case report. *Aus Dent J*, Jun;45(2):131-3.

[3] Rishiraj, B., Epstein, J. B., Fine, D., Nabi, S., and Wade, N.K. (2005). Permanent vision loss in one eye following administration of local anesthesia for a dental extraction. *Int J Oral Maxillofac Surg*, Mar;34(2):220-3.

A-15. PESTICIDES IN PRODUCE: THE DIRTY DOZEN

Many conventionally grown vegetables and fruits contain toxic pesticides, some of which have been banned in Europe. Children are especially vulnerable to pesticides in food. Pesticides may impact thyroid functioning[1] and neurodegenerative diseases like Parkinson's.[2] Pesticides show up in breast milk. Babies in utero who have been exposed to organophosphorus pesticides display mental and reproductive dysfunction.[3]

We recommend that you try to use only organically grown produce, especially for juicing where these toxins would be concentrated. At a minimum, stay away from produce known as the "dirty dozen."

The following information on the dirty dozen, comes from www.EWG.org:[4]

1. **Strawberries**. One third of all conventional strawberry samples contain 10 or more pesticides.
2. **Spinach**. 97% of conventional spinach samples contain pesticide residues, especially permethrin, a neurotoxic insecticide.
3. **Nectarines**. 94% of nectarine samples contain two or more pesticides; one sample contained 15.
4. **Apples.** 90% of apple samples have detectable pesticide residues. 80% contain diphenylamine, a pesticide banned in Europe.
5. **Grapes.** Grapes contain an average of five pesticides; more than 96% test positive.
6. **Peaches.** 99% of conventional peaches have detectable pesticide residues; an average of four different types.
7. **Cherries.** 30% of conventional cherries contain iprodione, a pesticide banned in Europe. It may cause cancer. Conventional cherries contain an average of five pesticides.
8. **Pears.** More than half of conventionally grown pears have residues of five or more pesticides in relatively high concentrations. This includes both insecticides and fungicides.
9. **Tomatoes.** The average conventionally grown tomatoes contain four pesticides; one sample had 15 pesticides and chemicals resulting from the breakdown of these pesticides.
10. **Celery.** More than 95% of conventional celery samples were positive for pesticides. One sample had 13 different chemicals.
11. **Potatoes.** Potatoes had more pesticide residues by weight than any other crop, especially chlorpropham.
12. **Sweet bell peppers.** 90% of conventional bell peppers have pesticide residues. They tend to have fewer pesticide residues than other foods, but these pesticides are more toxic to health.

You can find EWG's full list of pesticides in produce at www.ewg.org/foodnews/full-list.php. The next 20 items on the list are cherry tomatoes, imported snap peas, lettuce, blueberries, hot peppers, plums, kale/collards, and cucumber.

[1] Freire, C., Koifman, R.J., Sarcinelli, P.N., Simoes Rosa, A.C., Clapauch, R., et al. (2013). Long-term exposure to organochlorine pesticides and thyroid status in adults in a heavily contaminated area in Brazil. *Environ Res,* Nov;127:7-15.

[2] van der Mark, M., Vermeulen, R., Nijssen, P.C., Mulleners, W.M., Sas, A.M., et al. (2014). Occupational exposure to pesticides and endotoxin and Parkinson disease in the Netherlands. *Occup Environ Med,* Nov;71(11):757-64.

[3] Yu, Y., Yang, A., Zhang, J., Hu, S. (2013). Maternal exposure to the mixture of organophosphorus pesticides induces reproductive dysfunction in the offspring. *Environ Toxicol,* Sep;28(9):507-15.

[4] Shopper's Guide to Pesticides in Produce. (2018). Dirty Dozen. Retrieved Sep 12 2018 from https://www.ewg.org/foodnews/dirty-dozen.php.

A-16. EYE EMERGENCY CARE

Eye emergencies include cuts, scratches, objects in the eye, burns, chemical exposure, and blunt injuries to the eye or eyelid. Certain eye infections and other medical conditions, such as blood clots or glaucoma, may also need prompt medical care. Since the eye is easily damaged, any of these conditions can lead to vision loss if untreated.

Contact your eye doctor right away or seek emergency service if you experience any of the following:

- **Sudden vision loss or change**. Sudden vision loss could be caused by a problem with the blood supply to the eye or a problem with the retina (the tissue layers containing photoreceptor cells at the back of the eye that receive light). Optic nerve problems can also cause vision loss, but these are usually slower in onset.

  First Aid. See your doctor right away.

- **Sudden onset of double vision or loss of part of visual field.** This is potentially very serious and can represent a stroke.

  First Aid. Go the emergency room and/or call your eye doctor right away.

- **Severe eye pain**. Intense eye discomfort can be due to a variety of things such as foreign bodies, eye inflammation, or high eye pressure. Any severe pain should be evaluated.

  First Aid. Do not rub the eye. Check with your eye doctor right away. See the instructions for foreign body in eye.

- **Severe eyelid swelling or inability to open the eye.** This may be due to an infection of the tissues around the eye. The condition may require antibiotics and occasionally may be treated with surgery. An insect sting or other type of allergic reaction can also cause swelling.

  First Aid. Don't rub and check with your eye doctor.

- **Eye trauma**. Complete evaluation is essential after any type of eye injury. Anyone who sustains a serious injury to the eye, including scratches or blunt injuries, should be seen as soon as possible.

  First Aid. In the case of a serious eye injury, the injured eye should be covered with a protective shield and the injured person should not have anything to eat or drink because repair in the operating room may be required. An examination by a non-ophthalmologist emergency room physician does not replace a complete evaluation by a trained ophthalmologist.

- **Chemical injury.** A chemical injury to the eye can be caused by a work-related accident or by common household products such as cleaning solutions, garden chemicals, solvents, or other types of chemicals. Fumes and aerosols can also cause chemical burns.

    With **acid burns**, the haze on the cornea often clears and there is a good chance of recovery.

    Alkaline substances such as lime, lye, drain cleaners, and sodium hydroxide found in refrigeration equipment may cause permanent damage to the cornea and are potentially much more dangerous than an acid burn.

    First Aid. It is important to flush out the eye with large amounts of clean water or salt water (saline). This kind of injury needs medical care right away. If possible, wash eye out immediately, even before going to the hospital or eye doctor, then seek emergency care.

- **Small object in eye or eyelid.** Dust, sand, and other debris can easily enter the eye. Persistent pain, sensitivity to light, and redness are all signs that treatment is needed.

    First Aid. If dust, sand, or debris is most likely, don't rub the eye, wash your hands, and gently inspect the eye under the upper and lower lids. Don't touch the cornea (the white of the eye) with your finger. Gently pull on the eyelashes to open the eyelid(s) to inspect for debris. Your eye will naturally water, which may wash out the debris.

- **Foreign body in eye (high speed).** A foreign body in the eye may harm vision if the object enters the eye itself or damages the cornea or lens. Foreign bodies thrown at high speed by machining, grinding, or hammering metal have the highest risk of injuring the eye.

    First Aid. Bandage the eye, even bandage both eyes to lessen eye movement. Don't try to remove the object, but immediately seek emergency help from your eye doctor or emergency room. Do not use cotton swabs, tweezers, or anything else to try to remove the object. If the object is large, tape a clean paper cup over it to protect against being pressed upon. Try to keep the patient calm.

A-17. ALCOHOL AND YOUR EYES

Moderate alcohol usage is generally safe, such as the consumption of a glass of wine or a drink daily. Heavy drinking affects the health of the liver (which is related to eye health) over time and can lead to the following vision problems:

- Permanent blurry and double vision.
- Poor pupil constriction making it more difficult to drive at night.
- Loss of peripheral (side) vision.
- Inflammation of the optic nerve, resulting in poor side vision and loss of ability to distinguish colors.
- Involuntary excessive movement of the eyes back and forth.

Excessive alcohol consumption reduces the availability of **antioxidants** needed in the body for vision and overall health.[1] It increases the level of toxins and free radicals that interfere with fat digestion which are created when alcohol is broken down in the liver.[2]

Alcohol reduces protective **glutathione** levels because it interferes with liver functioning. Although red wine has been touted for its antioxidant benefit and heart health, "moderate" consumption has been associated with an increased risk of breast cancer.[3] Heavy drinking increases the risk of many diseases, including heart disease, anemia, cirrhosis, depression, seizures, hypertension, immune system suppression, nerve damage, and pancreatic disease.[4]

Most alcoholics are malnourished and suffer from vision-impacting deficiencies.

- **Vitamin A.** This is especially true of vitamin A,[5] which is essential for good vision.
- Alcoholics often exhibit **B1**,[6] **B6**,[7] and **vitamin B12** deficiency.
- **Glutathione**, a key antioxidant, is inhibited by excessive alcohol consumption.[8]
- **Vitamin D** deficiency is associated with excessive alcohol intake.[9]

Nutrient deficiencies and impaired functioning of the systems that support vision health mean that excessive drinking contributes to many vision diseases and conditions.

- **Cataracts.** Excessive use of alcohol significantly increases the risk of cataracts.[10]
- **Central serous choroidopathy.** Alcohol use is a risk factor.[11]
- **Colorblindness.** Alcoholics have a high rate of tritanopia. Excessive alcohol consumption is linked to a high rate of blue-yellow color errors as compared to red-green.[12]
- **Conjunctivitis.** Alcoholics have a higher concentration of staph and strep microflora in conjunctival tissue, than those who drink moderately.[13]
- **Macular edema.** Alcoholism significantly increases the risk of macular edema.[14]
- **Keratoconus.** Too much alcohol decreases magnesium levels,[15] causing elastic tissue thinning (as in the cornea).
- **Leber's disease.** Alcohol consumption increases the risk of developing Leber's and other neurodegenerative conditions linked to dysfunctional mitochondria:[16]

- **Poor night vision.** Alcohol intake impairs vitamin A absorption, needed for night vision.
- **Macular degeneration.** Heavy drinking increases the risk of macular degeneration.[17]
- **Ocular migraine.** Alcohol consumption may trigger ocular migraines.
- **Neurodegeneration.** Excess alcohol consumption is linked to toxic optic neuropathy, nutritional optic neuropathy (because it inhibits nutrient absorption),[18] and optic neuritis (because detoxification in the liver decreases glutathione levels).[19]
- **Sjogren's syndrome.** Those with Sjogren's should avoid alcohol because it dehydrates eye and other tissues.

Drink in moderation if desired, eat healthy and exercise regularly to improve your chances of retaining healthy vision.

---

[1] Van Gossum, A., Closset, P., Noel, E., Cremer, M., Neve, J. (1996). Deficiency in antioxidant factors in patients with alcohol-related chronic pancreatitis. *Dig Dis Sci,* June;41(6):1225-31.

[2] Lieber, C. (2003). Relationship between nutrition, alcohol use, and liver disease. *Alcohol Res Health,* 37(3):220-31.

[3] Brooks, P.J., Zakhari, S. (2013). Moderate alcohol consumption and breast cancer in women: from epidemiology to mechanisms and interventions. *Alcohol Clin Exp Res,* Jan;37(1):23-30.

[4] Freeman, D. 12 Health Risks of Chronic Heavy Drinking. Retrieved April 18 2018 from https://www.webmd.com/mental-health/addiction/features/12-health-risks-of-chronic-heavy-drinking#1

[5] Ibid. Lieber. (2003).

[6] Martin, P.R., Singleton, C.K., Hiller-Sturmhofel, S. (2003). The Role of Thiamine Deficiency in Alcoholic Brain Disease. *Alcohol Res Health,* 2003;27(2):134-42.

[7] Hoyumpa, A.M., (1986). Mechanisms of vitamin deficiencies in alcoholism. *Alcohol Clin Exp Res,* Dec;10(6):573-81.

[8] Yeligar, S.M., Harris, F.L., Hart, C.M., Brown, L.A. (2014). Glutathione attenuates ethanol-induced alveolar macrophage oxidative stress and dysfunction by downregulating NADPH oxidases. *Am J Physiol Lung Cell Mol Physiol,* Mar 1;306(5):L429-41.

[9] Wijnia, J.W., Wielders, J.P., Lips, P., van de Wiel, A., Mulder, C.L., et al. (2013). Is vitamin D deficiency a confounder in alcoholic skeletal muscle myopathy? *Alcohol Clin Exp Res,* Jan;37 Suppl 1:E209-15.

[10] Gong, Y., Feng, K., Yan, N., Xu, Y., Pan, C.W. (2015). Different amounts of alcohol consumption and cataract: a meta-analysis. *Optom Vis Sci,* Apr;92(4):471-9.

[11] Haimovici, R., Koh, S., Gagnon, D.R., Lehrfeld, T., Willik, S. (2004). Risk factors for central serous chorioretinopathy: a case-control study. *Ophthalmology,* Feb;111(2):244-9.

[12] Colblinder. Tritanopia - Blue-Yellow Color Blindness. Retrieved Nov 21 2017 from http://www.color-blindness.com/tritanopia-blue-yellow-color-blindness/.

[13] Gunduz, G., Gunduz, A., Polat, N., Cumurcu, B.E., Yakupogullari, Y. (2016). The Effect of Chronic Alcoholism on the Conjunctival Flora. *Curr Eye Res,* Jun;41(6):734-9.

[14] Acan, D., Calan, M., Er, D., Arkan, T., Kocak, N., et al. (2018). The prevalence and systemic risk factors of diabetic macular edema: a cross-sectional study from Turkey. *BMC Ophthalmol,* Apr 12; 18(1):91.

[15] Johnson, S. (2001). The multifaceted and widespread pathology of magnesium deficiency. *Med Hypotheses,* Feb;56(2):163-70.

16 Sadun, A., Carelli, V., Salomao, S.R., Berezovsky, A., Quiros, P.A., et al. (2003). Extensive investigation of a large Brazilian pedigree of 11778/haplogroup J Leber hereditary optic neuropathy. *Am J Ophthalmol,* Aug;136(2):231-8.

[17] Cederbaum, A. (1989). Role of lipid peroxidation and oxidative stress in alcohol toxicity. *Free Radic Biol Med,* 7:537–5394. Biologically, heavy drinking may cause oxidative damage to the retina leading to the development of AMD.

[18] Woon, C., Tang, R.A., Pardo, G. (1995). Nutrition and optic nerve disease. *Semin Ophthalmol,* Sep;10(3):195-202.

[19] Vogt, B.L., Richie, J.P. (2007). Glutathione Depletion and Recovery After Acute Ethanol Administration in the Aging Mouse. *Bio Chem Pharmacol,* May 15; 73(10): 1613–1621.

A-18. AUTHORS AND CONTRIBUTORS

Authors:

Marc Grossman, O.D., L.Ac., co-founder of Natural Eye Care, Inc. is best described as a holistic eye doctor. He uses a multi-disciplinary approach using nutrition, eye exercises, lifestyle changes, and Chinese Medicine. These provide him with a wide array of tools and approaches to tackle difficult eye problems. Dr. Grossman lectures nationally on natural vision care philosophy and method and teaches workshops for health care professionals including physical therapists, chiropractors and body workers, social workers, occupational therapists and other optometrists. He is a consultant to school systems, rehabilitation centers and the U.S. Military Academy at West Point.

Michael Edson, L.Ac., co-founder and President of Natural Eye Care, Inc., is an acupuncturist, and Qi Gong practitioner who manages the day-to-day operation of the corporation. With Dr. Grossman he conducts workshops on holistic vision care.

Other health professionals who contributed to this guide:

Sam Berne, O.D. has been in private practice in New Mexico for over 25 years where he works with patients to improve their vision and overall wellness through holistic methods. He specializes in the use of essential oils and in behavioral vision therapy. He has been awarded "The Special Awards" for Service from the Behavioral Optometrists in Mexico for his innovative and holistic work with children. His website is drsamberne.com.

Brett Bevell is an author who has practiced Reiki since 1995 and teaches Reiki trainings worldwide. His website is brettbevell.com.

Jason Elias, M.A., L.Ac., Dipl. O.M., is an acupuncturist and healer whose professional training includes work in psychology, the Alexander technique, massage therapy, bioenergetic therapy, Traditional Chinese Medicine, and herbal medicine, both Eastern and Western. He has studied with masters of aikido, acupuncture, ayurveda, and psychic healers. His website is fiveelementhealing.net.

Mark R. Filippi, D.C. has practiced behavioral chiropractic for the last 20 years in private practice. His work has always had an eclectic flavor and vitality that drives him to the cutting edge. In addition to being a peer-reviewed, published, clinical researcher, Dr. Filippi has been a field consultant and post-graduate instructor since 1997. His website is somaspace.org.

Scott Forman, M.D. is convinced that functional medicine, a holistic branch of medicine that joins nutritional biochemistry, life style, and genomics with other features of Integrative Medicine, is the future of medicine for the treatment of chronic medical disorders. He practices consultative neuro-ophthalmology, caring for both children and adults with complex ocular and neurologic disorders. He has studied neurobiology, craniosacral therapy, orthobionomy, visceral therapy, and is certified in functional medicine. He is Associate Professor of Ophthalmology, Neurology, and Neurosurgery at NY Medical College. His website is somerseye.com.

Phyllis R Freeman, Ph.D. is Senior Researcher at the Hudson Valley Healing Arts Center in Hyde Park, NY. She has a Ph.D. in Experimental and Psychological Psychology from Bryn Mawr. She has co-authored 11 studies including five on Lyme disease. She was Associate Professor and Dean of the graduate school of the State University of New York at New Paltz.

Damon Miller, M.D. has been in private practice in California since 1995 and is a board-certified medical doctor and also certified by the American Naturopathic Certification Board. His website is organicmd.com

David Nidorf, M.D. is an emergency medicine specialist practicing in the Hudson Valley, NY.

Daniel Orlansky, E-RYT 500, a yoga teacher since 1992, is certified in meridian yoga, kali ray triyoga, and kundalini yoga. He holds a master's degree in expressive art therapy/dance therapy from Lesley University and has been a visiting lecturer in movement studies at Tufts University. His website is yogaofenergyflow.com.

Ami Ranani, O.D., owner and optometrist at Somers Eye Center, has dedicated the last 38 years to serving his patients while largely based in Somers, NY. He received his Doctorate in Optometry from the Pennsylvania College of Optometry in 1976. His website is somerseye.com

Andy Rosenfarb, N.D., L.Ac. is the founder and clinical director of Acupuncture Health Associates in Westfield, NJ, and a world-renowned expert in the field of Chinese Medical Opthalmology. Since 1997, he has been leading the field in integrated treatment methods that combine Traditional Chinese Medicine, Naturopathic Medicine, and new cutting-edge therapies to help people who are suffering from debilitating eye diseases maintain and improve their eyesight. His website is acuvisiontherapy.com.

Jody Toyonaga, O.D., C.N.P., L.Ac. practices at the Seikinesis Eastern and Holistic Clinic in Yahud, Monsoon, Israel. She is a Canadian eye doctor, acupuncturist, and holistic nutritionist who is currently living and working in Israel. She specializes in eye disease as well as digestive health and emotional disorders, such as anxiety and depression. The Seikinesis website is seikinesis.com.

Ron Wish, M.D. is thoroughly trained in both modern medical science and complementary healing. He grounded himself in conventional family medicine and completed a three-year residency program at the University of Maryland Hospital. He specializes in craniosacral therapy and energy work. His website is drwishcraniosacral.com.

INDEX

nearsightedness (continued)
    signs, symptoms, causes, and risks, 7, 7*fig,* 268, 269–270
    treatment for, 270–273
    types of, 267–268
nerves of the eye
    defined anatomically, 1, 2*fig,* 3, 6
    see also optic nerve
niacin (B3), 90
night vision, poor, 519–528
    Chinese medicine and, 527–528
    defined, 519
    diet and lifestyle recommendations, 525–527
    formulas and products recommended for, 729
    nutrients for, 66, 74, 87, 118, **524–525**
    photoreceptors and, 520–521
    signs, symptoms, causes, and risks, 521–523
    treatment, complementary, 524–528
    types of, 521
    vitamin A deficiency and, 519, 523
nutrients
    absorption of, 715–718
    antioxidants and, 16, 17
    formulas and products recommended, 727–729
    inflammation reducing, 23
    juicing and, 165–166
    lack of as cause of eye conditions, 15
    oxidative stress impairing function and, 16
    vegetarians and, 37, 40, 53–56, 93
    vision protecting, 11
    see also specific carotenoids, bioflavonoids, vitamins, essential fatty acids, enzymes, amino acids, minerals, and herbs

O
ocular herpes, 665–672
    Chinese medicine and, 672
    defined, 665–666
    diet and lifestyle recommendations, 671
    juicing recipe for, 712
    nutrients for, 669–671
    signs, symptoms, causes, and risks, 668–669
    treatment, complementary, 669–672
    treatment, conventional, 669
    types of, 666–667, 666*fig*
    types of herpes viruses, 665
ocular rosacea, 675–680
    Chinese medicine and exercises, 678–679
    defined, 675
    diet and lifestyle recommendations, 678–679
    nutrients for, 677–678
    pathology of, 675–676
    signs, symptoms, causes, and risks, 676–677
    treatment, complementary, 677–680
    treatment, conventional, 677
omega-3 (ALA, EPA, DHA), 105–107, 105*fig*
omega-6 (LA, ARA, GLA), 105, 105*fig,* **107–108**
optic nerve
    brain and, 6
    defined, 1, 2*fig,* 3, 541, 553
    edema, 89
    formulas and products recommended for, 728
    juice recipe for, 712
    nutrients and, 92, 93, 125
    oxidative stress and, 15
    see also optic neuritis; optic neuropathy
optic nerve atrophy
    see optic neuropathy
optic neuritis, 553–560
    Chinese medicine and, 559–560
    defined, 553
    diet and lifestyle recommendations, 558–559
    incidence of, 553
    juicing recipe for, 712
    nutrients and, 556–558
    population incidence of, 553
    symptoms, causes, and risks, 554–555
    treatment, complementary, 555–560
    treatment, conventional, 555
    types of, 553–554
    see also optic neuropathy
optic neuropathy, 541–548
    Chinese medicine and, 548
    defined, 541
    diet and lifestyle recommendations, 547–548
    nutrients and, 91, 92, 93, 123, **544–546**
    signs, symptoms, causes, risks, 542–544
    stroke of optic nerve, inflamed optic nerve…, 541–542
    treatment, complementary, 544–548
    see also optic neuritis
orbit of the eye
    acupuncture and acupressure points around, 187–188, 187*fig*
    defined anatomically, 1
organic *vs.* non-organic food, 38, 167
organizations for eye care support, 755–756

reiki therapy, 737

resveratrol, **19,** 59, **78–79**

retina

acupuncture and, 149, 150, 155, 156

damage to or degeneration of, 203, 205, 219, 221, 615

with pets, 226, 229–230

see also specific eye conditions

defined anatomically, 2, 2*fig,* 3, 3*fig,* 480–481, 480*fig*

formulas and products recommended for, 729

juicing recipe for, 712–713

layers and detachment of, 563, 563*fig*

measuring inflammation in, 21

microcurrent stimulation, 169, 173, 175, 177

nutrients and, 65, 77, 98, 107, 118, 132

oxidative stress and, 22–23

processing light and, 5–7

see also chapter on nutrients and chapter on drugs (for visual side effects)

retinal bleeding, 141, 143, 145, 156, 159, **248**

retinal detachment, 563–567

Chinese medicine and, 567

diet and lifestyle recommendations, 566–567

exudative type, 564

layers of the retina and, 563, 563*fig*

nutrients for, 565–566

pets and, 230–231

research, upcoming, 567

rhegmatogenous type, 563

signs, symptoms, causes, and risks, 564

tractional type, 563

treatment, complementary, 565–567

treatment, conventional, 564–565

retinal pigment epithelium (RPE), 2–3*fig,* 74, 203

blue light damage and, 330–331

retinitis pigmentosa and other retinal conditions, 317, 317*fig,* 480, 480*fig,* 579, 603*fig*

retinal vein occlusion, 569–576

Chinese medicine and, 575–576

defined, 569, 569*fig*

diet and lifestyle recommendations, 574–575

incidence rate, 569

nutrients for, 572–574

related conditions, 571

signs, symptoms, causes, and risks, 570–571

treatment, complementary, 572–576

treatment, conventional, 571–572

types of, 569–570, 569*fig*

retinitis pigmentosa, 579–587

acupuncture and, 585

Chinese medicine and, 585

defined, 579

diet and lifestyle recommendations, 583–585

gene, drug, stem-cell, and other therapies, 585–587

gene mutation types, 579–581, 580*fig*

nutrients and, 87, 96, 97, **581–583**

photoreceptors, retinal epithelium, and genes, 579

signs, symptoms, causes, and risks, 580–581

treatment, complementary, 581–587

types of, 579–580, 580*fig*

Usher syndrome and, 615

riboflavin (B2), 89–90

rod-cone dystrophy

see cone-rod dystrophy

rods, 2*fig,* 3, 3*fig,* 5

blue light and, 330–331

disorders of, 341–347, **520–521,** 520*fig,* 579

rolfing therapy, 738

rutin, 59, **75–76**

S

saffron, 64, 131

sclera, defined anatomically, 1, 3*fig,* 74

selenium, 125

serrapeptase, 112–113

silymarin (milk thistle extract), 74

Sjogren's syndrome (SS), 591–599

Chinese medicine and, 598

defined, 369, **591**

diagnosis of, 593

diet and lifestyle recommendations, 597–598

nutrients for, 595–597

rate of occurrence, 591

research, upcoming, 599

signs, symptoms, causes, and risks, 592, 593–594

treatment, complementary, 595–598

treatment, conventional, 594

types of, 591–592

typical behavior of, 591

smoking, 162, 242

soaking and sprouting food, 33–35, 753–754

Stargardt disease, 481–482, 603–609

Chinese medicine and, 608